Holmes has done it again! This erudite and endlessly interesting book is a "must have" for all serious students of herbal medicine. Elegantly blending concepts from western vitalistic and traditional oriental systems, it provides a solid scientific explanation for the energetic properties of traditional chinese herbs. As an added bonus, it also gives direct applications to western clinical disease states. Perhaps the first truly cross-cultural herbal, *Jade Remedies* is destined to become a classic reference manual.

Chanchal Cabrera, MNIMH, AHG, President, Gaia Garden Herbal Apothecary, Vancouver

Jade Remedies is a valuable contribution to the 21st century model of Integrated Medicine. Every healer inspired to use plants wisely will be enriched by reading Peter Holmes' reference text.

Amanda McQuade-Crawford, MNIMH, author of *The Herbal Menopause Book*

Peter Holmes has produced a new volume filled with insight and satisfying detail for both the herbal enthusiast and the health care professional. *Jade Remedies* brings new clarity to the concepts of Chinese phytotherapy by explicating them in the context of the western vitalistic traditions. This is an important reference for both students and practitioners.

Dan Kenner, L.Ac., O.M.D., author of *Whole Systems Models*

Jade Remedies is an encyclopedia of therapeutic knowledge ... a highly thought-provoking discussion of Chinese herbal medicine. Peter Holmes is a creative voice in the development of East Asian botanical medicine in the west.

Ted Kapchuk, O.M.D., author of *The Web That Has No Weaver*

Following *The Energetics of Western Herbs,* Peter Holmes has produced another unique gem that boldly explores herbal integration. Clear and enjoyable to read as it is detailed and comprehensive, this beautiful book offers us new maps for the journey towards the wise application of Chinese herbal medicine. It is a blessing that Peter Holmes' creative mind reaches out to make connections, where walls and separation tend to limit awareness and understanding.

Randall Barolet, O.M.D., co-author of *Chinese Herbal Medicine: Formulas & Strategies*

Peter Holmes is a pioneer in the process of Western medicine integrating with traditional Chinese medicine. His new book, *Jade Remedies,* will be an essential resource for health practitioners in every branch of the healing arts. It will help those of us with a Western mind (just about all of us) understand the beauty and intricacies of Chinese medicine. This will enable more Westerners to tap into the rich storehouse of experience and knowledge refined over 5,000 years that is traditional Chinese herbal medicine.

Christopher Hobbs, L.Ac., A.G.H., author of *Handbook for Herbal Healing*

Jade Remedies releases the Chinese materia medica from the shroud of Oriental mystique into a context that can be understood by the health care practitioner not trained in the nuances of Chinese medicine. Peter Holmes weaves a sensible new approach, synthesizing from both Eastern and Western traditions. The intrinsic nature of what works is presented in a format that brings the practical to the forefront. Most materia medicas are compilations of what has come before. Peter Holmes' thoughtful, fresh approach helps us look at Chinese herbs with new eyes and think about them as we never had before.

Steven Foster, author of *Herbal Emissaries: Bringing Chinese Herbs to the West*

Finaly, a Chinese herbal materia medica that successfully merges the Western scientific with the Chinese energetic approach. With the inclusion of the chemical constituents of the medicinals this book helps to make Chinese remedies accessable to a Western practitioner as it also demystifies the Chinese theoretical idiom. New uses of the medicinals can now be incorporated, based on scientific research. With this book a welcome and timely perspective is created on an ancient form of medicine. This can only expand one's knowledge of single medicinals.

Dagmar Ehling, D.O.M., author of *The Chinese Herbalist's Handbook*

JADE REMEDIES

A Chinese Herbal Reference for the West

Vol. 2

中药西说

JADE REMEDIES

A Chinese Herbal Reference for the West

PETER HOLMES

Vol. 2

Snow Lotus Press • Boulder

Important Notice

The information contained in this book is for educational purposes only. It is not intended to diagnose, treat or prescribe, and does not purport to replace the services of a trained practitioner or physician. The information presented herein is correct and accurate to the author's knowledge up to the time of printing. However, because herbal medicine, like everything else, is in constant development, it is possible that new information may cause future modifications to become neccessary.

Illustrations from *Zhi Wu Ming Shi Tu Kao* by Wu Qi-chun, 1848
Additional original illustrations by Mary Beth Jay
Oriental calligraphy throughout by Pan Hui-xiang, except for secondary remedy names by Chu Shi-xiong
Phytogeographic chart by Sarah Russell
Cover design by Peter Holmes and Vicky Londerville
Cover photographs by Paul Berg

FIRST EDITION

ISBN 1-890029-29-7

Published by Snow Lotus Press, Inc., Boulder, Colorado, U.S.A.
Manufactured in the United States of America

Contents, Vol. 2

PART TWO : The Materia Medica

PART THREE : Cross Indexes, Glossaries & Charts

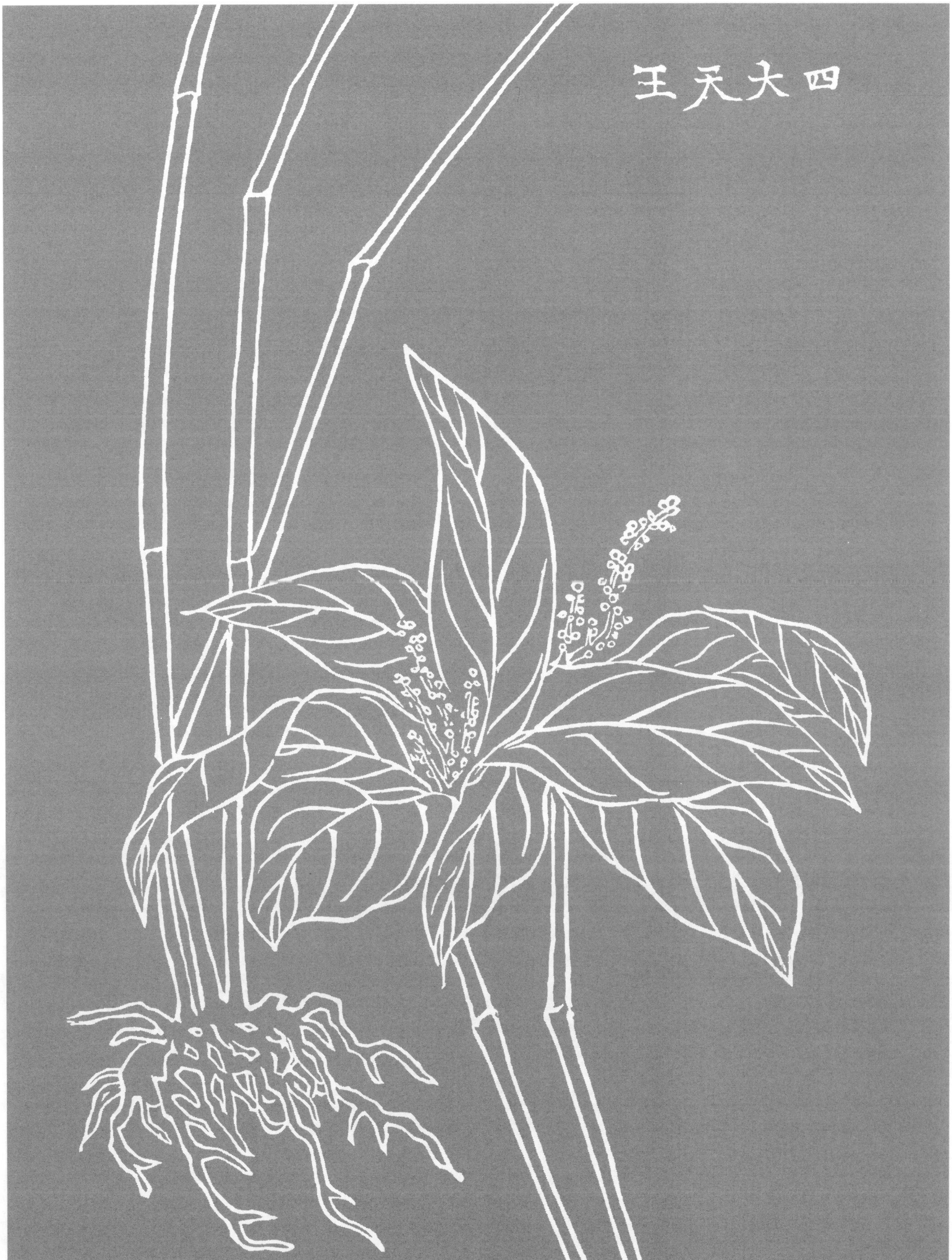
四大天王

肌肉骨骼系统用药

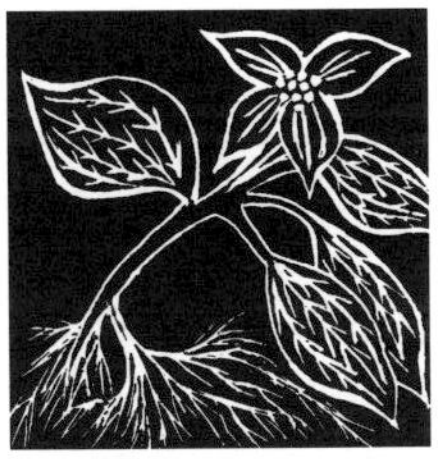

Remedies for the Musculoskeletal System

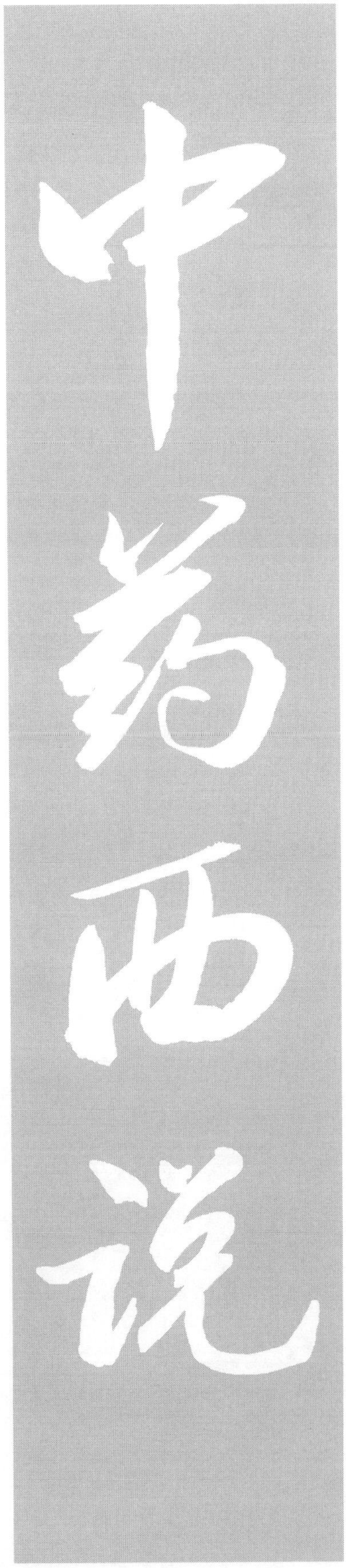

Oriental doctors avail themselves of a wide variety of remedies for treating disorders affecting the muscles, tendons, joints, bones and connective tissue—the whole physical framework that supports the organ systems. What is remarkable from the Western point of view is not just the sheer array of herbs available for relieving pain, inflammation and stiffness of the joints and sinews—impressive as this is—but rather the emphasis Chinese herbalists place on strengthening and functionally enhancing the tissues as a means of preventing disorders. Here again, and true to the fundamental tenets of their vitalistic healing system, the principle "tonification of deficiency" is given full expression in clinical practice.

In the traditional herbals, plants for musculoskeletal problems are found in the categories that "fortify the Yang" and "dispel wind damp." In this text these remedies are organized according to the fourfold *restore, relax, stimulate, sedate* classification of Western energetic herbal medicine. This not only makes the relationships between the type of remedy and type of condition clearer, but it also defines more clearly the exact functions of the herbs in each section—in Chinese as well as in Western terms.

The best example of this classification is those remedies found in the large traditional class of "remedies to fortify the Yang" that are primarily *restoratives* to the musculoskeletal system. In traditional Chinese terms, these *restoratives* actually "tonify the Liver and Kidney," rather than the Kidney Yang, as they address the syndrome "Liver and Kidney depletion." It is only by applying the concept *"musculoskeletal restorative"* to the category *"Yang tonics"* that we can define this particular group as *"Liver and Kidney restoratives."*

- ***Musculoskeletal restoratives*** treat deficiency conditions with connective tissue, bone, ligament or muscular weakness, presenting joint or limb weakness and soreness.
- ***Musculoskeletal stimulants*** treat deficiency conditions with chronic ligament or muscular deficiency, irritation or inflammation, displaying joint or limb pain and stiffness.
- ***Musculoskeletal relaxants*** treat excess conditions involving autonomic nervous stress, displaying muscular and peripheral spasms, cramps and tremors.
- ***Musculoskeletal sedatives*** treat excess conditions with acute ligament or muscular inflammation, accompanied by severe joint pain, swelling and discoloration, as well as fever.

Because the *relaxants* primarily work through nervous relaxation for their *spasmolytic* effects, they are presented in the nervous system section.

The Musculoskeletal Remedies

Restoratives

Musculoskeletal restoratives are effective for weakness and soreness of the bones, muscles and tendons, especially the legs, knees and lower back. Oriental practitioners speak of "tonifying the Liver and Kidney and strengthening the sinews and bones" with these remedies. Several of these remedies, such as Eucommia Du Zhong (the bark of the gutta-percha tree from alpine mid-China), are known to specifically strengthen the connective tissue itself. Western conditions that are helped by them include muscular dystrophy (atrophy), neurogenic arthropathy, degenerative arthritis, polymyositis and myasthenia gravis.

The syndrome **musculoskeletal deficiency,** describing the above symptoms, is proposed as a more literal Western naming of the traditional Chinese symptom pattern **Liver and Kidney depletion.** The true preventive value of *musculoskeletal restorative* herbs can be realized when it is understood **musculoskeletal deficiency** can be present long before any Western medical condition is diagnosed.

Musculoskeletal restoratives have a warm, dry effective quality, and contain a variety of chemical components, including alkaloids, glycosides, essential oils and organic acids. As a result, many possess related secondary uses. Some, such as Acanthopanax Wu Jia Pi (the root bark of a prickly shrub from Northeast China related to ginseng), have a *resolvent detoxicant* action with *diuretic, analgesic* and *anti-inflammatory* subactions. Such remedies address underlying **metabolic toxicosis** and thereby relieve the chronic joint and muscle pain of the presenting symptom picture **wind/damp/cold obstruction**. Other remedies, like Dipsacus Xu Duan (the root of the common Japanese teasel), have an *astringent* and *mucostatic* effect on urogenital functions, relieving such symptoms as vaginal discharge and urinary and seminal incontinence.

Stimulants

Most conditions of musculoskeletal deficiency involve chronic ligament and muscular inertia or chronic joint irritation or inflammation. Typical symptoms include limited joint movement and painful joints and muscles. The traditional symptom picture encapsulating these complaints is **wind/damp/cold obstruction.** This syndrome may be found, for example, in rheumatoid arthritis, osteoarthritis, Paget's disease, progressive systemic sclerosis and rheumatic myalgia.

Circulatory stimulation (i.e., increased blood flow to the joints and muscles) is the specific treatment recommended for the above conditions. *Musculoskeletal stimulants* are said to "dispel wind, damp and cold from the channels, invigorate the collaterals and relieve painful obstruction" through their pungent, bitter, warm and stimulating effective qualities. The majority of these *stimulants* are therefore also *diaphoretic* and are often used in formulas for upper respiratory infections. However, it is their additional *analgesic, muscle relaxant* and *anti-inflammatory* actions that make them particularly useful for these chronic, cold arthritic and rheumatic conditions.

These *antiarthritics* and *antirheumatics* include the frequently used Ledebouriella Fang Feng (Wind-protector root, an umbellifer from China's grasslands), Cassia Gui Zhi (Cassia cinnamon twig from South China and Vietnam) and Notopterygium Qiang Huo (Notopterygium root, a high alpine umbellifer from East China). The majority contain essential oils and other important constituents, such as glycosides, furanocoumarins and steroidal saponins, all of which contribute to their well-rounded effect. Because some of these *stimulants* include a considerable *nervous sedative* and *muscle relaxant* effect as part of their action, they are also frequently used to treat painful inflammatory conditions such as tendinitis, bursitis, epicondylitis, carpal tunnel syndrome and torticollis.

Sedatives

Musculoskeletal sedatives are primarily *antiarthritic* herbs that treat acute inflammatory and painful conditions accompanied by fever. They relieve pain by "dispelling wind damp heat." Instances include acute rheumatoid arthritis or gout, tendinitis, bursitis, osteomyelitis, ankylosing spondylitis, rheumatic fever and lupus. The typical symptoms of these conditions—painful, stiff, swollen red joints and low-grade fever—are aptly summarized in the syndrome **wind/damp/heat obstruction.**

In conformity with the dynamic physiological effects of their energetic qualities, the majority of these *analgesic, anti-inflammatory* and *antipyretic* remedies are bitter, pungent and cool in nature. They relieve acute pain and inflammation involving tendons or joints, and most, like Aristolochia Guang Fang Ji (Fangchi birthwort root from China's subtropics) and Gentiana Qin Jiao (Large-leaf gentian root from northeast China and Korea), also reduce fever.

中药西说

REMEDIES TO RESTORE THE SINEWS AND BONES, AND RELIEVE WEAKNESS

➧ TONIFY THE LIVER AND KIDNEY, AND STRENGTHEN THE SINEWS AND BONES

Musculoskeletal restoratives, detoxicants

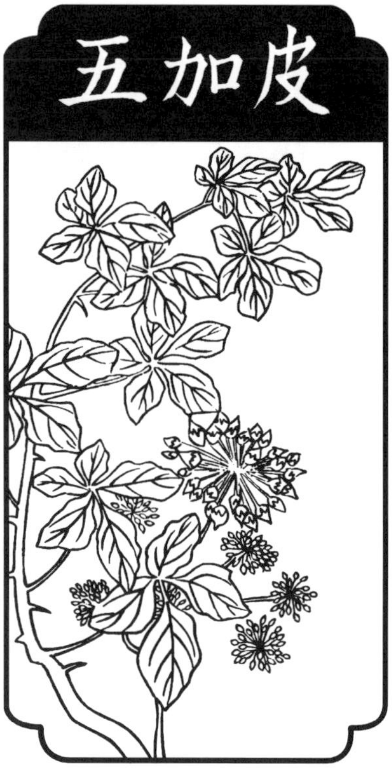

Acanthopanax Wu Jia Pi

Five Additions Root Bark *

Botanical source: *Acanthopanax gracilistylus* W.W. Smith or *A. spinosus* Miquel or *A. sessiliflorus* (Rupr. et Maxim.) Seem or *A. henryi* Harms (Araliaceae)
Pharmaceutical name: Cortex radicis Acanthopanacis
Chinese names: Wu Jia Pi, Wu Jia, Chai Zi (Mand); Ng Ga Pei (Cant)
Other names: Gokahi; *A. spinosus:* Ukogi, Kuko (Jap)
Habit: Deciduous spiny shrub from East and North China, growing on depleted slopes and in shrub thickets; in early summer, small umbels of greenish white axillary/terminal flowers appear.
Part used: the root bark .

Therapeutic category: mild remedy with minimal chronic toxicity
Constituents: methoxysalicylaldehyde, beta sitosterol, arachic/linoleic/palmitic acids, syringin, isofraxidin, flavonoids (incl. syringin, isofraxidin), essential oil, calcium oxalate, tannic acid, vitamins A, B1
Effective qualities: pungent, warm, dry
restoring, stimulating, decongesting
Tropism: musculoskeletal, urinary systems
Liver, Kidney channels
Air, Fluid bodies

Actions and Indications

musculoskeletal restorative, connective tissue restorative: bone, ligament and muscle weakness (esp. of back and knees), connective tissue weakness; osteoporosis, muscular dystrophy (atrophy)
detoxicant, anti-inflammatory: metabolic toxicosis with rheumatism, chronic arthritis, eczema, syphilis
draining diuretic: dysuria, general and leg edema
antipruritic: genital pruritus
Miscellaneous: beriberi, retarded walking in children

Symptom Pictures

musculoskeletal deficiency (Liver and Kidney depletion): weak, sore legs and knees, general weakness
metabolic toxicosis (wind/damp/cold obstruction): muscle and joint pain, malaise, fatigue, skin rashes

Preparation

Use: The root Acanthopanax Wu Jia Pi is decocted or used in tincture form. Traditionally, wines and liqueurs are also prepared with it.
Dosage: Decoction: 8-14 g
Tincture: 2-4 ml
Caution: Use sparingly in empty heat due to Yin deficiency.

Notes

Five additions root bark is a major traditional remedy for skeletal and muscular deficiencies. The remedy is given when rheumatic or arthritic conditions appear together with an underlying connective tissue weakness. From the Western perspective, two factors support this traditional usage. First is the content in salicylaldehyde *(analgesic)* and calcium oxalate *(bone-streng thening).* Second, the fact that, based on its total symptom profile, it is also a systemic *diuretic detoxicant* addressing chronic conditions of metabolic toxicosis (called fluids dyskrasia in traditional Greek medicine) presenting wind/damp/cold obstruction in the muscles and joints.

Although the name Wu Jia Pi—literally "Five additions bark"—is applied to a variety of *Acanthopanax* species, it most often refers to *Acanthopanax gracilistylus.* It properly no longer refers to Eleuthero ginseng, now renamed Ci Wu Jia, which, because of its numerous other properties, must be carefully distinguished from it. Ci Wu Jia is found in the Endocrine and Immune section.

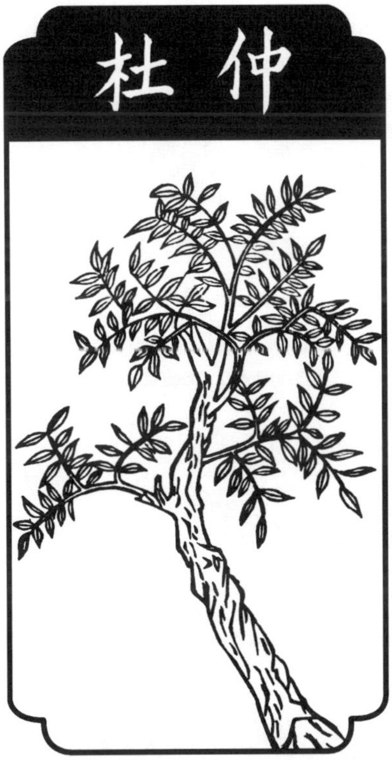

Eucommia Du Zhong

Eucommia Bark

Botanical source: *Eucommia ulmoides* Oliver (Eucommiaceae)
Pharmaceutical name: Cortex Eucommiae
Chinese names: Du Zhong, Si Xien, Si Zhong, Mu Mian (Mand); Dou Jung (Cant)
Other names: Gutta-percha tree; Tochu (Jap)
Habit: Tall, hardy deciduous tree from Central China's mountain regions, cultivated in the South China plains; pale green flowers appear in spring.
Part used: the bark

Therapeutic category: mild remedy with minimal chronic toxicity
Constituents: flavonoid and other glycosides (incl. pinoresinol diglucoside), iridoids (incl. aucubin, geniposide, harpagide, ajugoside, ulmoside, retoside), nonacosane, triacontanol, betulin, phytosterols (incl. sitosterol, daucosterol), liriodendrin, organic acids (incl. betulic/ursolic/vanillic acid), tannin, 15 lignans, alkaloids, resin 7% (incl. gutta-percha 2-6.5%), potassium, chlorogenic and geniposidic acid, organic acids, vitamin C
Effective qualities: sweet, a bit pungent and astringent, warm, dry
restoring, astringing, relaxing, softening, stabilizing, solidifying
Tropism: muskuloskeletal, reproductive, urinary, cardiovascular systems
Liver, Kidney, Heart, Dai, Yin Qiao channels; Fluid, Air bodies

Actions and Indications

musculoskeletal restorative, connective tissue restorative: bone, ligament and muscle weakness, connective tissue weakness; osteoporosis, fatigue from miscarriage
detoxicant: diuretic, analgesic, anti-inflammatory: metabolic toxicosis with back, knee and joint pain; rheumatoid arthritis, lumbar osteoarthrosis
antilipemic: hypercholesterolemia
urogenital mucostatic astringent: incontinence with enuresis, leucorrhea, spermatorrhea, genital pruritus, impotence; atonic bladder dysfunctions
vasodilator, hypotensive, nervous sedative: hypertension with dizziness, unrest
fetal relaxant, antiabortive: fetal unrest, threatened miscarriage
immunostimulant: infections in general
interferon inducent

Symptom Pictures

musculoskeletal deficiency (Liver and Kidney depletion): weak and sore lower back and knees, fatigue, frequent urination

metabolic toxicosis (cold obstruction): chronic joint pain and stiffness, cold extremities

genitourinary damp cold (Kidney Yang deficiency with **damp):** urinary dribbling, clear vaginal discharges, seminal incontinence, sexual disinterest

Preparation

Use: The bark Eucommia Du Zhong is decocted or used in tincture form.

Dosage: Decoction: 8-16 g (up to 30 ml for hypertension)
Tincture: 2-4 ml

Caution: Forbidden in Yin deficiency conditions with heat signs.

Notes

Named after the semi-legendary Daoist sage Du Zhong, Eucommia bark has an impeccable reputation as a *musculoskeletal* and *urogenital restorative.* To this we should add, from a Western viewpoint, that the remedy is a *connective tissue strengthener* with a good *detoxicant* action for cold arthritic conditions, and a *toning* action in atonic urinary dysfunctions, including incontinence. The three traditional symptom pictures listed epitomize the practical therapeutic applications of these essential functions, which become more valuable with advancing years.

Since the mid-1950s, however, both the bark and the leaf of this tree have emerged as leading remedies for hypertension, involving *vasodilatant, cholesterol-lowering* and *nervous sedative* mechanisms of action. The diglucoside pinoresinol is thought to be the main *hypotensive* agent. In addition, according to more recent theoretical and clinical research, **Eucommia leaf, Du Zhong Ye** (Mand.) or **Do Chong Yip** (Cant.), can be used effectively as a substitute for the bark in most of its clinical indications (Chang and But 1987).

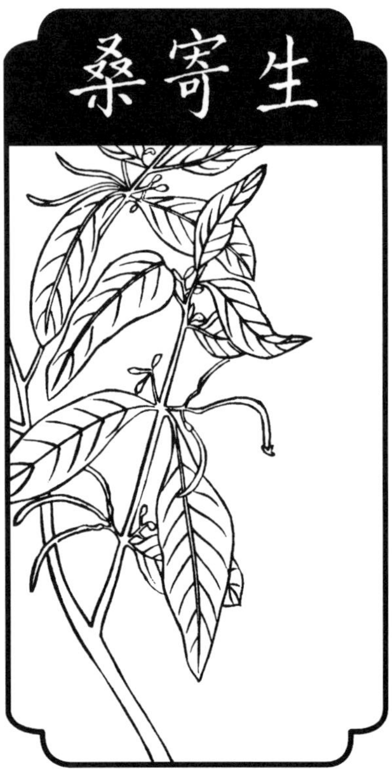

Loranthus Sang Ji Sheng

Asian Mistletoe Twig

Botanical source: *Loranthus parasiticus* Merr. or *L. yadoriki* Siebold (Loranthaceae)
Pharmaceutical name: Ramulus Loranthi
Chinese names: Sang Ji Sheng, Sang Shang Ji Sheng, Bei Sang Ji, Guang Sang Ji (Mand); Song Gei Sang (Cant)
Other names: "Mulberry parasite"; Sokisei (Jap)
Habit: Evergreen temperate East Asian semiparasitic shrub growing on tree branches; blooms with yellow or red small single flowers.
Part used: the twig and leaf

Therapeutic category: medium-strength remedy with some chronic toxicity
Constituents: quercetrin-arabinoside avicularin, flavonoid quercetrin, viscotoxins, choline, acetylcholine, histamine, aminobutyric acid, fatty acids, inositol, triterpenes, phospholipids
Effective qualities: sweet, a bit bitter, neutral
restoring, calming, relaxing, solidifying, stabilizing
Tropism: musculoskeletal, nervous, urogenital, cardiovascular systems
Liver, Kidney, Heart, Yang Wei, Yin Wei , Yin Qiao channels

Actions and Indications

musculoskeletal restorative: bone, ligament, muscle weakness (esp. of lower back and knees); muscular atrophy
detoxicant, diuretic, anti-inflammatory: metabolic toxicosis with chronic muscular rheumatism (myalgia), fibrositis, arthritis, paresthesia of lower extremities, eczema, skin rashes or scales
dermatropic: dry or lackluster skin
nervous sedative, analgesic: unrest, irritability, epilepsy, neuralgia
hypotensive cardiac relaxant: hypertension, neurocardiac syndrome with arrhythmia, angina pectoris, coronary disease
fetal relaxant, antiabortive: fetal unrest, threatened miscarriage
uterine hemostatic: menorrhagia, uterine bleeding during pregnancy
galactagogue: insufficient breast milk
hair-growth stimulant: hair loss
anti-frostbite (topically)
antitumoral
antiviral, phagocyte stimulant

Symptom Pictures

musculoskeletal deficiency (Liver and Kidney depletion): weak and sore lower back and legs, fatigue

metabolic toxicosis (wind/damp/cold obstruction): pain in leg muscles and tendons, skin rashes

heart Qi constraint with **nerve excess:** anxiety, feeling stressed, palpitations, chest pains

Liver Yang rising: palpitations, dizziness, headache, ringing in ears, restlessness

Preparation

Use: The leafy twig Loranthus Sang Ji Sheng is decocted or used prepared in a tincture.
Dosage: Decoction: 10-20 g
Tincture: 0.5-2 ml
Caution: In some people, idiosyncratic sensitivity to this medium-strength remedy may occur, displaying malaise, appetite loss, abdominal distension and mild diarrhea. Dosages should not be exceeded. Avoid longterm use of this remedy in large unalloyed doses.

Notes

The epiphytic Asian mistletoe grows upon various trees, such as the mulberry, peach, willow, oak, Taiwan maple and elm. The action of the twig has much in common with both European and American mistletoe as *cardiovascular relaxant, nervous sedative* and *antitumoral. Viscum coloratum* contains the same *antitumoral* viscotoxins as *Viscum album,* for example. Tense or constrained Qi conditions affecting neurocardiac functions are here addressed, including stress angina, arrhythmia and coronary disorders.

Asian mistletoe twig is also often found in traditional and modern formulas that treat fetal unrest and threatened miscarriage during the early months of pregnancy. Here again, a *relaxant* action is evident.

However, traditionally it is this remedy's *restorative* and *antirheumatic* actions on bones and sinews that has been so prized. Asian mistletoe twig is indicated for traditional symptom patterns such as Liver and Kidney depletion and wind damp obstruction, the latter benefitting from its combined *analgesic, anti-inflammatory* and *detoxicant* actions. Asian mistletoe is also a specific remedy for dry skin in general, as well as for dry forms of eczema and dermatitis in particular. The pharmacological mechanisms involved still await research.

Two closely-related forms of mistletoe, *Viscum coloratum* (Komb.) Nakai and *V. album* L. are properly called **Hu Ji Sheng** (Mand.) or **Wu Gei Sang** (Cant.), and the remedy derived from these, **Viscum Hu Ji Sheng.** The species *Viscum album* is the type of mistletoe commonly used in Western herbal medicine. In Taiwan, the remedy Sang Ji Sheng is sourced from *Scurrula ritozanensis, Viscum liquidambaricolus* and *V. coloratum.*

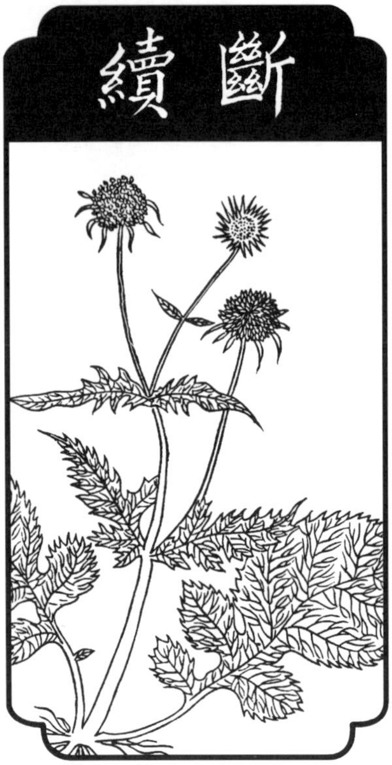

Dipsacus Xu Duan

Japanese Teasel Root

Botanical source: *Dipsacus japonica* Miquel or *D. asperoides* Wall. (Dipsacaceae)
Pharmaceutical name: Radix Dipsaci asperoidis
Chinese names: Xu Duan, Chuan Duan, Jie Gu, Shan Lo Bo, Liu Han (Mand); Juk Dyun, Chyun Dyun (Cant)
Other names: Sichuan teasel, "Solder fracture"; Zokudan (Jap)
Habit: Perennial temperate Asian herb found along roadsides and wild areas; blooms in autumn with racemes of magenta flowers.
Part used: the root

Therapeutic category: mild remedy with minimal chronic toxicity
Constituents: alkaloids (incl. lamine), benzene, phytosterol, essentialoil, vitamin E
Effective qualities: bitter, pungent, a bit sweet, warm, dry
restoring, astringing, solidifying, stabilizing, stimulating, decongesting
Tropism: muskuloskeletal, urogenital systems
Liver, Kidney, Dai, Yang Wei, Yin Qiao channels

Actions and Indications

musculoskeletal restorative/stimulant: bone, ligament and muscle weakness (esp. of lumbars, knees, legs); stiff joints
analgesic: lower back and knees soreness/pain; arthritis
urogenital mucostatic astringent: heavy white vaginal discharges (leucorrhea), spermatorrhea, enuresis
hemostatic: menorrhagia, passive intermenstrual bleeding (metrorrhagia), bleeding during pregnancy
uterine stimulant: amenorrhea, dysmenorrhea
fetal relaxant, antiabortive: fetal unrest, threatened miscarriage
vulnerary, detumescent: traumatic injuries with swelling; ruptured tendons, contusions, fractures, boils, carbuncles
antitumoral: tumors (incl. breast cancer)

Symptom Pictures

musculoskeletal deficiency (Liver and Kidney depletion): weak, sore or painful lower back and knees, weak legs, stiff joints

genitourinary damp cold (Kidney Yang deficiency with **damp):** white vaginal discharges, seminal incontinence, intermenstrual bleeding, heavy or painful menses

Preparation

Use: The root Dipsacus Xu Duan can be decocted or used as a tincture. Topical preparations are used for boils and tissue trauma of many types.
Dosage: Decoction: 8-14 g
Tincture: 1-4 ml
Caution: Forbidden during pregnancy without bleeding or threatened abortion present.

Notes

Being both *restorative* and *analgesic* to the musculature, Japanese teasel root excels where weakness and pain—especially of the lumbars—exist together. A tissue-toning *astringent* and *hemostatic,* another of its specialties is uterine bleeding of any kind, as well as all genital and urinary discharges caused by damp cold. The hard, small roots are also useful for treating fractures and various soft tissue traumas, hence the name Jie Gu, meaning "bone-mending."

Sichuan teasel root, Chuan (Xu) Duan Gen (Mand.) or **Chyun (Juk) Dyun Gan** (Cant.), from *Dipsacus asperoides,* has proven *anti-infective* against a gamut of bacteria and other microbes, including *Candida albicans.* In the West, teasel varieties are used as traditional remedies for liver and stomach stasis, and for promoting detoxification.

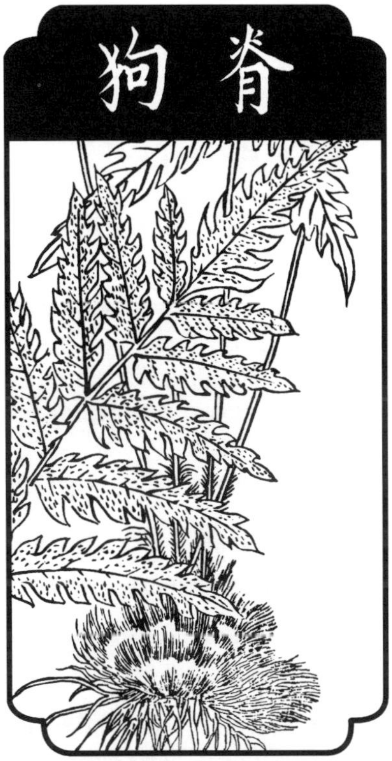

Cibotium Gou Ji

Dogspine Root *

Botanical source: *Cibotium barometz* J. Smith (Cyatheaceae)
Pharmaceutical name: Rhizoma Cibotii
Chinese names: Gou Ji, Jin Gou Ji, Jin Mao Gou Ji (Mand); Gau Jek (Cant)
Other names: Chain fern, Scythian lamb, Lamb-of-Tartary; Kuseki (Jap)
Habit: Perennial large hairy tree fern from temperate and tropical South China and Malaysia; grows in damp, shady wooded areas with acidic soil, especially along canals.
Part used: the rhizome

Therapeutic category: mild remedy with minimal chronic toxicity
Constituents: diterpenes, triterpenes, alkaloids, tannins, starch, vitamin E
Effective qualities: bitter, sweet, astringent, warm, dry
restoring, astringing, calming
Tropism: musculoskeletal, nervous, urinary , digestive systems
Liver, Kidney channels
Fluid body

Actions and Indications

musculoskeletal restorative: bone, ligament and muscle weakness (esp. of spine, back, legs and knees); muscular dystrophy (atrophy)
analgesic: rheumatoid myalgia, neuralgia, arthralgia, lumbago; acute rheumatoid arthritis
urogenital astringent mucostatic: incontinence with enuresis, leucorrhea, nocturnal spermatorrhea
laxative: constipation

Symptom Pictures

musculoskeletal deficiency (Liver and Kidney depletion): weak and sore legs, knees, back and spine
wind/damp/cold obstruction: muscle or joint pain, soreness or numbness
genitourinary damp cold (Kidney Yang deficiency): dribbling urination, vaginal/seminal discharges

Preparation

Use: The root Cibotium Gou Ji is decocted or used in tincture form. In Taiwan, *Cyathea* species represent this remedy.
Dosage: Decoction: 6-14 g
Tincture: 2-4 ml
Caution: Use cautiously in Yin deficiency syndromes with empty heat, and in conditions with difficult, obstructed urination (dysuria, stranguria).

Notes

With its bristling, hairy filaments, the spine-like appearance of this root has given rise to the name "dog-spine." Dogspine root is a straightforward *restorative* working on both neuromuscular and urogenital tissues, especially when the legs are affected or with atonic incontinence present. The remedy is additionally *analgesic* in painful arthritic and rheumatic conditions.

REMEDIES TO RELAX THE SINEWS AND RELIEVE JOINT AND MUSCLE PAIN

➤ DISPEL WIND/DAMP/COLD, INVIGORATE THE COLLATERALS AND RELIEVE PAINFUL OBSTRUCTION

Diaphoretic and analgesic antirheumatics, antiarthritics

防風

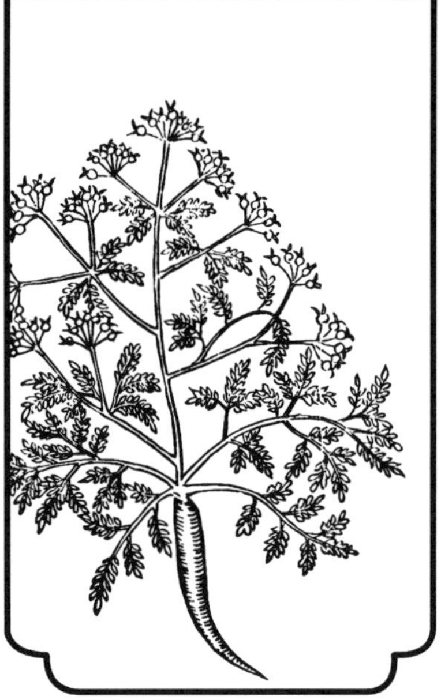

Ledebouriella Fang Feng

Wind-Protector Root *

Botanical source: *Ledebouriella divaricata* (Turcz.) Hiroe or *L. seseloides* (Hoffm.) Wolff (syn. *Siler divaricatum* Bentham et Hooker f. and *Saposhnikovia divaricata* [Turcz.] Schischkin) and spp. (Umbelliferae)
Pharmaceutical name: Radix Ledebouriellae
Chinese names: Fang Feng, Guan Fang Feng, Che Fang Feng (Mand); Fong Fung (Cant)
Other names: Laserwort; Bofu (Jap)
Habit: Perennial herb from Northeast and Central China's grasslands and slopes; compound umbels of small white blossoms flower in summer.
Part used: the root

Therapeutic category: mild remedy with minimal chronic toxicity
Constituents: essential oil oil (incl. methylbutenol, pinene, hexanal, pentanol, octanal, hendecanoic acid, phenols), mannitol, bitter glycosides, organic acids, polysaccharides
Effective qualities: pungent, sweet, warm, moist
stimulating, relaxing, dispersing, eliminating
Tropism: musculoskeletal, digestive systems
Liver, Spleen, Bladder channels; Warmth, Air bodies

Actions and Indications

circulatory and muscular stimulant/relaxant: deficient and spasmodic musculoskeletal conditions with rheumatic pain and stiffness; stiff neck
stimulant diaphoretic, anti-infective: common cold, flu (esp. onset), fever, rheumatic fever
anti-infective: antiviral, antibacterial, antifungal, phagocyte stimulant: infections in general
antidotal: poisoning from plants, arsenic
neuromuscular sedative: analgesic, anti-inflammatory: rheumatic myalgia, fibrositis, headache, migraine, body aches, abdominal pain
spasmolytic, anticonvulsant: diarrhea, colitis; tetany, seizures, lockjaw

Symptom Pictures

wind/damp/cold obstruction: sore, painful stiff muscles, cold extremities

external wind cold/heat: sneezing, headache, aches and pains, stiff neck, chills, feverishness

Preparation

Use: The root Ledebouriella Fang Feng is decocted in the standard way, or may be used in tincture form.
Dosage: Decoction: 3-10 g
Tincture: 2-4 ml
Caution: Use cautiously in metabolic deficiency with spasms, and in Yin deficiency syndromes with deficiency heat.

Notes

"Wind-protecting" is the literal translation of this remedy's name, Fang Feng, and refers both to the wind of rheumatic pain and the wind of the onset of influenza. With its *circulatory stimulant, spasmolytic* and strong *antiviral* properties, this pungent-sweet umbellifer treats both types of wind, endogenous and exogenous. In inflammatory rheumatic disorders such as fibromyalgia, good *anti-inflammatory* and *analgesic* actions come into play. With infections, Wind-protector root's polysaccharides appropriately provide additional immune stimulation.

This remedy may safely be used for long-term treatment. It is neither drying like other *diaphoretics* when used in formulas for viral infections, nor excessively *stimulating* in rheumatic conditions—unlike many other herbs in this section.

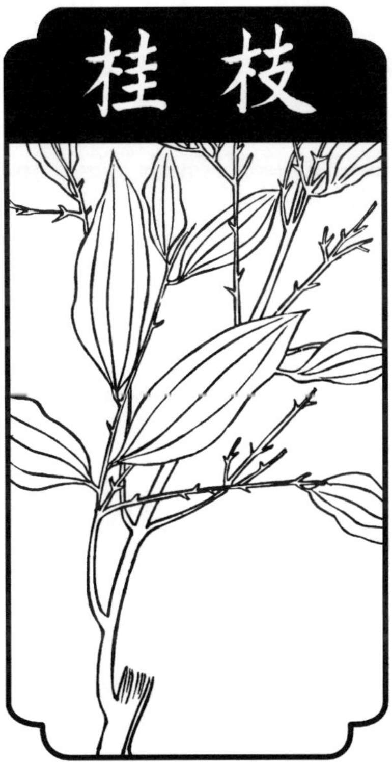

Cinnamomum Gui Zhi

Cassia Cinnamon Twig

Botanical source: *Cinnamomum cassia* Blume (Lauraceae)
Pharmaceutical name: Ramulus Cinnamomi cassiae
Chinese names: Gui Zhi, Rou Gui Zhi (Mand); Gwai Ji (Cant)
Other names: Saigon cinnamon; Keishi (Jap)
Habit: Evergreen cultivated subtropical tree from Guangxi, Guangdong, Hainan, Taiwan and Vietnam; flowers in early summer with yellow-white cymose blossom panicles.
Part used: the twig

Therapeutic category: mild remedy with minimal chronic toxicity
Constituents: essential oil 1-2% (incl. cinnamic aldehyde, cinnamic acid, cinnamyl acetate, phenylpropyl acetate), tannin, resin, mucilage
Effective qualities: pungent, sweet, warm, dry
stimulating, dispersing, decongesting, relaxing
Tropism: respiratory, reproductive, digestive systems
Lung, Bladder channels
Warmth, Air bodies

Actions and Indications

circulatory and muscular stimulant/relaxant: deficient and spasmodic musculoskeletal conditions with rheumatic or arthritic pain; arterial deficiency with cold extremities
stimulant diaphoretic, anti-infective (antiviral, antibacterial, antifungal): onset of cold and flu
neuromuscular sedative: analgesic, spasmolytic: rheumatic myalgia, arthralgia, headache, body aches, shoulder joint and abdominal pain, dysmenorrhea, chest pain
cardiotonic: chronic heart deficiency with palpitations
uterine stimulant, emmenagogue, parturient: delayed menses, amenorrhea, retained placenta
draining diuretic: edema
immune regulator, antiallergic: immune stress with cytotoxic allergies
antitumoral

Symptom Pictures

wind/damp/cold obstruction: pain in joints or muscles, cold hands and feet

external wind cold: sneezing, fear of cold, sweating, chills, feverishness, head and muscle aches, fatigue

uterus cold: delayed or stopped menstruation, menstrual cramps, difficult scanty flow

Preparation

Use: The twig Cinnamomum Gui Zhi may be decocted in the standard way or taken in tincture form. The latter has a greater *stimulating* and *warming* effect. The essential oil of Cassia cinnamon leaf is required to bring out the herb's full *anti-infective* potential, but, because of its tissue irritant effect, must only be taken orally in a gelatin capsule (1-2 drops with olive oil) (see also Holmes 1989).

Dosage: Decoction: 3-10 g
Tincture: 1-3 ml

Caution: Forbidden in all excess or deficient hot conditions, during pregnancy, in menorrhagia and throat problems.

Notes

Cassia cinnamon twig is much used in formulas that treat arthritic and rheumatic conditions presenting chronic pain. Being an *arterial stimulant*, this warming *diaphoretic* remedy is also standard for the onset of flu or cold with chills, aches and pains and slight sweating—external wind cold conditions in Chinese medicine. In distinction to Cassia cinnamon bark (a *cardiovascular stimulant*), Cassia twig addresses external, not internal, cold conditions affecting the superficial circulation of the muscles and extremities. Because it provides a *warming, stimulant* touch, this remedy is often added to a formula that is too cooling or insufficiently dispersing.

Cinnamon bark, Gui Pi (M.) or **Gwai Pei** (C.) is derived from species such as *Cinnamomum japonicum, C. burmanii* and *C. wilsonii.* Its *arterial stimulant, spasmolytic, analgesic* and *uterine stimulant* actions are considered similar to but less strong than Rou Gui, Cassia cinnamon bark.

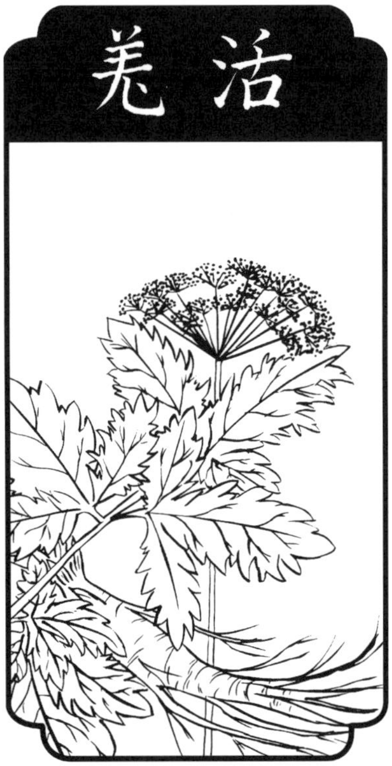

Notopterygium Qiang Huo

Notopterygium Root

Botanical source: *Notopterygium incisum* Ting Mss. or *N. forbesii* Boissier or *N. francherii* Boissier (Umbelliferae)
Pharmaceutical name: Rhizoma et radix Notopterigii
Chinese names: Qiang Huo (Mand); Geung Wut (Cant)
Other names: Kyokatsu (Jap)
Habit: Perennial herb from Central and West China's high mountain regions; grows among other herbs and shrubs; the umbels bloom in late summer.
Part used: the rhizome and root

Therapeutic category: mild remedy with minimal chronic toxicity
Constituents: essential oil (incl. angelical), palmitic/stearic/oleic/linoleic acids, alkaloids
Effective qualities: pungent, bitter, warm, dry
stimulating, dispersing, eliminating, relaxing, calming
Tropism: muscular, respiratory, urinary, reproductive systems
Bladder, Kidney channels
Air body

Actions and Indications

circulatory and muscular stimulant/relaxant: deficient and spasmodic musculoskeletal conditions with stiff, painful shoulder and neck joints
stimulant diaphoretic, anti-infective (antiviral): onset of cold and flu, fever
neuromuscular sedative, analgesic: rheumatoid myalgia (esp. of upper trunk), neuralgia, arthralgia, lower backache, headache, rheumatoid arthritis
interferon inducent, antifungal

Symptom Pictures

wind/damp/cold obstruction: joint pain and swelling, cold hands and feet, muscle numbness and pain, esp. in shoulders, neck and arms

external wind cold: sneezing, aches and pains in head and muscles, chills, feverishness, no sweating

Preparation

Use: The root Notopterygium Qiang Huo is decocted or used in tincture form for best results.

Dosage: Decoction: 3-10 g
Tincture: 2-4 ml

Caution: Notopterygium root should not be used in Blood (metabolic) or Yin deficiency or exterior deficiency syndromes. Being a strong *diaphoretic* like Ephedra Ma Huang, it should be reserved for the above conditions only.

Notes

A pungent, warm, dry-natured umbellifer from the Western Chinese provinces of Gansu and Sichuan furnishes this *stimulant* and *analgesic* remedy. Primarily employed in formulas for neuromuscular, rheumatic and arthritic conditions of the wind/damp/cold type, Notopterygium root excels with numbness and pain present, especially in the upper back. Its *diaphoretic* and *anti-infective* actions serve upper respiratory infections presenting muscle aches and pains.

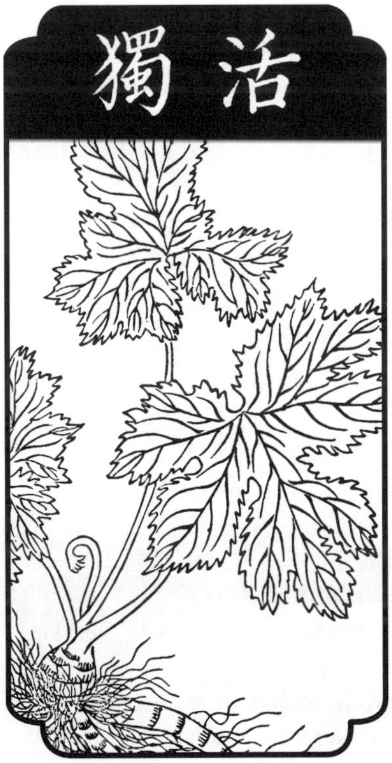

Angelica Du Huo

Hairy Angelica Root *

Botanical source: *Angelica pubescens* Maximowicz or *A. laxiflora* Diels and spp. (Umbelliferae)
Pharmaceutical name: Radix Angelicae pubescentis
Chinese names: Du Huo, Qiang Huo, Du Yao Cao (Mand); Duk Wut (Cant)
Other names: Downy/Furry/Pubescent angelica, "Self-moving"; Dokkatsu (Jap)
Habit: Perennial mountain herb from Central and North China, especially Sichuan and Hubei, growing in ravines and thickets; compound umbels of terminal white flowers appear in summer.
Part used: the root

Therapeutic category: mild remedy with minimal chronic toxicity
Constituents: essential oil, alkaloids (incl. scopoletin), flavonoids, coumarins and furanocoumarins (incl. angelol, angelicol, osthol, umbelliferone, bergapten, isoangelol, anpubesol, columbianadin, columbianadin acetate, columbianetin, xanthotoxin, isoimperatorin), glabralactone, angelic/palmitic/tiglic/stearic/linolenic/oleic/aminobutyric acids, phytosterols, glucose
Effective qualities: pungent, bitter, warm, dry
stimulating, dispersing, relaxing, calming, decongesting
Tropism: muscular, nervous, circulatory, respiratory, reproductive systems
Bladder, Kidney, Lung, Ren channels; Air, Fluid, Warmth bodies

Actions and Indications

circulatory and muscular stimulant/relaxant: deficient and spasmodic musculoskeletal conditions with chronic paresthesia and contraction of extremities

stimulant diaphoretic, anti-infective: common cold, flu (esp. with aching muscles and headache)

neuromuscular sedative: analgesic, anti-inflammatory: arthralgia, myalgia, neuralgia, neuritis, dysmenorrhea, lumbar pain, headache, toothache; rheumatoid arthritis

nervous sedative, spasmolytic: unrest, irritability, muscle spasms
uterine stimulant, emmenagogue: amenorrhea, prolonged pregnancy, retained placenta or lochia
draining diuretic: edema
stimulant/relaxant expectorant: chronic bronchitis with coughing and wheezing
photosensitizer
antibacterial, interferon inducent: infections generally; abscesses

Symptom Pictures

wind/damp/cold obstruction: limb, muscle or joint pain; numb, stiff lower back and legs, cold hands and feet,

lung phlegm cold: coughing with production of white sputum, wheezing, chills, sneezing, headache

Preparation

Use: The root Angelica Du Huo is used in a decoction or tincture.

Dosage: Decoction: 3-10 g
Tincture: 1-4 ml

Caution: Forbidden in Yin deficiency conditions with empty heat and in Blood (metabolic) deficiency syndromes. Also forbidden during pregnancy because of its *uterine stimulant* action.

Notes

This pubescent *Angelica* species from the montane wilds of Sichuan is loaded with a rich assortment of essential oils, alkaloids and glycosides, including a wide spectrum of coumarins. It addresses a large variety of painful (wind, damp and cold) rheumatic and arthritic conditions. Hairy angelica's pungent-bitter qualities are both *stimulant* and *relaxant* on the circulatory and neuromuscular level, and somewhat *sedative* on the central nervous level. The remedy is ideal for chronic arthritic and neuralgic pain with joint numbness and stiffness. Predictably for an *Angelica,* other conditions presenting cold stagnation (including amenorrhea and dysmenorrhea) are treated through its tropism for female reproductive and bronchial functions.

威靈仙

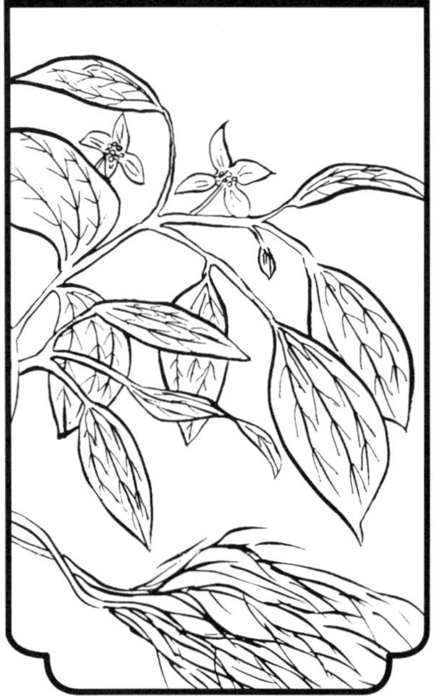

Clematis Wei Ling Xian

Chinese Clematis Root

Botanical source: *Clematis chinensis* Osbeck or *C. hexapetala* Pallas and spp. (Ranunculaceae)
Pharmaceutical name: Radix Clematis
Chinese names: Wei Ling Xian, Mian Tuan Tie Xian Lian (M); Wai Ling Sin (C)
Other names: Vase vine, Asian virgin's bower, Six-petal clematis, "Terrible spiritual immortal"; Ireisen (Jap)
Habit: Perennial woody climbing herb from Southeast Asia, growing on hillsides, roadsides and streamsides; in summer, panicles of pale green terminal/axillary flowers appear.
Part used: the rhizome and root

Therapeutic category: mild remedy with minimal chronic toxicity
Constituents: glycosides anemonin & protoanemonin 0.25%, anemonol, sterols, saponins, phenols, oleanolic acid
Effective qualities: pungent, a bit bitter, salty and sweet, warm, neutral
stimulating, relaxing, calming, decongesting
Tropism: muscular, nervous, urinary, reproductive, digestive systems
Bladder, Liver channels; Air, Fluid, Warmth bodies

Actions and Indications

muscular stimulant/relaxant: deficient and spasmodic musculoskeletal conditions with joint stiffness, paresthesia of limbs
neuromuscular sedative, analgesic: rheumatic myalgia, fibrositis, neuralgia, arthralgia, backache, lumbar pain or muscular strain, knee pain, headache
anti-inflammatory: acute neuritis, mastitis, tonsilitis, laryngitis; chronic cholecystitis
uterine stimulant, parturient, arbortive: dysmenorrhea, amenorrhea (esp. due to cold); stalled or painful labor, uterine dystocia; miscarriage, retained placenta
draining diuretic: edema
cholagogue: gallbladder congestion, jaundice
antibacterial, antifungal: candidiasis, psoriasis, filariasis
Miscellaneous: dissolves small fish bones stuck in the esophagus

Symptom Pictures

wind/damp/cold obstruction: stiff painful joints, muscle aches or numbness, backache

uterus cold: difficult, painful or stopped menses, easily chilled

Preparation

Use: The root Clematis Wei Ling Xian is decocted or used in tincture form.
Dosage: Decoction: 4-16 g
Tincture: 1-4 ml
Caution: Forbidden in Qi or Blood (metabolic) deficiency syndromes, especially with spasms, and, being a *uterine stimulant*, during pregnancy.

Notes

A variety of actions coalesce to produce the excellent *antineuralgic* and *antirheumatic* effects Clematis root is so well known for, especially when applied with joint stiffness and joint or muscle pain present. Focusing primarily on the striped muscles and joints, the remedy's time-tested *analgesic, anti-inflammatory* and *diuretic* actions arise from a collection of various glycosides.

The same actions are also much used in menstrual and obstetrical formulas for treating spasmodic dysmenorrhea, amenorrhea and uterine dystocia with hypertonic contractions—essentially whenever relaxation and stimulation are needed simultaneously. In the third stage of labor, Clematis root will help expell the placenta.

Clematis root is often used in hospitals in the People's Republic for labor induction, with apparent 95% effectiveness: The fresh root, water-cleaned and sterilized, is introduced into the uterine cavity until resistance is felt; 2 cm of the root is left outside the cervix and fixed with gauze. Labor usually occurs within 24-48 hours (Chang and But 1987).

The *antifungal* action of Clematis root's phenol content is noteworthy in light of candidiasis and other fungal infections.

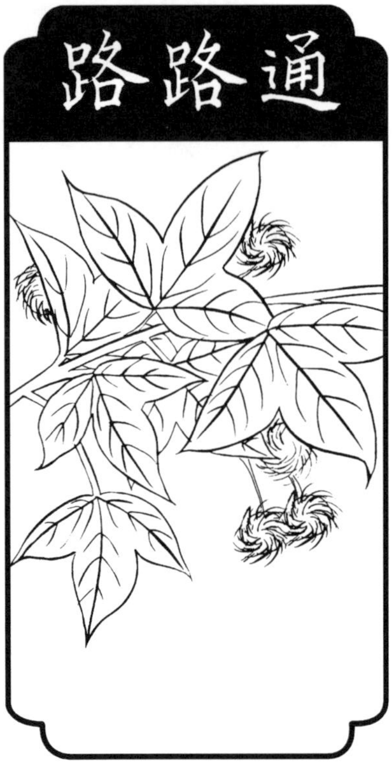

Liquidambar Lu Lu Tong

Taiwan Maple Fruit *

Botanical source: *Liquidambar taiwaniana/formosana* Hance (Hamamelidaceae)
Pharmaceutical name: Fructus Liquidambaris
Chinese names: Lu Lu Tong (Mand); Lou Lou Tung (Cant)
Other names: Fragrant maple, Sweetgum/Liquidambar fruit; Rorotsu (Jap)
Habit: Tall deciduous tree from Taiwan and South China found at forest outskirts, on hillsides, in sparse woods and shrubby places; also cultivated.
Part used: the fruit

Therapeutic category: mild remedy with minimal chronic toxicity
Constituents: essential oil (incl. camphene, dipentene, terpene, borneol), cinnamic acid, resin, benzine, triterpenic acid (liquidambaric acid) and lactone
Effective qualities: bitter, pungent, neutral
stimulating, relaxing, decongesting
Tropism: muscular, nervous, urogenital, digestive systems
Liver, Stomach, Bladder, Ren channels
Air, Fluid bodies

Actions and Indications

muscular stimulant/relaxant: deficient and spasmodic musculoskeletal conditions with limb contraction, muscular paresthesia and pain
neuromuscular sedative: analgesic, spasmolytic: rheumatic myalgia, arthralgia, neuralgia, dysmenorrhea, strangury, epigastric pain, intestinal colic with irregular stool, IBS
uterine stimulant, emmenagogue: amenorrhea, oligomenorrhea
galactagogue: insufficient breast milk
draining diuretic: anuria, edema
antiallergic, dermatropic: allergic disorders; dermatitis, urticaria, measles

Symptom Pictures

wind/damp obstruction: painful and numb muscles, esp. of lumbars and knees, stiff limbs

uterus Qi constraint: menstrual cramps, irregular, scanty or absent menses

intestines Qi constraint with **food stagnation:** epigastric or abdominal pain with distension, irregular and inconsistent bowel movement

kidney fluid congestion: water retention, difficult or scanty urination

Preparation

Use: The fruit Liquidambar Lu Lu Tong is decocted or used in tincture form (which is more *stimulating* and *analgesic*).
Dosage: Decoction: 3-10 g
Tincture: 2-4 ml
Caution: Being a *uterine stimulant*, this remedy is contraindicated during pregnancy.

Notes

The fruits of a beautiful maple tree variety from southern China—once gracing the imperial palace grounds of the Forbidden City—furnishes this remedy. Taiwan maple fruit's essentially *stimulating* and *relaxing* actions serve neuromuscular conditions typified by contraction, numbness and pain—in traditional terms, wind and damp obstructing the channels.

Painful, spasmodic menstrual and intestinal conditions are also relieved through the *analgesic, spasmolytic* effect of Taiwan maple's pungent-bitter effective qualities.

The resin extracted from the Taiwan maple fruit, called **Bai Jiao Xiang,** is used like the crude fruit itself. The tree resin is called **Feng Xia Zhi, Chinese storax** or **Formosa sweet gum;** it is used in a similar way to **Levant storax, Su He Xiang,** from *Liquidambar orientalis.*

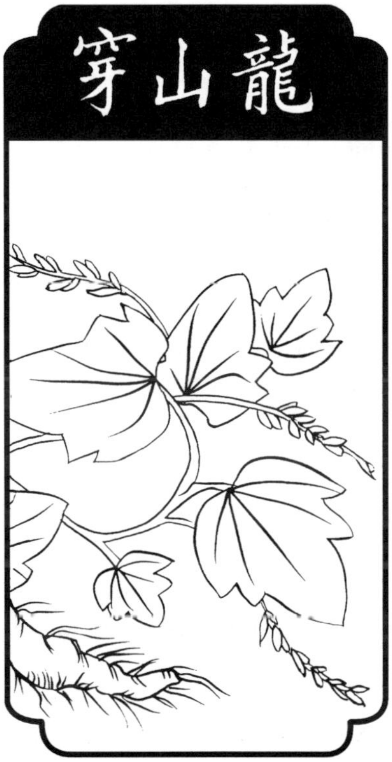

Dioscorea Chuan Shan Long

Nippon Yam Root

Botanical source: *Dioscorea nipponica* Makino (Dioscoreaceae)
Pharmaceutical name: Rhizoma Dioscoreae nipponicae
Chinese names: Chuan Shan Long (Mand); Chyun Saan Lung (Cant)
Other names: Uchiwadokoro, Yumoridokoro (Jap)
Habit: Perennial temperate East Asian twining vine, preferring cold climates and loose, sandy soil (although very adaptable); yellow-green single flowers hang down from axils.
Part used: the root

Therapeutic category: mild remedy with minimal chronic toxicity
Constituents: steroidal saponins (incl. dioscin, diosgenin, diostadiene)
Effective qualities: a bit bitter and sweet, warm, moist
stimulating, relaxing, decongesting, dissolving
Tropism: musculoskeletal, nervous, cardiovascular, respiratory, urinary systems
Kidney, Lung channels
Air, Fluid bodies

Actions and Indications

muscular relaxant: spasmodic musculoskeletal conditions with joint stiffness, muscular paresthesia
neuromuscular sedative: analgesic, anti-inflammatory: rheumatoid arthritis, rheumatic myalgia
coronary restorative: antilipemic, anticoagulant: coronary deficiency/disease, angina pectoris, cerebral arteriosclerosis; hyperlipidemia
hypotensive: hypertension
stimulant expectorant, antitussive: chronic bronchitis, cough
radiation-protective: radiation damage/sickness
antibacterial, diuretic: chronic brucellosis

Symptom Pictures

wind/damp/cold obstruction: painful, stiff joints; muscle pains and numbness
heart blood and Qi stagnation: chest tightness/pain, palpitations, difficult breathing

Preparation

Use: The root Dioscorera Chuan Shan Long is decocted or used in tincture form.
Dosage: Decoction: 10-30 g
Tincture: 2-4 ml
Caution: Contraindicated during pregnancy.

Notes

Containing a string of steroidal saponins, Nippon yam root is an effective and currently much used *antiarthritic, antirheumatic* and *coronary restorative* remedy. The protective effect that it provides against damage from radiation is also noteworthy.

Piper Hai Feng Teng

Kadsura Pepper Stem

海风藤

Botanical source: *Piper kadsura* (Choisy) Ohwi or *P. hancei* var. *hancei* or *P. hancei* var. *squamiglandiferum* Maximowicz (Piperaceae)
Chinese names: Hai Feng Teng, Shan Ju, Ju Bing Teng, Shi Nan Teng (Mand); Hoi Fung Tang (Cant)
Other names: "Sea wind vine"; Kaifuto (Jap)
Habit: Evergreen climbing vine from Southeast China and Taiwan, growing along the coast or in deep mountain woods; blooms in early summer with spikelets of single flowers.

Category: mild remedy with minimal chronic toxicity
Constituents: essential oil (incl. pinenes, limonene, sabinene, camphene, isoasarone, bornyl acetate), futoxide, futonenone, glycosides (incl. futoquinol, sitosterol, stigmasterol)
Effective qualities: pungent, bitter, warm, dry; stimulating, dispersing, relaxing
Tropism: muscular, nervous, respiratory, digestive systems; Liver, Kidney, Spleen, Lung channels

Actions: *Circulatory stimulant, diaphoretic, anti-infective, expectorant, antitussive, analgesic, spsmolytic, antitumoral*
Indications: Deficient and spasmodic musculoskeletal conditions with contracted/stiff/numb/ligaments and joints (wind/damp/cold obstruction syndrome); colds, coughs; bronchitis with lung wind cold and lung phlegm cold; rheumatic myalgia, arthralgia, lumbar pain, abdominal and epigastric pain (esp. with intestines damp cold); diarrhea, colitis; tumors.
Dosage: Decoction: 8-20 g
Tincture: 2-4 ml
Caution: Forbidden during pregnancy.
Notes: Similar in nature to Hairy angelica root, but even more *dispersing,* Kadsura pepper stem from South China is another essential oil-based remedy for symptom pictures presenting wind/damp/cold painful obstruction.

Recent pharmacognosical and ecological studies indicate that *Piper hancei* var. *squamiglandiferum* from southern Fujian province (a remedy now called **Xian Lin Ju**) was traditionally the source of the remedy Hai Feng Teng.

Sarcandra Jiu Jie Feng

Smooth Sarcandra Herb

九节风

Botanical source: *Sarcandra glabra* (Thunb.) Nakai (Chloranthaceae)
Chinese names: Jiu Jie Feng, Ju Jie Cha, Zhong Jie Feng (Mand); Gau Jit Fung (Cant)
Part used: the herb; also the root and entire plant
Category: mild remedy with minimal chronic toxicity

Constituents: flavonoids, cyanophoric glycosides, essential oil (incl. coumarins, lactones)
Effective qualities: bitter, a but pungent, cool, dry; stimulating, calming
Tropism: musculoskeletal, nervous, digestive, immune systems; Bladder, Spleen, Large Intestine channels

Actions: *Analgesic, vulnerary, antitussive, antitumoral, broad-spectrum anti-infective, detoxicant, antiulcer*
Indications: Rheumatoid arthritis, lumbar pain, leg pain, trauma pain; bone fractures; dizziness, headache; injuries from TB, cough; tumors (incl. cancer of pancreas, liver, stomach, rectum, esophagus, bladder, colon, gallbladder; leukemia, Hodgkin's disease); infections (incl. flu, encephalitis B, pneumonia, bacillary dysentery, gastroenteritis, tonsillitis, stomatitis); esp. *Staphylococcus aureus, Shigella, Salmonella, Proteus, Pseudomonas;* furunculosis, acute appendicitis, psoriasis; gastric and duodenal ulcer.
Dosage: Decoction: 15-30 g
Tincture: 2-4 ml
Caution: Occasional dizziness or tiredness has been reported from the use of this herb.
Notes: Smooth sarcandra herb is an important *anticancer* remedy in China.

Alangium Ba Jiao Feng

Alangium Root

八角枫

Botanical source: *Alangium chinense* (Lour.) Rehder (Alangiaceae)
Chinese names: Ba Jiao Feng (Gen) (Mand); Baat Gok Fung (Cant); "Eight-sided Alangium"
Part used: the root or root bark
Category: medium-strength remedy with some chronic toxicity
Constituents: alkaloids, anabasine, phenols, glycosides, cardiac glycosides, amino acids, resin
Effective qualities: pungent, warm, dry
Tropism: musculoskeletal, nervous, digestive, cardiovascular systems; Bladder, Spleen channels

Actions: *Muscle relaxant, analgesic, nervous sedative, vulnerary, cardiac stimulant, antivenomous*
Indications: Chronic rheumatic myalgia, rheumatoid arthritis, paresthesia (wind/damp/cold obstruction syndromes); anesthesia; muscle tension, traumatic injuries, contusions, sprains, fractures; fever, snakebite, flatulence.
Dosage: Decoction: 3-10 g
Tincture: 1-3 ml
The root hairs, being more toxic than the root itself, should be scraped off before use.
Caution: Not to be used continuously on its own for over three weeks because of its medium-strength nature. Fatigue and dizziness are signs of mild intoxication.
Notes: Alangium root is often used for surgical anesthesia, alongside acupuncture.

Sargentodoxa Da Xue Teng

Sargentodoxa Stem

大血藤

Botanical source: *Sargentodoxa cuneata* (Oliv.) Rehder et Wilson (Sargentodoxaceae)
Chinese names: Da Xue Teng, Jiu Jie Feng, Ju Jie Cha, Zhong Jie Feng, Hong Teng (Mand); Daai Hyut Tang (C)
Habit: Perennial vine common throughout China in open mountain forests; yellow raceme blossoms bloom in spring.
Category: mild remedy with minimal chronic toxicity
Effective qualities: bland, a bit bitter, astringent, warm, dry; stimulating, relaxing, calming, decongesting
Tropism: musculoskeletal, reproductive, digestive systems; Liver, Large Intestine channels

Actions: *Analgesic, emmenagogue, hemostatic, draining diuretic, detoxicant, anthelmintic, antibacterial*
Indications: Arthritis, rheumatism, muscular numbness from wind/damp obstruction; traumatic injury; amenorrhea, dysmenorrhea, menorrhagia, miscarriage; edema; appendicitis, filariasis, ancylostomyasis (hookworm), ascariasis (roundworm).
Dosage: Decoction: 15-30 g
Tincture: 2-4 ml. The wine treated stems and the tincture are more *stimulant* and *analgesic.*
Caution: None

Chaenomeles Mu Gua

Chinese Quince Fruit

木瓜

Botanical source: *Chaenomeles lagenaria* (Loisel.) Koidz. or *C. speciosa* (Sweet) Nakai and spp. (Rosaceae)
Chinese names: Mu Gua, Chuan Mu Gua (Mand); Muk Gwa, Chyun Muk Gwa (Cant)
Other names: Japanese/Flowering quince; Mokka (Jap)
Habit: Deciduous spiny cultivated shrub from North China, India. Carmine flower clusters appear in spring.
Category: mild remedy with minimal chronic toxicity
Constituents: saponins, flavonoids, tannin, tartaric/malic/citric acid, fructose, vitamin C
Effective qualities: sour, a bit pungent, warm, dry; relaxing, decongesting, restoring, astringing
Tropism: muscular, digestive, urinary systems; Liver, Spleen channels

Actions: *Spasmolytic, analgesic, astringent, antiemetic, draining diuretic*
Indications: Spasmodic and deficient musculoskeletal conditions with cramping pain of joints in extremities (damp/cold obstruction syndrome); lower back and leg weakness; arthralgia, myalgia, severe abdominal pain, pain from roundworms; calf muscle cramps; diarrhea; vomiting, dyspepsia, leg edema, beriberi, cholera.
Dosage: Decoction: 4-12 g
Tincture: 1-4 ml
Caution: Forbidden in external conditions, and not to be used continuously because of its potential damaging effect to teeth and bones.
Notes: Chinese quince is a special *relaxant* remedy from the Chang Jiang (Yangze) river provinces. It is most often used in formulas for arthritic pain of the extremities and intestinal colic.

Luffa Si Gua Luo
Spongegourd

丝瓜络

Botanical source: *Luffa cylindrica* L. or *L. acutangula* Roxburgh (Cucurbitaceae)
Chinese names: Si Gua Luo (M); Sei Gwa Lou (C)
Category: mild remedy with minimal chronic toxicity
Constituents: B rutenone, xylan, xylose, galactan
Effective qualities: sweet, neutral; calming, relaxing
Tropism: musculoskeletal, reproductive, digestive, respiratory systems; Lung, Liver, Stomach channels

Actions: *Analgesic, anti-inflammatory, detoxicant, expectorant, antitussive, detoxicant, diuretic, emmenagogue, antipyretic, galactagogue*
Indications: Painful conditions, e.g. arthralgia with swollen joints, myalgia (wind/damp obstruction syndrome); chest and flank soreness, breast pain and swelling, testicle pain and swelling (orchitis), traumatic injury; breast abscess, acute bronchitis (lung phlegm heat syndrome) with coughing, difficult expectoration, fever and chest pain; food poisoning (summer heat syndrome) with fever and oliguria; insufficient breast milk in nursing mothers; amenorrhea.
Dosage: Decoction: 6-14 g
Tincture: 2-4 ml
Caution: None.
Notes: The **ashes** of **baked Luffa sponge** are *astringent* and *hemostatic;* they are given for enteritis, blood in the stool and urine, uterine bleeding, cancerous swellings and hemorrhoids.

Morus Sang Zhi
Mulberry Twig

桑枝

Botanical source: *Morus alba* L. (Moraceae)
Chinese names: (La) Sang Zhi (Mand); Song Ji (Cant)
Other names: White mulberry; Soshi (Jap)
Habit: Deciduous tree, both wild and cultivated; flowers in May with stalked hanging catkins.
Category: mild remedy with minimal chronic toxicity
Constituents: mulberrin, mulberrochromene, cyclomulberrin, betulinic abid, morin, dihydromorin, cudranin, tetrahydrostilbene, dihydrokaempferol, maclurio, fructose, glucose, saccharose, tannins
Effective qualities: a bit bitter and sweet, cool, dry; relaxing, stimulating, decongesting
Tropism: muscular, nervous, urinary, immune systems; Liver channel

Actions: *Analgesic, draining diuretic, immunostimulant, hair growth stimulant*
Indications: Joint and muscle pain and stiffness in wind/damp obstruction syndrome; myalgia, arthralgia, water retention (esp. in legs); low lymphocyte transformation rate, infections in general; slow or deficient hair growth.
Dosage: Decoction: 15-30 g
Tincture: 2-5 ml
Caution: None.

Pinus Song Jie

Knotty Pine Wood Shaving

松节

Botanical source: *Pinus tabulaeformis* Carrington or *P. massoniana* Lamb or *P. yunnanensis* Franchet (Pinaceae)
Chinese names: Song Jie, Ou Song Jie (Mand); Chung Jit (Cant)
Category: mild remedy with minimal chronic toxicity
Constituents: turpentine, resin, essential oil
Effective qualities: bitter, warm, dry; calming, relaxing
Tropism: musculoskeletal, digestive, respiratory systems; Liver, Kidney channels

Actions: *analgesic, anti-infective, digestant*
Indications: Arthritic joint soreness and pain from wind/damp/cold, traumatic pain, toothache; colds, nausea, dyspepsia.
Dosage: Decoction: 10-16 g
Tincture: 2-4 ml
Caution: Use cautiously in Yin and Blood deficiency conditions.
Notes: **Pine pollen, Song Hua Fen,** is given as a *blood cell stimulant* and general *restorative,* especially to the heart and lungs. The nutritious **pine kernel** is called Song Zi.

Bombyx Can Sha

Silkworm Dropping

蚕砂

Zoological source: *Bombyx mori* L.
Chinese names: Can Sha, Wan Can Sha, Yuan Can Sha (Mand); Chan Sa (Cant)
Other names: Sansha (Jap)
Category: mild remedy with minimal chronic toxicity
Constituents: phytol, sitosterol, cholesterol, ergosterol, tetracosanol, lupenol, carotene, vitamin B1
Effective qualities: sweet, pungent, warm, dry; relaxing, stimulating
Tropism: musculoskeletal, digestive systems; Liver, Spleen, Stomach channels

Actions: *Analgesic, spasmolytic, anti-inflammatory, antiemetic, hemostatic, hypoglycemiant*
Indications: Spasmodic musculoskeletal conditions with pain and stiffness of joints or muscles (wind/damp obstruction syndrome); arthralgia, myalgia; calf muscle spasm, severe abdominal pain and diarrhea in intestines Qi constraint syndrome; colic, nausea, vomiting, headache; hyperglycemia, diabetes.
Dosage: Decoction: 10-18 g
Tincture: 2-4 ml.

The tincture or wine is especially good for treating uterine bleeding.

A hot compress of the toasted remedy is applied in hemiplegia, to stiff or paralyzed muscles, hands, feet and joints, and to numbness in the skin.

Caution: None.

REMEDIES TO REDUCE INFLAMMATION AND RELIEVE JOINT PAIN AND SWELLING

➤ DISPEL WIND/DAMP/HEAT AND RELIEVE PAINFUL OBSTRUCTION

Anti-inflammatory, analgesic, antipyretic antiarthritics

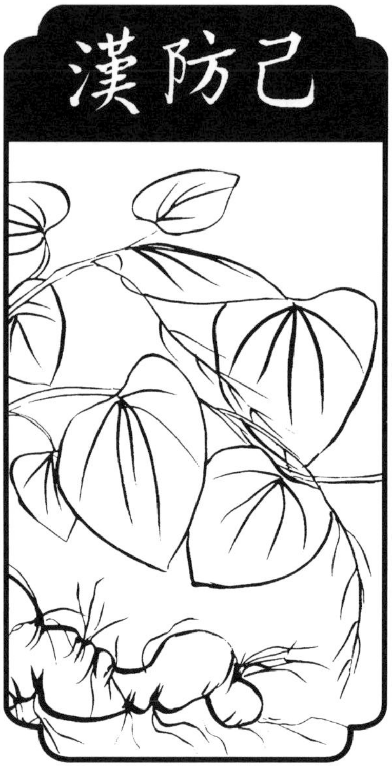

Stephania Han Fang Ji

Stephania Root

Botanical source: *Stephania tetrandra* S. Moore (Menispermaceae)
Pharmaceutical name: Radix Stephaniae tetrandrae
Chinese names: Han Fang Ji, Fen Fang Ji, Fang Ji (Mand); Haan Fong Gei, Fong Gei (Cant)
Other names: Kanpoi (Jap)
Habit: Perennial twining vine from Central China, Zhejiang and Anhui; found on hillside bush and along roads in humid, shady conditions; small, pale yellow, four-petaled single capitate flowers open in early summer.
Part used: the root

Therapeutic category: mild remedy with minimal chronic toxicity
Constituents: alkaloids (incl. tetrandrine, dymethyltetandrene, cyclanoline, fangchinoline, stephenanthrine, oxofangchirine), flavonoids (incl. menisine, menisidine), essential oil (incl. phenols), organic acids
Effective qualities: bitter, a bit pungent, cold, dry
calming, relaxing, stimulating, decongesting
Tropism: muscular, nervous, urinary, digestive systems
Bladder, Kidney, Spleen, Lung channels
Fluid, Air, Warmth bodies

ACTIONS AND INDICATIONS

neuromuscular sedative/relaxant: analgesic, anti-inflammatory: acute musculoskeletal conditions with pain and contraction; acute arthritis, neuralgia, rheumatic myalgia (incl. fibromyalgia), lower back pain; muscular paresthesia, acute gastroenteritis, dysentery
antipyretic: fevers
draining diuretic, spasmolytic: generalized or leg edema, ascites; dysuria, oliguria, strangury; spastic neurogenic bladder, urge incontinence
coronary dilator, hypotensive: hypertension, angina pectoris, arrhythmia
muscle relaxant: anesthesia
immune regulator, antiallergic: immune stress with immediate allergies (incl. rhinitis, asthma)
antitumoral, interferon inducent: tumors (incl. cancer; esp. of liver and blood)
leukocytogenic: leukopenia
antibacterial, antiamoebic
Miscellaneous: carbuncles, scabies, peptic ulcer, beriberi

SYMPTOM PICTURES

wind/damp/heat obstruction: fever, thirst; painful, swollen, hot red joints, stiff hands and feet

kidney and liver fluid congestion: lower limb or generalized water retention, abdominal distension, difficult or scanty urination

Preparation

Use: The root Stephania Han Fang Ji is decocted or used in tincture form.

Dosage: Decoction: 6-12 g
Tincture: 2-4 ml

Caution: Contraindicated in internal damp conditions and to be used cautiously in Yin deficiency patterns.

Notes

With its bitter-cold qualities, Stephania root is equally effective as a *sedative/relaxant* for the musculoskeletal system (in acute forms of arthritis, neuralgia and rheumatic conditions) and as a *stimulant/relaxant diuretic* (edema, spastic neurogenic dysuria and urge incontinence).

Stephania's main alkaloid tetrandrene has shown good *analgesic, anti-inflammatory, hypotensive, antiallergic, antimicrobial* and *antitumoral* activity. Since then, the root (or its extracted alkaloid) has assumed a high-profile, becoming a standard remedy in the treatment of conditions such as neuralgia, hypertension, cardiac arrhythmia, immediate allergies and cancer.

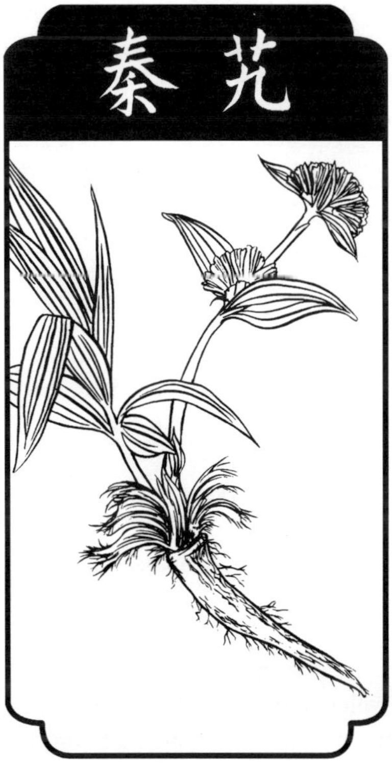

Gentiana Qin Jiao

Large-Leaf Gentian Root *

Botanical source: *Gentiana macrophylla* Pallas or *G. tibetica* or *G. dahurica* Fischer or *G. crassicaulis* Duthie ex Burkhill or *G. straminea* Maximowicz (Gentianaceae)
Pharmaceutical name: Radix Gentianae macrophyllae
Chinese names: Qin Jiao (Mand); Cheun Gau (Cant)
Other names: Jingyo (Jap)
Habit: Perennial temperate mountain herb from Northeast Asia; purple flowers open in summer.
Part used: the root

Therapeutic category: mild remedy with minimal chronic toxicity
Constituents: alkaloids (incl. gentianine, gentianidine, gentianol), glycosides (incl. gentiopicroside, gentialutine, gentiatibetine, gantianaine, gentioflavine, sweroside, tetraacetyl swertiamarin), essential oil
Effective qualities: pungent, bitter, cool, moist
calming, relaxing, decongesting, sinking
Tropism: nervous, cardiovascular, hepatic systems
Liver, Stomach, Gallbladder channels
Air, Warmth bodies

Actions and Indications

neuromuscular sedative/relaxant: analgesic, anti-inflammatory: acute musculoskeletal conditions with pain, stiffness, contraction and spasms; neuralgia, arthralgia, tendinitis; rheumatoid arthritis, neuritis, cerebrospinal meningitis
antipyretic: remittent fever (esp. in lung TB and infantile malnutrition)
hepatic diuretic: jaundice (esp. acute, infantile), liver congestion
hypotensive: hypertension
demulcent laxative: constipation with dryness
hemostatic, decongestant: hematuria, hemorrhoids
antiallergic, antihistaminic: immediate allergies (incl. rhinitis, urticaria)
antifungal, antibacterial, interferon inducent

Symptom Pictures

wind/damp (heat) obstruction: stiffness or swelling in joints of extremities, muscle pains and spasms

liver damp heat: fatigue, right flank pain, yellowing of skin

Preparation

Use: The root Gentiana Qin Jiao is used in decoction or tincture form.

Dosage: Decoction: 4-12 g
Tincture: 1-4 ml

Caution: Contraindicated in diarrhea from intestinal deficiency, frequent urination and chronic pain with emaciation.

Notes

Whereas the digestive remedy Gentiana Long Dan Cao is botanically and therapeutically very similar to the Western Gentian root, Large-leaf gentian root is distinct from both. It possesses pungent, relaxing qualities as well as bitter, calming and cooling ones. This wind/damp/heat-clearing remedy is mainly used for acute, inflammatory, painful, contracted arthritic conditions and acute forms of liver congestion with jaundice and generally dysbiotic/subinfectious terrain.

Loaded with an exceptionally rich assortment of alkaloids and glycosides, the Large-leaf gentian also exerts a *relaxing* influence that extends to a *hypotensive* effect on the circulation. The alkaloid gentianine in particular has shown *antihistamine* activity.

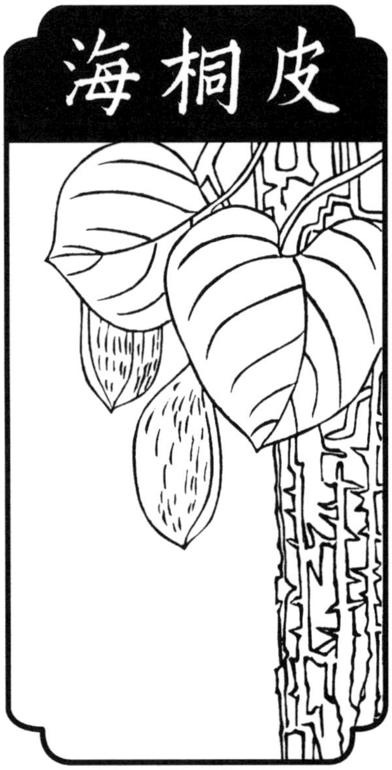

Erythrina Hai Tong Pi

Asian Coral Tree Bark

Botanical source: *Erythrina variegata* L. var. *orientalis* Merril (Leguminosae)
Pharmaceutical name: Cortex Erythrinae
Chinese names: Hai Tong Pi (Mand); Hoi Tung Pei, Hung Tung Pei (Cant)
Other names: Indian coral tree, Cockspur; Kaitohi (Jap)
Habit: Tall spinous shade tree from South China and Southeast Asia with brilliant red flowers.
Part used: the bark

Therapeutic category: mild remedy with minimal chronic toxicity
Constituents: alkaloids erythraline and hypaphorine, amino acids, organic acids
Effective qualities: bitter, pungent, cool, dry
relaxing, calming, stimulating, decongesting
Tropism: muscular, nervous, digestive, repiratory, cardiovascular, reproductive systems
Liver, Spleen, Kidneys channels; Air, Fluid bodies

Actions and Indications

neuromuscular sedative: analgesic, anesthetic: acute musculoskeletal conditions with acute or chronic pain; rheumatic myalgia, arthralgia (esp. lower back/knees), muscle spasm/pain, toothache, neuralgia; neurodermatitis
cholagogue, draining diuretic: jaundice, hepatic deficiency, edema
stimulant expectorant: bronchitis
uterine stimulant, astringent: amenorrhea, menorrhagia
anti-infective, dermatropic: antifungal, antipruritic: fungal skin infections, yeast infections with vaginitis,

pruritus, scabies, pruritic skin lesions, chronic dermatitis (incl. neurogenic)
anthelmintic: intestinal parasites

Symptom Picture

wind/damp/heat obstruction: aching, pain and swelling in lower back and knees, painful swollen joints

Preparation

Use: The bark Erythrina Hai Tong Pi is decocted or used in tincture form. Compresses, douches, suppositories, etc. can be prepared for pruritic skin infections and vaginitis, and a gargle of the decoction is used for toothache.

Dosage: Decoction: 6-16 g
Tincture: 2-5 ml

Caution: Contraindicated in Blood (metabolic) deficiency, and during pregnancy.

Notes

The bark of the common Asian coral tree is traditionally given in acute lower back and leg pain of an arthritic or muscular nature. Today this remedy is notable for the treatment of fungal and neurogenic skin conditions. With its additional *astringent* action, it also addresses fungal forms of pruritic vaginitis, including candidiasis.

雷公藤

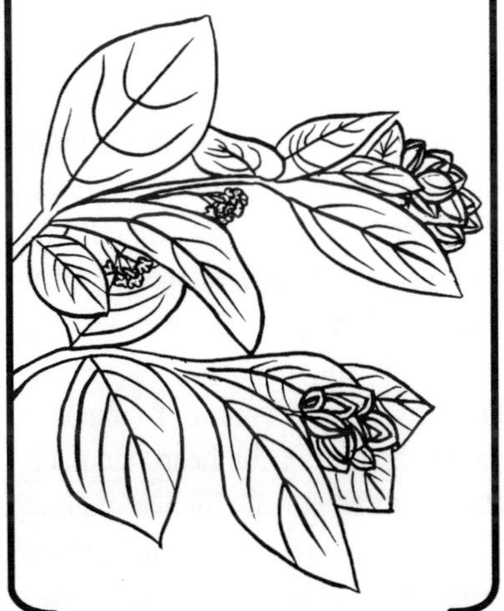

Tripterygium Lei Gong Teng

Yellow Vine Root Pith

Botanical source: *Tripterygium wilfordii* Hooker f. (Celastraceae)
Pharmaceutical name: Medulla radicis Tripterygii
Chinese names: Lei Gong Teng, Cai Chong Yao, Huang Teng, Zi Jin Pi (Mand); Leui Gung Tang (Cant)
Habit: Perennial climbing vine from subtropical Southeast China and Taiwan; grows on shady, damp hillsides and along wooded streamsides and mountain valleys; prefers cloudy, damp weather and fairly fertile soil; flowers in May/June with panicles of small white blossoms.
Part used: the root xylem (pith)

Therapeutic category: medium-strength remedy with both cumulative and some acute toxicity
Constituents: tripterygium alkaloids (incl. wilfordine, wilforgine, wilfortrine, wilforzine, wilforine), macrocyclic alkaloids (incl. celacemine, celabenzine, celafurine, celacinnine), sesquiterpene alkaloid (wilfornine), epoxyditerpenes (incl. triptolide, tripdiolide, triptonide, triptonolide, triptophenolide, hypolide), diterpines (incl. tripterine [celastrol], triptonoterpene and its methyl ether, triptolidenol), dulcitrol, glycosides (incl. 5 triterpenoids [incl. triptotriterpenic acid, orthosphenic acid, wilforlides A and B]), tripchlorolide, vitamin C
Effective qualities: pungent, cold
calming, stimulating, dissolving
Tropism: musculoskeletal, urinary, integumentary systems
Liver, Bladder channels; Warmth, Air bodies

Actions and Indications

musculoskeletal sedative/relaxant: analgesic, anti-inflammatory: acute musculoskeletal conditions with joint pain, swelling and stiffness; rheumatoid arthritis, neuralgia, lupus, lepra reaction, vasculitis, polymyositis
immune regulator (immunosuppressant), antiallergic: immune stress with allergic and autoimmune

disorders (incl. rheumatoid and psoriatic arthritis, lupus, psoriasis, Behcet's syndrome, ankylosing spondylitis, Sjögren's syndrome, Reiter's syndrome, dermatomyositis, allergic purpura, allergic vasculitis, multiple sclerosis)
dermatropic, antipruritic: skin and mucosal disorders (incl. eczema, dermatitis, intractable pruritus, pustulosis, erythema multiforme, pustular psoriasis, dermatomyositis, Sweef syndrome, pityriasis, pemphygus, alopecia aerata)
renal restorative: glomerulonephritis, purpuric nephritis, infantile nephrotic syndrome, albuminuria
antitumoral, resolvent: tumors (incl. cancer); uterine and breast cancer, chronic breast disease (fibroadenoma), progressive systemic sclerosis (scleroderma), mixed connective tissue diseases
contraceptive, spermicidal (reversable): contraception
antifungal: ringworm (tinea)
anthelmintic, antibacterial: parasites
pesticidal, insecticidal: worms, maggots, wrigglers, rodents; larvae
anti-inflammatory detoxicant (topically): rheumatoid arthritis, snakebites
Miscellaneous: lung TB, bronchial asthma, cerebral thrombosis, thromboangiitis, menopausal menorrhagia

Symptom Picture

wind/damp/heat obstruction: painful, discolored, numb or swollen joints, skin rashes, itching skin

Preparation

Use: The root pith Tripterygium Lei Gong Teng is decocted or used in tincture form. When using this fairly toxic remedy internally, it is important to use the least toxic part of the plant, namely the root xylem or pith: Two layers of root bark (outer and inner bark) must be entirely removed before the pith becomes available. Additionally, the older the root pith the better, because its toxicity dissipates with age. The decoction time should be at least 3 hours.

For best and safest results, internal treatment with this botanical should be prolonged and intermittent (see also below). Maximal effect is usually obtained after three months of treatment, after which a maintenance dose of about one-third of the initial dose is given. Relapses are also successfully treated with this remedy.

The whole plant is also employed in topical applictions for conditions such as arthritis, snake bites, skin itching, eczema, etc. The leaves or the root bark are used to kill maggots, wrigglers, larvae, rats, etc.

Dosage: Long decoction (3 hours or more): 6-20 g
Tincture: 1-3 ml

Caution: Tripterygium Lei Gong Teng should only be used under professional supervision. Because of its medium-strength status, doses should begin small and only be increased after a two-week course of treatment, if still ineffective at that time. Continuous courses of treatment should be interrupted every two weeks for several days, depending on the patient's reaction and the severity of the disorder. Generally, a break of 7-10 days should be taken after a one-month course. Side effects can be minimized if the remedy is taken after meals and together with vitamin B6 or an antacid tablet. Monitoring progress and side-effects with blood tests is advised during treatment. The remedy should be discontinued at any time that side-effects become too severe, followed by large doses of vitamin B4 and C.

Forbidden during pregnancy and in hemorrhage. Cautious use is advised in diseases of the heart, stomach, spleen, liver and kidneys, and when treating young women. The adverse reactions to this remedy include nausea, upper abdominal discomfort, appetite loss, vomiting, loose stool, palpitations, dizziness, erosion and bleeding of the lips and mouth mucosa, sore throat, skin itching, amenorrhea and other menstrual disorders. Extreme toxic reactions include renal failure, contact dermatitis, spleen and liver injury and damage to spermatogenic epithelium.

Notes

A highly alkaloidal plant from the Southern provinces and Taiwan, Yellow vine root pith has emerged during the last decade as *the* major Chinese remedy for various hypersensitivity conditions. The fact that, despite its drawback of side-effects, it is consistently employed in most of today's known autoimmune disorders, for instance, attests to its high degree of efficacity.

For these conditions, which include those affecting the musculoskeletal system (rheumatoid arthritis, lupus, multiple sclerosis, among others), Yellow vine shows strong *analgesic, anti-inflammatory* and *antipruritic* actions that complement its *immunosupressant* effect. These effects have been shown to operate by an inhibition of both cellular and humoral immunity. On one hand, the remedy inhibits interleukin 2 production, thereby lowering T-lymphocyte transformation especially. On the other hand, it inhibts humoral immunity, especially thymus dependant, antigen-induced antibody formation (Xu Yue-lin and Kang Ke-fei 1988). These *immune-inhibiting* actions are needed in types II through V hypersensitivity conditions to stop immune functions from injuring or destroying healthy cells.

Yellow vine root pith is also considered highly effective for both acute and chronic renal conditions, and produces encouraging results in many forms of cancer.

Aristolochia Guang Fang Ji

广防己

Fangchi Birthwort Root

Botanical source: *Aristolochia fangchi* Wu or *A. westlandii* Hemslow (Aristolochiaceae)
Chinese names: Guang Fang Ji, Fang Ji (Mand); Gwong Fong Gei, Fong Gei (Cant)
Other names: Koboi (Jap)
Habit: Twining, thick woody deciduous vine from subtropical South China; small flower racemes bloom in spring.
Category: mild remedy with minimal chronic toxicity
Constituents: aristolochic acids, aristolactam
Effective qualities: very bitter, pungent, cold, dry; calming, relaxing, decongesting
Tropism: musculoskeletal, nervous, respiratory, urinary systems; Bladder, Spleen, Kidney, Lung channels

Actions: *Analgesic, anti-inflammatory, antipyretic, draining diuretic, detoxicant, astringent*
Indications: Acute musculoskeletal conditions with pain (wind/damp/heat obstruction syndrome); myalgia, neuralgia, arthralgia, rheumatoid arthritis, neuritis, fever; edema (general or facial); gonorrhea, cholera.
Dosage: Decoction: 4-12 g
Tincture: 1-4 ml
Caution: Use cautiously in Yin deficiency conditions.

Cocculus Mu Fang Ji

木防己

Three-Leaf Cocculus Root *

Botanical source: *Cocculus trilobus* (Thunb.) De Candolle (Aristolochiaceae)
Chinese name: Mu Fang Ji, Tu Fang Ji, Fang Ji (Mand); Mut Fong Gei, Fong Gei (Cant)
Other names: Koboi (Jap)
Habit: Twining, woody deciduous vine from South and Central China; grows among shrubs and scrub, on slopes and roadsides; flowers in summer with cymes of small, white single terminal flowers.
Category: mild remedy with minimal chronic toxicity
Constituents: alkaloids trilobine, homotrilobine, magnoflorine, trilobamine, coclobine, menisarine, normenisarine
Effective qualities: bitter, pungent, cold; calming, relaxing
Tropism: musculoskeletal, nervous, urinary, respiratory systems; Bladder, Lung, Spleen, Kidney channels

Actions: *Analgesic, anti-inflammatory bronchial relaxant, antiasthmatic, antipyretic, detoxicant, antivenomous, antitumoral, hypotensive*
Indications: Acute musculoskeletal conditions with pain (esp. wind/damp/heat syndrome); myalgia, neuralgia, neuritis, arthralgia, rheumatoid arthritis; bronchial asthma, nephritis, urinary tract infections, fever; sores, boils; snake and insect bites; hypertension, beriberi, paralysis.
Dosage: Decoction: 6-12 g
Tincture: 1-4 ml
Caution: Use with caution in Yin deficiency conditions.
Notes: Of the four main plants that go under the remedy name Fang Ji, *Cocculus trilobus* is specifically called Mu Fang Ji. This is an alkaloidal plant whose component trilobine has received some research. Although similar in action to its companions in this section, Cocculus Mu Fang Ji enjoys the reputation for being the most generally effective for treating painful acute arthritic conditions.

Menispermum Bei Dou Gen
Siberian Moonseed Root

北豆根

Botanical source: *Menispermum dauricum* De Candolle (Menispermaceae)
Chinese names: Bei Dou Gen, Bian Fu Gen (Mand); Pan Dau Gan (Cant)
Category: medium-strength remedy with chronic toxicity
Constituents: alkaloids 1-2% (incl. menisperine, tetrandrine, dauricine, sinomenine, daurinoline, dauricolin, daurisoline, acutumine, magnoflorine)
Effective qualities: bitter, cold, dry; calming, relaxing, sinking
Tropism: neuromuscular, respiratory systems; Bladder, Lung, Heart channels

Actions: *Analgesic, neuromuscular (and muscle) relaxant, analgesic, anti-inflammatory, antipyretic, hypotensive, stimulant expectorant, antitussive, detoxicant, detumescent, anti-infective*
Indications: Acute musculoskeletal conditions with pain (wind/damp/heat obstruction); myalgia, neuralgia, neuritis, acute and chronic arthritis; acute laryngitis and pharyngitis, fever; hypertension; acute and chronic bronchitis with cough, pneumonia; esp. *Hemophilus influenzae* and *Diplococcus pneumoniae*; swollen, red boils; cancer; skin allergies.
Dosage: Decoction: 4-12 g
Tincture: 1-3 ml
Caution: Do not use continuously on its own at maximum dosage because of some cumulative toxicity.
Notes: Because of its *analgesic* action, this remedy (or its total extracted alkaloids) is also used in surgical anaesthesia, usually together with regular anesthetics.

Trachelospermum Luo Shi Teng
Star Jasmine Stem

络石藤

Botanical source: *Trachelospermum jasminoides* (Lindl.) Lemaire (Apocynaceae)
Chinese names: Luo Shi Teng, Shi Long Teng, Bai Hua Teng (Mand); Lok Sek Tang (Cant); "Enmesh stone vine"
Habit: High-climbing woody vine from South China
Category: mild remedy with minimal chronic toxicity
Constituents: acrtiin, tracheloside, nortracheloside, sitosterol, matairesonoside, nortracheloside, dambonitol, cymarose, tannins, resin
Effective qualities: bitter, cool
Tropism: musculoskeletal, nervous systems; Liver, Kidney, Heart channels

Actions: *Analgesic, anti-inflammatory, detoxicant, antipyretic, hypotensive, antibacterial, emmenagogue*
Indications: Inflamed, swollen joints; contracted, stiff ligaments; wind/damp/heat obstruction syndrome; muscle spasms, pain and numbness; arthritis, rheumatic myalgia, lumbar pain, fevers; fire toxins such as abscesses, boils, sore throat; hypertension; amenorrhea.
Dosage: Decoction: 10-16 g
Tincture: 2-4 ml
Caution: Forbidden during pregnancy.
Notes: **Star jasmine leaf** and **root** are used in a similar way to the stem.

Lonicera Jin Yin Teng

Japanese Honeysuckle Stem and Leaf

金银藤

Botanical source: *Lonicera japonica* Thunberg (Caprifoliaceae)
Chinese names: Jin Yin Teng, Ren Dong Teng, Yin Hua Teng (Mand); Gam Gan Tang, Yan Dong Tang (Cant)
Category: mild remedy with minimal chronic toxicity

Constituents: lonicerin, flavonoids, tannins, lutolin-rhamnoglucoside
Effective qualities: sweet, cold, dry; calming, dissolving, astringing
Tropism: musculoskeletal, epidermal systems; Heart, Lung channels

Actions: *Anti-inflammatory, antiarthritic, spasmolytic, broad-spectrum anti-infective (immunostimulant, antibacterial, antiviral, antifungal)*

Indications: Acute rheumatoid arthritis with hot, swollen joints (wind/damp/heat obstruction); acute infections (incl. common cold, influenza, enteritis, bacillary dysentery with melena, pneumonia, hepatitis, infected wounds).

Dosage: Decoction: 10-30 g
Tincture: 2-5 ml

Caution: Forbidden in deficient cold conditions.

Periploca Gang Liu Pi

Silk Vine Root Bark

杠柳皮

Botanical source: *Periploca sepium* Bunge (Asclepiadaceae)
Chinese names: Gang Liu Pi, Xiang Jia Pi, Bei Wu Jia Pi (Mand); Gong Lau Pei, Heung Ga Pei (Cant)
Category: medium-strength remedy with some chronic toxicity

Constituents: cardiotonic glycosides (incl. periplocin, periplocymarin), alpha-amyrin, sitosterol, glycosides G and K, salicylaldehyde
Effective qualities: sweet, warm, dry; restoring, calming
Tropism: musculoskeletal, cardiovascular, nervous systems; Heart, Kidney channels

Actions: *Analgesic, aphrodisiac, coronary and cardiac restorative*

Indications: Rheumatic myalgia; lumbar, bone, rheumatic and arthritic pain; impotence; congestive heart failure.

Dosage: Decoction: 3-8 g
Tincture: 0.5-2 ml

Caution: Only to be used for a few days at a time. Do not exceed doses nor use continuously as its medium-strength nature causes cumulative toxicity.

Notes: This remedy is sometimes used to adulterate or substitute for Acanthopanax Wu Jia Pi, Five Additions root bark. One of its names is Bei Wu Jia Pi, "Northern five additions bark." Research has shown, however, that it possesses none of that remedy's *restorative* action on muskuloskeletal tissues. In this respect, Silk vine root bark is a simple *analgesic.*

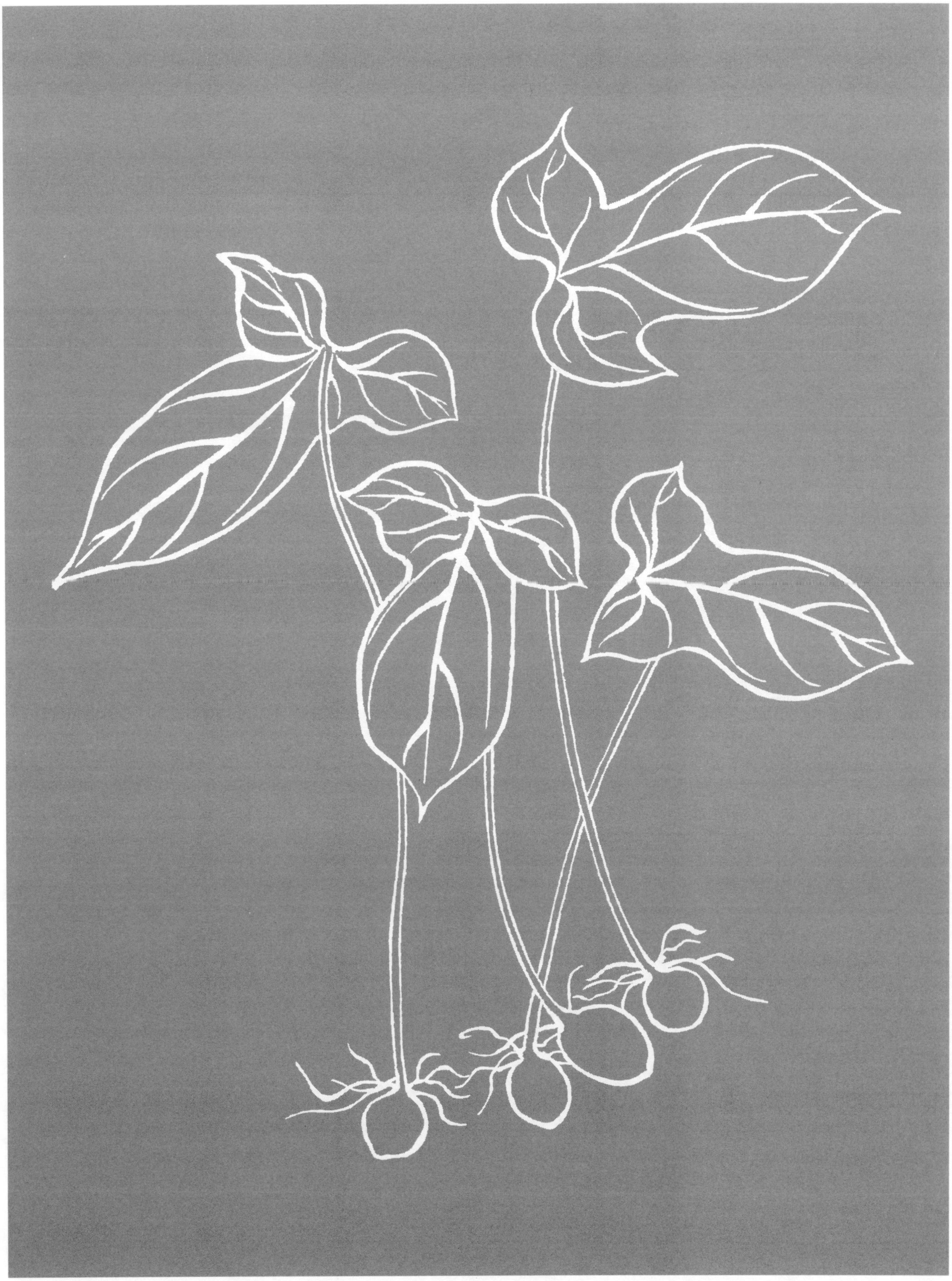

神經系统用药

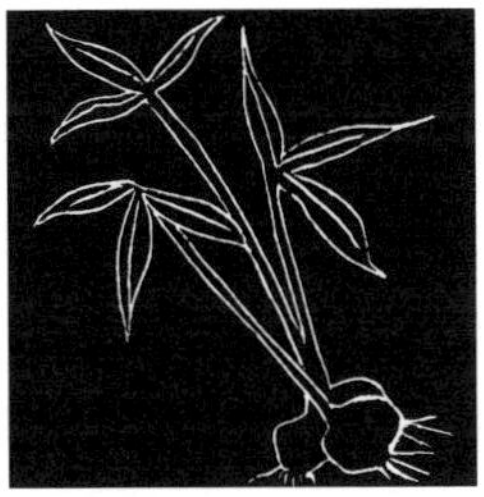

Remedies for the Nervous System

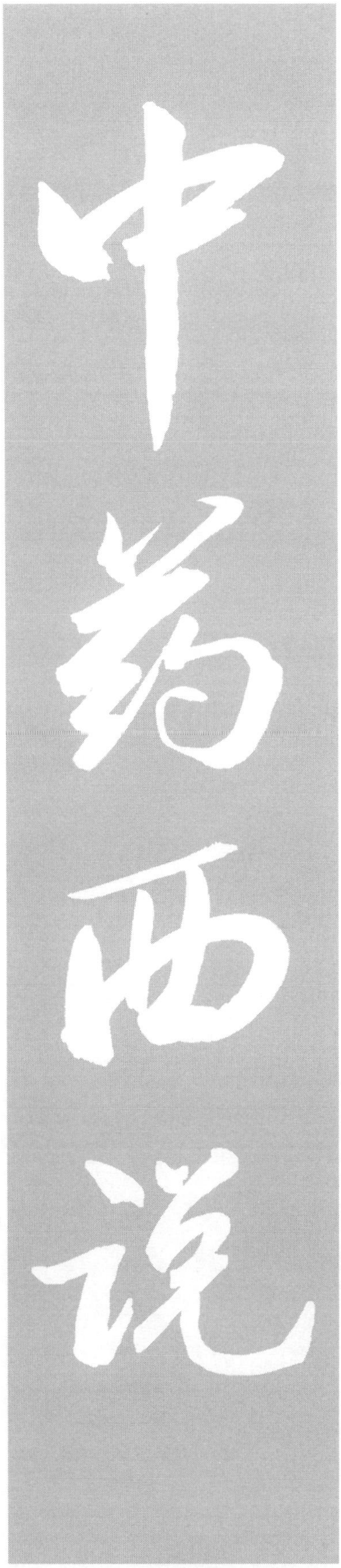

As part of a complete system of medicine, the Oriental pharmacopeia contains numerous herbal, mineral and animal remedies for treating nervous system disorders. They are useful for conditions of chronic neurological deficiency involving depression, fainting or sensory loss, as well as for acute excess conditions including spasms, agitation or pain.

Traditional Chinese medicine has no concept of "nerves" and the nervous system as such. Nevertheless, based on a vitalistic system of pathology, Chinese doctors over milleniums have developed highly refined treatment strategies and corresponding remedies for neurological disorders.

To find these nervous system remedies, however, one must delve into several traditional herb categories. All *nervous stimulants,* for example, are found in the herb class that "opens the orifices and revives the senses," that is, revives consciousness. The majority of *nervous relaxants,* on the other hand, are derived from the category that "extinguishes internal wind and stops spasms." *Nervous sedatives* like Ursus Xiong Dan (Bear gallbladder) are taken from the class that "quells fire," while other *nervous sedatives,* such as Ligusticum Gao Ben (Chinese lovage root) and Bupleurum Chai Hu (Asian buplever root), come from the category that "releases the exterior." Others still are found elsewhere in the Materia Medica; for instance, Corydalis Yan Hu Suo (Chinese corydalis root), which because of its *analgesic* effect is traditionally classed among the remedies that "vitalize the Blood."

Some Asian plant remedies are now generally accepted as working on the nervous system, and are routinely used for neurological disorders in modern clinics throughout the Chinese-speaking world. However, there remain many more remedies with a nervine tropism than are generally known. The main way we define an Oriental herb as possessing neurological activity is through analyzing its uses for traditional symptom pictures, as well as those complaints it is popularly used to relieve. As supporting evidence, we can also look to its chemical constituents, as well as contemporary pharmacological research from China, Taiwan and Hong Kong. Comparative evidence from Western botanicals with similar pharmacologies and uses will, in some cases, also prove very fruitful.

There is a more general approach that can help us understand the description of nervous system disorders in Chinese medicine. We can learn from looking at the functional organ/channel networks that present neurological pathology, along with the herbal remedies that treat them. Specifically, much of the symptomatology of the Liver, Pericardium, Heart, Bladder and Governing (Du) channels is neurological by nature. Consequently, remedies addressing the symptom pictures of these channels are clear candidates for the nervous system category.

Remedies having a primary affinity with the nervous system can be organized according to the four basic therapeutic actions: *restoring, stimulating, relaxing* and *sedating*. This allows us to match the herbs to the corresponding nervous condition, as described by Western vitalistic physiopathology.

- ***Nervous restoratives*** treat deficiency nervous conditions involving cerebral and nervous weakness, presenting chronic depression and fatigue.
- ***Nervous stimulants*** address deficiency and cold nervous conditions with severe cerebral and nervous weakness, accompanied by mental stupor and coma.
- ***Nervous relaxants*** treat excess nervous conditions such as nervous tension, displaying spasms and convulsions.
- ***Nervous sedatives*** treat excess nervous conditions involving either:
  - nervous tension presenting pain and agitation.
  - nervous tension with fever presenting heat, spasms and agitation.

The Nervous Remedies

Restoratives

By restoring central nervous functions, the *restorative* remedies address conditions of chronic nervous (especially cerebral) deficiency. Sometimes also known as neurasthenia, this deficiency crystallizes around the syndrome **nerve and brain deficiency.** When used over time, *central nervous restoratives* will relieve symptoms of chronic depression, fatigue, mental stupor, memory loss, absent-mindedness, dizziness, headache, and often certain types of paralysis and paraplegia. These *restoratives* are important for such conditions as Huntington's disease, Parkinson's disease, Alzheimer's disease, Guillain-Barré syndrome, myelitis and peripheral neuritis. Because in the long run they lift the spirit, the *restorative* herbs are sometimes called *antidepressants.*

In Oriental medicine, most nervous and cerebral functions are subsumed under the functions of the Liver and Kidney. When the essence of these channel networks is depleted, symptoms such as those above may appear. Hence, the traditional naming of the symptom picture **nerve and brain deficiency** is **Liver and Kidney Essence deficiency** (and sometimes **Liver and Kidney Yin deficiency).**

Among the outstanding *nervous restoratives* available to us in Oriental medicine are Polygonum He Shou Wu (the root of the Flowery knotweed, a fairly common scrambling vine), Ligustrum Nu Zhen Zi (the berry of the South Chinese mountain shrub, Glossy privet) and Centella Ji Xue Cao (Gotu kola herb, found in the subtropics worldwide). Because they help restore actual nerve cells, these can be qualified as *trophorestorative.* These *restoratives* are not uniform in either effective qualities or chemical constituents. In traditional Chinese terms the majority are known to "tonify the Liver and Kidney and benefit the Essence."

Other significant *central nervous restoratives,* such as Panax Ren Shen (Asian ginseng root from Northeast Asia) and Schisandra Wu Wei Zi (the berry of the climber Chinese magnolia vine) are found in other sections, notably the endocrine and immune systems.

Stimulants

Central nervous stimulants are required when cerebral and other nervous functions need a "jump start." This is the case in severe **nerve and brain deficiency** syndromes characterized by symptoms of drowsiness, stupor, catatonia, vertigo, fainting, coma, collapse, paresthesia and paralysis. Because of their consciousness-reviving and consciousness-enhancing effects, these remedies are sometimes called *analeptics* and *psychogenics,* respectively. In traditional Chinese medical terms, they are described as "aromatic remedies that open the orifices and revive the senses."

Nervous stimulants are used in chronic conditions such as long-term catatonia, paralysis and numbness, as well as in more acute conditions, to revive consciousness and regain movement. They can therefore assist in disorders such as Yin-type schizophrenia, concussion, cerebral contusion, the sequelae of cerebrovascular accident, heat exhaustion, myelitis, ataxic cerebral palsy, Bell's palsy, Guillain-Barré syndrome, myasthenia gravis and peripheral neuritis.

Analeptics and *psychogenics* include Acorus Shi Chang Pu (Rock sweet flag root, a water plant and cousin of the Western Calamus) and Dryobalanops Bing Pian (Borneo camphor from Southeast Asia). The majority operate through their high essential oil content and are pungent and warm in quality.

Relaxants

Nervous relaxants essentially treat tense conditions of the autonomic-visceral nervous system, termed **nerve excess,** or more traditionally, **Liver Qi constraint** and **Liver Yang rising.** Keynote symptoms here are restlessness, irritability, headache, dizziness, ringing in ears and sleep loss. When these conditions worsen, signs of peripheral nervous stress arise, pictorially described in Chinese medicine as **internal wind.** This condition manifests as tremors, spasms, agitation and seizures. **Internal wind** may lead to such conditions as **wind phlegm obstruction,** manifested by paralysis, hemiplegia and opisthotonos.

Nervous relaxants are specifically *spasmolytic* and *anticonvulsant,* traditionally described as "extinguishing internal wind and clearing wind phlegm." Through their systemic *relaxant* effect on both central visceral and peripheral nervous functions, they treat conditions such as chronic stress, heat cramps, spastic and athetoid cerebral palsy, epileptic convulsions, tetany, cerebrovascular accident, hypocalcemia, Huntington's disease (chorea) and Parkinson's disease. Alkaloids figure prominently in the chemical profile of these *relaxants,* as in the important remedies Uncaria Gou Teng (Gambir vine twig from the woods of Central China) and Gastrodia Tian Ma (Celestial hemp root, a variety of alpine orchid).

Typically, more animal remedies are found in this section of the Materia Medica than in any other. Tortoise shell, turtle shell and the horns of ruminants such as the antelope, water buffalo and goat are very high in calcium, through which they exert significant *spasmolytic* and *sedative* actions.

Moreover, because autonomic nervous functions inform every body system, each system has its own type of *relaxant remedies* that serves that particular group of smooth muscles. *Respiratory relaxants,* for example, are *nervous relaxants* causing bronchodilation, an effect used in the spasmodic bronchial condition called asthma. Likewise, *uterine relaxants* are *nervous relaxants* that loosen the uterine cramps of spasmodic dysmenorrhea. The "relaxants" section in the introduction to each system therefore describes the various and numerous applications of *nervous relaxants.*

Sedatives

Sedative remedies for the nervous system are divided into two types:

- *depressant analgesics* and *hypnotics* that reduce nervous tension and relieve pain and agitation.
- *depressant antipyretics* and *spasmolytics* that reduce nervous tension, reduce fever and relieve spams and agitation.

The first type of *sedative* is *nervous depressants* with *analgesic* and *hypnotic* effects. They treat the syndrome **Qi constraint with nerve excess,** presenting symptoms of pain, agitation, sleep loss and dizziness. Traditionally these symptoms are also ascribed to the syndrome **Liver Yang rising.** Because they relieve a wide spectrum of pain, these *sedatives* can be indispensable in managing conditions ranging from flu with painful throat and muscle pains, to peripheral neuritis, arthritis, neuralgia, bone pain (ostalgia), toothache, and abdominal, lumbar, biliary, menstrual and renal pain.

Analgesics and *hypnotics* on the whole are pungent and warm-natured. They carry a variety of constituents, including glycosides, essential oils and alkaloids, that participate in their pain-relieving effect. This class includes highly effective botanicals such as Siegesbeckia Xi Xian Cao (Hairy siegesbeckia, a common Southeast Asian herb), which focuses on bone and muscle pain, Bupleurum Chai Hu (Asian buplever root, a much used umbellifer from Northeast Asia), used in a variety of painful conditions, and Tribulus Bai Ji Li (Caltrop fruit from Central China's lowlands), with its tropism for painful, pruritic skin conditions.

The second type of *sedative* remedy is simultaneously *sedative* and *relaxant* to the nerves, and has an additional *antipyretic* or temperature-lowering effect. While today these remedies are defined as *spasmolytics, anticonvulsants* and *antipyretics,* in traditional terms they "quell fire, extinguish wind and calm the spirit." Their primary use is in febrile conditions resulting in the syndrome **nerve excess.** Here the central nervous system is stressed—causing agitation, insomnia, and so on, along with disruption of peripheral functioning. Febrile tremors, contractures, spasms and convulsions are possible results. Such symptoms might be seen in Western medical conditions including heat syndrome, meningitis, encephalitis, eclampsia, tetanus and rheumatic fever.

The primarily bitter, salty, cold energetic nature of these *depressants* derives from their mineral, bile salt and amino acid content. They can effectively relieve the fever, delirium, pain and spasms found in such hot/febrile syndromes as **Liver fire, Pericardium fire** and **Heart fire.** This category of remedies contains numerous animal remedies, one mineral remedy and one botanical remedy. Among the animal remedies, Bubalus Shui Niu Jiao (Water buffalo horn) and Ursus Xiong Dan (Bear gallbladder) should be singled out for their fairly wide usage. The mineral remedy Gypsum Shi Gao (Gypsum from Central China) is likewise often used because of its reliable *antipyretic, spasmolytic* and *analgesic* actions combined.

REMEDIES TO RESTORE THE NERVES AND BRAIN, AND RELIEVE DEPRESSION

➤ TONIFY THE LIVER AND KIDNEY, AND BENEFIT THE ESSENCE

Antidepressant central nervous restoratives

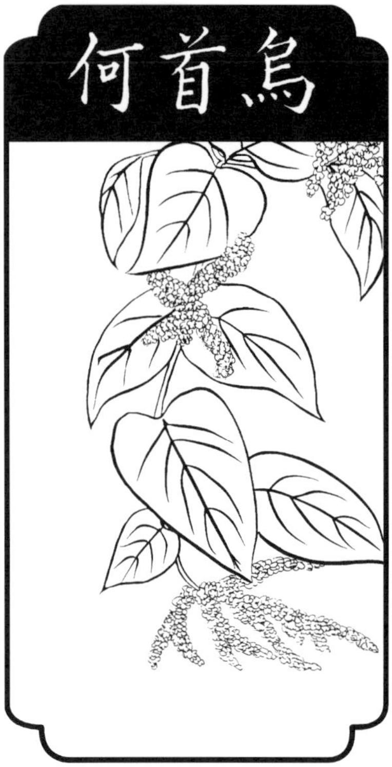

Polygonum He Shou Wu

Flowery Knotweed Root

Botanical source: *Polygonum multiflorum* Thunberg (Polygonaceae)
Pharmaceutical name: Radix Polygoni multiflori
Chinese names: He Shou Wu, Shou Wu (Mand); Ho Sau Wu, Sao Wu (Cant)
Other names: Climbing knotweed, Tuber fleeceflower, Chinese cornbind, Fo-ti, "Black-haired Mr. He"; Kashuu (Jap)
Habit: Perennial deciduous twining vine found throughout China (except the northeast), Taiwan, Japan and Vietnam; grows along roads and streams, in valley shrub thickets and among rock crevices; fond of warm, moist conditions and loose, fertile sandy soil; blooms in autumn with slender panicle clusters of small green-white axillary/terminal flowers.
Part used: the root

Therapeutic category: mild remedy with minimal chronic toxicity
Constituents: glucoside 1.2%, anthraquinones (incl. rhein, emodin, chrysophanol, chrysophanic acid, physcion), lecithin 3.7%, allantoin, chrysarobin, rhapontin, chelidonic acid, fats, tannin, starch 45%, trace elements
Effective qualities: sour, astringent, a bit sweet, neutral, dry
restoring, astringing, raising, stimulating, decongesting, dissolving, diluting
Tropism: neuromuscular, reproductive, vascular, lymphatic, digestive systems
Liver, Kidney, Du, Dai channels; Air, Fluid bodies

Actions and Indications

central nervous trophorestorative: antidepressant: cerebral and nervous deficiency with mental and physical fatigue, depression; chronic stress, nervous breakdown, neurasthenia, schizophrenia, paraplegia, peripheral neuritis, sleep disorder, Huntington's disease, Alzheimer's disease, Guillain-Barré syndrome, myelitis, somnambulism
musculoskeletal restorative: weak back and knees; muscular dystrophy
antioxidant (free radical inhibitor), aging retardant: toxicosis, premature senility
immune enhancer: low resistance with chronic infections (includ. AIDS)
reproductive restorative: infertility, low sperm count, sexual disinterest
mucostatic astringent: incontinence with spermatorrhea, diarrhea; leucorrhea, menorrhagia, hemorrhoids
detoxicant, antilipemic: metabolic toxicosis with eczema, rheumatic myalgia, sore extremities; atherosclerosis, hyperlipidemia
lymphatic decongestant, dissolvent: lymphadenitis (incl. scrofula), lymph gland TB, fibrocystic breasts; boils, carbuncles, sores
stimulant laxative: chronic constipation
antibacterial, antiviral, antigenic, lymphocyte stimulant: infections in general
interferon inducent

Symptom Pictures

nerve and brain deficiency (Kidney Essence deficiency): depression, exhaustion, sleeping problems, loss of memory and concentration, dizziness, early hair graying

genitourinary damp cold: white vaginal discharges, premature ejaculation, sexual disinterest, heavy menses

metabolic toxicosis: malaise, swollen lymph glands, skin rashes, boils

Preparation

Use: The root Polygonum He Shou Wu is either decocted or used in tincture form. Steel pans of any kind should not be used for the decoction. The raw, not steam-processed root must be used to obtain the *detoxicant* effect.

Dosage: Decoction: 10-25 g
Tincture: 2-4 ml

Caution: Use cautiously with diarrhea present.

Notes

The first extant Oriental text written about a single herb, the He Shou Wu Lu of the year 813, records the fortuitous discovery of Flowery knotweed's virtues. This sour-astringent root is traditionally considered a fortifier to two of the three Yin components of the body, namely the Essence and Blood. The plant's very name, "Black-haired Mr. He," is witness to its systemic rejuvenative powers. The story goes that in 812, a fifty-six year old, heirless, silver-haired Mr. He fathered a son and regained a youthful complexion along with a full head of strong, black hair after eating this root as a vegetable for a whole year. To this day the remedy is used to slow down signs of aging, especially the most conspicuous of all—grey hair.

Flowery knotweed today is specifically known for its *restorative* actions on the urogenital, muscular and nervous systems. It has always been esteemed as one of the main remedies for increasing male sperm, and as a good *reproductive restorative* for both men and women's reproductive and sexual deficiencies. The root's moderate astringency extends application to vaginal and seminal discharges of many types.

However, it is Flowery knotweed's new guise as a *nervous* and *cerebral restorative* that is currently receiving the most attention. And here this remedy remains a unique phenomenon still. Clinical successes with this botanical across China in chronic cerebral insufficiency conditions—from sleep disorders and depression to active forms of schizophrenia—leave no doubt that Flowery knotweed root should be considered an important *nervous trophorestorative.* Already in 1975 the remedy's lecithin content was advanced as the main factor implicated in directly nourishing nerve tissue on one hand and increasing the growth and development of erythrocytes on the other. In terms of Western physiology, its tropism for the nervous system certainly helps explain usage for the traditional syndrome Kidney Essence deficiency.

When Flowery knotweed root's systemic *detoxicant, antioxidant* and *immune enhancing* actions are added to the *tonifying* effects, the resultant gestalt is clearly one that holds promise for the treatment of many of today's chronic, multifactorial disorders. These so often entail aspects of endogenous and exogenous toxicosis, a general free radical burden and compromised neural functioning—the list of these is long. Although current claims for Flowery knotweed being an *adaptogen* are inaccurate (if we are to stick to Brehckman's original definition of an adaptogen), the remedy's impressive therapeutic profile certainly justifies its consistent characterization, prevalent in both professional and popular Chinese medicine, as a premier longevity remedy.

In Taiwan another plant is often used to represent the remedy He Shou Wu, namely the tuber of the **potato yam,** *Dioscorea bulbifera.* In most other countries where Chinese medicine is practised, however, this is considered a distinct remedy, commonly known as **Huang Yao Zi.** In this text Dioscorea Huang Yao Zi is found under the *cardiovascular restoratives* as an *astringent hemostatic.*

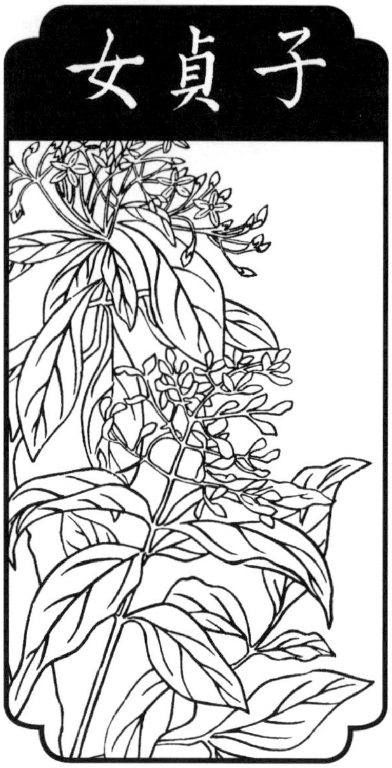

Ligustrum Nu Zhen Zi

Glossy Privet Berry *

Botanical source: *Ligustrum lucidum* Aiton (Oleaceae)
Pharmaceutical name: Fructus Ligustri
Chinese names: Nu Zhen Zi, La Shu, Dong Qing (Mand); Neui Jing Ji (Cant)
Other names: Japanese wax privet, Chinese privet, "Girl chaste"; Joteishi (J)
Habit: Large evergreen mountain shrub from Central and South China Korea and Japan; likes a humid, warm climate and moist, fertile, sandy soil on plains and hillsides; also cultivated; blooms in summer with fragrant, small white flowers on branch ends.
Part used: the fruit

Therapeutic category: mild remedy with minimal chronic toxicity
Constituents: organic acids (incl. oleanolic, linoleic, acetyloleanolic, palmitic), betulin, ligustrazine, lupeol, mannitol, glucose, salidroside, invertin
Effective qualities: a bit sweet, astringent and bitter, neutral
restoring, raising, decongesting
Tropism: nervous, urinary, respiratory, immune systems
Kidney, Liver, Lung, Du channels; Air, Fluid bodies

Actions and Indications

central nervous restorative: parasympathetic nervous stimulant: cerebral and nervous deficiency with chronic mental and physical fatigue; chronic stress, neurasthenia, sleep disorder, tinnitus, Parkinson's disease
vision restorative: poor or blurred eyesight; retinal (macular) degeneration, cataract, central retinitis
antioxidant (free radical inhibitor), aging retardant: premature aging, vision loss, toxicosis
immune enhancer: low resistance with frequent or chronic infections; immunodeficiency disorders
leukocytogenic, lymphocyte stimulant: low WBC count (leukopenia, incl. due to chemotherapy); infections in general
immune regulator, antiallergic: immune stress with immediate allergies (incl. rhinitis, angioedema, urticaria, otitis, atopic dermatitis, asthma); immune complex disorders (incl. food allergies, chronic hepatitis, arthritis)
anti-inflammatory
antitumoral: cancer (incl. cervical)
draining diuretic: edema, metabolic toxicosis
laxative: constipation
Miscellaneous: chronic bronchitis

Symptom Picture

nerve and brain deficiency (Liver and Kidney Essence deficiency): dizziness, spots in vision, ringing in ears, absent-mindedness, fatigue, sleeping difficulties, premature graying hair, loose teeth

Preparation

Use: The berry Ligustrum Nu Zhen Zi is decocted or used in tincture form.
Dosage: Decoction: 8-16 g
Tincture: 2-4 ml
Caution: Forbidden in Yang deficiency syndromes, including cold in the intestines.

Notes

The bitter-sweet, shiny black berry of the Glossy privet tree is an ancient emblem of female chastity, and an early Daoist remedy for life-extension. Its reputed *anti-aging* action can be mainly explained by its *immune-enhancing* and *antioxidant* properties. However, with its similarities of symptomatology to both Schisandra berry and Flowery knotweed, Glossy privet also demonstrates a *restorative* effect on the central nervous system. This is a remedy to forestall signs of both chronic stress and advancing years, such as lowered immunity, graying hair, ear ringing and failing vision. Glossy privet's well-known effect on vision disorders such as macular degeneration also makes sense in light of its combined *antioxidant* and *detoxicant diuretic* actions. Here it acts much like Bilberry leaf and Ginkgo leaf, although the exact pharmacology involved is still missing.

Today Glossy privet berry is also finding application in the treatment of hypersensitivity disorders, showing an *immune regulating* action in various allergic and immune complex conditions.

In Europe, other species of Privet berry were used medicinally up to the 1800s.

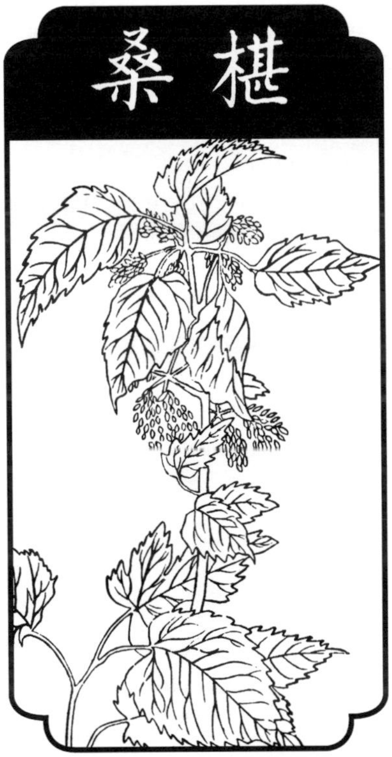

Morus Sang Shen

Mulberry Fruit

Botanical source: *Morus alba* L. (Moraceae)
Pharmaceutical name: Fructus Mori
Chinese names: Sang Shen, Sang Shen Zi (Mand); Song Sam (Cant)
Other names: White mulberry; Sojin (Jap)
Habit: Deciduous temperate East Asian tree, much cultivated for silkworm culture; flowers in May with stalked hanging catkins.
Part used: the fruit spike

Therapeutic category: mild remedy with minimal chronic toxicity
Constituents: thiamine, riboflavin, glucose, fructose, oleic/stearic/linoleic/tannic/malic acid, isoquercitin, cyanidin, tannin, calcium, trace minerals (incl. phosphorus, iron, copper, zinc), vitamin B1, B2, C, carotene
Effective qualities: sweet, sour, cool, moist
restoring, raising, nourishing
Tropism: nervous, digestive systems
Heart, Liver, Kidney channels
Air, Fluid bodies

Actions and Indications

central nervous restorative: cerebral and nervous deficiency with mental and physical fatigue; chronic stress, neurasthenia, convalescence, nervous breakdown, tinnitus
vision restorative: vision impairment
nutritive, hemogenic: anemia; fatigue, dizziness
secretory: thirst, dehydration (incl. diabetic)
demulcent laxative: constipation, dry hard stool

Symptom Pictures

nerve and brain deficiency (Liver and Kidney Essence deficiency): poor concentration and memory, ringing in ears, dizziness, sleeping problems, poor eyesight, early hair graying

Blood and fluids deficiency: fatigue, dizziness, blurred vision, thirst, constipation, sleep loss

Preparation

Use: The fruit Morus Sang Shen is briefly decocted or used in tincture form.
Dosage: Decoction: 15-30 g
Tincture: 2-4 ml
Caution: Contraindicated in diarrhea and Kidney Yin deficiency with empty heat.

Notes

Mulberry fruit is a much-used *moistening restorative* and *nutritive* remedy acting both on the nerves and blood. Particular conditions relieved by this *cerebral* and *vision tonic* (with a raising effect) are symptoms of mental fatigue or incapacity, poor eyesight and thirst.

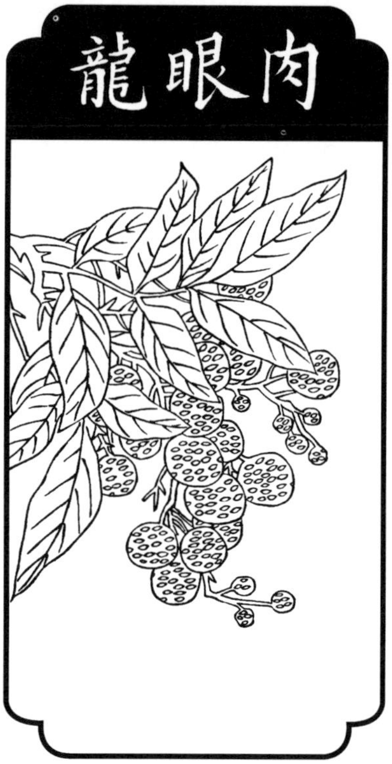

Euphoria Long Yan Rou

Longan Fruit

Botanical source: *Euphoria longan* (Lour.) Steud. (Sapindaceae)
Pharmaceutical name: Arillus Euphoriae
Chinese names: Long Yan Rou, Gui Yuan Rou, Li Zhi Nu, Gui Yuan Rou (Mand); Lung Ngaan Yuk (Cant)
Other names: "Dragon eye flesh"; Ryuganniku (Jap)
Habit: Subtropical evergreen tree cultivated in South China, Malaysia, Réunion and Mauritius; flowers in spring with small cream white flowers.
Part used: the aril or fruit pulp

Therapeutic category: mild remedy with minimal chronic toxicity
Constituents: adenine, choline, glucose, sucrose, proteins, fats, calcium, phosphorus, iron, riboflavin, niacin, ascorbic and tartaric acid, vitamins A, B
Effective qualities: sweet, warm, moist
restoring, raising, nourishing
Tropism: nervous, digestive systems
Heart, Spleen channels
Air, Fluid bodies

Actions and Indications

central nervous restorative: cerebral and nervous deficiency with chronic mental and physical fatigue; amnesia, chronic stress, neurasthenia, convalescence, nervous breakdown, menopause
nutritive: weakness, postpartum debility
anthelmintic, detoxicant

Symptom Pictures

nerve and brain deficiency: memory and concentration loss, fatigue, sleeping problems, blurred vision

heart Blood deficiency: palpitations, dizziness, fatigue, sleep loss

Preparation

Use: The fruit Euphoria Long Yan Rou is infused or briefly decocted; it may also simply be eaten.
Dosage: Infusion and decoction: 8-14 g
Caution: Forbidden with intestines mucous damp and signs of heat present.

Notes

Like the Mulberry, Longan fruit is primarily *restorative* to the nervous system and brain; in the past it was also called Yi Zhi because of its repute for enhancing mental faculties. Again like Mulberry fruit, the sweet Longan is very *nutritive,* a fact confirmed by its high mineral content.

This tasty fruit from China's tropical South boasts a variety of other popular uses that now include the menopause. Its intake is said to render the skin diaphanous, the eye radiant and sexuality vibrant. The best historical testimony is that of the celebrated imperial concubine Yang Gui-fei. This Tang court star is said to have daily consumed Longan fruits for these purposes.

旱蓮草

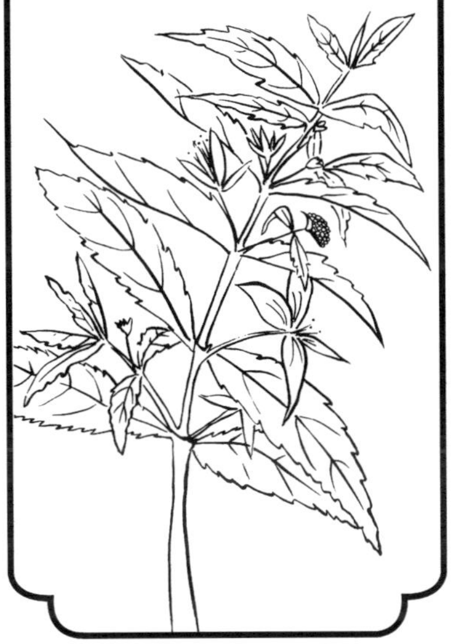

Eclipta Han Lian Cao

Field Lotus Herb *

Botanical source: *Eclipta prostata* L. or *E. alba* Hasskarl (Compositae)
Pharmaceutical name: Herba Ecliptae
Chinese names: Han Lian Cao, Mo Han lian, Li Chang (Mand); Hon Lin Chou, Mak Hin Lin (Cant)
Other names: Ink plant; Kanrenso (Jap); Bhringaraj (Sans)
Habit: Annual erect or spreading temperate Asian herb growing in grassland, by roadsides, streamsides and among shady, damp grass thickets; summer sees small white axillary or terminal flowerheads appearing.
Part used: the herb

Therapeutic category: mild remedy with minimal chronic toxicity
Constituents: saponins (incl. ecliptine, terthienylmethanol, thiophene derivates), wedelolactone, nicotine, tannin, vitamin A
Effective qualities: sweet, sour, astringent, cool, dry
restoring, raising, astringing, relaxing
Tropism: nervous, vascular, digestive, respiratory systems
Liver, Kidney, Du channels; Air, Fluid bodies

Actions and Indications

central nervous restorative: cerebral and nervous deficiency with depression; chronic stress, neurasthenia, sleep disorder, nervous breakdown
hair restorative: premature hair graying, hair loss, balding
hemostatic, coagulant: hemorrhage with blood in stool, urine or spittle; vomiting blood, nosebleed, uterine bleeding
astringent, vulnerary, styptic: diarrhea, eczema, ulcers, injuries with bleeding
anti-infective, anti-inflammatory: diphtheria, hepatitis, gastroenteritis, dysentery, conjunctivitis, urinary tract infection, rice-field dermatitis, tinea pedis, lung TB, abscesses
hepatic: liver cirrhosis, chronic hepatitis, liver and spleen enlargement
Miscellaneous: infantile malnutrition

Symptom Pictures

nerve and brain deficiency (Liver and Kidney Essence deficiency): blurred vision, dizziness, ringing in ears, premature hair graying, sleeping problems, memory loss, loose teeth

Blood heat: bleeding from upper or lower orifices, uterine bleeding

Preparation

Use: The herb Eclipta Han Lian Cao is infused or prepared in tincture form. However, when decocting a formula, it is fine to decoct this herb in with other remedies, as it doesn't contain any volatile essential oils. Topical swabs or compresses are also prepared for bleeding from injuries or sores, and for eczema.
Dosage: Infusion/decoction: 15-30 g
Tincture: 2-4 ml
Caution: Contraindicated in digestive or urogenital deficiency with cold.

Notes

In the literate tradition of Chinese medicine, Field lotus herb is valued as the main *Yin tonic* without an oily quality—and hence appreciated by the digestion. As with the similar remedy Ligustrum Nu Zhen Zi (Glossy privet berry), its symptomatology clearly suggests a *restorative* action on the central nervous system. The herb's reputation for preventing, or at least slowing down, the signs of aging is even greater in Ayurvedic medicine.

In the Chinese folk tradition, Field lotus herb was and is used mainly for stopping bleeding of any kind—a more acute use of this *astringent* remedy.

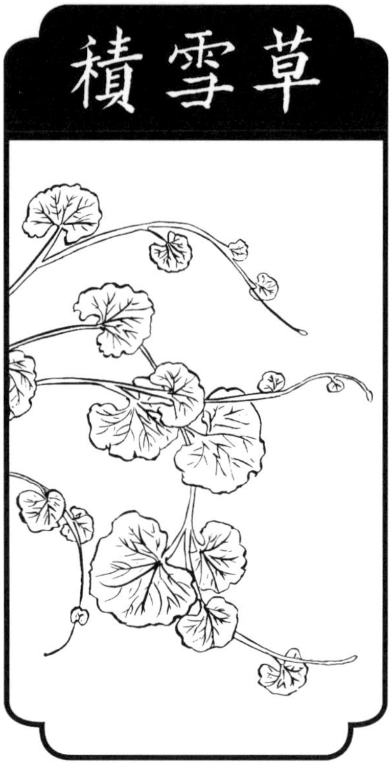

Centella Ji Xue Cao

Gotu Kola Leaf

Botanical source: *Centella asiatica* (L.) Urban (syn. *Hydrocotyle asiatica* L) (Umbelliferae)
Pharmaceutical name: Folium Centellae
Chinese names: Ji Xue Cao, Luo Di Da, Peng Da Wan, Han Ke Cao (Mand); Jik Syut Chou, Pang Daai Yan, Gam Hok Chou (Cant)
Other names: Asian centella, Indian pennywort; Brahmi (Sans)
Habit: Perennial spreading herb from temperate and subtropical regions, including China, Malaysia, India, West Africa, the West Indies and Hawai'i; inhabits fields, meadows, roadsides, stream banks and shady hillsides; umbels of small purple or yellowish axillary flowers bloom in spring.
Part used: the leaf or herb

Therapeutic category: mild remedy with minimal chronic toxicity
Constituents: glycosides (centelloside, asiaticoside), alkaloid (hydrocotylin), catechol and epicatechol (traces), bitter vellarine, triterpenic acids (asiatic acid, asiatoside, madecassic acid), hydrocyanic acid, peptic acids, resins, tannins
Effective qualities: a bit sweet, bitter and pungent, cool, dry
restoring, raising, astringing, solidifying, calming
Tropism: nervous, respiratory, urinary, digestive systems
Lung, Bladder, Kidney, Du, Yang Qiao, Dai channels; Fluid, Air bodies

Actions and Indications

central nervous restorative: cerebral/nervous deficiency with chronic mental and physical fatigue, depression; chronic stress, nervous breakdown, epilepsy
aging-retardant: premature senility/aging
adrenocortical restorative: chronic fatigue, low stamina; adrenocortical deficiency; menopausal syndrome
immune enhancer: chronic or frequent infections; immunodeficiency conditions
venous decongestant, astringent restorative: venous deficiency with varicose veins, hemorrhoids, pelvic congestion
connective tissue restorative: cellulite, varicose veins, hypermobile joints
detoxicant: dermatropic, diuretic, antivenomous: metabolic toxicosis with chronic eczema, pruritus, psoriasis, leprosy, syphilis; boils, furunculosis, lymphadenitis, snake bite
broad-spectrum anti-infective, anti-inflammatory: infectious conditions; acute respiratory infection (incl. bronchitis), tonsillitis, laryngitis, common cold, hepatitis, urinary tract infection, measles, food poisoning; pleuritis, vaginitis, cervicitis
antipyretic: fevers (esp. remittent fevers)
vulnerary: bleeding wounds

Symptom Pictures

nerve and brain deficiency (Kidney Essence deficiency): fatigue, depression, poor memory and concentration, early hair graying

metabolic toxicosis: fatigue, malaise, skin rashes, fetid urine, chronic boils

venous blood stagnation: varicose veins, spider veins, hemorrhoids, fatigue, heavy periods with premenstrual downward pressure

lung phlegm heat: coughing, production of yellow/green purulent sputum

Preparation

Use: The herb Centella Ji Xue Cao is infused, decocted along with other remedies or taken in tincture form. The fresh juice is applied to sores and ulcers. Topical applications in general are excellent for most chronic skin diseases, chronic boils, wounds and insect and animal bites.

Dosage: Infusion and decoction: 10-30 g. High doses are used mainly for acute infections.
Tincture: 2-5 ml

Caution: An aggravation of skin itching may occasionally be experienced at first when treating this condition. Very large and continuous doses of this remedy may cause headache, dizziness or temporary fainting.

Notes

Although primarily used in traditional China for acute bronchial infections and first-aid purposes, Gotu kola leaf today has achieved worldwide status as an important *nervous restorative.* Like its companion remedies in this class, Gotu cola is not a *cerebral stimulant;* nor does it contain any alkaloids related to this action. The notion arose because the herb was confused with the *nervous stimulant* Kola nut, *Cola vera,* which contains over 1.25% caffeine (Mowrey 1986). Gotu kola is a "down-home" *nerve* and *brain builder* useful for such boldface symptoms as memory loss and chronic tiredness, both mental and physical. In Chinese medical terms, Kidney Essence is the energetic function tonified.

This is not to say that we're not looking at a complex herb: We are. Gotu kola has also shown excellent *restorative* actions on the connective tissue and venous circulation (triterpenic acids operative). The remedy also enjoys a massive reputation as a deep systemic, i.e., *resolvent detoxicant,* especially as regards chronic skin eruptions.

Nevertheless, it is hard not to feel that there is a missing piece to the intriguing Gotu kola puzzle. Indian texts authoritatively claim major *gland restorative, fatigue-reducing* and *anti-aging* actions for this remedy. These effects cannot solely be explained by its currently known activities. There is at least one missing piece of information. It could be that Gotu kola is downright *adaptogenic,* or *antioxidant,* or *pituitary-adrenocortical stimulant* ... or all of those things. The remedy deserves more research than it has received to-date.

Sesamum Hei Zhi Ma

Black Sesame Seed

黑芝麻

Botanical source: *Sesamum indicum* De Candolle (Pedaliaceae)
Chinese names: Hei Zhi Ma, Hu Ma Ren (Mand); Hak Ji Ma (Cant)
Category: mild remedy with minimal chronic toxicity
Constituents: oleic/linoleic/palmitic/arachid acids, glycerol, sesamolin, arginine, choline, globulin, lecithin, phytin, pentosane, resinoid sesamin, calcium, trace minerals, vitamins E, A and B.
Effective qualities: sweet, a bit pungent, neutral, moist; restoring, raising, nourishing, calming
Tropism: nervous, digestive systems; Liver, Kidney ch.

Actions: *Nervous restorative, hemogenic, adrenocortical restorative, demulcent laxative*

Indications: Nervous deficiency with tiredness, blurred vision, tinnitus, dizziness, headache, paresthesia; Blood and Yin deficiency syndromes; fatigue, stamina loss, convalescence, postpartum exhaustion; adrenal cortex deficiency; constipation from dryness.

Dosage: Decoction: 10-30 g
Tincture: 2-5 ml

Caution: Use carefully in diarrhea from digestive deficiency.

REMEDIES TO STIMULATE THE NERVES AND BRAIN, AND REVIVE CONSCIOUSNESS

➤ OPEN THE ORIFICES AND REVIVE THE SENSES WITH AROMATIC REMEDIES

Analeptics, psychogenics

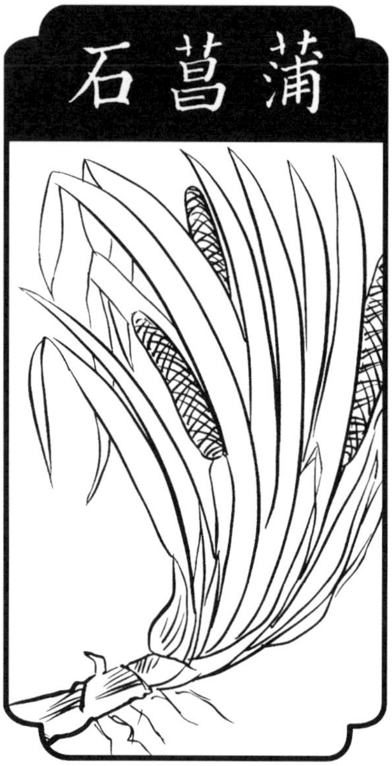

Acorus Shi Chang Pu

Rock Sweet Flag Root

Botanical source: *Acorus gramineus* Solander (Araceae)
Pharmaceutical name: Rhizoma Acori graminei
Chinese names: Shi Chang Pu, Chang Pu, Chang Yang (Mand); Sek Cheung Pou (Cant)
Other names: Chinese sweet grass, Grass-leaf sweet flag; Shobu (Jap)
Habit: Perennial evergreen water herb from mid China; grows in lowland marshes and swamps among wet rocks and in mountain gullies and creeks; minute viridian flowers form a slender spike that blooms in summer.
Part used: the rhizome

Therapeutic category: medium-strength remedy with slight chronic toxicity
Constituents: essential oil 0.5-0.9% (incl. asarone, euasarone, sekishone, propenyl-veratrone, methylchavicol, asarylaldehyde, humulene, caryophyllene, phenols), amino acid, saccharides, organic acids (incl. palmitic acid)
Effective qualities: pungent, warm, dry
stimulating, raising, relaxing
Tropism: nervous, digestive, respiratory systems
Liver, Heart, Spleen, Lung, Du channels; Air body

Actions and Indications

central nervous stimulant: psychogenic, analeptic: acute or chronic cerebral and nervous deficiency; amnesia, coma, catatonia, deafness; concussion, cerebral contusion
nervous relaxant/sedative, spasmolytic: unrest, delirium, seizures; cerebral palsy, epilepsy, chorea
pungent digestant, spasmolytic, analgesic: dyspepsia, epigastric/abdominal fullness, intestinal colic; acid dyspepsia, anorexia, chronic gastroenteritis, colitis, IBS
stimulant expectorant: bronchitis
antimalarial, vermicidal: malaria, intestinal parasites
detoxicant: Euphorbia species intoxication
anti-infective: antibacterial, antifungal: intestinal fermentation/dysbiosis
dermal (topically): carbuncles, wet ulcers

Symptom Pictures

nerve and brain deficiency (Heart phlegm damp obstruction): mental depression and dullness, memory loss, catatonic stupor, disorientation, deafness

Qi constraint with **nerve excess (Liver Yang rising):** dizziness, ringing in ears, sleep loss, agitation, spasms

intestines Qi constraint: feeling stressed or tense, indigestion, abdominal pain, diarrhea or constipation

intestines mucous damp (Spleen damp): indigestion, abdominal pain, poor appetite, epigastric distension

lung phlegm damp/cold: coughing, expectoration of abundant white sputum, tight chest

Preparation

Use: The root Acorus Shi Chang Pu is decocted or used in powder, pill or tincture form. To preserve its volatile oils, the sliced or chopped root should be added to a decoction only 10 minutes before removal from heat. The larger the dose, the more *nerve relaxant* and *sedative* its effect.

Dosage: Decoction, pill or powder: 3-9 g
Tincture: 1-3 ml

Caution: Use with care in Yin deficiency conditions with empty heat, irritability with much perspiration, vomiting blood and seminal incontinence. Being a medium-strength remedy, never use indefinitely on its own at high doses.

Notes

There is much overlap between this and the other variety of Sweet flag, *Acorus calamus*, **Shui Cheung Pu** (Mand.) or **Seui Cheung Pou** (Cant.). Both remedies are used primarily for the same conditions, namely damp cold and spasmodic conditions affecting the chest, digestive and reproductive organs. However, whereas Acorus Shui Chang Pu is used more for its *digestive* and *bronchial stimulant* and *mucostatic* actions, the pungent-warm Acorus Shi Chang Pu is applied more for its bivalent *nervous stimulant/relaxant* effect. It is the remedy of choice when cerebral deficiency and systemic nervous tension occur simultaneously.

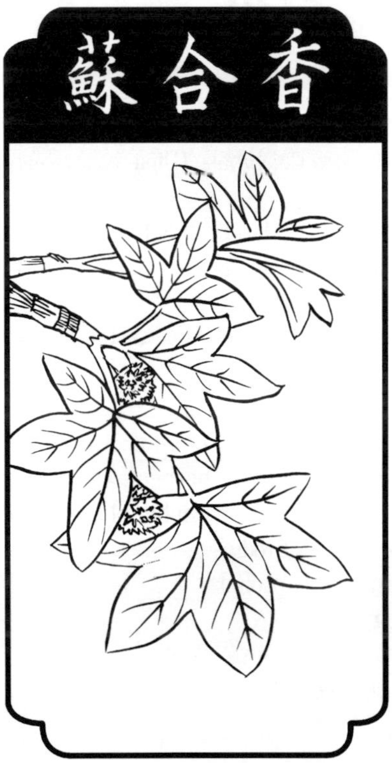

Liquidambar Su He Xiang

Storax Resin

Botanical source: *Liquidambar orientalis* Miller (Hamamelidaceae)
Pharmaceutical name: Styrax Liquidis
Chinese names: Su He Xiang (Mand); Sou Hap Heung (Cant)
Other names: Rose maloe resin, Oriental sweet gum, "Revive and meet aromatic"; Rassamala (Jav), Sogoko (Jap)
Habit: (Sub)tropical Asian and African tree
Part used: the resin expressed from the tree

Therapeutic category: mild remedy with minimal chronic toxicity
Constituents: essential oil (incl. cinnamic/oleanonic/epioleanonic acids, esters, alcohols), resin
Effective qualities: sweet, pungent, warm, dry
stimulating, raising, relaxing
Tropism: nervous, digestive systems
Heart, Spleen, Du channels
Air, Fluid bodies

Actions and Indications

central nervous stimulant: psychogenic, analeptic: acute cerebral and nervous deficiency with fainting; stroke, concussion, cerebral contusion, coma, catatonia
nervous relaxant: analgesic, anticonvulsant: chest and abdominal pain; seizures, epilepsy
coronary restorative: coronary deficiency/disease, angina pectoris
anti-infective, antiparasitic, antivenomous, antidotal: epidemic infections, scabies, malaria, poisoning
vulnerary, antiseptic (topical): wounds, ulcers, frostbite; ringworm, tinea
astringent mucostatic: leucorrhea, gonorrhea
stimulant expectorant: bronchitis, cough
antitumoral: cancer

Symptom Picture

nerve and brain deficiency (Heart phlegm damp obstruction): mental depression, dullness or stupor, disorientation, drowsiness, faintness

Preparation

Use: The resin Liquidambar Su He Xiang is used in powder or tincture form. Topical applications are also prepared for various external conditions.

Dosage: Powder and pill: 0.3-1 g
Tincture: 0.15-0.5 ml

Caution: Contraindicated in high fever, collapse and spontaneous sweating. Use cautiously during pregnancy.

Notes

Storax resin derives from a large tree that originates in the Middle East. It has been used in Asia and the West for many a century. Both comatose and painful convulsive conditions benefit from its comprehensive *cerebral* and *nervine stimulant* action.

Sweetgum resin from North America, Mexico and Central America is derived from the related sweetgum tree, *Liquidambar styraciflua*, and is used similarly to Storax resin.

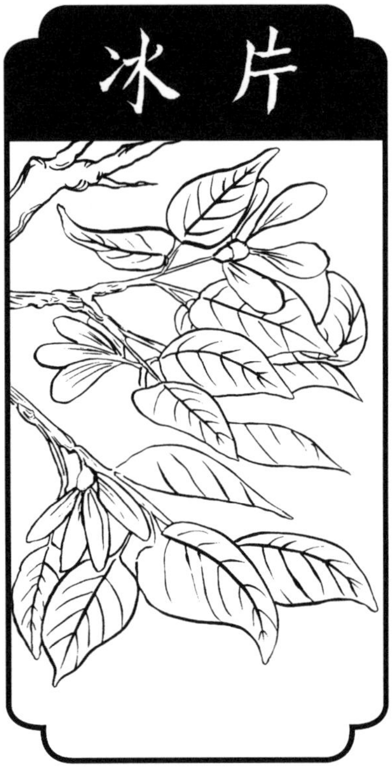

Dryobalanops Bing Pian

Borneo Camphor

Botanical source: *Dryobalanops camphora* Colebrooke (Dipterocarpaceae)
Pharmaceutical name: Borneolum
Chinese names: Bing Pian, Long Nao (Xiang) (Mand); Bing Pin (Cant)
Other names: Malayan/Sumatran camphor, Borneol, "Ice slice"; Hyohen (Jap)
Habit: Large, tall tropical evergreen tree from Southeast Asia.
Part used: the stearopten resin distilled from the tree trunk, or the product synthesized from turpentine or camphor

---

Therapeutic category: mild remedy with minimal chronic toxicity
Constituents: essential oil (incl. monoterpenols [borneol, camphol], sesquiterpenes [humulene, elemene, caryophyllene, camphene]), dipterocarpol, hydroxydammarenone, dryobalanone, erythrodiol
Effective qualities: pungent, bitter, astringent, cool, dry
stimulating, raising, relaxing
Tropism: nervous, cardiovascular, epidermal systems
Heart, Lung, Du, Yang Qiao channels
Air, Warmth bodies

Actions and Indications

nervous stimulant: psychogenic, analeptic: acute or chronic cerebral and nervous deficiency with fainting, depression; catatonia, coma, shock, stroke with mouth spasm, heatstroke, concussion, cerebral contusion, peripheral neuritis
nervous relaxant: spasmolytic, anticonvulsant: spasms, seizures
anti-inflammatory, analgesic, detumescent, antipruritic: conjunctivitis, tonsilitis, pharyngitis, stomatitis, dermatitis, arthralgia, toothache; sores, boils, pruritus, hemorrhoids, ulcers (incl. mouth)
antibacterial, antifungal: infections (incl. fungal skin infections), scabies
adrenocortical stimulant: adrenocortical deficiency
preservative
Topically for photophobia, excessive tearing, congested eyes, corneal opacity, nasal polyp

Symptom Picture

nerve and brain deficiency (Heart phlegm damp obstruction): mental depression and dullness, disorientation, fainting, catatonic stupor

nerve excess with **internal wind (wind phlegm obstruction):** tremors, cramps, convulsions

Preparation

Use: The resin Dryobalanops Bing Pian is used in powder or tincture form, or given in external applications for traumatic, inflammatory, fungal, optic and miscellaneous other conditions.

Dosage: Powder, pill: 0.03-0.1 g
Tincture: 0.03-0.1 ml

Caution: Forbidden in Qi and Blood deficiency, and in cerebral excess. Use cautiously during pregnancy.

Notes

Related to Camphor from the laurel camphor tree, Borneo camphor has always been prized for its healing properties in a region stretching from Sumatra and Borneo (where it originates) to the Mediterranean countries. The secondary Chinese name of this pungent-bitter resinous exudate, Long Nao Xiang, "Dragon brain aromatic," attests to its high value to the Chinese for a variety of purposes, including medicine, perfumery and environmental fragrancing.

In medicine Borneo camphor is a frequent ingredient in patent remedies for both deficient and spasmodic nervous conditions. Phlegm damp obstructing the Heart and wind phlegm obstruction are the two main Chinese medical syndromes treated in this respect. The remedy-achieves a *consciousness-reviving,* or *psychogenic,* action by stimulating higher brain centers. Note the presence of monoterpenoid alcohols, in this respect, that also contribute *anti-infective* actions. Borneo camphor's sesquiterpenes, on the other hand, determine the *anti-inflammatory* and *analgesic* applications, both oral and topical, for which the remedy is also much valued.

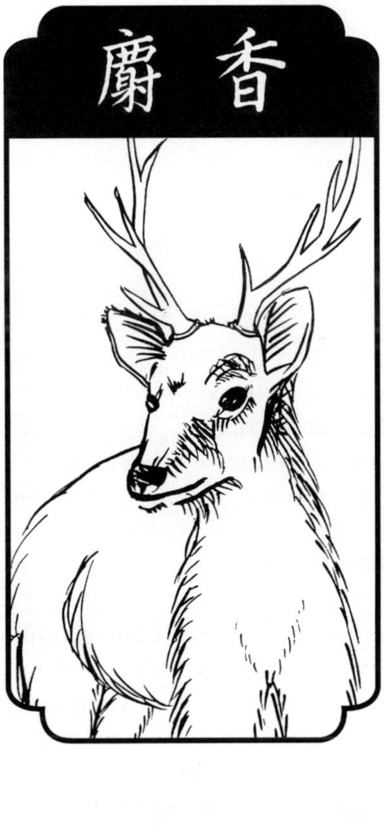

Moschus She Xiang

Musk

Zoological source: *Moschus berezovskii* Flerov or *M. sifanicus* Przewalski or *M. moschiferus* L. (Cervidae)
Pharmaceutical name: Secretio Moschi
Chinese names: She Xiang (Mand); Se Heung (Cant)
Other names: Jako (Jap)
Habitat: Eastern China, including Tibet, Yunnan and Sichuan.
Part used: the navel secretions from the preputial follicles of the Asian musk deer, or the synthesized product

---

Therapeutic category: mild remedy with minimal chronic toxicity
Constituents: alkaloid muscone 0.5-2%, normuscone, muscopyridine, androstane derivatives, amino acids, cholesterol, calcium carbonate phosphate, proteins, wax, lipids cholesterol, bile, protein, sterol, inorganic salts, ketone
Effective qualities: pungent, warm with cooling potential
stimulating, raising, decongesting, relaxing
Tropism: nervous, cardiovascular, digestive, reproductive systems
Liver, Heart, Spleen, Du, Yang Qiao, Yin Qiao channels
Air, Warmth body

Actions and Indications

nervous stimulant: psychogenic, analeptic: acute or chronic cerebral and nervous deficiency with exhaustion; coma of stroke or high fever, shock, collapse, cerebral contusion, concussion, catatonia, paresthesia, paralysis, anosmia

nervous relaxant: spasmolytic, anticonvulsant: febrile delirium, heat cramps, hysteria, seizures, spasmodic cough, spasmodic lumps; CVA, cerebral palsy, peripheral neuritis, chorea, whooping cough, spasms of the glottis

analgesic: sharp thoracic, epigastric, abdominal or uterine pain, limb pain, sciatica

cardiovascular/central circulatory stimulant, sympathetic nervous stimulant, hypertensive: hypothermia, cardiac deficiency, low blood pressure, circulatory collapse, congestive heart failure, angina pectoris, heatstroke

cerebral vasodilator: vascular headache, migraine

uterine stimulant, parturient, abortive: intractable amenorrhea, uterine dystocia, miscarriage, placental retention

androgenic, aphrodisiac: sexual disinterest, impotence

resolvent detoxicant, detumescent: pyogenic infections (incl. boils, sores, carbuncles), tuberculous lymphadenitis

antitumoral: early and middle stage of cancer

antipyretic, diuretic: fever (low or high)

vulnerary, anti-inflammatory: injuries, wounds, skin ulcers (esp. suppurating); vitiligo

antibacterial

Symptom Pictures

nerve and brain deficiency (Heart phlegm damp obstruction): exhaustion, mental stupor, depression, confusion, disorientation

nerve excess with **internal wind (wind phlegm obstruction):** tremors, spasms, pains, convulsions

Pericardium fire: delirium, high fever, convulsions, fainting

Heart and Kidney Yang deficiency (Yang deficiency): prostration, cold limbs, mental stupor, purple lips

devastated Yang: chills, cold limbs, diarrhea with undigested food, prostration, collapse, fainting

Preparation

Use: Because of wildlife preservation (and cost) factors, synthetic Moschus She Xiang should always be used in preference to the animal remedy. Although usually taken as powder or pill, it may also be used in tincture form.

Dosage: Powder or pill: 0.06-0.1 g
Tincture: 5-7 drops

Smaller doses are more *stimulant,* and larger ones more *relaxant* to the nervous system.

Caution: Forbidden in pregnancy, Yin deficiency heat, hypertension, sympathetic CNS, cerebral hyperactivity and cerebral congestion.

Notes

Deer musk is a classic, highly effective *stimulating/relaxing* remedy that has many emergency-room type of traditional uses confirmed by modern research. As a *stimulant* to both the nervous and cardiovascular systems, Musk will treat any form of coma or collapse, regardless of its origin or dynamic (e.g., stroke, concussion, fever, hypothermia, congestive heart failure, etc.). Note its *sympathetic stimulant* and *hypertensive* actions, in this respect. As a fairly systemic *nervous relaxant,* on the other hand, Musk addresses spasmodic, convulsive and painful disorders of many types. However, its long-term *anti-migraine* effect may paradoxically be due to a cerebral *vasodilatant* action.

The remedy's main chemical compound is the alkaloid muscone, which has been synthesized and is also found in other animal secretions such as the civet, *Viverricula indica,* and the muskrat, *Ondatra zibethica.* Fortunately, the synthetic product has proven as effective as deer musk itself, thereby making the many superlative benefits of Musk available without endangering this unique deer species. In recent years, moreover, farms in Shaanxi, Anhui and Sichuan have been successfully breeding domesticated musk deers with higher yields of secretions.

馬銭子

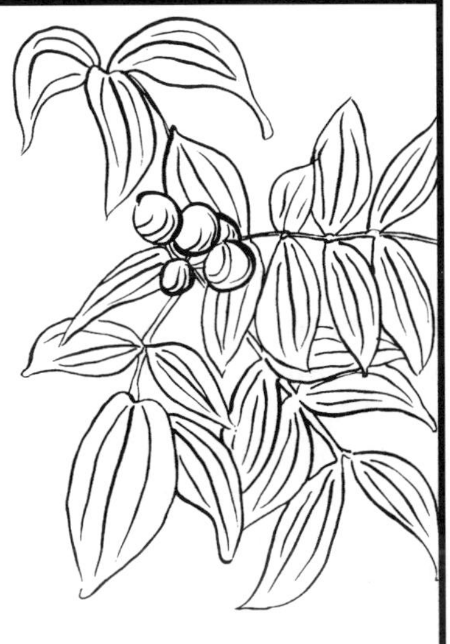

Strychnos Ma Qian Zi

Prepared Vomit Nut

Botanical source: *Strychnos pierrana* A.W. Whill. or *S. nux-vomica* L. or *S. wallichiana* Steud. ex De Candolle (Loganiaceae)
Pharmaceutical name: Semen Strychnotis preparatae
Chinese names: Ma Qian Zi, Fan Mu Bie (Mand); Ma Chin Ji (Cant)
Other names: Nux Vomica, "Horse money"; Basenchi (Jap)
Habit: Climbing (sub)tropical Asian shrub or tree growing on hillsides, slopes and in roadside woods; flowers in spring with white flowers.
Part used: the seed prepared through baking

Therapeutic category: medium-strength remedy with some chronic toxicity
Constituents: alkaloids (incl. strychnine, brucine c. 1%, vomicine, novacine, pseudostrychnine, pseudobrucine, brucidine, colubrine, tetrahydrostrychnine, strychinicine), fixed oil, proteins, chlorogenic acid, monoterpenoid loganine
Effective qualities: bitter, cool, dry
restoring, raising, stimulating, relaxing
Tropism: nervous (incl. medulla), musculoskeletal, digestive, hepatobiliary, urinary, reproductive systems
Liver, Spleen, Kidney, Heart, Du channels; Air, Fluid bodies

Actions and Indications

central nervous stimulant: psychogenic, antidepressant: cerebral and nervous deficiency with chronic depression and fatigue; chronic stress, neurasthenia, catatonic schizophrenia, convalescence, nervous breakdown
neuromuscular stimulant: paralysis and paraplegia (general and local, incl. flaccid medullary, infantile, laryngeal, alcoholic, post-diphtherial, of bladder/uterus/intestines); paresthesia, ataxia, myelitis, Guillain-Barré syndrome, peripheral neuritis, hemiplegia; sequelae of poliomyelitis, barbiturates, alcohol and opium intoxication, shock; atonic neurogenic bladder with incontinence/enuresis, nocturia; spermatorrhea, cholera, dysentery, typhoid
musculoskeletal restorative: bone, muscle and tendon weakness; hypotonic limbs and body; myasthenia gravis, rheumatism, rheumatoid arthritis, ataxia, muscular dystrophy; antalgic gait
uterine stimulant, parturient: hypotonic uterine dystocia
gastrointestinal/digestive stimulant: appetite loss, chronic dyspepsia, umbilical pain, diarrhea; anorexia, convalescence, malabsorption syndrome, malnutrition
liver decongestant, chologogue: chronic jaundice, right flank pain; liver and spleen congestion
antiemetic: nausea, vomiting from any cause
anti-inflammatory: laryngitis
vulnerary, detumescent: injury from falls, fractures, contusions, cold ulcers, carbuncles
anti-infective, anthelmintic: lymph gland and lung TB, hookworm
antitumoral: cervical cancer
Miscellaneous: chronic aplastic anemia

Symptom Pictures

nerve and brain deficiency (Heart phlegm damp obstruction): exhaustion, depression, mental stupor

neuromuscular and skeletal deficiency (Liver and Kidney depletion): weakness, weak bones and muscles, muscle tingling and soreness

wind/damp/cold obstruction: muscle and joint numbness, stiffness or pain, exhaustion

liver, gallbladder and stomach Qi stagnation: right subcostal pain or fulllness, flatulence, umbilical pain, sallow yellow complexion and skin, constipation

Preparation

Use: Because of its fairly toxic nature, the seed Strychnos Ma Qian Zi is usually used pre-prepared through baking. It is used in powder (and in derivatives such as pills) or tincture form. Topical applications—such as plasters and pastes—for facial paralysis, hemiplegia, myelitis, etc. are very successful, while laryngeal insufflation (blowing the powder down the throat) is practiced for throat conditions.

Dosage: ***The prepared seed,*** Strychnos **Zhi Ma Qian Zi:**

Powder or pill: 0.6-1.2 g
Tincture: 3-18 drops

The raw seed, Strychnos **Ma Qian Zi:**

Powder or pill: 0.2-0.3 g, i.e. 0.6-0.9 g per day
Tincture: 1-6 drops, i.e. 3-18 drops per day

Caution: Only to be used under professional supervision. Dosages must not be exceeded. Contraindicated in children and weak people, during pregnancy and breastfeeding, and in excess or deficiency heat conditions, including high fever, inflammation and cerebral blood congestion. Also forbidden in hypertension, severe liver and kidney lesions, cerebral or medullary hyperactivity, and paralysis with contractions or spasms. Avoid using this remedy in acute conditions and when there is tissue irritation present, or compensate with other remedies.

If only the raw seed (Ma Qian Zi) is available, it is best to start with a low dose and gradually increase it over a week or two. Signs of cumulative toxicity include dizziness, headache, dry mouth, indigestion, irritability and apprehension.

Notes

The bitter Vomit nut from India and the East Indies is regarded as a valuable medicine in all three major medical systems: Chinese, Indian and Greek/European. Operating through nervous stimulation, the remedy has essentially *stimulant* and *restorative* actions.

North American Eclectic practitioners of the last century got closer to the essence of its many indications than anyone by stating that "the keynote to its use is atony" (King 1889). Deficiency conditions involving the nervous, musculoskeletal and digestive systems are Vomit nut's terrain. While the underscored symptomatology includes nervous depression, paralysis, numbness, weak limbs, anorexia and constipation, the remedy's actions are consistently effective in all conditions and syndromes presented here.

Styrax An Xi Xiang
Benzoin

安息香

Botanical source: *Styrax benzoin* Dryander (Styracaceae)
Chinese names: An Xi Xiang (M); Ngon Sik Heung (C)
Other names: Gum Benjamin, "Tranquility aromatic"
Habit: Perennial (sub)tropical tree found throughout Asia.
Part used: the tree resin
Category: mild remedy with minimal chronic toxicity

Constituents: essential oil (incl. sumaresinolic acid, cinnamyl cinnamate, styracin, styrene, benzaldehyde, benzoic acid, cinnamic acid), vanillin
Effective qualities: bitter, pungent, warm; stimulating, raising, calming
Tropism: nervous, respiratory, reproductive, musculoskeletal systems; Liver, Heart, Spleen, Lung, Du channels

Actions: *Analeptic, psychogenic, analgesic, stimulant expectorant, diuretic, mucostatic, antiseptic*
Indications: Fainting (incl. from postpartum blood loss), stroke, concussion, cerebral contusion; chest and abdominal pian, arthritic pain, bronchitis with productive coughing, leucorrhea.

Topically for skin irritation, cracked skin, sores, wounds.

Dosage: Decoction: 1.5-3 g
Tincture: 0.2-1.5 ml

Caution: Forbidden in Yin deficiency and full heat conditions.
Notes: Benzoin was another "aromatic" (*xiang*) commonly used in perfumery and medicine.

Securinega Yi Ye Qiu
Securinega Shoot and Root

一叶萩

Botanical source: *Securinega suffruticosa* (Pall.) Rehder (Euphorbiaceae)
Chinese names: Yi Ye Qiu, Ye Di Zhu (Mand); Yat Yip Chau (Cant)
Category: medium-strength remedy with chronic toxicity

Constituents: alkaloids securinine, allosecurinine, dihydrosecurinin
Effective qualities: bitter, pungent, warm; stimulating, raising, calming
Tropism: nervous, musculoskeletal, reproductive systems; Liver, Kidney channels

ACTIONS: *Analeptic, psychogenic, arterial stimulant, cardiotonic, hypertensive, reproductive restorative*
INDICATIONS: Nervous paralysis (incl. facial), stroke, cerebral contusion, concussion, hemiplegia, paraplegia, rheumatic lumbar pain, paresthesia, poliomyelitis, multiple sclerosis, ataxia; menopausal syndrome, impotence.
Dosage: Decoction: 2-6 g
Tincture: 0.5-1.5 ml
Caution: Being medium-strength, do not take on its own over a three-week period.

REMEDIES TO RELAX THE NERVES AND STOP SPASMS

➤ EXTINGUISH INTERNAL WIND, STOP SPASMS AND CLEAR WIND PHLEGM

Spasmolytics, anticonvulsants

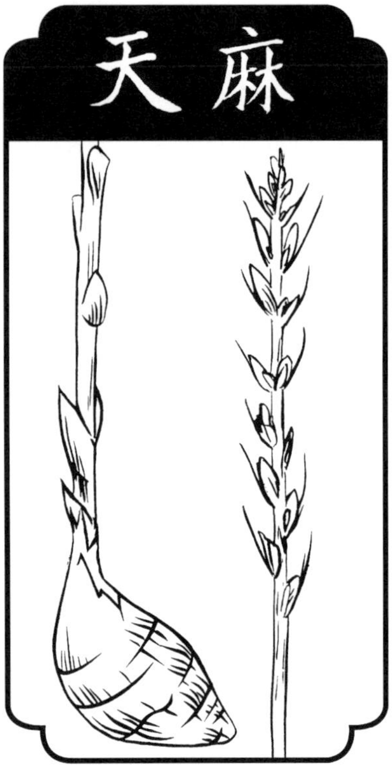

Gastrodia Tian Ma

Celestial Hemp Corm *

Botanical source: *Gastrodia elata* Blume (Orchidaceae)
Pharmaceutical name: Rhizoma Gastrodiae
Chinese names: Tian Ma, Chi Jian, Ming Tian Ma (Mand); Tin Ma (Cant)
Other names: Tenma (Jap)
Habit: Saprophytic temperate alpine herb from Central and Southwest China, Korea and Japan; grows in damp, shady places beneath shrubs and trees; blooms in summer with numerous small orange terminal flower clusters.
Part used: the rhizomatous corm

Therapeutic category: mild remedy with minimal chronic toxicity
Constituents: glycosides, alkaloids (incl. gastrodine), vanillyl alcohol, vanillic aldehyde, vanilline, mucilage, antifungal protein (GAFP), vitamin A, trace minerals (incl. manganese, cobalt, lithium, molybdanum)
Effective qualities: sweet, a bit pungent, neutral
relaxing, calming
Tropism: nervous, muscular, cardiovascular, digestive systems
Liver, Pericardium, Yin Wei channels; Air body

ACTIONS AND INDICATIONS

nervous relaxant: spasmolytic, anticonvulsant: spasmodic nervous conditions with spasms and seizures (esp. infantile; tetany, hemiplegia, opisthotonos, epilepsy, cerebral palsy, chorea
neuromuscular sedative, analgesic: agitation, headache, migraine, rheumatic and arthritic neuralgia, lumbar pain
hypotensive: hypertension (esp. with paresthesia or paralysis of extremities), migraine, vertigo, blurred vision; essential hypertension
cholagogue
antifungal
interferon inducent

SYMPTOM PICTURES

nerve excess with **internal wind (wind phlegm obstruction):** agitation, tremors, cramps, convulsions

Qi constraint with **nerve excess (Liver Yang rising):** irritability, unrest, dizziness, ringingin ears, headache

wind damp obstruction: pain and numbness of lower extremities and back

PREPARATION

Use: The corm Gastrodia Tian Ma is decocted or used in tincture form.
Dosage: Decoction: 3-10 g
Tincture: 2-4 ml
Caution: None.

Notes

An orchid from the Central China plains furnishes this valuable remedy. Celestial hemp corm is a widely used *relaxant* and *sedative* to the nervous system, with no cumulative toxicity. Wind phlegm and Liver Yang rising are the traditional patterns treated. The sweet corm is a specific remedy for cramps and spasms of the extremities and pain of the lower limbs and back. Traditionally, this botanical is also believed to sharpen the memory and promote strength.

Gastrodia elata is known to grow in proximity to another plant, the polypore mushroom *Armillaria mellea* (Vabi ex Fr.) Quehl (Polyporaceae), **Mi Huan Jun**, the honey mushroom. It is thought that the metabolites of this companion plant contribute to the actions of Gastrodia Tian Ma. Following promising pharmacological studies on Armillaria Mi Huan Jun, clinical assays have been conducted successfully employing this fungus as a substitute for Gastrodia Tian Ma.

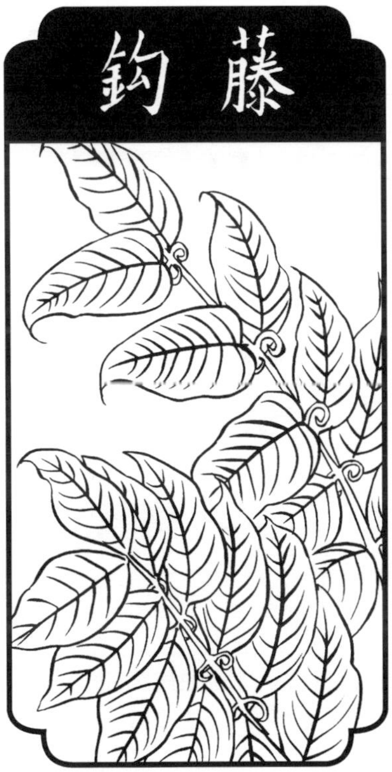

Uncaria Gou Teng

Gambir Vine Twig

Botanical source: *Uncaria rhynchophylla* (Miq.) Jackson, *U. hirsuta* Haviland, *U. macrophylla* Waller, *U. sinensis* Havil. and spp. (Rubiaceae)
Pharmaceutical name: Ramulus et uncus Uncariae
Chinese names: Gou Teng, Shuang Gou Teng, Diao Teng, Gou Gou (Mand); Ngau Tang, Sheung Ngau Tang, Sheung Ngau (Cant)
Other names: Sharp-leaf gambir vine, White cutch, "Hook vine"; Koto (Jap)
Habit: Evergreen climbing shrub or vine from South China and Japan; inhabits wooded mountain valley slopes, ravines and stream banks; ball-shaped terminal flowerheads of small, pale green blossoms open in summer.
Part used: the twig and thorn

Therapeutic category: medium-strength remedy with some chronic toxicity
Constituents: indole and oxindole alkaloids (incl. rhynchophylline, corynoxeine, isocorynoxeine, hirsutine, hirsuteine, isorhynchophylline, dihydrocorynantheine, corynantheine, geissoschizine,akuammigine), nicotinic acid
Effective qualities: sweet, bitter, cool
relaxing, calming
Tropism: nervous, muscular, cardiovascular, reproductive systems
Liver, Pericardium, Yin Wei channels; Air body

Actions and Indications

nervous relaxant: spasmolytic, anticonvulsant: spasmodic nervous conditions with spasms and seizures (esp. infantile); epilepsy, stroke, hemiplegia, paralysis (incl. due to stroke), paresthesia, chorea, cerebral palsy, infantile nystagmus; intestinal colic
nervous sedative: headache, unrest, irritability, insomnia, delirium
sympathetic inhibitor, peripheral vasodilator, hypotensive: hypertension (with dizziness), sympatheticotonia
fetal relaxant: fetal unrest, threatened miscarriage
antipyretic: fevers in general (incl. in children)
anti-inflammatory: eye inflammation

Symptom Pictures

nerve excess with **internal wind (wind phlegm obstruction):** agitation, tremors, convulsions

Qi constraint with **nerve excess (Liver Yang rising):** dizziness, ringing in ears, headache, irritability

external wind heat: fever, headache, red eyes, restlessness

Preparation

Use: The twig Uncaria Gou Teng should be decocted for 10-15 mimutes, no longer. Over 20 minutes' decoction destroys the alkaloids' action. A tincture may also be used. The larger the dose, the more *sedative* its action.

Dosage: Short decoction: 8-16 g
Tincture: 2-4 ml

Caution: Because of its medium-strength status, do not use continuously alone at maximum dose for longer than four weeks. Like most other Oriental remedies, this remedy too is normally used in combination with others.

Notes

Gambir vine, a shrub from the mountains of Central and South China, is distinguished by its small, ox-blood red twigs shaped like ram's horns. These "recurvent stipules" comprise a much-used alkaloidal remedy that is routinely included in formulas treating nervous hyperfunctioning, both central and neuromuscular. Spasmodic disorders involving the striped muscles are its focus, including those involving the foetus during pregnancy. In reducing hypertension, Gambir vine's systemic *relaxant* action also involves cardiovascular functions.

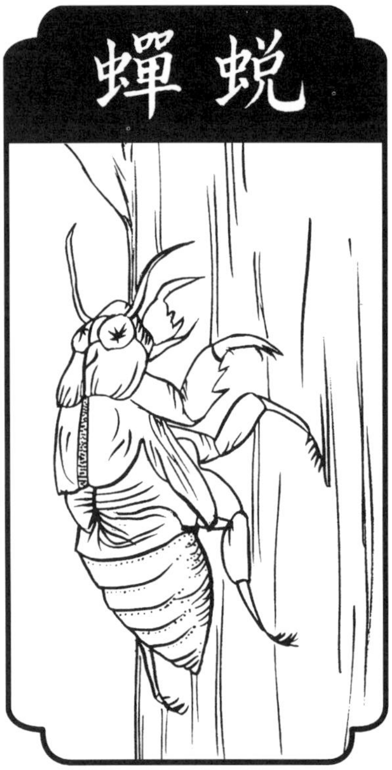

Cryptotympana Chan Tui

Cicada Slough

Zoological source: *Cryptotympana atrata* Fabricius (Cicadidae)
Pharmaceutical name: Periostracum Cryptotympanae
Chinese names: Chan Tui, Chan Yi, Chan Tuo (Mand); Sim Teui (Cant)
Other names: Sentai (Jap)
Habitat: Predominantly Shandong, Jiangsu, Henan, Hebei
Part used: the cicada nymph slough

Therapeutic category: mild remedy with minimal chronic toxicity
Constituents: amino acids (incl. threonine, alanine, valine, isoleucine, serine, aspartic acid, glutamic acid), keratin, chitin, chlorine, 2 nitrogenous substances, phenols
Effective qualities: sweet, salty, cold
relaxing, calming, sinking
Tropism: nervous, respiratory systems
Liver, Lung channels
Air, Warmth bodies

Actions and Indications

nervous relaxant: spasmolytic, anticonvulsant: spasmodic nervous conditions with spasms and seizures; epilepsy, tetany, chorea, lockjaw, infantile night-crying, cerebral palsy
nervous sedative, analgesic: irritability, insomnia, nervous tension, pain in general
antipyretic, anti-inflammatory: fever, heatstroke, inflammations (esp. red swollen eyes); conjunctivitis, laryngitis, rhinitis; voice loss
vasorelaxant diaphoretic: onset of infections with fever
rash-promoting, antipruritic: noneruptive measles, chickenpox, etc.; pruritus of measles
antiallergic, dermatropic, antipruritic: allergic and pruritic skin conditions (incl. atopic dermatitis); nettle rash, eczema, drug rashes, paint allergy, otitis
anticataract: nebula, cataract, corneal opacity
interferon inducent, antitumoral

Symptom Pictures

nerve excess with **internal wind:** tremors or spasms of extremities, pain, agitation

Qi constraint with **nerve excess (Liver Yang rising):** feeling stressed, unrest, dizziness, sleep loss

external wind heat: fever, irritability, painful swollen throat, voice loss

Preparation

Use: The slough Cryptotympana Chan Tui is decocted.
Dosage: Decoction: 3-6 g
Caution: Contraindicated in external deficiency. Use cautiously during pregnancy.

Notes

Cicada slough is one of the main remedies used in contemporary China for the treatment of tetanus, corneal opacity (e.g., cataract) and allergic and pruritic skin conditions. Being both *relaxing* and *sedating* to the whole nervous system, the remedy treats spasmodic and painful conditions known in Chinese medicine as internal wind.

Cicada slough's *heat-clearing* property makes it suitable for the onset of infections, especially with inflammation, pain and irritability present—wind heat conditions, in short. Inflammations of both infectious and allergic origin are well controlled with its use.

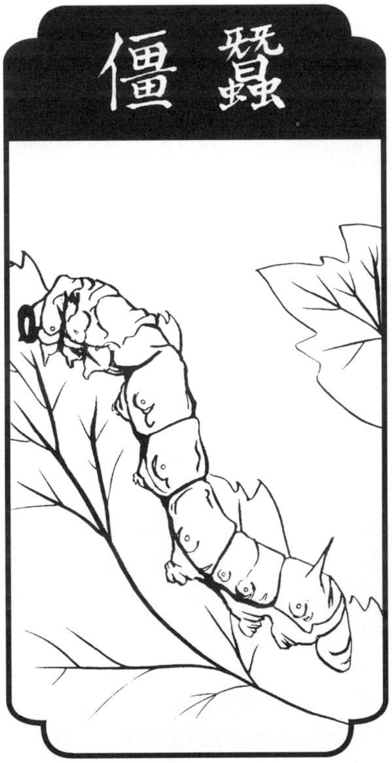

Bombyx Jiang Can

Silkworm Larva

Zoological source: *Bombyx mori* L. (Bombycidae) infected with *Beauvaria bassiana* (Bals.) Vuill. (Moniliaceae)
Pharmaceutical name: Bombyx batryticatus
Chinese names: Jiang Can, Bai Jiang Can (Mand); Geung Chaam (Cant); Jiang Yong (Mand) is the silkworm pupa artificially infected with *B. bassiana*
Other names: Kyosan (Jap)
Source: Produced in Jiangsu, Zhejiang, Sichuan and Guangdong provinces
Part used: the dried infected silkworm larva

Therapeutic category: mild remedy with minimal chronic toxicity
Constituents: ammonium oxalate, proteins, pyridine dicarboxylic acid, oxalic acid, destruxin, chitinase, bassianins, fibrinolysin, beauverician, fat
Effective qualities: pungent, salty, neutral
relaxing, dissolving
Tropism: nervous, epidermal, urinary, lymphatic systems
Liver, Lung, Stomach channels
Air, Warmth bodies

Actions and Indications

nervous relaxant: spasmolytic, anticonvulsant: spasmodic nervous conditions with spasms and seizures (incl. infantile); facial paralysis, Bell's palsy, cerebral palsy, epilepsy, MS
nervous sedative, hypnotic, analgesic: intermittent headache, toothache, agitation, night crying
anti-inflammatory, antipyretic: laryngitis, pharyngitis, parotitis, sore throat, voice loss; encephalitis and sequelae, erysipelas, rubella, psoriasis
resolvent detumescent, lymphatic decongestant: lymphadenitis (incl. cervical), lymph gland TB
antipruritic: urticaria (hives), dermatitis, pruritus (incl. scrotal, vaginal)
antidiabetic: diabetes mellitus (mild to moderate)

urinary: enuresis, nephritis, hematuria
hepatic: chronic liver disease
adrenocortical stimulant
antitumoral
antibacterial

Symptom Pictures

nerve excess with **internal wind:** agitation, pain, dizziness, tremors, spasms

external wind heat: painful swollen throat, headache, feverishness, unrest, blood-shot eyes

Preparation

Use: The stiff white larva Bombyx Jiang Can is decocted or used in powder or tincture form.
Dosage: Decoction: 3-10 g
Powder: 1-3 g
Tincture: 2-4 ml
Caution: Forbidden in anemic conditions.

Notes

Because of its essentially *relaxant* action on the nervous system, Silkworm larva is much used in pediatric formulas for convulsions of any type. Acute fevers and inflammations presenting pain and agitation (not only in children) are other typical indications for this time-tested remedy. Silkworm larva is also successful in resolving various skin conditions (inflammatory, pruritic, lymphatic) and is a renowned special remedy for various throat problems.

The silkworm pupa artificially infected with *Beauvaria bassiana* becomes the remedy **Jiang Yong;** it is often used to replace the naturally infected form Jiang Can.

天南星

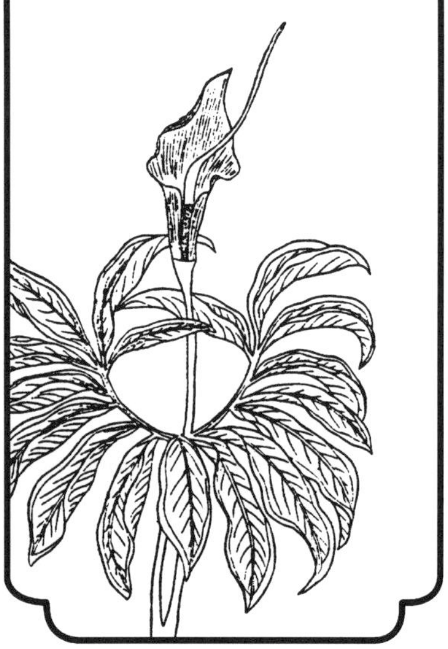

Arisaema Tian Nan Xing

Prepared Dragon Arum Corm

Botanical source: *Arisaema consanguineum* Schott or *A. amurense* Maximowicz or *A. heterophylla* Blume or *A. japonicum* Blume or *A. thunbergii* Blume and spp. (Araceae)
Pharmaceutical name: Rhizoma Arisaemae preparatae
Chinese names: Tian Nan Xing, Nan Xing, Hu Zhang; Zhi Nan Xing (Mand); Tin Naam Sing, Jek Naam Sing (Cant)
Other names: Jack-in-the-pulpit, Wild turnip, "Heaven South star"; Tennansho (Jap)
Habit: Perennial herb from eastern mid China, Korea, Japan; grows on damp shady slopes, in woods and forests; a greenish spadix flower spike forms in spring.
Part used: the prepared rhizomatous corm

Therapeutic category: medium-strength remedy with mild chronic toxicity
Constituents: triterpenoid saponins, benzoic acid, mannitol, amino acid, starch
Effective qualities: bitter, pungent, warm, very dry
relaxing, calming, stimulating
Tropism: nervous, respiratory systems
Liver, Lung, Spleen, Yin Qiao, Yin Wei channels
Air, Fluid bodies

Actions and Indications

nervous relaxant and neuromuscular stimulant: spasmolytic, anticonvulsant: spasmodic nervous conditions with spasms, tremors of extremities, seizures; facial paralysis, stroke with eye and mouth deviation, hemiplegia, epilepsy, tetany, opisthotonos, chorea, Bell's palsy, cerebral palsy

nervous sedative: analgesic, anti-inflammatory: unrest, insomnia, neuralgia; neurodermatitis, neuritis, pain and paresthesia of shoulder and extremities

stimulant expectorant: chronic bronchitis

detoxicant, detumescent, anti-inflammatory, antivenomous: inflammations, boils, carbuncles, abscesses, snakebite

antitumoral: tumors, cancer (incl. cervical)

antibacterial, antifungal

Symptom Pictures

nerve excess with **internal wind (wind phlegm obstruction):** feeling stressed, dizziness, limb numbness, spasms of hands and feet, facial paralysis, convulsions

lung phlegm damp: chest constriction and fullness, chronic cough, expectoration of copious white sputum

Preparation

Use: The sun-dried, untreated Dragon arum corm is called **Tian Nan Xing** or **Sang Nan Xing** (Mand.), or **Tin Naam Sing** or **Song Naam Sing** (Cant.). When processed with fresh ginger and alum to nullify its somewhat toxic nature, it is called **Zhi Nan Xing** (Mand.) or **Jek Naam Sing** (Cant.). This prepared remedy is decocted or used in tincture form. It is also ground and mixed with vinegar for topical applications for boils, abscesses, etc.

Dosage: Decoction: 4-10 g
Tincture: 1-3 ml

Caution: Even though prepared and detoxified, the remedy Zhi Nan Xing should not be used continuously because of very mild cumulative toxicity. Being pungent, dry and warm natured, this remedy is contraindicated in Yin deficiency, lung dry heat, lung Yin deficiency and lung phlegm dryness syndromes, as well as during pregnancy.

Notes

Prepared dragon arum corm combines reliable *relaxant* and *sedative* effects on the entire nervous system. Consisting of *spasmolytic, anticonvulsant, analgesic* and *anti-inflammatory* actions, these properties are especially effective for spasmodic disorders of the striped muscles, spasms, seizures and the like, as well as for painful inflammatory peripheral nerve conditions such as neuritis.

The other side of Prepared dragon arum corm is a *stimulant* one. The remedy's *neuromuscular stimulant* action is frequently made use of in formulas addressing the sequelae of stroke, hemiplegia and other forms of paralysis. Chronic bronchial disorders presenting tightness in the chest, abundant sputum and cough are managed through its reliable *bronchial stimulant* effect. The corm's uses are reflected in the related North American species, *Arisaema triphyllum,* which is also employed for asthma, productive bronchitis and sore throat.

Dan Nan Xing (Mandarin) or **Daam Naam Sing** (Cantonese) or Pulvis Arisaemae Cum Felle Bovis (pharmaceutical) is another variation on this remedy in addition to the ones described under Preparation above. This remedy consists of powdered Prepared dragon arum corm mixed with bovine bile. It has a bitter, cool energetic nature. It belongs to the medium-strength category of remedies because of its mild cumulative toxicity. Arisaema Dan Nan Xing is used for spasms, convulsions and strokes, especially those arising from children's fevers. The dosage is 3-6 g by decoction, 0.5-2 ml by tincture.

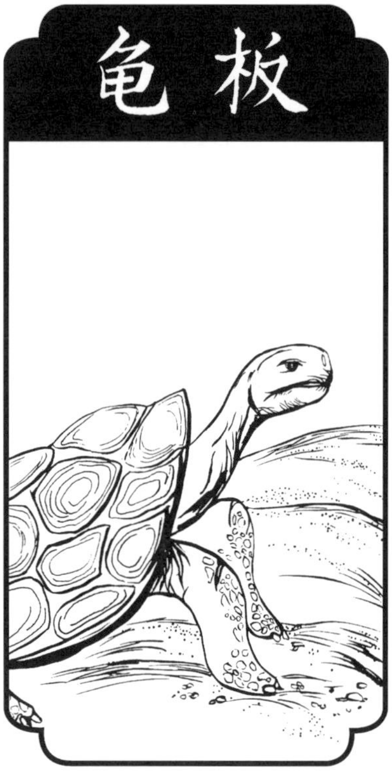

Chinemys Gui Ban

Tortoise Shell

Zoological source: *Chinemys reevesii* Gray (Testudinidae)
Pharmaceutical name: Plastrum Chinemis/testudinis
Chinese names: Gui Ban, Gui Jia (Mand); Gwai Baan (Cant)
Other names: Terrapin; Kixoban (Jap)
Source: Produced mainly in Zhejiang, Anhui, Hubei and Hunan provinces
Part used: the ventral shell (plastron)

Therapeutic category: mild remedy with minimal chronic toxicity
Constituents: keratin, gelatin, lipids, calcium, phosphorus, trace elements (incl. zinc, selenium, cadmium), 17 amino acids
Effective qualities: salty, sweet, neutral
relaxing, nourishing, restoring, solidifying, astringing
Tropism: nervous, musculoskeletal, urogenital, respiratory, endocrine systems
Liver, Kidney, Lung, Heart, Chong channels
Air, Fluid, Warmth bodies

Actions and Indications

nervous relaxant: spasmolytic: spasmodic nervous conditions with dizziness, tremors of extremities; hypoparathyroidism, hypocalcemia, tinnitus, facial spasms, tetany
relaxant parturient: stalled or difficult labor (uterine dystocia) with hypertonic contractions
antipyretic: low-grade fevers, sensation of heat in bones, night sweats, hot spells
musculoskeletal (tropho)restorative: bone, sinew and cartilage weakness, lumbar pain, weak legs/arms; osteomalacia, rickets, myelitis, osteoporosis, hypercalcemia, neurogenic arthropathy, muscular dystrophy, Paget's disease
protein anabolism stimulant, growth stimulant: poor or delayed bone development in babies and children, nonclosure of fontanelles; protein metabolism deficiency (incl. osteoporosis)
lung restorative: chronic cough, faint or weak voice
hemostatic, mucostatic: uterine bleeding, menorrhagia, leucorrhea, hemorrhoids, chronic dysentery/diarrhea
vulnerary: chronic ulcers, sores, ulcers, rectal fistula

Symptom Pictures

Liver and Kidney Yin deficiency with **nerve excess** and **internal wind:** spasms of hands, feet or calves, ringing in ears, dizziness, restlessness, hot spells

Yin deficiency: afternoon hot spells, fatigue, thirst, night sweats, low fever

musculoskeletal deficiency (Liver and Kidney depletion): fatigue, weakness in lower back, knee and legs

Preparation

Use: The shell Chinemys Gui Ban is decocted for at least 1 hour. When part of a formula, as is usual, it should be sliced and first decocted on its own for 30 minutes before any other ingredients are added.
Dosage: Long decoction: 10-30 g
Caution: Contraindicated during pregnancy, in indigestion, diarrhea due to intestines cold, and all external conditions.

Notes

Thought of in Chinese medicine primarily as a deep-acting *Yin tonic*, Tortoise shell shows versatile *restorative* and *relaxant/spasmolytic* properties. These are adapted to treating a variety of neurological, musculoskeletal and gynecological conditions arising from internal deficiency. The three symptom pictures indicating its use clearly spell this out. For pediatrics, Tortoise shell's special *growth-stimulant* activity, like that of Velvet deer antler, should be noted. The *parturient* action during labor and *hemostatic* action postpartum are often applied in obstetrics.

Amyda Bie Jia 鱉甲

Asian Soft-Shell Turtle Shell

Zoological source: *Amyda sinensis* Wiegman, *Trionix sinensis* Wiegmann and spp (Trionychidae)
Chinese names: Bie Jia (Mand); Bit Gaap (Cant)
Part used: the soft dorsal shell
Category: mild remedy with minimal chronic toxicity

Constituents: iodine, vitamin D, gelatin, colloid, keratin
Effective qualities: salty, neutral, moist; relaxing, restoring, stimulating, softening, dissolving
Tropism: nervous, reproductive, lymphatic systems; Liver, Spleen channels

ACTIONS: *Spasmolytic, anticonvulsant, antipyretic, emmenagogue, hemostatic, resolvent, dissolvent, lymphatic decongestant, laxative*
INDICATIONS: Spasms, night sweats, hot spells, unrest and chronic low-grade fever from Yin deficiency; infantile seizures, hypocalcemia; chronic malaria with intermittent fever/chills; amenorrhea, menorrhagia, uterine bleeding; hard epigastric and abdominal lumps; lymphadenitis, hard nodules; liver and spleen enlargement; urinary gravel.
Dosage: Decoction: 9-30 g. Decoct separately for about 30 minutes before adding other ingredients in a formula. Roasting or toasting the shell, or baking it in vinegar increases its *softening* and *dissolving* effects for lumps, hard glands and organ enlargement.
Caution: Use with caution during pregnancy, and in diarrhea and impotence. Do not use during an infection.

Eretmochelys Dai Mao 玳瑁

Hawksbill Turtle Shell

Zoological source: *Eretmochelys imbricata* (L.) (Chelonidae)
Chinese names: Dai Mao (Mand); Doi Mou (Cant)
Part used: the ventral shell of the turtle.
Category: mild remedy with minimal chronic toxicity

Constituents: keratin, gelatin, trace minerals
Effective qualities: sweet, salty, cold; relaxing, stimulating
Tropism: nervous, cardiovascular systems; Liver, Heart channels

ACTIONS: *Spasmolytic, anticonvulsant, analeptic, antipyretic, anti-inflammatory, detoxicant, antidotal, laxative*
INDICATIONS: Infantile seizures, delirium, mania, epilepsy, stroke, coma, hypocalcemia, the sequelae of fever; wind phlegm obstruction syndrome; acute arthritis, boils, abscesses; excessive tearing; herb poisoning; constipation.
Dosage: Decoction: 3-7 g
Caution: None.

Haliotis Shi Jue Ming 石决明

Abalone Shell

Zoological source: *Haliotis diversicolor* Reeve or *H. discus* Hannai Ino and spp. (Haliotidae)
Chinese names: Shi Jue Ming, Bao Yu (Jia) (Mand); Sek Kyut Ming (Cant)
Other names: Sea ear; Sekketsumei (Jap)
Source: China's southeast and northeast coast

Category: mild remedy with minimal chronic toxicity
Constituents: calcium tricarbonate c. 87-94%, chlorides, phosphates, iron, magnesium, trace minerals (incl. silicon), 17 amino acids
Effective qualities: salty, cool; calming, restoring, sinking
Tropism: nervous system, eyes; Liver, Kidney channels

Actions: *Spasmolytic, anticonvulsant, hypotensive, antipyretic, vision restorative, optitropic*
Indications: Nervous hyperfunctioning with spasms, seizures, stress, unrest, headache, dizziness, tinnitus, chronic insomnia; hypocalcemia, Qi constraint with nerve excess (Liver Yang rising) syndrome; hypertension, fevers; photophobia, blurred vision, pterygium, nebula or other visual obstructions (incl. due to glaucoma and cataract).
Dosage: Decoction: 10-30 g
Powder: 0.5-2 g

The shell Haliotis Shi Jue Ming is decocted for a minimum of 1 hour. The finely ground or powdered shell may also be used straight, preferably in a gelatin capsule.
Caution: None.
Notes: Abalone shell is a commonly used *nervous relaxant* and *sedative* for chronic Qi constraint or Liver Yang rising syndromes. The remedy has a special reputation for treating essential hypertension involving failing kidneys.

The shell's ultimately *restorative* effect on the whole system relies for its action on calcium, other minerals and an array of amino acids.

Pinellia Zhang Ye Ban Xia
Pedatisect Pinellia Corm

掌叶半夏

Botanical source: *Pinellia pedatisecta* Schott (Araceae)
Chinese names: Zhang Ye Ban Xia, Wu Zhang Nan Xing (Mand); Jeung Yip Bun Ha, Fu Jeung Lam Sing (Cant)
Habit: Perennial herb from temperate China, Japan and Korea, found on damp, shady slopes and beneath trees; minute flowers open within a tall spadix.
Category: mild remedy with minimal chronic toxicity
Effective qualities: pungent, warm, dry; relaxing, calming
Tropism: nervous, musculoskeletal systems; Liver, Bladder channels

Actions: *Spasmolytic, anticonvulsant, analgesic, expectorant, antitussive, detumescent, lympatic decongestant, antitumoral, antivenomous*
Indications: Spasmodic nervous conditions with spasms, cramps, tremors of muscles; stroke, infantile seizures, tetany; rheumatic myalgia, chest and abdominal pain; bronchitis, cough; lymphadenitis; tumors, cancer (esp. cervical and lymphatic); snake bite.
Dosage: Decoction: 3-10 g
Tincture: 1-2.5 ml

This remedy is also often used topically for snake bites.
Caution: None.

Agkistrodon Bai Hua She
Multibanded Krait

白花蛇

Zoological source: *Agkistrodon acutus* Gunther and *Bungarus multicinctus* Blythe (Viperidae)
Chinese names: Bai Hua She, Qi She (Mand); Baak Fa Se (Cant)
Other names: Embroidered pit viper; Hakkada (Jap)
Part used: the whole snake body
Category: medium-strength remedy with some chronic toxicity
Constituents: glycoprotein thrombin, lipase, bungarotoxin, coagulase
Effective qualities: sweet, salty, warm, dry; relaxing, calming
Tropism: nervous, musculoskeletal, cardiovascular, epidermal systems; Liver, Spleen channels

Actions: *Spasmolytic, anticonvulsant, neuromuscular sedative, hypnotic, analgesic, hypotensive, dermatropic antifungal, interferon inducent*

Indications: Spasmodic nervous conditions with spasms, cramps, tremors of muscles and tendons, infantile fright seizures; paresthesia and weakness of limbs, paralysis of face and extremities; wind phlegm obstruction syndrome; tetany, chorea, cerebral/Bell's palsy, hemiplegia; reslessness, anxiety; pain in general; neuralgia, myalgia, arthralgia from wind damp obstruction; hypertension; fungal skin conditions (incl. scabies); neurogenic eczema, scabies.

Dosage: Decoction and powder: 2-5 g
Tincture and medicated wine: 0.25-2 ml
Ointments are prepared for external use.

Caution: Contraindicated in Blood and Yin (metabolic/nutritional) deficiencies with empty heat signs. Do not use on its own continuously due to some cumulative toxicity.

Notes: This animal remedy, a variety of pit viper, is an effective *nervous relaxant* and *sedative,* providing relief from spasms, seizures and pain in a variety of neurological and muscular conditions. Traditionally, Multibanded krait is also held to strengthen the bones and sinews.

Zaocys Wu Shao She

Black Grass-Snake

乌梢蛇

Zoological source: *Zaocys dhumnades* Cantor (Viperidae)
Chinese names: Wu Shao She (Mand); U Sau Se (C)
Other names: "Black stripe snake;" Ushooda (Jap)
Part used: the entire animal
Category: mild remedy with minimal chronic toxicity

The actions, indications of this remedy are the same as for the previous remedy, Agkistrodon Bai Hua She. Zaocys Wu Shao She is milder in effect, however.

Dosage: Decoction: 3-10 g
Powder: 3 g

Caution: Forbidden in Yin deficiency with empty heat. Use cautiously in Blood (meatbolic) deficiency syndromes.

Elephe She Tui

Snake Slough

蛇蜕

Zoological source: *Elephe taeniurus* Cope, *E. carinata* Gunther and *Dinodon rufozonatum* Cantor (Viperidae)
Chinese names: She Tui, She Tuo, Long Zi Yi (Mand); Se Toi (Cant)
Part used: the slough or molt of various snakes
Category: mild remedy with minimal chronic toxicity
Constituents: collagen
Effective qualities: salty, sweet, neutral; relaxing
Tropism: nervous, dermal systems; Liver channel

Actions: *Spasmolytic, anticonvulsant; anti-inflammatory dermatropic, detoxicant, antifungal, fetal relaxant*

Indications: Infantile convulsion, epilepsy; mastitis, laryngitis, mouth ulcers, carbuncles, hemorroids, fistula, scabies, skin lesions, fungal infections; corneal disorders, pterygium, hordeolum; brain cysticercosis, epidemic parotitis.

Dosage: Decoction: 1-3 g
Powder: 0.3-0.6 g

Caution: Contraindicated during pregnancy, but used to correct transverse presentation at childbirth.

Buthus Quan Xie

全蝎

Scorpion

Zoological source: *Buthus Martensi* Karsch and spp. (Buthidae)
Chinese names: Quan Xie, Quan Chong (Mand); Chyun Kit (Cant)
Other name: Zenkatsu (Jap)
Part used: the entire animal
Category: medium-strength remedy with chronic toxicity
Constituents: buthotoxin (katsutoxin), trimethylamine, taurocholic acid
Effective qualities: sweet, pungent, neutral; relaxing, calming
Tropism: nervous, lymphatic systems; Liver channel

ACTIONS: *Spasmolytic, anticonvulsant, analgesic; resolvent detoxicant, anti-inflammatory, detumescent, hypotensive vasodilator, diuretic*

INDICATIONS: Spasmodic nervous conditions with spasms, cramps, tics, seizures (incl. infants'); nerve excess with internal wind (wind phlegm obstruction) syndrome; lockjaw, tetany, stroke, epilepsy, hemiplegia, opisthotonos, facial paralysis, cerebral palsy, CVA, chorea, deafness; severe headache, migraine, severe arthritic and rheumatic pain, trigeminal neuralgia, sciatica, hernia; purulent boils, sores, scrofula, lymphadenitis, abscesses, malaria, leucorrhea, uterine prolapse; anuria, jaundice, urinary stones, strangury.

Dosage: Decoction: 3-5 g
Powder: 0.6-1 g

Scorpion tail: Powder and decoction: 0.25-1.5 g

Buthus Quan Xie is also applied externally for infected sores, etc.

Caution: Only to be used for acute conditions and never continuously because of its cumulative toxicity. Contraindicated with internal wind (spasms) caused by metabolic or nervous deficiency (Yin and Blood deficiency).

NOTES: One of the most potent *nervous relaxant, spasmolytic* and *analgesic* remedies in the Oriental pharmacy, Scorpion is a good example of a *relaxant* that is not actually a *nervous sedative.*

Traditional Greek medicine (Tibb Unani) also uses Scorpion as a remedy for some of the conditions above.

Scolopendra Wu Gong

蜈蚣

Centipede

Zoological source: *Scolopendra subspinipes mutilans* Koch (Scolopendridae)
Chinese names: Wu Gong, Chuan Zu (M); Ng Gung (C)
Other names: Gosho (Jap)
Habitat: Southwest China, other (sub)tropical locations
Part used: the whole animal
Category: medium-strength remedy with chronic toxicity
Constituents: taurine, hydroxylysine, histamine-like substance, hemolytic protein, fatty oil, formic acid, amino acids, androgen, cholesterol
Effective qualities: pungent, warm; relaxing, calming
Tropism: nervous, lymphatic, immune, epidermal systems; Liver channel

ACTIONS: *Spasmolytic, anticonvulsant, analgesic, detumescent, detoxicant, antivenomous, antifungal, antitumoral*

INDICATIONS: Spasmodic nervous conditions with spasms, seizures (incl. in infants); nerve excess with internal wind (wind phlegm obstruction) syndrome; lockjaw, facial paralysis, opisthotonos, epilepsy, tetany, leg cramps; chronic headache, arthralgia; lymphadenitis, scrofula, swollen boils, sores, carbuncles, erysipelas, diphtheria; poisonous snake/insect bites; fungal skin conditions (incl. ringworm).

Dosage: Decoction: 2-4 g
Powder: 0.6-1 g
Tincture: 0.5-1 ml

Caution: Not to be used continuously on its own, and forbidden during pregnancy.

Chloris Qing Meng Shi

Chlorite

青礞石

Geological source: Chloris
Chinese names: Qing Meng Shi (Mand);
Ching Mung Sek (Cant)
Source: Central China, Sichuan
Category: mild remedy with minimal chronic toxicity

Constituents: magnesium, aluminum, iron, silicon
Effective qualities: sweet, salty, neutral; relaxing
Tropism: nervous, respiratory, digestive systems; Liver, Lung channels

ACTIONS: *Spasmolytic, anticonvulsant, bronchodilatant, expectorant, digestant, antitumoral*
INDICATIONS: Spasms, seizures (incl. from epilepsy and infantile); cough with profuse viscous sputum; wheezing, asthma; overnight food stagnation; gynecological tumors.
Dosage: Decoction: 10-15 g (place inside a cheesecloth bag first).
Powder: 3-6 g
Caution: During pregnancy.

REMEDIES TO SEDATE THE NERVES AND RELIEVE PAIN

➤ CALM THE SPIRIT AND RELIEVE PAIN

Depressant analgesics and hypnotics

豨薟草

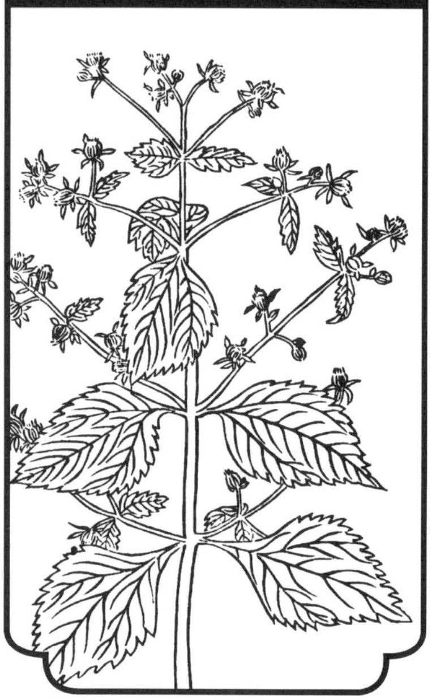

Siegesbeckia Xi Xian Cao

Hairy Siegesbeckia Herb

Botanical source: *Siegesbeckia pubescens* Makino or *S. orientalis* L. or *S. glabrescens* Makino (syn. *Minyranthus heterophylla* Turcz.) (Compositae)
Pharmaceutical name: Herba Siegesbeckiae
Chinese names: Xi Xian Cao, Xi Lian (Mand); Hei Lim Chou (Cant)
Other names: Divine herb, St. Paul's wort; Kirenso (Jap)
Habit: Annual pilose herb from China, Phillipines, Java and India, growing on roadsides and waste ground; in autumn, bright yellow terminal flowers appear on racemes in panicle formation.
Part used: the herb

Therapeutic category: mild remedy with minimal chronic toxicity
Constituents: bitter diterpenoid glycosides (incl. darutoside, darutigenol, dihydroxykauranoic acid), alkaloids, essential oil (incl. phenol), salicylic acid, amino acids, organic acids, saccharides
Effective qualities: bitter, pungent, a bit sweet, cool, dry
calming, relaxing, restoring
Tropism: nervous, musculoskeletal, cardiovascular, hepatobiliary systems
Liver, Spleen, Kidney, Yin Wei channels; Air, Warmth bodies

Actions and Indications

nervous and muscular sedative: analgesic, anti-inflammatory: nervous hyperfunctioning with pain, agitation, muscle tension; neuralgia, rheumatic myalgia, ostalgia, osteomyelitis, rheumatoid arthritis, insomnia
sympathetic nervous inhibitor, hypotensive, vasodilator: unrest, irritability, tension; hypertension, stress
neuromuscular stimulant: poor memory, facial and limb paralysis, hemiplegia, numbness/weakness of back/legs
resolvent detoxicant, antiseptic, antivenomous: skin infections, mastitis, boils, furuncles, ulcers; acute infectious hepatitis, malaria, animal and insect bites
dermatropic detoxicant, antipruritic: weeping eczema, pruritus

Symptom Pictures

Qi constraint with **nerve excess (Liver Yang rising):** headache, dizziness, blurred vision, feeling stressed, irritability, unrest, sleeping difficulties, tense muscles

wind damp obstruction: facial and limb muscle pain and numbness, weak back and legs

Preparation

Use: The herb Siegesbeckia Xi Xian Cao is briefly decocted or infused in the normal way. The tincture is a good alternative. Swabs, compresses, etc., are prepared for topical use.
Dosage: Short decoction and infusion: 10-25 g. High doses of 45 g of the herb are used for malaria.
Tincture: 1-4 ml
Caution: Forbidden in Blood or Yin (metabolic or adrenal) deficiency conditions.

Notes

Siegesbeckia herb is unique in being one of the very few remedies with both *sedative* and *restorative* actions on the brain, nerves and muscles. The herb's specific *draining* effect on the sympathetic nerves makes this one of the best for Qi constraint of a chronic nature. Often seen today as a result of chronic overwork and unproductive stress, sympathetic CNS hyperfunctioning also often includes hypertension, insomnia and various painful conditions—all of which will respond to this remedy.

Muscular pain and numbness in themselves are frequently treated with formulas that engage Siegesbeckia's *analgesic* and *anti-inflammatory* neuromuscular actions—justifiably, in view of the salicylic acid content on one hand, and its bitter, pungent, cool qualities on the other.

The plant is named after Johann Sigesbeck, director of the St. Petersburg, Russia, botanic gardens in the 1730s.

In Taiwan the species *Anisomeles ovata* (Labiatae) is sourced for the remedy Xi Xian Cao.

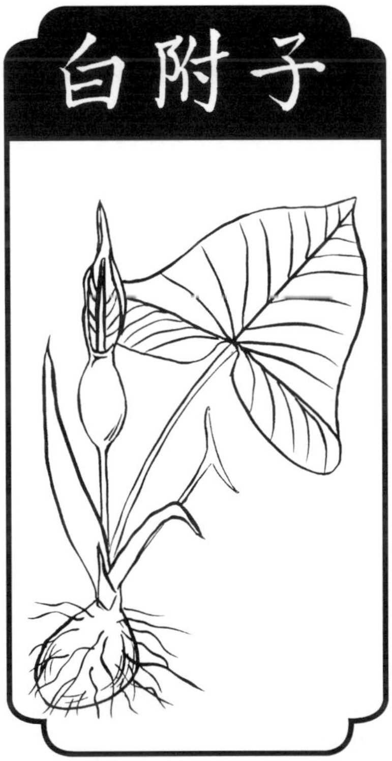

Typhonium Bai Fu Zi

Prepared Giant Typhonium Root

Botanical source: *Typhonium giganteum* Engler (Araceae) and *Aconitum coreanum* (Lvl.) Raipaics. (Ranunculaceae)
Pharmaceutical name: Rhizoma Typhonii seu Aconiti coreani
Chinese names: Bai Fu Zi; *T. gig.*: Yu Bai Fu, Du Jiao Lan; *A. cor.*: Guan Bai Fu (Mand); Baak Fu Ji, Duk Gok Lin (Cant)
Other names: "White appendage;" *A. cor.*: Korean aconite; Byakubushi (Jap)
Habit: Perennial temperate East Asian herb growing in moist, fertile ground; blooms in late summer and autumn with a spadix of purple flowers.
Part used: the root

Therapeutic category: mild remedy with minimal chronic toxicity
Constituents: *T. gig.*: saponin, beta-sitosterol, inositol, mucilage, saccharose
A. cor.: alkaloids (incl. hypaconitine)
Effective qualities: pungent, sweet, warm, dry
calming, relaxing, stimulating, dissolving
Tropism: nervous, muscular systems
Liver, Stomach, Yang Qiao channel
Air body

Actions and Indications

nervous sedative: analgesic: nervous hyperfunctioning with pain in the head and face (esp. lateral headache); migraine, vertigo; myalgia, neuralgia
nervous relaxant: spasmolytic, anticonvulsant: spasms, seizures; epilepsy, tetany, hemiplegia, chorea
neuromuscular stimulant: facial paralysis, hemiplegia, stroke with deviation of eyes and mouth; peripheral neuritis, Bell's palsy, paresthesia
lymphatic decongestant: lymphadenitis with swollen glands
antitubercular: tuberculosis
antifungal, antiparasitic, antivenomous: fungal skin infections, scabies, ulcers, scrofula, genital pruritus, snake bites

Symptom Pictures

wind (phlegm)/damp/cold obstruction: dizziness, lateral headache, facial and head pain, numbness
Qi constraint and nerve excess with **internal wind:** agitation, spasms, pain, convulsions

Preparation

Use: To nullify its toxic nature, the root Typhonium Bai Fu Zi can only be used in processed form. The prepared root is decocted or used in tincture form. Externally, liniments, compresses and the like are used for parasitic and fungal infections, ulcers and vaginal pruritus.

Dosage: Decoction: 2-6 g
Tincture: 0.5-2.5 ml

Caution: Forbidden during pregnancy and in Yin deficiency with empty heat.

Notes

Both Giant typhonium root and Korean aconite root are used to provide the remedy Bai Fu Zi. Whatever the botanical source, this remedy is a classic *nervous sedative, relaxant* and *stimulant* all at once. The main uses for its *analgesic* action include severe lateral headache, migraine and neuralgia, while the *stimulant* aspect addresses hemiplegia and the sequelae of stroke.

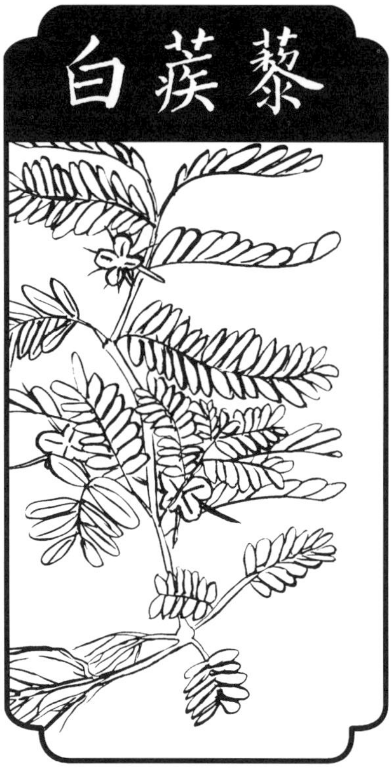

Tribulus Bai Ji Li

Caltrop Fruit

Botanical source: *Tribulus terrestris* L. (Zygophyllaceae)
Pharmaceutical name: Fructus Tribuli
Chinese names: Bai Ji Li, Ci Ji Li, Zhi Xing (Mand); Baak Jat Lai (Cant)
Other names: Puncture vine, Ground burnut, Goat's head; Gokshura, Shvadamstra (Sans); Burra Gokhru (Hi); Byakujitsuri (Jap)
Habit: Low perennial herb from Central China, North India, Australia and Africa growing on low ground by roadsides and in pastures; yellow and purple flowers appear in midsummer.
Part used: the fruit

Therapeutic category: mild remedy with minimal chronic toxicity
Constituents: essential oil (incl. kaempferol), sapogenins (chlorogenin, diosgenin, togogenin, hecogenin, gitogenin), glucoside, alkaloids harman and harmine, tribuloside, fixed oil with acids, tannins, diastase, peroxydase, potassium nitrate, phlobaphenes, vitamin A
Effective qualities: a bit sweet, bitter and pungent, astringent, cool
calming, relaxing, softening, restoring
Tropism: nervous, cardiovascular, respiratory, epidermal, urinary, systems
Liver, Lung, Bladder, Ren channels; Air, Warmth bodies

Actions and Indications

nervous sedative: analgesic: nervous hyperfunctioning with unrest, pain; stress, headache, neuralgia (incl. sciatica), lumbar and shoulder pain, premature ejaculation
dermatropic, antipruritic: neurogenic dermatitis, eczema, urticaria, vitiligo, shingles, pruritus
hypotensive: hypertension (esp. with dizziness)
intestinal relaxant: neurogenic dyspepsia, colic, IBS
bronchodilator: asthmatic breathing, cough
urinary demulcent relaxant/restorative: urinary dryness with dysuria, oliguria, strangury; spastic neurogenic bladder, chronic urinary tract infection, urge incontinence, nephritis, metabolic acidosis
resolvent diuretic, urinary antilithic: urinary gravel and stones
anti-inflammatory: cystitis, acute conjunctivitis, stomatitis, mastitis
reproductive restorative: impotence, infertility, seminal deficiency (incl. low sperm count), amenorrhea

astringent: bleeding in general, hemorrhoids
galactagogue: loss of breast milk (lactation)
antibacterial, antiparasitic: intestinal parasites

Symptom Pictures

Qi constraint with **nerve excess (Liver Yang rising):** feeling stressed, chest or flank pain and distension, headache, unrest, dizziness, itching skin, skin rashes, red irritated eyes

bladder Qi constraint: difficult, painful or scanty urination, dry itchy skin

intestines Qi constraint: abdominal pain and distension, appetite loss, flatulence

Preparation

Use: The fruit Tribulus Bai Ji Li is decocted or used in tincture form.
Dosage: Decoction: 6-12 g
Tincture: 2-4 ml
Caution: Use with care during pregnancy and in Qi or Blood (metabolic) deficiency conditions.

Notes

Found in the herbal pharmacies of both China and India, Caltrop fruit is a complex remedy with a wide variety of constituents to show for its large range of potential actions. The remedy's effects are *sedative, relaxant* and *restorative,* respectively affecting the nervous system, smooth muscles and urogenital organs.

The main conditions that Caltrop fruit addresses are those entailing pain, especially when stress or nervous tension is involved. They include urinary pain and urge incontinence, especially from spastic bladder or metabolic acidosis. The skin will also benefit from the dual *nervine* and *detoxicant diuretic* action. In this respect, Caltrop fruit should be a leading remedy in formulations addressing neurogenic skin disorders.

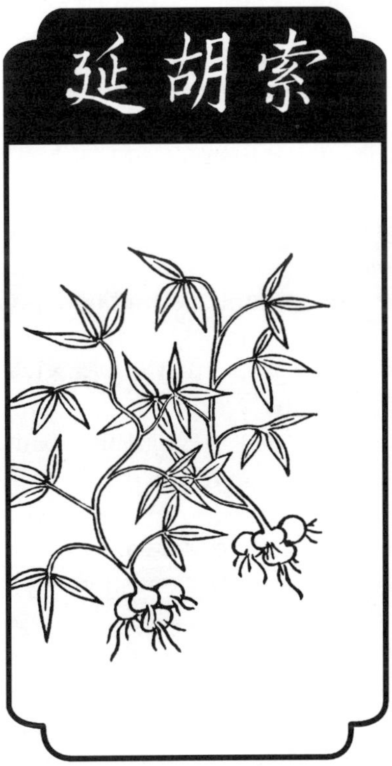

Corydalis Yan Hu Suo

Asian Corydalis Corm

Botanical source: *Corydalis turtschaninovii* Bess. f. or *C. yanhusuo* Y.H. Chow et C.C. Hsu or *C. ambigua* Chamisso et Schlechtendal var. *amurensis* Maximowicz or *C. remota* Fischer et Maximowicz (Papaveraceae)
Pharmaceutical name: Rhizoma Corydalis
Chinese names: Yan Hu Suo, Yuan Hu, Yan Hu, Xuan Hu (Suo) (Mand); Yin Wu Sok, Yin Wu, Yun Wu (Cant)
Other names: Chinese fumewort; Engosaku (Jap)
Habit: Perennial herb from Northeast China, Siberia, Japan; also cultivated in the sandy soil of the mid-coastal province Zhejiang; racemes of pale magenta flowers open in spring.
Part used: the rhizomatous corm

Therapeutic category: mild remedy with minimal chronic toxicity
Constituents: isoquinoline alkaloids (incl. corydaline, tetrahydropalmatine, protopine, allocryptopine, dehydrocorydaline, tetrahydrocoptisine, tetrahydrocolumbamine, corybulbine, corydalmine, glaucine, stylopin, homochelidonine, coptisine, columbamine, palmatine, dehydroglaucine, methyllaurotetanine, tetrahydroprotoberberine [yuanhunine])

Effective qualities: bitter, a bit pungent, warm; calming, relaxing
Tropism: nervous, cardiovascular, digestive, respiratory, genital, endocrine systems
Liver, Heart, Pericardium, Stomach, Lung, Yang Wei, Yang Qiao channels
Air, Fluid bodies

Actions and Indications

nervous sedative: hypnotic, analgesic: nervous hyperfunctioning with unrest, pain, anxiety; insomnia, pain in chest, epigastrium, abdomen, joints, all colic pain, postpartum abdominal pain, menstrual pain (dysmenorrhea), headache, hernial pain, neuralgia; neurocardiac syndrome, anxiety states, chronic stress
muscle relaxant: muscle tension, Meniere's disease
hypotensive coronary vasodilator: early stage of hypertension, coronary disease, angina pectoris, myocardial infarct; hypothermia
hemostatic: uterine bleeding
antacid antisecretory: gastric hyperacidity, peptic ulcer, chronic gastritis
pituitary-adrenal stimulant
anticontusion: injuries from impact, fractures, sprains, strains
anesthetic: minor surgery
interferon inducent

Symptom Pictures

Qi constraint with **nerve excess:** feeling stressed or anxious, chest or abdominal pain, menstrual pain, headache, tight muscles, insomnia

heart Qi constraint and **heart blood and Qi stagnation:** palpitations, labored breathing, chest tightness and pains, dizziness, anxiety

Preparation

Use: The corm Corydalis Yan Hu Suo is decocted or used in tincture form. One traditional practice is to decoct the corms first in vinegar before adding them to other remedies in a formula for decoction.
Dosage: Decoction: 4-11 g
Tincture: 2-4 ml
Caution: Contraindicated during pregnancy.

Notes

Originating in Siberia, Asian corydalis is derived from various species of the poppy or bleeding-heart family. The small corm is a well-researched alkaloidal remedy and one of the few that, amazingly, can still be classed as a mild remedy, i.e., one without any known cumulative toxicity. Asian corydalis is used mainly for its reliable *central nervous sedative, analgesic* and *cardiac relaxant* properties. Its *vasorelaxant, hypotensive* action, for example, is routinely put to use in formulas treating coronary deficiency with hypertension, angina and myocardial infarct. Pain involving most tissues and regardless of origin will respond to the remedy's *analgesic* action. However, in the managment of conditions involving chronic pain, other remedies are still often combined with Asian corydalis in a prescription to create a greater focus on the location and type of pain presenting. Epigastric pain from peptic ulcer in particular will benefit from its additional proven *antacid* action.

In energetic terms, Asian corydalis corm releases constrained Qi, with a particular focus on promoting the smooth circulation of Qi and blood in the chest. The coronary circulation, with all its vital functions, is thereby maintained and enhanced. In this connection, the asterisk symptoms relieved are anxiety and chest pain—especially when arising from high levels of long-term unproductive stress.

Asian corydalis should be clearly distinguished from the related European *Corydalis cava*, a *neuromuscular sedative*, and the North American *Corydalis formosa*, or Turkey corn, a *gastric stimulant* and *diuretic*.

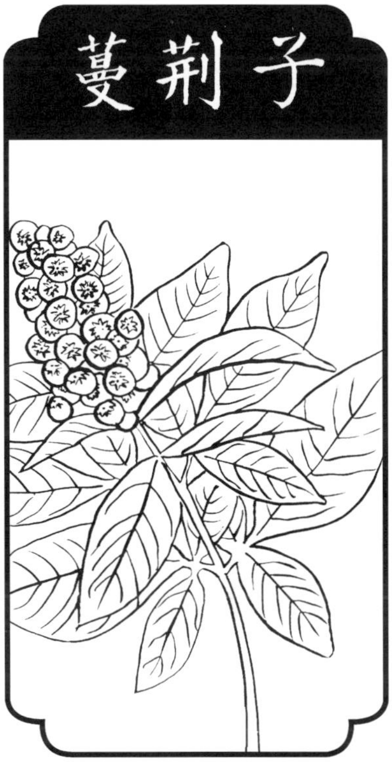

Vitex Man Jing Zi

Seashore Chastetree Berry *

Botanical source: *Vitex rotundifolia* or *V. trifolia* L. (Verbenaceae)
Pharmaceutical name: Fructus Viticis rotundifoliae
Chinese names: Man Jing Zi, Mian Jing Zi (Mand); Maan Ging Ji, Ging Ji (Cant)
Other names: Mankeishi (Jap)
Habit: Deciduous shrub from coastal China found on beaches, oceansides and lakesides; flowers in summer with racemes of small pink flowers.
Part used: the fruit

Therapeutic category: mild remedy with minimal chronic toxicity
Constituents: essential oil (incl. camphene, pinene), flavonoids (incl. vitexicarpin, casticin, aucubin, agnuside, orientin, luteolin), vitamin A
Effective qualities: bitter, pungent, cool
calming, relaxing
Tropism: nervous, musculoskeletal systems
Liver, Stomach, Bladder channels
Air, Fluid bodies

Actions and Indications

nervous and muscular sedative: analgesic: nervous hyperfunctioning with pain; headache (incl. due to tension and hypertension), migraine, rheumatic myalgia, neuralgia, arthralgia
muscle relaxant: muscle spasm/tension; stiff, numb muscles and joints
relaxant diaphoretic: onset of flu or cold with headache
anti-inflammatory: red, painful, swollen eyes; conjunctivitis
optitropic: spots in vision, cataract, watery eyes
antitumoral, interferon inducent: breast cancer
Miscellaneous: insufficient beard growth

Symptom Pictures

Qi constraint with **nerve excess (Liver Yang rising):** feeling stressed, headache, dizziness, unrest, irritability, muscle tension and pain, muscle and joint stiffness or numbness

external wind heat: headache, muscle aches and pains, feverishness, chills, unrest, red painful tearing eyes

Preparation

Use: The berry Vitex Man Jing Zi should be used in a short decoction or in tincture form.
Dosage: Decoction: 6-10 g
Tincture: 2-4 ml
Caution: Use cautiously in eye conditions and headaches due to Blood or Yin deficiency.

Notes

Like the Mediterranean Chasteberry, this Chinese littoral variant of the *Vitex* genus is a *nervous sedative* that releases constrained Qi and relieves the various neurological symptoms arising therefrom. These essentially consist of either neuralgic or myalgic types of pain. In traditional Chinese medical practice, however, the bitter-pungent berry is mainly utilized as an *analgesic* back-up in *relaxant diaphoretic* formulas treating wind heat onset of infections.

Today, Seashore chastetree berry is also a common ingredient in *relaxant* and *analgesic* prescriptions addressing various rheumatic and eye conditions (inflammatory or otherwise).

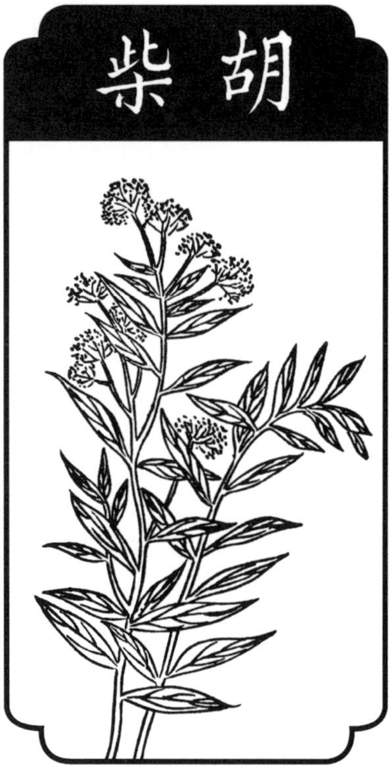

Bupleurum Chai Hu

Asian Buplever Root

Botanical source: *Bupleurum chinense* De Candolle, *B. falcatum* L., *B. longiradiatum* Turchaninov and spp. (Umbelliferae)
Pharmaceutical name: Radix Bupleuri
Chinese names: Chai Hu, Bei Chai Hu (Mand); Chaai Wu (Cant)
Other names: Hare's ear, Thoroughwax, "Kindling barbarian"; Saiko (Jap)
Habit: Fragrant perennial Northeast Asian herb growing on sunny slopes, waste ground and roadsides; in late summer and autumn, compound umbels of small, yellow terminal/axillary flowers appear.
Part used: the root

Therapeutic category: medium-strength remedy with some chronic toxicity
Constituents: triterpenoid saponins (incl. sapogenin, daikogenin, saikosaponins, saikogenins), phytosterols (spinasterol, furfurol, bupleurumol, stigmasterols), hexanoic and pentanoic acids, adonitol, angelicin, oleic/linoleic/palmitic/stearic/lignoceric acids, polysaccharides, essential oil (incl. ketone)
Effective qualities: bitter, a bit pungent and astringent, cool, very dry
calming, relaxing, astringing, solidifying, stabilizing
Tropism: nervous, cardiovascular, digestive, reproductive, respiratory systems
Liver, Gallbladder, Pericardium, Yang Wei channels; Air, Warmth b.

Actions and Indications

nervous sedative: analgesic, anti-inflammatory, spasmolytic: nervous hyperfunctioning with unrest and pain; headache, dysmenorrhea, intercostal neuralgia, myalgia, dyspepsia, peptic ulcer, biliary and intestinal colic, IBS, cholecystitis, cholangitis, spasmodic coughing, deafness
hypotensive (mild): hypertension
antipyretic: remittent fevers, infantile fevers, malaria
anti-infective: antiviral, antibacterial, antigenic, interferon inducent: acute and chronic infections in general (incl. common cold, flu, infectious hepatitis, pleurisy, peptic ulcer, polio, other chronic viral infections)
immune regulator, antiallergic: immune stress with immediate allergies (incl. rhinitis, otitis media, urticaria, bronchial asthma, some food allergies)
liver protective: toxicosis (all types), liver infections
radiation protective: radiation damage
pituitary-adrenocortical stimulant
astringent, antiprolapse: hemorrhoids, rectal or uterine prolapse, acute diarrhea

Symptom Pictures

Qi constraint with **nerve excess:** feeling stressed, unrest, chest pain and tightness, menstrual pain, headache, painful digestion with bloating, allergies

gallbladder fire: irritability, sharp right subcostal pain, chest fullness, fever, jaundice

Shao Yang heat: intermittent fever, vomiting, bitter taste in mouth, irritability, nausea

Preparation

Use: The root Bupleurum Chai Hu is decocted or used in tinture form.
Dosage: Decoction: 3-10 g
Tincture: 1-3.5 ml
Caution: Contraindicated in Rising Liver Yang causing dizziness, tinnitus or headache, or in Yin and fluids deficiency causing symptoms of dryness. Because of its medium-strength status, do not use on its own continuously.

Notes

Asian buplever root, an umbellifer from North China, is a classic remedy for acute nervous, biliary and febrile disorders. Loaded with active saponins, acids, essential oil and phytosterols, the bitter root's *nervous sedative/relaxant* effect serves to systemically reduce pain, spasm and inflammation. Acute tense digestive conditions such as cholecystitis and colic respond especially well to it. Acute infections generally will benefit not only from Asian buplever's good *anti-inflammatory* and *antipyretic* actions, but also from its *anti-infective* effect, which includes immediate immune stimulation *à la* Echinacea. Appropriately for one of today's major chronic disease predisposing factor, toxicosis, the remedy's famed *liver-protectant* action serves all types of toxicosis in general as well as hepatobiliary infections in particular.

Several anticomplementary polysaccharides have recently turned up in this remedy, indicating new applications such as immediate allergies (Yamada and Kiyohara 1989).

Ligusticum Gao Ben

Chinese Lovage Root

藁本

Botanical source: *Ligusticum sinense* Oliver or *L. jeholense* Nakai et Kitag (Umbelliferae)
Chinese names: Gao Ben, Gui Qing, Wei Heng (Mand); Gou Bun (Cant)
Other names: Straw-weed; Kohon (Jap)
Habit: Perennial herb from mid China's mountain valleys; blooms in summer with white blossomed umbels.
Category: mild remedy with minimal chronic toxicity
Constituents: essential oil (incl. cnidilide, neocnidilide, butylidene phthalide, limonene, elemicin, terpineol, pinene, terpinolene, cnidilide, myristicin), palmitic acid, sucrose
Effective qualities: pungent, warm, dry; calming
Tropism: nervous, muscular, reproductive systems; Bladder, Liver, Du channels

Actions: *Analgesic, spasmolytic, emmenagogue, anti-inflammatory, antipyretic, resolvent dermatropic detoxicant, antiviral, antifungal*

Indications: Nervous hyperfunctioning with vertexal headache, dizziness, neuralgia (incl. trigeminal); wind damp cold obstruction syndrome with headache (esp. at vertex) and stiff neck; toothache, myalgia, acute lumbar pain, acute rheumatoid arthralgia, abdominal pain, dysmenorrhea; amenorrhea; eczema, influenza.

Dosage: Decoction: 3-10 g
Tincture: 2-4 ml

Caution: Because of its very dry nature, this remedy is contraindicated in Blood or Yin deficiency patterns.

Notes: Chinese lovage root is most often used as a supportive *analgesic* remedy in influenza and mylagic or neuralgic conditions, where its *fever* and *inflammation-lowering* actions work appropriately. Historically it was also widely used for menstrual conditions and cosmetic preparations.

Chinese lovage root should be differentiated from other *Ligusticum* species such as **Sichuan lovage root,** *Ligusticum wallichii*, the **Western lovage root,** *L. levisticum*, and **Osha root,** *L. porterii*. Most of these species have little therapeutic use in common.

Paederia Ji Shi Teng

Chicken Dung Vine Root and Stem

鸡矢藤

Botanical source: *Paederia scandens* (Lour.) Merrill var. tomentosa (Bl.) Handel-Mazetti (Rubiaceae)
Chinese names: Ji Shi Teng, Ji Xiang Teng, Chou Teng, Qing Teng (M); Gai Niu Tang, Gai Heung Tang (C)
Category: mild remedy with minimal chronic toxicity
Habit: Perennial twining vine from Mid and South China, growing in thickets, wild areas and hillsides; pink terminal flowers open in August.
Constituents: paederoside, scandoside, paederosidic acid, asperuloside, alkaloids (g-sitosterol, oleanolic acid), ess. oil
Effective qualities: sweet, pungent, warm; calming, relaxing, dissolving
Tropism: nervous, musculoskeletal, digestive, respiratory, reproductive systems; Bladder, Liver, Lung channels

Actions: *Analgesic, anesthetic, spasmolytic, antirheumatic, hypotensive, digestant, liver decongestant, uterine stimulant (emmenagogue, parturient), expectorant, vulnerary, anti-infective, resolvent detoxicant*
Indications: Arthritis, rheumatism, toothache, abdominal pain, biliary pain, labor pains, trauma pain, fractures, strains, contusions; dyspepsia, cholecystitis, jaundice, flatulence, infantile malabsorption and malnutrition, alcoholism; stalled labor, prolonged pregnancy; leukopenia; bronchitis, whooping cough, lung TB; epidemics, hepatitis, dysentery; herpes, intestinal parasites; abscesses, boils, ulcers, phosphorus poisoning, snakebites, eczema, pruritus, leprosy.
Dosage: Decoction: 15-60 g
Tincture: 2-5 ml
Preparations are made for topical application.
Caution: Forbidden during pregnancy. The botanical may cause a typical odor on the breath and in the urine.
Notes: Excellent results in labor induction have also been achieved with this wide-acting remedy.

Cynanchum Xu Chang Qing
Panicled Dogbane Root and Herb *

徐长卿

Botanical source: *Cynanchum paniculatum* (Bunge) Kitagawa, syn. *Pycnostelma paniculatum* (Bunge) K. Schumann (Asclepiadaceae)
Chinese names: Xu Chang Qing, Yao Ju Xiao (Mand); Cheui Cheung Hing
Category: mild remedy with minimal chronic toxicity

Constituents: deacylcynanchogenin, paenol 1%, alkaloids sarcostin and tomentogenin, flavone
Effective qualities: pungent, dry, neutral; calming, relaxing, decongesting
Tropism: nervous, musculoskeletal, digestive, reproductive, epidermal systems; Bladder, Liver channels

Actions: *Analgesic, hypotensive, liver decongestant, draining diuretic, vulnerary, detoxicant, antilipemic, antibacterial*
Indications: Rheumatic and arthritic pain, abdominal/lumbar/menstrual pain, toothache; acute gastroenteritis; herpes zoster; edema, ascites, cirrhosis; irregular menstruation; eczema, neurodermatitis, urticaria; traumatic injury, snakebite.
Dosage: Decoction: 8-12 g
Tincture: 2-4 ml
Caution: None.

Schefflera Qi Ye Lian
Taiwan Schefflera Leaf and Stem

七叶莲

Botanical name: *Schefflera arboricola* Hayata or *S. kwangsiensis* Merr. ex H.L. Li or *S. venulosa* (Wight et Arn) Harmslow (Araliaceae)
Chinese names: Qi Ye Lian, Qi Jia Pi (Mand); Chat Yip Lin (Cant)
Habitat: Epiphytic herb from Southeast Asia
Category: mild remedy with minimal chronic toxicity

Constituents: organic acids (incl. fumaric/succinic/hydroxybutyric/malic/citric/tartaric/aconitic acids), alkaloids, amino acids, phenols, saponins, resins
Effective qualities: bitter, sweet, warm; calming, relaxing
Tropism: nervous, musculoskeletal, digestive systems; Spleen, Bladder, Liver channels

Actions: *Hypnotic, analgesic, spasmolytic, vulnerary, detumescent, bronchodilator*
Indications: Painful conditions, incl. rheumatoid arthralgia, lumbago with wind/damp/cold; various types of headache, migraine, neuralgia (all types); traumatic injury with pain and bleeding, sprains, fractures; insomnia, abdominal and biliary pain, asthma.
Dosage: Decoction: 16-35 g internally and externally.
Tincture: 2-4 ml
Caution: Contraindicated during pregnancy because of some *uterine stimulant* effect.

Aconitum Chuan Wu

Prepared Sichuan Aconite Root Tuber

川乌

Botanical source: *Aconitum carmichaeli* Debeaux (Ranunculaceae)
Chinese names: Chuan Wu, Wu Tou (Mand); Chyun Wu, Wu Toi (Cant)
Part used: the processed one year old primary root tuber
Category: medium-strength remedy with chronic toxicity
Constituents: alkaloids (incl. aconitine, hypaconitine, mesaconitine, talatisamine)
Effective qualities: pungent, hot, dry; calming, stimulating
Tropism: nervous, muscular, cardiovascular, digestive systems; Spleen, Liver, Heart channels

ACTIONS: *Analgesic, anti-inflammatory, anesthetic*
INDICATIONS: Rheumatic and arthritic pain (wind damp cold syndrome); acute abdominal and chest pain, hemiplgia, vascular headache (incl. migraine).
Dosage: Decoction: 2-8 g
Tincture: 0.5-2 ml
The tincture is also used as a local surgical *anesthetic.*
Caution: Do not overdose or use over one week at a time. Forbidden during pregnancy and in Yin deficiency conditions with false cold and true heat.
NOTES: Although toxic in its crude state, this root when properly processed has very low toxicity. Chuan Wu and Cao Wu (below) are the two types of **Wu Tou** (Aconite root) currently differentiated.

Aconitum Cao Wu

Prepared Wild Aconite Root Tuber

草乌

Botanical source: *Aconitum chinense* Paxton, *A. kusnezoffii* Reichenbach, *A. delavayi* Franchet, *A. japonicum* Thunberg, *A. triphyllum* Nai. (Ranunculaceae)
Chinese names: Cao Wu, Bei Wu Tou (M); Chou Wu (C)
Part used: the processed one year old primary root tuber
Category: mild remedy with minimal chronic toxicity
Constituents: alkaloids (incl. aconitine)
Effective qual.: pungent, hot, dry; calming, stimulating
Tropism: nervous, musculoskeletal, digestive, cardiovascular systems; Spleen, Kidney channels

ACTIONS: *Analgesic, anti-inflammatory, detoxicant, anesthetic*
INDICATIONS: Rheumatic and arthritic pain (wind damp cold syndrome), lower back and leg pain, neuralgia, paralysis of stroke; boils, furunculosis, deep-rooted ulcers at early stage.
Dosage: Decoction: 2-8 g
Tincture: 0.5-2 ml
The tincture is also used for local anesthesia.
Caution: Do not overdose. Prepared wild aconite root is forbidden during pregnancy and in Yin deficiency conditions.

Sinomenium Qing Feng Teng

Sinomenium Root

青风藤

Botanical source: *Sinomenium acutum* Rehder et Wilson (Menispermaceae)
Chinese names: Qing Feng Teng, Qing Teng, Fang Ji (Mand); Ching Fung Tang (Cant)
Habit: Deciduous vine from Central China, growing in hills and sparse forests among shrub thickets; blooms in summer with small, pale green flower panicles.
Category: mild remedy with minimal chronic toxicity
Constituents: alkaloids (incl. acutimine, disinomenine, diversine, convulsine, paralysine, sinactine, tuduranine)
Effective qualities: bitter, pungent, cold, dry; calming, relaxing, decongesting
Tropism: nervous, musculoskeletal, urinary systems; Bladder, Liver channels

ACTIONS: *Analgesic, muscle-relaxant, draining diuretic*
INDICATIONS: Arthritis, rheumatoid myalgia, lumbar pain; wind/damp/cold syndrome; water retention; beriberi.
Dosage: Decoction: 10-16 g
Tincture: 2-4 ml
Caution: None.

Citrus Ju He
Tangerine Seed

橘核

Botanical source: *Citrus reticulata* Blanco (Rutaceae)
Chinese names: Ju He (Mand); Gwat Hat (Cant)
Category: mild remedy with minimal chronic toxicity
Constituents: essential oil (incl. limonene), obakulactone, nomilin, lipids, protein
Effective qualities: bitter, neutral; relaxing, calming
Tropism: nervous, digestive, reproductive systems; Liver, Kidney channels

ACTIONS: *Analgesic, spamolytic, detumescent*
INDICATIONS: Gastric, abdominal, joint, muscle, lower back and testicle pain; testicle swelling, hernia, mastitis.
Dosage: Decoction: 3-10 g
Tincture: 1-3 ml
Caution: Forbidden in Qi deficiency conditions.

REMEDIES TO SEDATE THE NERVES, REDUCE FEVER AND STOP SPASMS

➤ QUELL FIRE, EXTINGUISH WIND AND CALM THE SPIRIT

Depressant antipyretics and spasmolytics

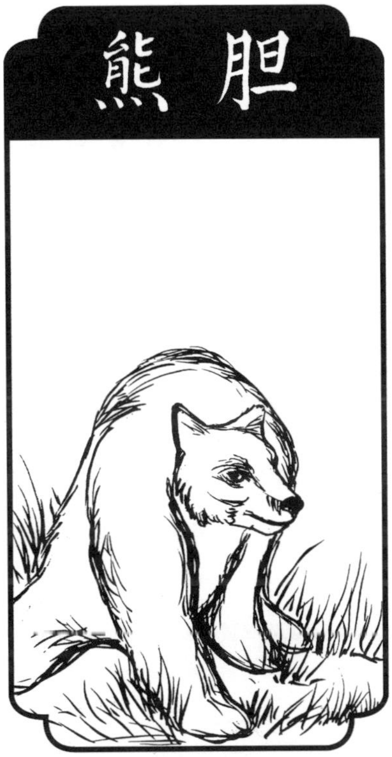

Ursus Xiong Dan

Bear Gallbladder

Zoological source: *Ursus arctos* L. and *Selenarctos thibetanus* G. Cuvier (Ursidae)
Pharmaceutical name: Fel Ursi
Chinese names: Xiong Dan (Mand); Hung Daam (Cant)
Other names: Yutan (Jap)
Part used: the dried gallbladder with bile

Therapeutic category: mild remedy with minimal chronic toxicity
Constituents: bile (incl. ursodeoxycholic/chenodeoxycholic/cholic/deoxycholic/tauroursodesoxy acids), cholesterol, taurine, bilirubin, trace elements
Effective qualities: bitter, salty, cold
calming, sinking, relaxing, stimulating, dissolving
Tropism: nervous, hepatobiliary, digestive, respiratory systems
Gallbladder, Liver, Heart, Spleen, Stomach channels
Warmth, Air bodies

Actions and Indications

nervous sedative/relaxant: spasmolytic, anticonvulsant: spasmodic nervous hyperfunctioning with pain, agitation, spasms; delirium from fever or burns; febrile and infantile seizures, intestinal colic; encephalitis, meningitis, rheumatic fever, tetany
antipyretic: high fever (incl. epidemic fevers), heatstroke
anti-inflammatory: acute infections (incl. cholelithiasis, cholangitis, hepatitis, conjunctivitis, pharyngitis, optic neuritis, dermatitis)
choleretic, cholagogue, cholelitholytic, anti-bacterial: acute biliary tract infection, acute jaundice, acute gallstone attack
bronchodilator, antitussive: asthma with paroxysmal cough, whooping cough
hypotensive: renal hypertension
detumescent, analgesic, detoxicant: trauma with swelling, boils, sprains, fractures, hemorrhoids
optitropic: corneal nebula, corneal opacity
antiallergic
Miscellaneous: coma due to hepatitis or trauma; strychnine poisoning; sequelae of infantile nephritis

Symptom Pictures

Qi constraint with **nerve excess** and **internal wind (Liver Yang rising** and **Liver Fire):** irritability, sleep loss, fever, red swollen eyes, painful spasms, convulsions

gallbladder fire: sharp right subcostal pain, vomiting, jaundice, dizziness, bitter mouth taste, feverishness, unrest

lung Qi constraint: severe wheezing, coughing, chest constriction

Preparation

Use: The gallbladder Ursus Xiong Dan is decocted or used in capsules or pills; the latter are particularly useful for avoiding the remedy's fishy taste, which may cause nausea and vomiting. Externally, compresses, ointments, etc., are often prepared.

Dosage: Decoction, capsule, pill: 1.5-3 g

Caution: Caution during pregnancy and in liver diease. Avoid combining with Rehmannia Sheng Di Huang and Aristolochia Guang Fang Ji.

Notes

Bear gallbladder with its content in dried bile is classified and graded into three types and qualities, according to their color: translucent amber, yellowish green and dark brown or dark green—the first being the top grade.

This bitter, salty and cold natured remedy has a long history of reliable use in Asia for treating fever and convulsions. The overall neurological profile of Bear gallbladder is *sedative* and *relaxant,* with outstanding *anti-inflammatory* effects. Today these actions are especially applied for treating or preventing gallstone attacks, as its acids content actually dissolves gallstones.

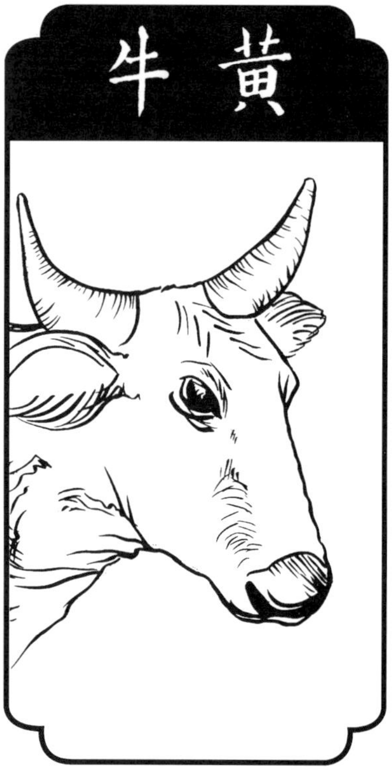

Bos Niu Huang

Ox Gallstone

Zoological source: *Bos taurus domesticus* Gmelin and *Bubalis bubalis* L. (Bovidae)
Pharmaceutical name: Calculus Bovis
Chinese names: Niu Huang (Mand); Ngau Wong (Cant)
Other names: Ox/cow bezoar; *B. bub*.: Water buffalo gallstone; "Cattle yellow"
Part used: the gallstone with dried bile, or the composite artificial product

---

Therapeutic category: mild remedy with minimal chronic toxicity
Constituents: bilirubin 10-15%, bile (incl. cholic/deoxycholic/chenodeoxycholic/lithocholic acids), cholesterol, ergosterol, carotenoid, acidic peptides (SMC), amino acids, sodium, potassium, calcium, magnesium, iron, copper, zinc, phosphorus
Effective qualities: sweet, a bit bitter, cool
calming, sinking, sedating, relaxing, stimulating, dissolving
Tropism: nervous, cardiovascular, digestive, muscular systems
Heart, Liver channels
Air, Warmth bodies

Actions and Indications

nervous sedative/relaxant: spasmolytic, anticonvulsant: spasmodic nervous hyperfunctioning with agitation and spasms; delirium from fever or burns; febrile and infantile seizures; epilepsy, tetany, lockjaw
hypotensive: renal hypertension
central nervous stimulant: febrile coma, heatstroke
digestive stimulant: choleretic, cholagogue, enzymatic digestant, laxative: biliary and pancreatic dyspepsia, poor fat digestion, jaundice, constipation
stimulant expectorant, antiasthmatic: chronic bronchitis, bronchial asthma
cholelitholytic: cholecystitis, gallstones (cholelithiasis)

antipyretic, antiviral, antibacterial, phagocyte stimulant: high fever, encephalitis, whooping cough, infections in general
anti-inflammatory, detoxicant, detumescent: acute infections (incl. pharyngitis, laryngitis, stomatitis, otitis media, tonsilitis, conjunctivitis, cholangitis, purulent skin inflammations), boils, furunculosis, deep-rooted ulcers
antiallergic: food allergies (esp. clam)
hemogenic: low red blood cell count; anemia

Symptom Pictures

Qi constraint with **nerve excess** and **internal wind (Liver Yang rising):** irritability, sleep loss, fever, allergies, painful spasms

gallbladder and stomach Qi stagnation: slow, painful digestion, epigastric discomfort and distension, constipation

lung Qi constraint: spasmodic coughing, wheezing, irritability

Preparation

Use: Preparations of Bos Niu Huang are usually based on the powdered gallstone.
Dosage: Powder, pill or decoction: 0.15-0.5 g
Caution: Contraindicated during pregnancy, in phlegm cold conditions and in digestive deficiency with cold.

Notes

In Chinese, Ayurvedic and Greek traditional medical systems, the bezoar, a mineral concretion found in the fourth stomach of various ruminant animals, was possibly the most highly prized animal remedy of all. Ancient Pan-Asian trade routes such as the Silk Road routinely saw bezoars from Shandong province on China's northeast coast reach Persia, Bagdhad and, later, even Venice. From there they were distributed to many a court or up-scale town pharmacy throughout Europe for use in traditional Greek medicine. The lucky apothecaries could pride themselves on having obtained an extraordinary remedy for nervous and digestive disorders—extraordinary because of its distant source, its rarity value and its manifest effectiveness.

Most bezoars used in traditional times, however (and certainly those used today), are actually gallstones from the gallbladders of oxen, cattle and water buffaloes, as the name Niu Huang, "ox yellow," attests. Today, the pharmacology of the bile acids, bilirubin, trace minerals, and so on, that comprise the gallstones of these and other ruminants is well researched, making traditional experience more precise. Chinese medicine currently defines three types of Ox gallstone: the yellow (highest in cholic acids), the dark brown (highest in bilirubin) and the brown (with moderate amounts of cholic acids and bilirubin).

The overall character of Ox gallstone is both *draining* and *stimulating,* sharing some properties with Bear gallbladder and Musk. Sweet-bitter and cooling by nature, the remedy's *draining* effect is evident in its *central nervous sedative, antipyretic* and *anti-inflammatory* actions. These actions are put to use for constrained Qi and febrile (hot) conditions that lead to internal wind, i.e., spasms and convulsions. The *stimulating* effect of Ox gallstone, on the other hand, notably affects the central nerves, exocrine pancreas, gallbladder and bronchi. The comprehensive *digestive stimulant* action is especially used to treat digestive conditions entailing enzymatic and biliary insufficiency, notably with loss of fat breakdown and food allergies present. Ox gallstone thereby possesses a good preventive effect in the formation of gallstones. Moreover, like Bear gallbladder, it also possesses a direct *dissolving* effect on these. A wide variety of combining possibilities clearly exists with this remedy.

For cost reasons, an artificial remedy is also prepared from the bile acids of cattle, sheep and pigs. Here the bile acids are combined with cholesterol, bilirubin, inorganic salts (magnesium sulfate, ferrous sulfate, calcium phosphate) and starch. The effect of this **composite gallstone** has shown to be completely comparable to that of the natural ox or cattle gallstone.

羚羊角

Saiga Ling Yang Jiao

Antelope Horn

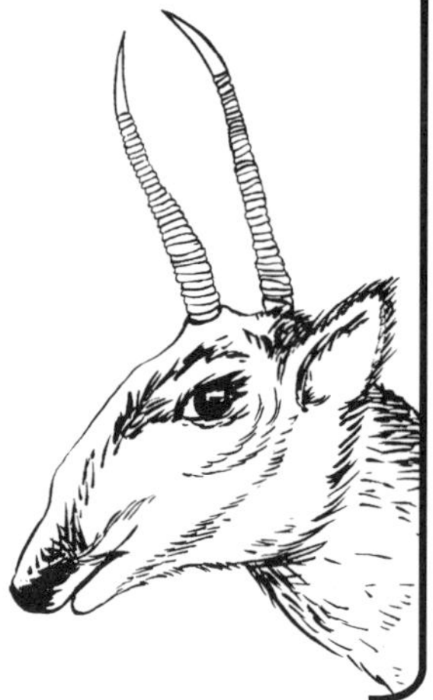

Zoological source: *Saiga tatarica* L. (Bovidae)
Pharmaceutical name: Cornu Saigae
Chinese names: Ling Yang Jiao (Mand); Ling Yeung Gok (Cant)
Other names: Japanese serow, Goat antelope; Reiyokaku (Jap)
Habitat: Gansu, Inner Mongolia, Northeast China, Sichuan
Part used: the horn

Therapeutic category: mild remedy with minimal chronic toxicity
Constituents: keratin, calcium tetraphosphate, inorganic salts, vitamin A
Effective qualities: salty, cold
relaxing, calming, sinking
Tropism: nervous, cardiovascular, hepatic systems
Liver, Heart, Pericardium channels
Air, Warmth bodies

Actions and Indications

nervous sedative/relaxant: spasmolytic, anticonvulsant, hypnotic: nervous hyperfunctioning with spasms, seizures (incl. due to fever, heat syndrome); delirium, mania, vertigo, coma; hypocalcemia, epilepsy, tetany, encephalitis, meningitis, rheumatic fever, colic
antipyretic: high fever, heatstroke
anti-inflammatory, analgesic: acute conjunctivitis, headache, corneal opacity, photophobia
hypotensive
oxygen metabolism inhibitor

Symptom Pictures

nerve excess with **internal wind (wind phlegm obstruction):** dizziness, headache, blurred vision, spasms

Pericardium fire with **nerve excess:** fever, manic behavior, delirium, fainting

Preparation

Use: The horn Saiga Ling Yang Jiao is used mainly in powder form, occasionally in decoction
Dosage: Powder and pill: 1-4 g
Decoction: 1-5 g. Decoct separately and strain in a coffee filter before adding to another decoction.
Caution: None.

Notes

The calcium-rich Antelope horn is the remedy of choice when an average strength, general-use *nervous sedative* and *heat-clearing* remedy is required.

In addition to the above uses, Antelope horn in the past was also deemed useful in dysentery, erysipelas, postpartum infection and depression. Continual use was said to strengthen the bones and muscles, and increase male potency.

Goat horn, Shan Yang Jiao (Mand.), **San Yeung Gok** (Cant.) and **Ram horn, Gu Yang Jiao** (Mand.), **Gung Yeung Gok** (Cant.) are often used as a less expensive substitue for Antelope horn. They are similar but less effective than Antelope horn. 10-18 g of the powdered horn is cooked separately for about 30 minutes and then added to another herb decoction if needed.

水牛角

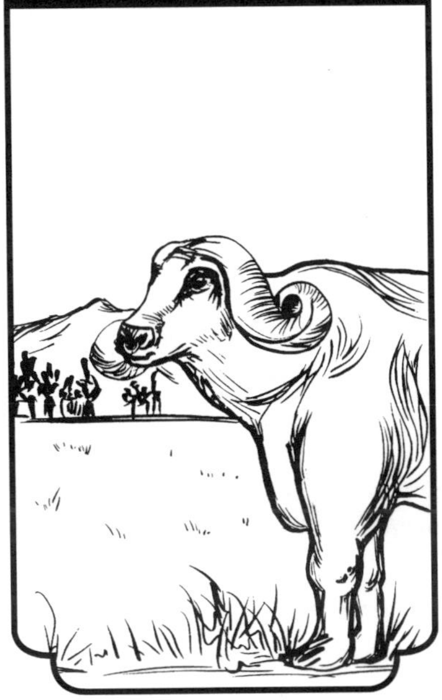

Bubalus Shui Niu Jiao

Water Buffalo Horn

Zoological source: *Bubalus bubalis* L. (Bovidae)
Pharmaceutical name: Cornu Bubali
Chinese names: Shui Niu Jiao (Mand); Seui Ngau Gok (Cant)
Other names: Suigyu No Tsuno (Jap)
Habitat: Southeast China, Southeast Asia
Part used: the horn

Therapeutic category: mild remedy with minimal chronic toxicity
Constituents: cholesterol, amino acids (incl. alanine, arginine, aspartic acid, cystine, proline, tyrosine, histidine, valine), guanidine derivatives, keratin
Effective qualities: bitter, salty, cold
calming, sinking, relaxing, astringing
Tropism: nervous, cardiovascular systems
Liver, Heart, Yin Qiao channels
Air, Warmth bodies

Actions and Indications

central nervous sedative/relaxant: analgesic, spasmolytic, anticonvulsant: nervous hyperfunctioning with pain, agitation, spasms; seizures, headache, coma, tetany, heat exhaustion, hypocalcemia
antipyretic (mild): high fever, heatstroke
anti-inflammatory, phacocyte stimulant: acute pharyngitis, laryngitis with pain
hemostatic: hemorrhage, vomiting blood, nosebleed, purpura
pituitary-adrenal stimulant

Symptom Pictures

Blood and Nutritive level heat: agitation, insomnia, fever, bleeding, coma, skin rashes, bleeding from upper orifices
nerve excess with **Heart (phlegm) fire:** fever, agitation, delirium, spasms, convulsions

Preparation

Use: The horn Bubalus Shui Niu Jiao is decocted or used in powder form.
Dosage: Decoction: 30-90 g
Powder: 4-20 g
Caution: Only to be used in excess conditions. Use with caution during pregnancy. Contraindicated in skin rashes without high fever present.

Notes

With its bitter, salty, cold qualities, Water buffalo horn treats both excess heart spirit conditions such as Heart fire, and febrile spasmodic conditions (with or without active bleeding). The remedy's excellent *anti-inflammatory* effects, most likely due to a *stimulating* action on the pituitary-adrenocortical system, are frequently used for acute throat infections with severe pain.

Other bovine horns are also similarly used under the standard remedy name Shui Niu Jiao.

Rhinoceros horn, Xi Jiao, should no longer be used for these conditions, as it is derived from a currently endangered species. This remedy has the same functions and uses as Water buffalo horn, except that it is not a *pituitary-adrenal stimulant* and is only mildly *anti-inflammatory*. Its *antipyretic* and *nervous relaxant* effects are considered stronger, however.

Gypsum Shi Gao

Gypsum

石膏

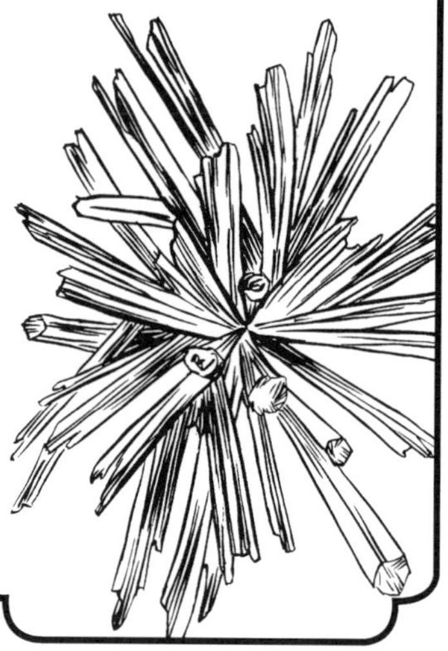

Geological source: *Gypsum*
Pharmaceutical name: Gypsum fibrosum
Chinese names: Shi Gao (Mand); Sek Gou (Cant)
Other names: Native calcium sulphate, selenite, alabaster; Sekko (Jap)
Source: The hard white mineral is mined primarily in the eastern provinces Shandong, Henan, Anhui and Hubei.
Part used: the mineral

Therapeutic category: mild remedy with minimal chronic toxicity
Constituents: calcium sulfate dehydrate (with 32.5% calcium dioxide); contaminants clay, sand, organic and sulfur compounds (sulfur dioxide 46.6%); traces of iron and magnesium, usnic acid, 20.9% water
Effective qualities: sweet, pungent, very cold
calming, astringing, sinking
Tropism: nervous, respiratory, digestive systems
Lung, Stomach channels
Warmth, Air bodies

Actions and Indications

nervous sedative/relaxant: spasmolytic, anticonvulsant: nervous hyperfunctioning with spasms; delirium, seizures (incl. from fever, heat syndrome, hypocalcemia)
analgesic: headache, acute toothache, osteitis deformans , osteoarthritis with pain, stiffness; osteomyelitis
antipyretic, anti-inflammatory: high fever, heatstroke; burns, scalds, gingivitis, pyogenic inflammations
secretory: dry throat, thirst
antitussive: chronic coughing, wheezing; asthma
vulnerary, dermatropic: wounds, ulcerated sores, eczema, burns, abscesses

Symptom Pictures

Yang Ming stage/Qi level heat: high fever without chills, heavy sweating, thirst, irritability, agitation

lung heat: thirst, dehydration, coughing, wheezing

stomach fire: headache, swollen or painful gums, toothache

Preparation

Use: The mineral Gypsum Shi Gao is decocted. It should be broken up and cooked alone for 20-30 minutes before any other herbs are added. When powdered and calcined (and usually mixed with other herb powders), it is used topically for sores, ulcers, burns, etc. The calcined remedy is called **Duan Shi Gao.**
Dosage: Decoction: 10-30 g. Up to 90 g may be decocted for spiking/dangerous high fever (up to 30 g in children).
Caution: Contraindicated in Yang deficiency syndromes, with a weak stomach and when the pulse is very weak.

Notes

The mineral Gypsum is a *nervous sedative* with good *analgesic* effects. Because it is also very cooling, however, in clinical practice the remedy is used primarily for treating high fever and heatstroke with nervous excess. Chinese researchers attribute Gypsum's powerful *antipyretic* action to its secondary constituents, not the calcium sulfate itself. More likely, it is the synergy of all its constituents together that create this action.

Gypsum's success in the treatment of osteoarthritis, osteitis and other metabolic skeletal disorders that present pain and stiffness is said to lie mainly in its sulfur and magnesium content.

Pheretima Di Long

Earthworm

地龙

Zoological source: *Pheretima aspergillum* E. Perrier (Megascolecidae) and *Allolobophora caliginosa* (Savigny) *trapezoides* Ant. Deges (Lumbricidae)
Chinese names: Di Long, Di Long Gan, Guang Di Long, Qiu Yin (Mand); Dei Lung (Cant)
Other names: Jiryu (Jap)
Part used: the whole animal
Category: mild remedy with minimal chronic toxicity
Constituents: lumbrofebrine, lumbritin, hypoxanthine, adenine, terrestrolumbrylysin, xanthine, guanine, guanidine, choline, amino acids (histidine, arginine, lysine, valine, alanine), enzyme
Effective qualities: salty, cold; relaxing, decongesting, sinking
Tropism: nervous, musculoskeletal, respiratory, cardiovascular, urinary systems; Liver, Spleen, Lung, Kidney channels

ACTIONS: *Spasmolytic, anticonvulsant, antipyretic, muscular relaxant, bronchial relaxant, hypotensive, vasodilatant, anti-inflammatory, diuretic, antiseptic, hemolytic, anticoagulant, vulnerary* (topical)
INDICATIONS: Spasmodic nervous hyperfunctioning with spasms, seizures (esp. in febrile disease or heat syndromes), Qi level heat with internal wind syndrome; hemiplegia from stroke, epilepsy, tetany, meningitis, encephalitis, high fever, heatstroke; painful/stiff/numb extremities from arthritis or stroke; chronic bronchitis, bronchial asthma, whooping cough; hypertension, vascular headache, cerebral thrombosis; acute conjunctivitis, pharyngitis, tracheitis; peptic ulcer, chronic prostatitis; urinary infections, strangury, dysuria, jaundice, edema, leg ulcers, eczema, burns, erysipelas, filariasis.
Dosage: Decoction: 4-14 g
Caution: Forbidden in hypertension or shock.
NOTES: Earthworm is essentially a *relaxant* remedy with *heat-clearing* properties that act on the temperature regulating center. As such, it is best adapted for spasmodic febrile and inflammatory conditions of the musculature or bronchi—such as one finds in asthma, for example. Lumbrofebrine and other constituents have long demonstrated *antipyretic* and *bronchodilatant* activity in Japanese research.

Traditional Greek medicine also made use of Earthworm for the majority of above complaints. The remedy enjoyed a great reputation for treating the respiratory conditions listed.

Naja She Dan

Viper Gallbladder

蛇胆

Zoological source: *Naja naja atra* and *Bungarus fasciatus* and *Elaphe radiata* and spp. (Viperidae)
Chinese names: She Dan (Mand); Se Daam (Cant)
Category: medium-strength remedy with chronic toxicity
Constituents: bile acids, cholesterol, trace minerals
Effective qualities: sweet, bitter, cold relaxing
Tropism: nervous, respiratory, digestive systems; Liver, Spleen channels

ACTIONS: *Spasmolytic, anticonvulsant, analgesic, antipyretic, hemostatic, antiseptic, anthelmintic*
INDICATIONS: High fever in children, infantile seizures, hemiplegia due to stroke; heatstroke; whooping cough, rheumatic pain, diarrhea, bloody dysentery, abdominal pain, eye pain, blurred vision, hemorrhoids, gum bleeding, toothache; skin infections (incl. acne), conjunctivitis, pinkeye; intestinal parasites.
Dosage: Decoction: 1-3 g
Caution: None.
NOTES: The best remedy is the gallbladder collected in spring and summer. Over 15 species of snake furnish this remedy, but the three viper species listed are considered highest in quality.

Phyllostachys Tian Zhu Huang
Tabasheer

天竹黄

Botanical source: *Phyllostachys nigra* Munro var. *henonis* Stapf, *P. reticulata* K.Koch, *Bambusa textilis* McClure, *Indosasa crassiflora* McClure (Gramineae)
Chinese and other names: Tian Zhu Huang (Mand); Ting Juk Wong (Cant); "Heavenly bamboo yellow"
Part used: the hardened siliceous secretion found within the joints of bamboo

Category: mild remedy with minimal chronic toxicity
Constituents: silicon 70-90%, potassium hydroxide 1%, potassium/aluminum/ferric oxides, crystals (incl. mannitol, stearic acid, hypocrellines)
Effective qualities: sweet, cold; calming, relaxing
Tropism: nervous, cardiovascular, respiratory systems; Liver, Lung, Heart, Triple Warmer channels

Actions: *Spasmolytic, anticonvulsant, antipyretic, hypotensive, expectorant*
Indications: Spasms, febrile and infantile seizures, stroke from hypertension; acute bronchitis with difficult expectoration and dry cough in lung phlegm heat syndromes.
Dosage: Decoction: 3-10 g
Powder: 0.7-1 g
Tincture: 1-3 ml
Caution: None.
Notes: The bamboo concretion Tabasheer is used in Chinese, Malaysian, Indian and Greek medicine alike.

Sus Zhu Dan
Pig Gallbladder

猪胆

Zoological source: *Sus scrofa domestica*
Chinese names: Zhu Dan (Mand); Ju Daam (Cant)

Category: mild remedy with minimal chronic toxicity

Notes: This remedy possesses the same nature, functions and uses as Ursus Xiong Dan, Bear gallbladder (see above). However, it is not *cholagogue* and *hypotensive* in action, and therefore cannot treat indigestion from biliary deficiency, and hypertension.

梅地落

内分泌及免疫系统用药

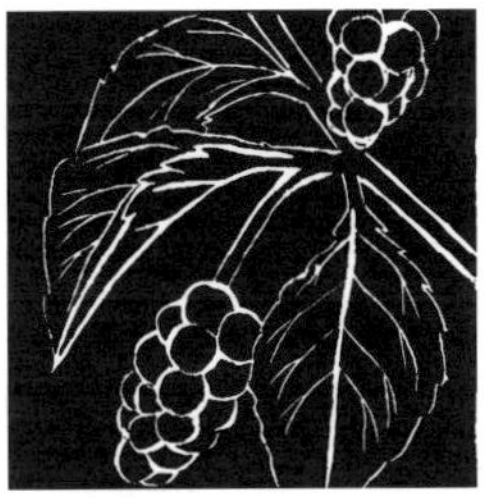

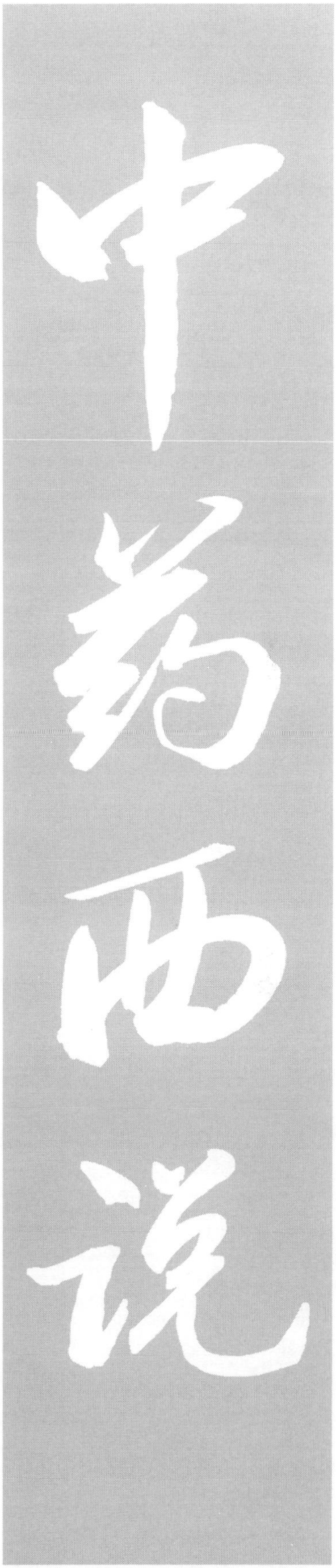

Remedies for the Endocrine and Immune Systems

In Asian medicine there is a class of remedies that promote greater vitality, disease resistance and longer life. China's oldest herbal, the Shennong Ben Cao, classifies them as "imperial remedies," as they have the safest, most beneficial, most profound and longest-lasting effects known. These superior herbs have been used for millenniums by all who could afford them. To this day, the common person in the Far East takes for granted the powerful yet subtle life-enhancing effects of remedies such as Asian ginseng root, Wolfberry, Deer antler, Astragalus root and Reishi mushroom. They are an inextricable part of the culture, as commonplace as rice and silk. Disease prevention and health maintenance with these *tonics* is, in fact, big business in Asia.

Today, most of these imperial remedies are known to act on the endocrine and immune systems, through which they unfold a hidden yet all-pervasive influence on the whole human organism. Although *tonics* of this kind are found throughout this materia medica, several have such a comprehensive effect on endocrine and immune functions that they require a special category to themselves. This is made especially so considering that their *restoring* and *regulating* actions on endocrine and immune functions is interwoven with a further effect: that of enhancing individual adaptation to stress.

Because of the nature of today's primary health needs—chronic deficiency conditions involving stress, fatigue, compromised immunity and viral infections—the remedies in this section have become increasingly important in the clinic and increasingly popular with the public. They play a growing role in both curative herbal medicine and preventive natural health care methods. The use of these herbs has spread to nearly every corner of the globe in a large variety of forms, ranging from the crude plant to such processed and packaged products as syrups, tablets, capsules and various liquid extracts.

The Endocrine and Immune Remedies

Remedies in this section are known as *endocrine restoratives, immune enhancers* and *adaptogens* because their essential effect on the system is to strengthen the endocrine glands, balance hormonal secretions, enhance or potentiate immune functions and generally improve the individual's adaptation response to stress (*adaptogenic* simply means "adaptation-generating"). Most of them also include *restorative* and *balancing* actions on the nervous system (including the brain), an integral complement to the endocrine system. These remedies then act to either enhance vitality and resistance, improve energy or reduce the negative effects of chronic and unproductive stress on the individual. For this reason, they have also been called "harmony remedies" (Fulder 1982), as the concept of harmony—on both a physiological and ontological level—is central to achieving greater vitality and longevity.

Oriental practitioners traditionally classify these super-remedies as *Qi tonics, Yang tonics, Blood tonics* and *Essence tonics,* and employ them for "increasing the righteous energies in order to dispel the depraved energies" (*fu zhen qu xie*) and for "generating the pulse" (*sheng mai*). This points to their primary use as preventive and maintenance remedies rather than curative ones, designed to treat deficiency, not excess, and chronic rather than acute conditions. *Adaptogenic endocrine* and *immune restoratives* are the remedies of choice for conditions involving long-term stress, recurrent infections, chronic disease, slow recovery from sickness, postpartum exhaustion and trauma (including postoperative and emotional), especially when accompanied by low vitality and endurance. These remedies are routinely used in both the East and the West in formulations for chronic fatigue and weakness (whether from internal deficiency or viral disease), cancer, weight loss, appetite loss, sexual disinterest, impotence, blood pressure disorders and allergic/hypersensitivity disorders. Because a weak, fine or deep pulse is typical of such chronic deficiency conditions, these *restoratives* implement the treatment method known as "generating the pulse."

The Endocrine Aspect

The endocrine functions restored by these herbs include those of the pituitary, adrenals, thyroid, pancreas and gonads. It is likely, although not yet scientifically confirmed, that some of these *endocrine restoratives* operate directly on the main controlling gland of the lower brain itself, the hypothalamus. In any case, the majority of them not only strengthen, but also regulate these glands. They are actually able to rebalance glandular functions and their hormonal secretions, regardless of whether these are deficient or stressed. Eleutherococcus Ci Wu Jia (Eleuthero ginseng root) is an outstanding case in point. It regulates thyroid, adrenal and pancreatic functions, and can be used in deficiency or stress conditions of these glands. Likewise, it has proven to normalize the cerebral circulation in cases of either constricted or inadequate blood supply, as well as to balance blood pressure, low or high. It is by harmonizing metabolic functions to regain internal balance that *endocrine restoratives* obtain the polyvalent healing effects that we call *adaptogenic*.

Endocrine restoratives can best be described as having a triggering action on the system. The axiom that herbs operate in conjunction with the human life force, or Qi, is here clearly exemplified. These remedies—like other organic medicinals belonging to the mild and medium-strength therapeutic category—act like "spark plugs" for glandular functions. Essentially, the herb gives the body a certain amount of information, and the body's life force utilizes it according to the requirements of a particular condition at any given time. Synthetic drugs, however, exert a direct, linear, controlling effect on target glands and their secretions (hence the epithet "magic bullets"). The herbs in this section inform and suggest rather than directing and controlling, and the body responds spontaneously according to need. Moreover, the remedy informs the whole system rather than merely one or several of its parts, which is why *adaptogens* in particular address the most influential and all-pervasive system of all, the endocrine system. These are important criteria for us in understanding the nature and dynamics of these *adaptogenic* remedies.

The Adaptogenic Aspect

As noted above, the *adaptogenic* action of remedies in this section is interwoven with their *restorative* action on hormonal and neural functions. With their deep, cumulative *normalizing* action on endocrine, nervous and metabolic processes, *adaptogens* increase the individual's capacity to cope with and adapt to systemic and localized stress. Consequently, they liberate more life energy for the individual.

Stress is a part of life, and individuals normally are able to respond to stress in an attempt to regain a state of internal balance. When the individual cannot meet stress with an intrinsic vital response, however, damaging effects ensue. Any internal deficiency—whether physiological, affective or mental—can make stress overwhelming, life-eroding and energy-sapping. It exhausts adaptation energy by calling on glandular and nervous reserves. In this case, however, the available energy for adaptation gradually becomes depleted as the individual unsuccessfully strives for homeostatis. The person literally becomes "stressed-out."

The individual's energy potential for adaptation is determined by genetics (Selye 1976). Because adaptation energy is finite and cannot be increased, it should not be drawn upon excessively nor squandered. However, the rate at which it is used up—for used up it must be—can itself be controlled. And the key to slowing down the consumption of adaptive energy lies in improving the quality of our adaptation to stress.

Because *adaptogens* make extreme or continual stress less damaging to the whole system, thereby tending to conserve the expenditure of finitely available adaptive energy, they can also be qualified as *rejuvenative* and *aging-retardant*. They enhance and prolong human life.

Interestingly, although the energy potential for adaptation has not yet been successfully defined, let alone quantified, the Oriental physiological concept of *yuan Qi*, "source/original energy," corresponds to it very exactly. The question then arises whether *adaptogenic* remedies are seen in Oriental medicine to enhance, protect or somehow boost the *yuan Qi*. The answer is a definite "yes." Asian ginseng, for example, is described as "greatly increasing the Original Qi." Moreover, the majority of Oriental *adaptogens* are said in Chinese texts to tonify the Yang, the Qi, the Blood and the Essence—an extremely wide area of application. Through circumstantial evidence, this again points to *adaptogenic* effects, because the balance-promoting *adaptogens* are uniquely able to treat a wide variety of conditions and symptoms, sometimes opposing conditions. It is their hallmark.

It may well seem that the remedies in this section are "cure-alls"; the endless list of their actions and indications seems to include most of the known ills of humankind. However, there is a reason for this. The reason, as already touched on, lies in an ability that *adaptogens* alone possess: that of *regulating* or *normalizing* physiological functions under stress. In Western terms, this is the fundamental property that defines a remedy as *adaptogenic*. All remedies in this section, without exception, fit this definition. As Fulder (1982) states:

> Drugs which locate their action in the middle of the flux of hormones would easily have the range of powers the Chinese claim for them. They would be effective during the course of multitudes of diseases, for diseases appear only halfway through a play in which disharmonies hold the stage for the first act. They would be precious, for restoration of inner homeostasis is a hard-won goal. Many, many medicines are known to change bits of the body machinery, but there are few indeed that can increase the smooth running of the whole.

Adaptogens are "harmony remedies" in every sense of the word.

The Immune Aspect

When taken daily over a period of time, *adaptogenic endocrine restorative* remedies also exert an *immune-enhancing* effect. By harmoniously restoring the whole system deeply, gently and cumulatively, and by facilitating glandular and neural adaptation responses to stress, they can gradually increase nonspecific resistance to disease and thereby reduce the risk of infection or immune disorders. Their *immune-enhancing* activity can be validated experimentally, especially through *in vivo* statistical trials, as has been done in China with all remedies in this section.

The concept of the ground or terrain can help us understand the relationship of *endocrine restoratives* to immunity. Our outlook on life, thoughts, feelings and actions, the integrity of our endocrine and nervous systems, the intestinal flora and metabolism—these all constitute our individual ground. It is the internal harmony and vigor of our ground that determines the integrity of the immune system, that is, its resistance to the microbe's ability to infect us. Being essentially opportunistic, pathogens cannot thrive in a healthy ground. Because *adaptogenic endocrine restoratives* build up our ground on endocrine/nervous/humoral foundations, they are therefore necessarily *immune enhancers* as well.

What are the physiological dynamics of *immune enhancers?* Backed by millenniums of traditional common wisdom, the budding science of psychoneuroimmunology is increasingly able to demonstrate those inseparable links between an individual's outlook on life, and endocrine, nervous and immune functions. The health and integrity of one set of functions will directly affect the other. This fact is confirmed daily when individuals are able to rise above and overcome serious disabling or chronic diseases such as AIDS, cancer and chronic fatigue syndrome. Informed at a template level by the individual's basic life attitude, hormonal neurotransmitters travel to every cell to affect immune functions, while immunotransmitters, conversely, affect nerve functions. The endocrine, central nervous and immune systems have close three-way connections mediated by numerous feedback mechanisms—many of them not yet clearly understood—which directly affect humoral and cellular immunity. In short, *endocrine restoratives,* most of which are also *nervous restoratives,* exert a sufficiently global and long-lasting action on the whole system, thereby building up immune functions on a long-term basis. The result is increased vitality, improved resistance to infection and speedier recovery when infection does occur.

Immune enhancement is not to be confused with immune stimulation. While immune enhancement denotes a gradual, cumulative, deep-level tonification of nonspecific resistance, immune stimulation refers to an immediate, short-lived stimulation of defense activities—such as lymphocyte phagocytosis and reticuloendothelial functioning—with no long-term immune potentiation. Clearly, *immune enhancers* should be used in times of relative good health to bolster resistance, and *immune stimulants* in cases of acute infection.

Immune enhancers are also given for chronic infections (never acute ones) of a bacterial, viral or parasitic nature (including the retroviral infections HIV, EBV, CMV and HHV, as well as Lyme's disease). This is because chronic infections can be either dormant and asymptomatic or active and symptomatic, depending on the vitality of the ground. *Immune enhancers* are able to shake off chronic, lingering or reactivated microorganisms by simply boosting the vitality of our hormonal, neural and humoral ground. Some of these botanicals, such as Astragalus Huang Qi (Astragalus root) and Eleutherococcus Ci Wu Jia (Eleuthero ginseng root), act directly on cellular metabolism and its energy-making mechanisms, thereby increasing available energy. Astragalus Huang Qi (Astragalus root), with its content in polysaccharides that have demonstrable *immunity-modulating* effects, is one of several botanicals much used in China and the West for both general immune enhancement and for treating chronic infections.

Three *immune enhancers* in this section definitely display *regulative* rather than simply restorative actions on the immune system. Ganoderma Ling Zhi (Reishi mushroom), Schisandra Wu Wei Zi (Schisandra berry) and Glycyrrhiza Gan Cao (Ural licorice root) are true *bivalent immunomodulators* that will assist immune functions to adjust in both deficiency and stress conditions. Ganoderma Ling Zhi (Reishi mushroom) in particular is used for treating both immune-deficient conditions with poor resistance and resultant infections, and immune-stress conditions with allergies, such as food and drug hypersensitivities, urticaria, atopic dermatitis, allergic rhinitis and allergic asthma. Moreover, this remedy addresses such autoimmune disorders as rheumatoid arthritis, lupus, multiple sclerosis, hemolytic anemia and psoriasis.

Summary of the Remedies' Actions

Eleutherococcus Ci Wu Jia (the root of Eleuthero ginseng, a spiny shrub from Northeast Asia), Panax Ren Shen (the root of Asian ginseng, a mountain plant from Taighur, Northeast China and Korea), Cervus Lu Rong (the young velvet horn of the sika deer from Inner Mongolia and North China) and Homo Zi He Chi (Human placenta) are premier *adaptogenic broad-spectrum endocrine restoratives* and *immune enhancers*. They systemically facilitate improved internal functioning by enhancing stress adaptation: They balance and tonify the majority of hormonal glands and, together with neural functions, core metabolic processes; they thereby also potentiate long-term immune functions.

Eleutherococcus Ci Wu Jia (Eleuthero ginseng root), Panax Ren Shen (Asian ginseng root), Schisandra Wu Wei Zi (Schisandra berry) and Ganoderma Ling Zhi (Reishi mushroom) are *adaptogens* that restore the nervous system in particular.

Astragalus Huang Qi (the root of several milkvetch species from north-central China and Inner Mongolia), Schisandra Wu Wei Zi (the berry of a woody climbing vine from China's temperate woods), Ganoderma Ling Zhi (Reishi mushroom, a polypore from coastal China and North America's Pacific Northwest) and Glycyrrhiza Gan Cao (Ural licorice root from Central and Southwest Asian grasslands) are *adaptogens* that primarily restore the adrenal cortex.

Schisandra Wu Wei Zi (Schisandra berry), Ganoderma Ling Zhi (Reishi mushroom), Panax Ren Shen (Asian ginseng root) and Glycyrrhiza Gan Cao (Ural licorice root) are noted in particular for excellent *immune-regulating* and *antiallergic* effects.

These are the "imperial remedies" of herbal preventive medicine today. It is these harmony remedies, more than any other type, that are able to prevent and treat some of the most prevalent and debilitating of modern disorders. Although for purposes of reducing stress and increasing vitality, harmony remedies are generally applicable, it is still neccessary to use them judiciously, not randomly. All *adaptogens* are not created equally. Likewise, the requirements of individual constitutions in their striving for optimum balance also vary considerably. It is always best to match the remedy's total characteristics with the individual's tendencies to imbalance as much as possible. Ultimately, harmony is the meeting of the right herb taken by the right constitution at the right time.

In general, once an appropriate remedy from this section has been found, it may be taken on a daily basis (with occasional breaks) as well as occasionally. Only Homo Zi He Chi (Human placenta) is not suitable for continuous use, as it possesses slight cumulative toxicity.

TONIFY THE RIGHTEOUS QI AND GENERATE THE PULSE

Endocrine restoratives, adaptogens, immune enhancers

刺五加

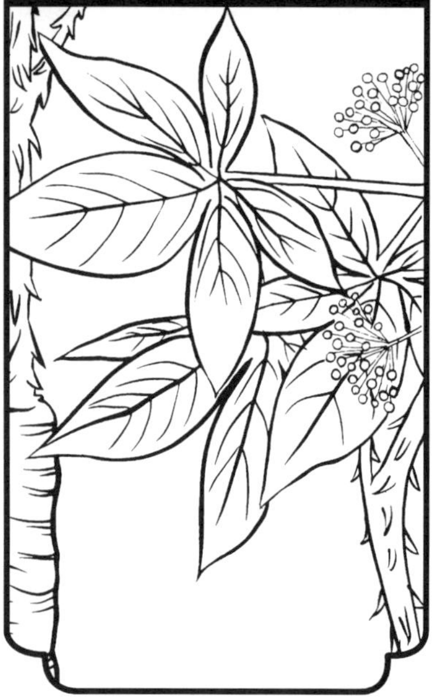

Eleutherococcus Ci Wu Jia

Eleuthero Ginseng Root

Botanical source: *Eleutherococcus senticosus* (Rupr. et Maxim.) Maximowicz, syn. *Acanthopanax senticosus* (Rupr. et Maxim.) Harmslow (Araliaceae)
Pharmaceutical name: Radix seu cortex radicis Eleutherococci senticosi
Chinese names: Ci Wu Jia (Gen Pi), Wu Jia Shen (Mand); Chi Ng Ga (Cant)
Other names: Siberian ginseng, Spiny ginseng, Russian root, Touch-me-not, Devil's bush; "Free-berried shrub"
Habit: Thorny deciduous perennial shrub from Northeast Asia (incl. Russia, China, Mongolia, Korea, Hokkaido); found in humid mountain regions at lower and middle elevations with slightly acidic, fertile alluvial or sandy soil; partial to sunny forest clearings and wood borders where it thrives in thickets and clumps; numerous yellowish white or pale violet terminal or clustered flowers open in June and July; clusters of black oval drupes appear in autumn.
Part used: the root and rhizome or the root bark

Therapeutic category: mild remedy with minimal chronic toxicity
Constituents: phenolic, resin, triterpenoid and oleanic acid glycosides c. 1% (incl. eleutherosides, senticosides); coumarins, lignans, sterols, polysaccharides, essential oil, saponins, isofraxidin, sucrose, glucose, beta-carotene, vitamins C and E, trace minerals (incl. copper)
Effective qualities: a bit pungent, bitter, neutral
restoring, raising, relaxing, calming, dissolving
Tropism: endocrine, nervous, immune, cardiovascular, respiratory, urinary, muskuloskeletal systems
Spleen, Liver, Kidney, Heart, Chong, Yin Wei, Ren, Yin Qiao, Du channels; Warmth, Air, Fluid bodies

Actions and Indications

broad-spectrum endocrine restorative/regulator/protective, adaptogenic: chronic adrenal, thyroid and pancreas insufficiency or excess/stress with chronic fatigue, low vitality, weakness, stamina loss; chronic stress, convalescence, trauma, surgery, hypothyroidism, diabetes, neurasthenia
antioxidant (free radical inhibitor), aging retardant: toxicosis, premature senility
nervous restorative: cerebral/nervous deficiency with insomnia, memory and concentration loss, depression; neurasthenia, sleep disorder
sense enhancer: poor vision and hearing
immune enhancer: low immunity with frequent or chronic infections; immunodeficiency disorders (incl. CFS, AIDS)

metabolic restorative/regulator: pituitary-adrenal stimulant, protein anabolism stimulant: metabolic disorders (incl. glycogen storage disorders, anemia, malabsorption, anorexia, toxicosis); anabolic and catabolic deficiencies with weight loss, stamina loss, debility; altitude sickness
hemogenic: anemia, amenorrhea

pancreas regulator: hypo/hyperglycemiant: hypoglycemia, hyperglycemia
oxygenator: hypoxia
muskuloskeletal restorative: weak or soft sinews and bones, loss of muscular strength, muscular dystrophy, retarded muscular development in children
reproductive restorative: pituitary-gonadal stimulant, androgenic, estrogenic, aphrodisiac: sexual disinterest, impotence, irregular menstruation
neurocardiac sedative: stress, anxiety, unrest, palpitations; anxiety states, neuroses, neurocardiac syndrome
blood pressure regulator: hyper/hypotensive: hypotension, moderate hypertension
coronary and cerebrovascular restorative/regulator, *vasodilator:* coronary deficiency/disease with angina; cerebral ischemia and thrombosis, vascular headaches, dizziness, cerebrovascular injuries, trauma to the head
resolvent detoxicant: metabolic toxicosis with arthritis, gout, myalgia, eczema
circulatory resolvent: antilipemic: hyperlipidemia, atherosclerosis
anti-inflammatory, analgesic: rheumatoid arthritis, rheumatic pain, backache
stimulant diuretic: oliguria, edema (esp. of lower limbs)
stimulant expectorant, antibacterial: chronic bronchitis, coughing, lung TB
immunostimulant anti-infective: infections in general (incl. EBV and HIV infection)
antitumoral, interferon inducent: tumors (incl. cancer)
radiation-protective: radiation damage/sickness (e.g. radiotherapy)

Symptom Pictures

neuroendocrine deficiency (Essence, Blood and Qi deficiency): exhaustion, low vitality and endurance, frequent or chronic infections, depression, dizziness, palpitations, poor sleep

liver, pancreas and adrenal Yin deficiency: loss of energy and stamina, somnolence, fatigue between meals, evening exhaustion, sweet cravings, anxiety, frequent infections, underweight

musculoskeletal deficiency (Liver and Kidney depletion): fatigue, sore back, weak legs and knees, loss of muscular strength

metabolic toxicosis with **wind/damp/cold obstruction:** dry skin, skin rashes, malaise, joint and muscle aches or pain (with or without muscle spasms)

Qi constraint: anxiety, feeling stressed, nervous behaviour, sleep loss

heart Qi constraint (heart Blood deficiency): anxiety, irritability, poor concentration, memory and sense perception, palpitations

Preparation

Use: The root or root bark of Eleutherococcus Ci Wu Jia is decocted, used in tincture form or taken powdered as tablets or capsules. The root bark is said to contain a higher percentage of active constituents than the whole root.

Dosage: Decoction: 4-16 g
Tincture: 1-5 ml
Powder: 1-6 g

Caution: To be used with some care, but not contraindicated, in Yin deficiency conditions presenting signs of empty heat (e.g., Yin deficiency diabetes where good results have been obtained from its use). Caution is also advised with severe hypertension, extrasystole and tachycardia.

Notes

Having a wider therapeutic catchment area than any other harmony remedy in this section, Eleuthero ginseng root tackles a large variety of challenges and ills generated by today's Western civilization. The amazing depth of its regulating and adaptogenic action deals radically with the key dynamics underpinning many modern disorders, such as immune deficiency, endocrine imbalance, tissue hypoxia and various forms of endogenous and exogenous toxicosis. These dynamics are all correlated causative factors of today's major complaint, fatigue.

Eleuthero ginseng is a relatively new find: It was only in 1854 that the Soviet botanist

Maximowicz (whose name is seen suffixing the numerous Asian plant species that he defined) identified the plant in the Ussuri region in the Russian Far East. As a remedy it had to await Brekhman's evaluation as an *adaptogen* in 1958.

Nevertheless, it is unfair to think of this fledgeling among the time-tested super-tonics only in terms comparative to Ginseng (the varieties of the *Panax* genus). Eleuthero ginseng has proved experimentally to exceed them in its adaptogenic capabilities and therefore potential fields of action and applications. Because it possesses more balanced and neutral qualities than other ginsengs, Eleuthero ginseng is ultimately a superior *adaptogen* and *immune enhancer*. In practice this also means that Eleuthero is easier to use in *any* situation. The first five symptom pictures indicated, involving essentially metabolic disorders, are the major conditions from a large variety of deficiencies that Eleuthero ginseng will address.

The normalizing action of Eleuthero ginseng root in the face of stress involves endocrine, nervous and cardiovascular systems in most of their metabolic functions: Thyroid, adrenal and pancreatic secretions are balanced and enhanced, nervous functions are harmonized, blood pressure is equalized and fluids and electrolytes are regulated. General anabolism is stepped up, resulting, for example, in increased lipid and protein metabolism and synthesis of the nucleic acids DNA and RNA. The oxygen-carrying capacity of the blood is improved. Available energy is further increased and fatigue reduced by Eleuthero ginseng's other actions on the cell. By optimizing hexokinase reactions, for instance, the remedy directly increases levels of cellular energy production.

Ye Zhi-shen's poem about this remedy, which he wrote in the Qing period, includes the line "I would rather a handful of Eleuthero than a cartload of gold and jewels." This sentiment could hardly be more appropriate than at the present time.

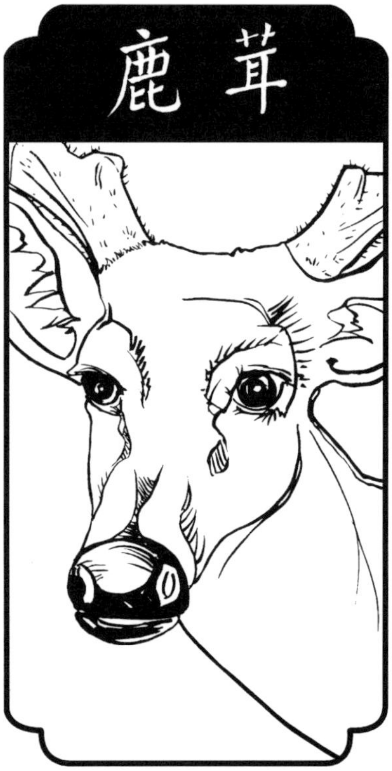

Cervus Lu Rong

Velvet Deer Antler

Zoological source: *Cervus nippon* Temminck or *C. elaphus* L. (Cervidae)
Pharmaceutical name: Cornu cervi parvum
Chinese names: Lu Rong, Rong Tou, Nen Lu Rong (Mand); Lok Yan (Cant)
Other names: Sika deer; Rokujo (Jap)
Habitat: Western and North China, Inner Mongolia and the mountains of Southwest China
Part used: the velvety, noncornified young horn

Therapeutic category: mild remedy with minimal chronic toxicity
Constituents: c. 50% amino acids (incl. tryptophane, threonine, valine, leucine, histidine, phenylalaline, arginine, proline, tyrosine, glutamic acid, serine, aspartic acid, proline), polyamines (putrescine, neuridine, spermidine), androgens, estrogens, sphingomyelin, cholesterol, ectosaponins, calcium phosphate/carbonate, magnesium, phosphorus, sphingmyelin, ganglioside, chondroitin A sulfate, choline analogues
Effective qualities: sweet, salty, warm, moist
restoring, astringing, nourishing, solidifying, thickening
Tropism: endocrine, immune, digestive, urinary, reproductive, skeletal systems
Spleen, Liver, Kidney, Chong, Dai, Ren, Yin Qiao channels
Fluid body

Actions and Indications

broad-spectrum endocrine restorative: adaptogenic, aging retardant: chronic hormonal deficiencies with long-term weakness, low vitality, stamina loss; chronic stress, convalescence, premature aging
immune enhancer: low immunity with frequent or chronic infections; immunodeficiency disorders (incl. CFS, AIDS)

---

metabolic restorative: pituitary-adrenal stimulant, protein anabolism stimulant: metabolic disorders, esp. anabolic deficiencies (incl. insufficient physical and mental growth in children, skeletal deformities [e.g. rickets], protein metabolism deficiency, glycogen storage disorders, malnutrition, anorexia)
anastative nutritive: chronic weight loss, mental retardation, debility
hemogenic: anemia, blood loss
oxygenator: poor oxygenation, tissue hypoxia; fatigue, reduced mental capacity, insomnia
sense enhancer: poor vision and hearing
muskuloskeletal restorative: skeletal and muscular weakness (esp. of lower back and legs); muscular dystrophy, hypercalcemia
reproductive restorative: pituitary-gonadal stimulant, androgenic, estrogenic, aphrodisiac: sexual disinterest, impotence, infertility
urogenital astringent/mucostatic restorative: incontinence with polyuria, enuresis, spermatorrhea, leucorrhea
renal restorative, diuretic: kidney deficiency
cardiovascular restorative, hypertensive: cardiac weakness in any condition; palpitation, arrhythmia, deficient circulation, hypotension
hemostatic: passive uterine bleeding (metrorrhagia)
vulnerary, cicatrisant: chronic indolent skin ulcers and boils; wounds, fractures

Symptom Pictures

neuroendocrine deficiency (Essence, Blood and Qi deficiency): chronic weakness, fatigue, poor concentration, appetite and sleep loss, chronic infection proneness

liver and adrenal Yin deficiency: early evening exhaustion, frequent infections, underweight, introversion

metabolic/Blood deficiency: pale complexion, spaceyness, cold extremities, dizziness, palpitations

genitourinary damp cold (Kidney Yang deficiency): sexual disinterest, impotence, frequent, copious, clear urination, white vaginal discharges

musculoskeletal deficiency (Liver and Kidney depletion): weakness of lower back and knees, fatigue

heart Yang deficiency: palpitations, fatigue, cold limbs, pale complexion, weak respiration, mental dullness or depression

Preparation

Use: The velvet deer antler Cervus Lu Rong is usually decocted alone in a double boiler, or taken in powder form. A tincture can also be prepared and is sometimes known as pantocrine.

Dosage: Decoction: 3-5 g
Powder: 1-3 g
Tincture: 1-2.5ml

Caution: Contraindicated in deficiency syndromes with empty heat.

Notes

Once a common medicinal item in the traditional Galenic apothecary in Europe, Velvet deer antler is also familiar in the Oriental pharmacy today. Under the scientific scrutiny of Chinese research, this emperor of traditional *Yang tonics* has consolidated its reputation as an outstanding *restorative, nutritive* and *rejuvenative* remedy. Its *immune-enhancing* action is a small but important part of these overall effects. Velvet deer antler has been found to increase oxygenation and therefore tissue metabolism in the major organs, to promote cellular regeneration through its ectosaponin content, to stimulate blood cell production in the bone marrow, to increase serum levels of erythrocytes, hemoglobin, leukocytes and reticulocytes, and to increase lymphocyte transformation (Chang and But 1987). Involving endocrine functions at the deepest level, these are some examples of the dynamics of the remedy's global *restorative* effect.

This remedy's extremely high amino acid content is cause for its primarily *anastative* and *nutritive* effect. In practice, this means that anabolic and metabolic states of deficiency, more than any others, will benefit from Velvet deer antler—those states especially found during childhood and old age. In vitalistic terms, not only are Blood and liver deficiency conditions tonified, but Essence, Qi and Yang deficiencies are also replenished—particularly those presenting cold and weakness.

紫河車

Homo Zi He Che

Human Placenta

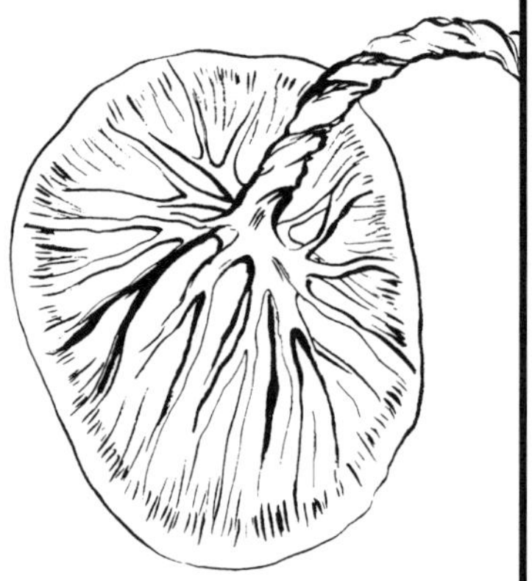

Zoological source: *Homo sapiens* L. (Hominidae)
Pharmaceutical name: Placenta Hominis
Chinese names: Zi He Che, Tai Yi, Tai Pan, Ren Bao (Mand); Ji Ho Je (Cant)
Other names: Shikasha (Jap)
Part used: the whole placenta

Therapeutic category: medium-strength remedy with some chronic toxicity
Constituents: hormones (incl. gonadotropins, prolactin, oxytocin, estrogen, progesterone, androgen, TSH, cortisone), interferon, urokinase, prostaglandins, hemoglobin, phosphorus, enzymes (incl. oxytocinases, histaminase, kininase, lysozyime, phospholipoprotein, saccharides, trace elements (incl. copper, zinc, iron, manganese, selenium, cadmium)
Effective qualities: sweet, salty, warm, moist
nourishing, restoring, thickening, relaxing
Tropism: endocrine, immune, reproductive, respiratory, vascular, systems
Liver, Kidney, Heart, Lung, Chong, Ren, Yin Qiao, Yang Wei channels; Fluid, Air bodies

Actions and Indications

broad-spectrum endocrine restorative, adaptogenic: chronic pituitary, spleen, adrenal, thyroid, gonadal deficiency with low stamina, low vitality, fatigue; debility, postpartum weakness, convalescence, insufficient lactation, uteruine and mammary deficiency
immune enhancer: low immunity with frequent or chronic infections; immunodeficiency disorders

---

metabolic restorative: pituitary-adrenal stimulant, anastative nutritive: metabolic disorders (incl. anemia, anorexia, malabsorption, malnutrition, delayed growth); anabolic deficiency with chronic weight loss, emaciation, debility
hemogenic: anemia, blood loss, amenorrhea
reproductive restorative, pituitary-gonadal stimulant, estrogenic, androgenic: infertility, impotence, habitual miscarriage
uterine trophorestorative: amenorrhea, undeveloped uterus, uterine atrophy
galactagogue: insufficient breast milk
demulcent respiratory restorative, bronchodilator: chronic lung conditions, chronic cough and wheezing, asthma (incl. allergic), lung TB
hemostatic, coagulant: bleeding, hemmorrhage (esp. uterine and postpartum)

dermatropic: skin conditions (incl. dermatitis, skin ulcers)
vulnerary: trauma, wounds
immunostimulant anti-infective, antigenic: influenza, measles, lung TB; infections in general

Symptom Pictures

endocrine deficiency (Essence, Blood and Qi deficiency): fatigue, weakness, loss of stamina, frequent or chronic infections, palpitations, sexual disinterest, underweight, daytime sweats

lung Yin deficiency: debility, emaciation, night sweats

adrenocortical deficiency (Lung and Kidney Yang deficiency): fatigue, loss of stamina, chronic cough and wheezing

Preparation

Use: Human placenta is usually used in powdered form, from which a tincture can also be made. It may also be deep-frozen to use as required. To best preserve the enzymes and other components, placenta should never be boiled or decocted. A small piece of fresh placenta blended with a red-colored juice (e.g., cherry, cranberry or dark grape) may be given to new mothers after delivery. In the experience of numerous midwives, this "placenta cocktail" is especially effective for reducing or stopping postpartum bleeding, boosting energies, relieving depression, preventing infection and generating adequate breast milk.

Dosage: Powder: 2-5 g
Tincture: 1-3 ml

Caution: Do not take continuously. Human placenta possesses some cumulative toxicity. Watch for signs of dryness which may indicate toxicity. Unlike other botanicals in this section, Human placenta is not recommended for general, long-term maintenance, especially without the presence of deficiency symptoms.

Notes

Human placenta is functionally *restorative* and substantially *nutritive* in addressing a wide range of endocrine, metabolic and immune deficiency conditions. Collectively these deficiencies are traditionally expressed in the syndromes Blood, Essence, Qi and Yang deficiency. Containing a wide variety of hormones, Human placenta is a generous *endocrine trophorestorative* and *adaptogenic* remedy. With its stimulation of interferon, gamma-globulin and antibodies, it also exerts specific *immune-potentiating* and *anti-infective* actions. Placenta is clearly a remedy for chronic deficiency conditions, regardless of whether they arose from poor lifestyle, chronic stress and overwork, chronic recurrent infections (especially with viral and fungal terrain), trauma or giving birth.

Placenta has been used for milleniums in China to treat deficiencies involving reproductive and respiratory functions. Chronic respiratory conditions with recurrent wheezing or systemic dryness, as in lung tuberculosis, are noted symptoms in this context. The remedy's *pituitary-adrenotropic* effect serves here not only to control the asthma, but also to reduce the deficiency heat arising from adrenal, or Yin, deficiency.

It makes sense that a remedy as intimately connected with human reproduction as the placenta should also be an outstanding *restorative* for infertility and impotence. Moreover, giving fresh placenta to a new mother following birth has become standard protocol among a growing number of midwives in the United States. By nourishing the blood and fluids, endocrine glands and organs, Placenta will not only help stop bleeding, but also speed up recovery, renew energies and relieve postpartum blues. In energetic terms, Placenta achieves this by replenishing the Chong, Ren and Yang Wei channels.

In a larger, bioenergetic context, Human placenta can be an individual's lifelong ally remedy from birth to death. It nourished you in the womb and can also be an invaluable support in times of stress or crisis, including everything from teething pain and school exams to divorce and bereavement. It is also helpful during the transitions from one phase of life to another, such as pre-adolescence, pre-adulthood, midlife and menopause.

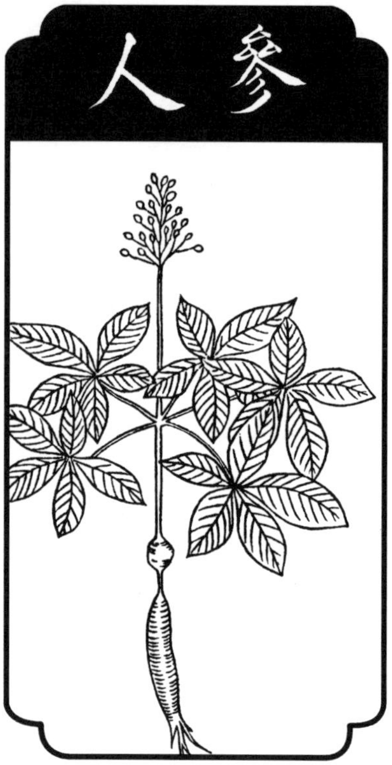

Panax Ren Shen

Asian Ginseng Root

Botanical source: *Panax ginseng* C.A. Meyer (Araliaceae)
Pharmaceutical name: Radix Panacis ginsengis
Chinese names: Ren Shen, Shen Cao, Tu Qing, Bai Shen, Xue Shen, Bian Tiao Shen, Bie Zhi Shen, Gao Li Shen, Hong Shen (Xu), Yuan Shen, Ye Shan Shen, Sheng Shai Shen, Yi Shan Shen, Shi Zhu Shen (Mand); Yan Sam (Cant)
Other names: "Human root," "Spirit herb," "Earth essence," "White root," "Blood root," "Life root," "Tartar root"; Ninjin (Jap)
Habit: Perennial mountain herb from Korea, Northeast China and Taighur, almost entirely cultivated; prefers shady, humid deciduous woods with rich moist loam; flowers in early summer with small terminal umbels of viridian blossoms.
Part used: the root

Therapeutic category: mild remedy with minimal chronic toxicity
Constituents: triterpenoid saponins (min. 31 ginsenosides 4%, incl. panaxosides), panaxadiol, panaxatriol, essential oil (incl. sesquiterpene panacene, elemenes, panaxynol), sterols (beta-sitosterol, stigmasterol, campesterol), maltol, triterpenes, flavonoids, organic acids, oleanolic acid, cholesterols, 17 amino acids, polyamines, nitrogenous compounds, nonacosane, tri/dipalmitin, linolein, enzymes, androgenic phytosterols, kaempferol, nicotinic acid, riboflavin, thiamine, glycopeptides, polysaccharides, polypeptide, mucilage, resin, vitamins, 20 trace minerals (incl. germanium, zinc, copper, iron, cobalt, manganese, vanadium)
Effective qualities: sweet, a bit bitter, warm, dry
restoring, nourishing, astringing, raising, relaxing, calming, stabilizing
Tropism: endocrine, nervous, respiratory, digestive, urogenital, cardiovascular systems
Spleen, Lung, Heart, Kidney, Chong, Ren, Dai, Yang Wei, Du, Yang Qiao

Actions and Indications

broad-spectrum endocrine restorative, adaptogenic: chronic glandular deficiencies with low stamina and endurance, low vitality, fatigue; chronic stress, neurasthenia, weight loss
antioxidant (free radical inhibitor), aging retardant: toxicosis, premature senility
central nervous trophorestorative, sympathetic stimulant: cerebral/nervous deficiency with depression, poor concentration, memory loss, chronic fatigue, insomnia, learning disability; nervous breakdown
immune enhancer: low immunity with frequent or chronic infections; immunodeficiency disorders (incl. CFS, AIDS)
immune regulator, antiallergic: immune stress with cell-mediated allergies (incl. chronic hepatitis, contact dermatitis, autoimmune disorders [incl. ulcerative colitis])

---

metabolic restorative/regulator: pituitary-adrenal stimulant: metabolic disorders (incl. glycogen storage disorders, anemia, anorexia, malabsorption, metabolic acidosis); anabolic and catabolic deficiencies with weight loss, low stamina, exhaustion, debility
anastative nutritive, liver restorative/protective: chronic liver disorders (incl. liver disease, toxicosis) with fatigue, weakness
hemogenic: anemia
hypoglycemiant, secretory: hyperglycemia, diabetes mellitus; thirst, dehydration
gastrointestinal restorative, sweet digestant: appetite loss, malnutrition, malabsorption

reproductive restorative: pituitary-gonadal stimulant: androgenic, estrogenic, aphrodisiac: sexual disinterest, impotence; androgen/estrogen deficiency conditions
urogenital astringent/mucostatic restorative: polyuria, enuresis, spermatorrhea, leucorrhea
cardiaovascular restorative/regulator (esp. *hypertensive*)*:* hypotension, hypertension, palpitations; loss of enthusiasm; senile heart, arrhythmia, myocardial deficiency/ischemia
psychogenic, analeptic: shock, collapse; circulatory collapse, hypovolemic and cardiogenic shock, cerebral ischemia
nervous relaxant: stress, unrest, tension, muscular tension, infantile seizures
respiratory restorative/relaxant: shallow breathing, poor stamina, wheezing; acute asthma
antilipemic: hyperlipidemia (incl. hypercholesterolemia)
hemostatic: asthenic/passive hemorrhage
immunostimulant anti-infective: antigenic, phagocyte/lymphocyte stimulant, leukocytogenic: infections in general (incl. EBV and HIV infection), low WBC count (leukopenia)
radiation-protective: radiation sickness (e.g. from radiotherapy)
Miscellaneous: organ prolapse, chronic low-grade fever

Symptom Pictures

neuroendocrine deficiency (Qi, Blood and Essence deficiency): long-term fatigue, weakness, chronic or frequent infections, forgetfulness, poor or absent sleep, depression

small intestine Qi and liver blood deficiency: fatigue, weakness, infection proneness, low stamina, palpitations, underweight

liver, pancreas and adrenal Yin deficiency: poor resistance, underweight, low physical stamina, somnolence, fatigue after or between meals, evening exhaustion, sweet cravings, anxiety spells

stomach/small intestine Qi deficiency (Spleen Qi deficiency): appetite/weight loss, fatigue, loose stool

heart Qi constraint with **nerve excess:** feeling stressed, anxiety, unrest, sleep loss, palpitations

Devastated Yang: cold limbs, shallow breathing, profuse sweating, fainting, collapse

lung Qi deficiency: shortness of breath, labored breathing, wheezing

Preparation

Use: The root Panax Ren Shen is taken in decoction or tincture form. The root is also traditionally steamed on its own in a double boiler. **Red ginseng root,** called **Hong Ren Shen** (Mand.) or **Hung Yan Sam** (Cant.), is prepared by steaming the whole or sliced root. It is considered somewhat more effective, or *stimulating,* than the uncured root.

Dosage: Decoction: 1-8 g. The average dose is 3 g.
Tincture: 0.25-3 ml. The average dose is 1 ml.
Large doses are required for treating shock, e.g. 10-30 g by decoction or 3-10 ml of tincture.

Caution: Asian ginseng root is forbidden in the following conditions: Yin deficiency with empty heat; all full heat conditions, high blood pressure with sympathetic nervous stress (Liver Yang rising), and extreme hypertension. Women should not use Asian ginseng at full dose on a daily basis for over 10 days or so because of its strongly *androgenic* effect which develops male characeristics physically and in character. Longterm use of Asian ginseng should entail low doses only and should be periodically interrupted for several days, as slight cumulative toxicity may occur. Typical symptoms of the Ginseng abuse syndrome include nervousness, agitation, euphoria, sleep loss, skin rashes, morning diarrhea and high blood pressure. This condition is enhanced by the concomitant intake of coffee.

Notes

With names like *Spirit herb, Life root* and *Earth essence*, this supreme Asian harmony remedy enjoys a long history of use in Northeast Asia among indigenous Russian, Korean and northeast Chinese peoples. The healing properties of this venerated root are indissolubly embedded in their cultural myths. The mysteries of Asian ginseng root are shrouded deep among the hoary tribal spiritual practices that originate in Earth-based shamanism.

Over the decades, extensive worldwide scientific research has merely continued the traditional focus placed on this botanical superstar, while stripping very little of its ancient mystery.

Modern pharmacology confirms Asian ginseng root's superb *adaptogenic, restorative* and *regulative* functions, which have been empirically known to northeast Asians since prehistoric times. These effects hinge primarily on its action on the pituitary-adrenal and adrenal-pancreas-liver axes. Being a powerful wide-spectrum *restorative,* primarily to endocrine, nervous, metabolic, immune and circulatory functions, Asian ginseng is considered in East Asia *the* foremost tonic.

This emperor of all ginsengs grows in the same general region as Eleuthero ginseng, and at first glance the two plants seem to have very similar applications. However, it is Asian ginseng root has a long tradition of native therapeutic use. The best way to differentiate Asian ginseng from Eleuthero ginseng is this: The Asian variety works more on the nervous system. It is a *stimulant* to the sympathetic nervous and cardiovascular systems and to adrenergic functions. In Chinese medical terms, Asian ginseng tonifies the Qi and the Yang. Eleuthero ginseng, on the other hand, works more on the metabolic system, called the Blood in Oriental terms. On the whole, it has a more *regulating* effect than the more *stimulating* actions of Asian ginseng. Because of the widespread preventive use of Asian ginseng in recent decades, this differentiation between these two ginseng types is worth remembering.

The different emphases of the two ginsengs explains why Asian ginseng root treats only deficiency, not excess conditions. Asian ginseng may actually aggravate excess conditions that involve stagnation or heat, such as liver congestion. Because many of today's major disorders often involve aspects of deficiency and excess together, self-medication with Asian ginseng is usually not a good idea. *Panax* is not—and in Northeast Asian tribal societies never was—the all-purpose panacea that its name makes it out to be.

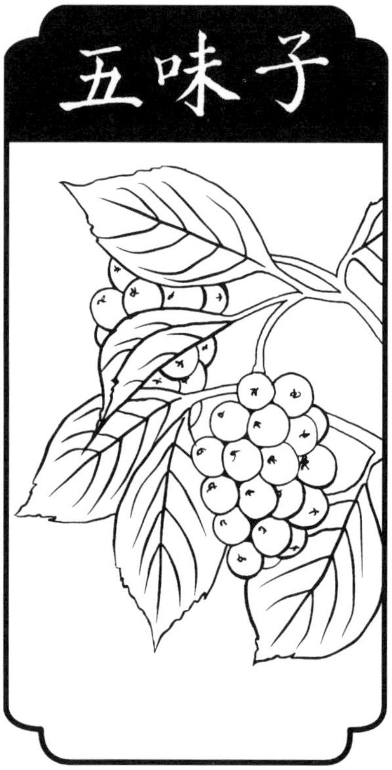

Schisandra Wu Wei Zi

Schisandra Berry

Botanical source: *Schisandra chinensis* (Turcz.) Baillon or *S. sphenanthera* Rehder et Wilson (syn. *Maximowiczia sinensis* Ruprecht) (Magnoliaceae)
Pharmaceutical name: Fructus Schisandrae
Chinese names: Wu Wei Zi, Wu Wei; *S. chin.:* Bei Wu Wei Zi; *S. sphen.:* Nan Wu Wei Zi, Hua Zheng Wu Wei Zi (Mand); Ng Mei Ji (Cant)
Other names: Chinese magnolia vine, "Five taste berry"; Gomishi (Jap)
Habit: Deciduous woody climbing vine from montane temperate China; grows in woods and thickets in rich loose soil and likes a cool or cold climate; blooms in May, June and July with pale yellow axillary flower clusters.
Part used: the fruit

Therapeutic category: mild remedy with minimal chronic toxicity
Constituents: essential oil 3% (incl. sesquicarene, bisabolene, beta-chamigrene, ylangene, citral), lignans (incl. schizandrin, deoxyschizandrine, wuweizisu C, wuweizichun B, schisantherins A, B, C, D, E, F, G, kadsuranin, gomisin A and B), triterpenopids (incl. schizandrol, schisanhenol, schisanhenrin, enshicine, epischisandrome, chicanine, enwuweizic acid, schisanlactone A), stigmasterol, citric/malic/tartaric acids, saccharides, sitosterol, tannins, resin, vitamins C, E, minerals (incl., phosphorus, manganese, silicon)
Effective qualities: sour, salty, astringent, warm, dry
restoring, raising, stimulating, astringing, stabilizing
Tropism: neuroendocrine, respiratory, digestive, cardiovascular, reproductive
Lung, Stomach, Heart, Kidney, Du, Yang Qiao, Chong, Dai, Yang Wei

Actions and Indications

adrenocortical restorative, adaptogenic, aging-retardant: adrenal cortex deficiency with chronic loss of stamina, fatigue; stress, overwork, chronic illness
central nervous trophorestorative: cerebral and nervous deficiency with memory loss, concentration loss, headache, dizziness, chronic mental and physical fatigue, insomnia; chronic stress, sleep disorder, nervous breakdown, psychosis, paralysis, cerebellar ataxia, peripheral neuritis, myelitis, Huntington's disease, Parkinson's disease, Menière's disease, Alzheimer's disease, Guillain-Barré syndrome, sequelae of CVA
sense enhancer: poor sense perception (incl. vision, hearing, touch)
immune enhancer: low immunity with frequent or chronic infections; immunodeficiency disorders (incl. CFS, AIDS)
immune regulator, antiallergic: immune stress with allergic skin conditions (incl. urticaria, atopic dermatitis); autoimmune disorders

---

metabolic restorative, oxygenator: metabolic disorders; shallow breathing, altitude sickness, tissue hypoxia
liver trophorestorative/protective, dermatropic: liver deficiencies (incl. glycogen storage disorders, hepatitis [all types], liver disease, metabolic toxicosis, dry/rough skin)
intestinal astringent, antibacterial, lymphocyte stimulant: diarrhea; acute enteritis, dysentery
gastric acidity regulator: dyspepsia from gastric hyper- or hypoacidity
respiratory restorative, expectorant, antitussive: coughing, wheezing; low respiratory capacity, asthma
urogenital restorative: astringent, mucostatic, aphrodisiac (mild): incontinence with enuresis, leucorrhea, spermatorrhea; sexual disinterest
uterine stimulant, emmenagogue, oxytocic: amenorrhea; prolonged pregnancy, stalled labor
blood pressure regulator: hypotension, hypertension
anhydrotic: excessive day or night sweating
interferon inducent

Symptom Pictures

neuroendocrine deficiency (Kidney Essence deficiency): headache, dizziness, absent-mindedness, forgetfulness, reduced vision or hearing, depression, fatigue, chronic or frequent infections, poor quality or little sleep

adrenocortical deficiency (Lung and Kidney Yang deficiency): fatigue, low endurance, daytime sweating, shallow breathing, wheezing, allergies

liver and adrenal Yin deficiency: low stamina, fatigue, exhaustion at night, introversion, frequent infections

genitourinary Qi deficiency (Kidney Qi deficiency): urinary and seminal incontinence, fatigue, sexual disinterest

intestines cold (Spleen and Kidney Yang deficiency): chronic diarrhea, esp. in the morning, fatigue

Preparation

Use: The berry Schisandra Wu Wei Zi is used in standard decoction or tincture form.
Dosage: Decoction: 4-10 g
Tincture: 2-4 ml
For respiratory conditions: Decoction: 1.5-3 g
Tincture: 1-2 ml
Caution: Forbidden in the early stages of cough or rashes, in full heat conditions and during pregnancy.

Notes

With its sour, mouth-puckering taste, the small, shrivelled purple drupe of the Chinese magnolia vine has come a long, long way. In olden days, Chinese doctors made extensive use of the "five-taste berry's" bracing *astringent tonic* effect on the respiratory, digestive and urogenital systems, treating such conditions as chronic cough and asthma, chronic diarrhea, and urinary and genital discharges, as well as general fatigue due to Qi deficiency.

Today, like several other east Asian botanicals now popular in the West, Schisandra berry is proving its renewed relevance by addressing major contemporary health problems. Foremost among its benefits are the *restorative* effects on the brain and central nervous system. More specifically, the remedy has proven to directly stimulate nerve cells, thereby increasing intellectual activity, coordination and sense perception. This action has recently been applied to a gamut of neurological conditions ranging from banal headache, sleep disorder and memory loss, to disorders such as psychoses, spastic paralysis and cerebellar ataxia. Interestingly, the overall symptomatology of these conditions strongly suggests a tonification, in Chinese medical terms, of Kidney Essence.

Several of Schisandra berry's major actions make it clear, however, that it is more than just a remedy for nervous deficiencies. They strongly suggest that the berry essentially operates in the same territory as the other remedies in this section—as an *adaptogen* that facilitates response to unproductive stress. As such, Schisandra is able to modulate endocrine and immune functions as well as neural ones. Through a tonification of the adrenal cortex and liver, it will treat chronic metabolic deficiency conditions causing symptoms such as fatigue, low endurance, frequent infections and blood sugar swings. All types of hepatitis, for example, have responded very favorably to Schisandra.

Some uncertainty still surrounds this remedy's *oxygenation-enhancing* effect. It may soon prove appropriate for some of today's worst chronic disorders, viral infections included: The implications of increased tissue oxygenation for the management of chronic viral infections are significant. Nonetheless, in China, Schisandra has become the major ingredient in formulas designed to reduce altitude sickness.

Schisandra berry's action on the immune system also bears highlighting, as it has been discovered not only to stimulate inadequate immune functions, but also to regulate them when they become disordered—as in allergic and autoimmune reactions. Lignans are known experimentally for their *immunosuppressant* activity. Schisandra has had a long string of lignans identified among its numerous components. The full extent of its *antiallergic* property, however, still remains unknown, and awaits investigation.

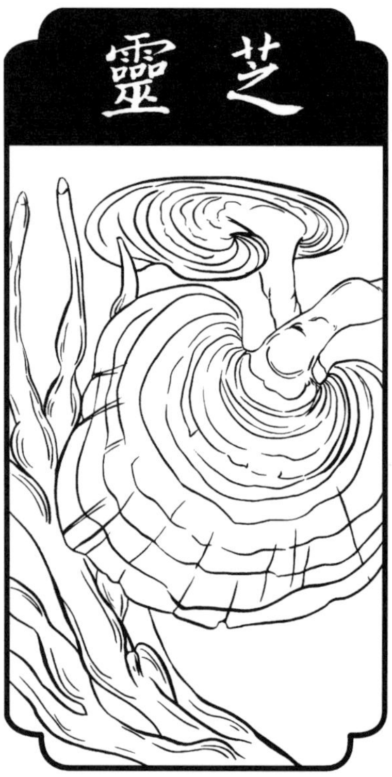

Ganoderma Ling Zhi

Reishi Mushroom

Botanical source: *Ganoderma lucidum* (Leyss. ex Fr.) Karsten or *G. japonicum/sinense* (Fr.) Lloyd or *G. capens* Lloyd or *G. applanatum* (Pers. ex Gray) Patrin or *G. tsugae* Murray (Polyporaceae)
Pharmaceutical name: Sclerotium Ganodermae
Chinese names: Ling Zhi, Ling Zhi Cao, Yang Shen Zhi, Chi Zhi, Dan Zhi, Qi Zhi (Mand); Ling Ji (Cant)
Other names: Ganoderma, "Spiritual/Shaman's mushroom," "Nourish spirit mushroom," "Red mushroom," "Cinnabar mushroom," "Red pill mushroom," "Soul mushroom"; Reishi (Jap)
Habit: Brown-black saprophytic fungus found in China's coastal provinces and in the Pacific Northwest of North America; grows on roots, trunks and rotting tree stumps of oak and other broad-leaved trees; also cultivated in sterilized sawdust media.
Part used: the fruiting body or cap

Therapeutic category: mild remedy with minimal chronic toxicity

Constituents: *(G. lucidum)* soluble proteins, 32 amino acids (incl. glutamic acid, alanine), polypeptides, fungal lysozyme, acid protease, sterols (ergosterol, llanosterol, sitosterol ganodosterone), lactones, alkaloids, triterpenes (incl. lucidenic/ganoderic/ganodermic acids), polysaccharides (incl. beta-D-glucans, ganoderans, GL-1, D-6), choline, betaine, stearic/palmitic/behenic/nonadecanoic/oleic acids, nucleotide adenosine, tetracosane, hentriacontane, cyclooctasulphur, potassium chloride, sulphur, trace minerals (incl. copper, iron, zinc, germanium)

Effective qualities: bland, a bit sweet and bitter, neutral
restoring, calming, relaxing, dissolving

Tropism: nervous, immune, endocrine, digestive, respiratory, cardiovascular systems
Lung, Spleen, Liver, Pericardium, Heart, Kidney, Liver, Chong, Yin Wei, Yang Wei channels; Air, Fluid bodies

Actions and Indications

adrenocortical restorative/regulator, adaptogenic: chronic deficiency conditions with fatigue, weakness, low stamina and vitality; chronic stress, convalescent debility
antioxidant (free radical inhibitor), aging-retardant: toxicosis, premature senility
neurocardiac restorative: cerebral/nervous deficiency, heart weakness, neurasthenia; memory loss, mental capacity loss
immune enhancer: low immunity with frequent or chronic infections; immunodeficiency disorders (incl. CFS, AIDS)
immune regulator, broad-spectrum antiallergic: immune stress with immediate allergies (incl. pollen and drug allergies, rhinitis, bronchial asthma, urticaria, purpura, angioedema, atopic dermatitis); cell and antibody-mediated allergies and immune complex disorders (incl. food allergies, atopic dermatitis, nephritis, chronic hepatitis, chronic bronchitis and pneumonia, autoimmune disorders [incl. hemolytic anemia, multiple sclerosis, serum sickness, rheumatoid arthritis, lupus, psoriasis, celiac sprue, Grave's disease, vasculitis, Crohn's disease])

---

metabolic restorative: metabolic disorders, esp. anabolic deficiencies (incl. debility, malnutrition, malabsorption, glycogen storage disorders, anorexia, muscular dystrophy, myasthenia gravis)
anastative nutritive, liver trophorestorative/protective, detoxicant: liver congestion; all chronic liver and spleen conditions (incl. hepatitis, liver degeneration/necrosis); loss of endurance and immunity, toxicosis
oxygenator: altitude sickness, shallow breathing, tissue hypoxia
neurocardiac sedative, hypotensive: nervous and cardiac stress with unrest and insomnia; neurocardiac syndrome, anxiety states, phobias, neurosis; hypertension
coronary restorative/dilator, antilipemic: coronary deficiency/disease, hyperlipidemia
hypotensive: hypertension
parasympathetic nervous antagonist
expectorant, antitussive: wheezing, coughing; acute bronchial asthma, chronic bronchitis
immunostimulant anti-infective: antibacterial, antiviral, phagocyte/lymphocyte stimulant: infections in general (incl. viral conditions, pneumonia [Strep. and Staph.], EBV and HIV infection)
antitumoral, interferon inducent: tumors, early stage of cancer
radiation-protective, leukocytogenic: radiation sickness (therapeutic or environmental), leukopenia

Symptom Pictures

liver and adrenal Yin deficiency (Blood and Qi deficiency): chronic or frequent infections, underweight, fatigue, loss of motivation and stamina, exhaustion at night

heart Qi constraint (heart Blood and Spleen Qi deficiency): unrest, sleep loss, palpitations, feeling stressed

heart blood and Qi stagnation: chest tightness or pain, palpitations, fatigue

lung Qi constraint: wheezing, tight chest, coughing, palpitations, allergies, feeling stressed

lung phlegm cold: chronic coughing with thin white sputum, wheezing, cold extremities

Preparation

Use: The mushroom Ganoderma Ling Zhi is decocted on low heat exactly at boiling point (without any bubbling) for at least two hours, until 1/3 of the water remains. Break up into small pieces, powder or liquidize the mushroom cap first (do not use the inactive stem). Tinctures are somewhat less effective, but still viable.

Taking vitamin C together with Reishi mushroom may increase Reishi's effectiveness in resolving viral infections and early cancers.

Dosage: Long decoction: 1-5 g. The single dosage generally reserved for more serious disorders is 4-5 g. All other conditions respond well to 1-3 g per dose.

For example, to make a three-day average supply (9 doses), use nine cups (just over 3 pints) of water to 27 g (just under 1 oz) of the dry Reishi mushroom cap. Through low heat decoction reduce the water down to three cups (just over 1 pint). Take a 1/3 cup dose three times a day on an empty stomach 20 minutes before eating. Refrigerate between use and reheat as needed.

Tincture: 0.5-2.5 ml (i.e. 12-70 drops)

Caution: As with most *detoxicant* remedies, very minor side effects (such as loose stool, dry mouth and skin rash) may occasionally be experienced because of the body's cleansing reaction.

Notes

There are several Chinese herbs that, being integral to the almost prehistoric shamanistic and alchemical practices of China's early Daoists, are hallowed with claims of their being elixirs of immortality. Today, these claims naturally arouse our skepticism or downright disbelief. Still, the hyperbolic reputation of some of these botanicals should not discourage us from keeping an open mind, especially when modern clinical research widely supports their stellar status.

Reishi mushroom is one such remedy. The various names given this particular fungus, for example—many of them code names for spiritual or yogic practices—clearly are a reflection of this. Its usefulness in treating a wide variety of today's most serious disorders is being increasingly realized. In my experience, conditions involving compromised metabolic and immune functioning are essentially its two target areas. Reishi's amino acids are important to its *nutritive* and *restorative* actions on the liver and metabolic processes in general. For example, the mushroom has specifically been shown to increase liver protein synthesis and nucleic acid and protein metabolism (Chang and But 1987). Here, as with many another Chinese super-remedy—be it an *Essence, Blood or Qi tonic*—the liver and adrenal cortex Yin functions are the hidden crucible of Reishi's *metabolic restorative* effects.

On the other hand, both long-term immune enhancement and immediate immune stimulation may be achieved through the use of this mushroom. Immune health is given a boost, not only to prevent infections, but also to the point of a preventive effect on cancer. The mushroom is a traditional folk remedy for early cancer. Its polysaccharides play a major role in modulating immunity for both immune deficiency and immune stress conditions, suggesting routine inclusion in treatment protocols for the entire range of today's elusive viral infections, as well as allergic and autoimmune disorders in general. At the current state of the herbal art, Reishi is the premier, if not the only, *antiallergic* remedy able to address the whole spectrum of hypersensitivity disorders (types I through V).

Beyond Reishi mushroom's *restoring* and *regulating* effects on metabolism and immunity, however, lies a deeper power. Its *adaptogenic* effect not only offers a wide range of protection from unproductive stress, but also directly modulates metabolic and immune functions themselves. By enhancing our adaptation response to stressors, Reishi will finely calibrate these intricate and delicate functions.

The name *ling* for this remedy, difficult though it is to translate, actually refers to the spiritual insight and potency achieved by shamans. It is very probable that the mushroom was traditionally used by early shamans and Daoists as an aid for journeying and meditation practices. Reishi generates a sense of inner calm and harmony, while also heightening mental perception, both logical and intuitive. Perhaps this is why Reishi can be seen as an elixir of immortality.

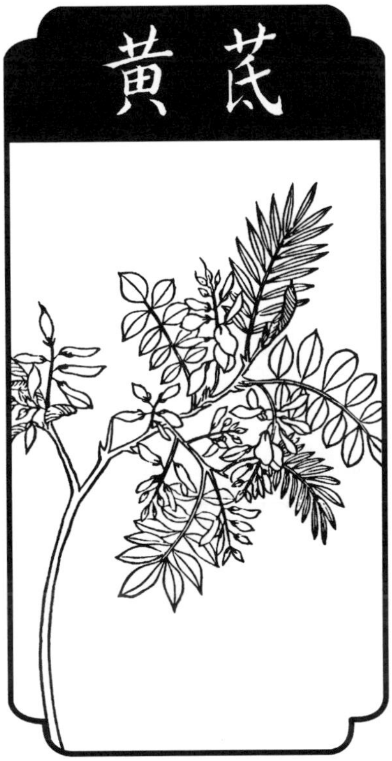

Astragalus Huang Qi

Astragalus Root

Botanical source: *Astragalus membranaceus* (Fischer) Bunge or *A. mongholicus* Bunge and spp. (Leguminosae)
Pharmaceutical name: Radix Astragali
Chinese names: Huang Qi, Bei Qi, Tai Shen, Ji Cao (Mand); Wong Kei, Baak Kei (Cant)
Other names: Membranous/Mongolian milkvetch, Yellow vetch; Ogi (Jap)
Habit: Perennial herb with long taproot from North-Central China and Inner Mongolia, growing on windy grassland, sunny slopes and by forest margins, brush and roadsides; likes warm or cool dry climate and thick, fertile, well-drained sandy humus soil; yellow flowers on axillary racemes appear in summer.
Part used: the root

Therapeutic category: mild remedy with minimal chronic toxicity
Constituents: flavonoids (incl. formononetin, astraisoflavone), choline, betaine, saponins (astramembrannins I and II, daucosterin, soyasaponins, astragalosides), triterpenoids, polysaccharides, folic/glucuronic acid, sitosterol, daucosterol, lupeol, aminobutyric acid, asparagine, androgen, 19 amino acids, kumatakenin, fatty acids, trace minerals (incl. selenium, molybdanum, uran.)
Effective qualities: sweet, a bit warm, dry
restoring, astringing, solidifying, stabilizing
Tropism: endocrine, immune, digestive, urinary systems
Spleen, Lung, Chong, Dai, Yang Wei channels
Air, Fluid bodies

Actions and Indications

adrenocortical restorative, adaptogenic, aging-retardant: adrenal cortex deficiency with low stamina; chronic fatigue, weakness, low vitality, endurance loss; premature aging
immune enhancer: low immunity with frequent or chronic infections; immunodeficiency disorders (incl. CFS, AIDS)
antiallergic

---

metabolic restorative: metabolic disorders (incl. glycogen storage disorders, malabsorption, metabolic toxicosis); catabolic and anabolic deficiencies with fatigue, debility, weight loss
liver restorative/protective, anastative nutritive: liver deficiencies (incl. liver disease, chronic hepatitis), malabsorption, malnutrition, lowered immunity
renal restorative, diuretic, detoxicant: chronic nephritis with edema, metabolic toxicosis, dysuria, oliguria
resolvent detoxicant: chronic boils, sores, carbuncles, abscesses
astringent, antisecretory, anhydrotic, antiprolapse: chronic diarrhea, excessive perspiration (incl. night sweats), uterine, rectal and gastrointestinal prolapse, rectocele
hemostatic: passive bleeding (esp. uterine bleeding)
vulnerary: chronic nonhealing wounds, sores and ulcers
immunostimulant anti-infective: antigenic, leukocytogenic, phagocyte stimulant, antibacterial: all infections (incl. liver and kidney infections, EBV and HIV infection); leukopenia
Misc.: ***interferon inducent, antitumoral, hypotensive***

Symptom Pictures

liver and adrenal Yin deficiency: evening exhaustion, poor endurance and motivation, increased appetite, frequent or chronic infections, underweight

stomach and small intestine Qi deficiency (Spleen Qi deficiency): fatigue, appetite and weight loss, daytime sweating, loose stool

kidney Qi stagnation with **metabolic toxicosis :** malaise, fatigue, scanty infrequent urination, dry skin, skin rashes, chronic boils

Preparation

Use: The root Astragalus Huang Qi is decocted or used in tincture form.

Dosage: Decoction: 10-20 g
Tincture: 2-4 ml

Caution: Forbidden in Yin deficiency with heat, in external full heat, Qi stasis with intestinal (Spleen) damp, the initial stage of boils, and in nursing mothers.

Notes

Traditional Chinese doctors have used Astragalus root since earliest times for treating deficiency conditions involving metabolic or digestive dysfunction. They summarised these in the concept "Qi deficiency." As a result of contemporary research, this remedy's reputation continues to spike among Chinese clinicians. Deservedly so. For example, Astragalus root has been shown to enhance cellular metabolism, thereby making more energy available on cellular and individual levels. This definitely qualifies as an *adaptogenic* function. Astragalus also enhances humoral immune functioning in several ways—including increasing leukocytic interferon production, reticuloendothelial phagocytic activity and lymphocytic rosette formation (Chang and But 1987). The root's polysaccharides content has been demonstrated to be active in this respect—not only on China's mainland.

On the other hand, flavonoids and amino acids are involved with Astragalus root's excellent *liver restorative* and *liver protective* actions. These actions entail enhanced hepatic assimilation and storage along with an increase in liver protein synthesis. Liver Yin deficiency syndromes—with their telltale symptoms of loss of stamina and evening exhaustion—stand to benefit here. They are also hormonally supported by a crucial tonification of the adrenal cortex.

Astragalus root's generous saponin content indicates a rejuvenating action on red blood cells and increased nutrient absorption by the intestines. This includes enhanced calcium and silicon utilization. Moreover the root also contains generous amounts of trace minerals, including the important trace elements selenium and molybdanum, which it collects from the soil and stores. Through these twin dynamics, Astragalus will increase overall vitality, energy and weight gain. The traditional syndrome Spleen Qi deficiency—a major indication for this remedy—embodies these restorative actions on the metabolism.

It becomes clear why the net result of these various actions has earned Astragalus root the status of *Qi tonic*, or *energy tonic*. This mildly sweet, warm, yet dry-natured botanical is a unique and invaluable component in most formulations addressing metabolic and immune deficiency conditions, with or without an overlay of infection.

Because Astragalus root entails a significant *detoxicant diuretic* effect (saponins at work again), adequate kidney functioning—especially elimination—is assured. Hence it is routinely included in China in botanical prescriptions for kidney disorders. The symptom pattern kidney Qi stagnation here encapsulates both the preclinical and organic kidney indication for this remedy in an elegant emblem.

Although the Pharmacopoeia of the Peoples' Republic currently only enumerates the two *Astragalus* species listed at the top as correct botanical source for the remedy Astragalus Huang Qi, traditionally and currently many other species serve as botanical source. Not only that, but a different genus, *Hedysarum,* with its own several species, also represents the remedy Huang Qi. Historically the main source for Huang Qi was probably *Hedysarum polybotris,* which has recently been renamed **Hong Qi.** Hedysarum Hong Qi has been found equally and similarly as therapeutic as Astragalus Huang Qi. For a full discussion of this, see p. 48 in Chapter 2.

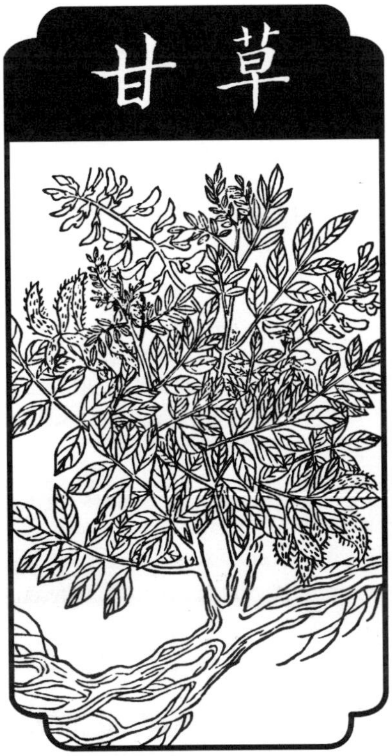

Glycyrrhiza Gan Cao

Ural Licorice Root *

Botanical source: *Glycyrrhiza uralensis* Fischer ex De Candolle or *G. glabra* L. or *G. glandulifera* Waldstein et Kitaibel (Papilionaceae)
Pharmaceutical name: Radix Glycirrhizae
Chinese names: Gan Cao, Mi Gan, Mi Cao (Mand); Gam Chou (Cant)
Other names: Manchurian/Asian licorice, "Sweet herb"; Kanzo (Jap)
Habit: Perennial glandular herb from the grasslands and sunny slopes of Central Asia, Siberia, West China and Inner Mongolia; prefers cool, dry, sunny places with rich, high calcium, sandy deep soil; blooms in summer with purple axillary flower clusters.
Part used: the root

Therapeutic category: mild remedy with minimal chronic toxicity
Constituents: flavonoids (liquiritin, isoliquiritin, liquiritigenin, liquiritigenin, licoflavone, licoricidin, licoricone, methylhydroxyisoflavone), steroids, triterpenoid saponins 6-14 % (glycirrhizine, glycyrrhetic acid, glyuranolide), ural-saponins A and B, neoglycitol, amino acids, resinous oil 15%, starch, glucose, (iso)-glycyrols, mannitol, apsaragin, asparanic acid
Effective qualities: very sweet, neutral, moist
restoring, relaxing, calming, softening
Tropism: endocrine, immune, respiratory, digestive, urinary, circulatory systems
Spleen, Lung, Yang Wei channels; Air, Warmth bodies

Actions and Indications

adrenocortical restorative: pituitary-adrenocortical stimulant: adrenal cortex deficiency with low stamina and endurance, chronic fatigue; adrenal failure, Addison's disease, menopausal syndrome
antioxidant (free radical inhibitor): toxicosis
immune regulator, antiallergic: immune stress with immediate allergies (incl. rhinitis, otitis, angioedema, bronchial asthma); cell-mediated allergies (incl. autoimmune disorders [e.g. ulcerative colitis, rheumatoid arthritis], contact dermatitis, chronic hepatitis)

---

liver protective: liver disorders (incl. jaundice, hepatitis)
hyperglycemiant: hypoglycemia
estrogenic: estrogen deficiency conditions (incl. menopause, PMS)
gastrointestinal restorative/relaxant: anastative digestant, demulcent, spasmolytic: malabsorption, malnutrition, anorexia; abdominal pain, colic, IBS
antacid antisecretory: gastric hyperacidity, peptic ulcer
bronchial demulcent, mucolytic expectorant: dry cough with scanty sputum, hoarseness; chronic asthma
urinary demulcent: urinary pain or irritation (all types)
antilipemic: hypercholesterolemia
anti-infective: immunostimulant, antibacterial, antiviral, antiseptic: bacterial and viral infections (incl. laryngitis, stomatitis, bronchitis, TB, pneumonia, whooping cough, enteritis, hepatitis, cystitis, conjunctivitis, dermatitis, chronic arthritis, EBV and HIV infection)
leukocytogenic: leukopenia
detoxicant, anti-inflammatory, antipyretic: boils, abscesses, carbuncles; fevers
antivenomous: poisoning from animal, mineral, herb or food source
antitumoral, interferon inducent: tumors (incl. granuloma, liver cancer)

Symptom Pictures

pancreas and adrenal Yin deficiency: fatigue after or between meals, afternoon somnolence, sweet or juice cravings, loss of stamina, early evening exhaustion

stomach and small intestine Qi deficiency (Spleen Qi deficiency): underweight, loose stool, weakness, epigastric pain, poor appetite

lung phlegm dryness: dry cough with scanty viscous phlegm, dry nose, mouth and throat

lung heat dryness: dry cough, fever, thirst, head and body aches

intestines Qi constraint: sharp abdominal pain, indigestion

Preparation

Use: The root Glycyrrhiza Gan Cao is decocted or used in tincture form (which makes it somewhat more warming.) Honey-fried Licorice root, **Zhi Gan Cao** (Mand.) or **Chek Gam Chou** (Cant.) is also more warming; it is used in preference to the raw root in conditions involving digestive (Spleen Qi) deficiency.

Dosage: Decoction: 3-14 g
Tincture: 1-4 ml

Caution: Contraindicated in nausea or vomiting due to intestines (Spleen) mucous damp, excess adrenal conditions such as hypertension and edema, hyperglycemic conditions, osteoporosis, and with excess secretions present generally.

Notes

Writing in 1871, Dr. Porter Smith, the respected British treaty-port medic of Hangzhou, noted that Ural licorice root was "the great corrective adjunct and harmonising ingredient in a large number of recipes." As one of several reviewers of the Maritime Customs' yearly Trade Reports who had access to inside information on the commerce of Chinese crude remedies, his statement carried much weight. It reflected not only the important role of this remedy in Oriental pharmacy, but also its specific therapeutic action. The situation remains unchanged today.

Like all remedies addressing endocrine and immune functions, Ural licorice root presents several distinct images. The remedy is indeed widely applicable for genuine therapeutic reasons, not merely because of its major sweetening effect on herbal formulas. As *endocrine* and *metabolic restorative*, Ural licorice mainly boosts adrenal and pancreatic weakness, especially those presenting functional blood sugar deficiencies. As a rare *immune regulating* remedy, the root has shown promising results in both immediate (type I) and cell-mediated (type IV) hypersensitivity conditions (Tsung 1989). As an *anastative digestive,* Ural licorice has been used since time immemorial for enhancing intestinal nutrient assimilation—see that cartel of saponins above in action. It is this application that has long earned it the central, indispensable role in countless herbal formulas of *Spleen Qi tonic*—like the Spleen itself being considered able of harmonizing and distributing the energies of other remedies throughout the whole system. And as a very smooth, thick *demulcent,* Ural licorice is valued for moistening dryness in the bronchial, digestive and urinary tracts. Clearly, no further justification is necessary for its inclusion in numerous formulas. But then again, how could we omit a mention of its superlative *anti-inflammatory, anti-infective* and *antivenomous* actions (flavonoids and saponins again involved)?

On the basis of both experimental and clinical evidence, there is no question that Western licorice, the species *Glycyrrhiza glabra,* shares the same therapeutic value as Asian licorice. The two kinds can therefore be exchanged in complete confidence whenever neccessary.

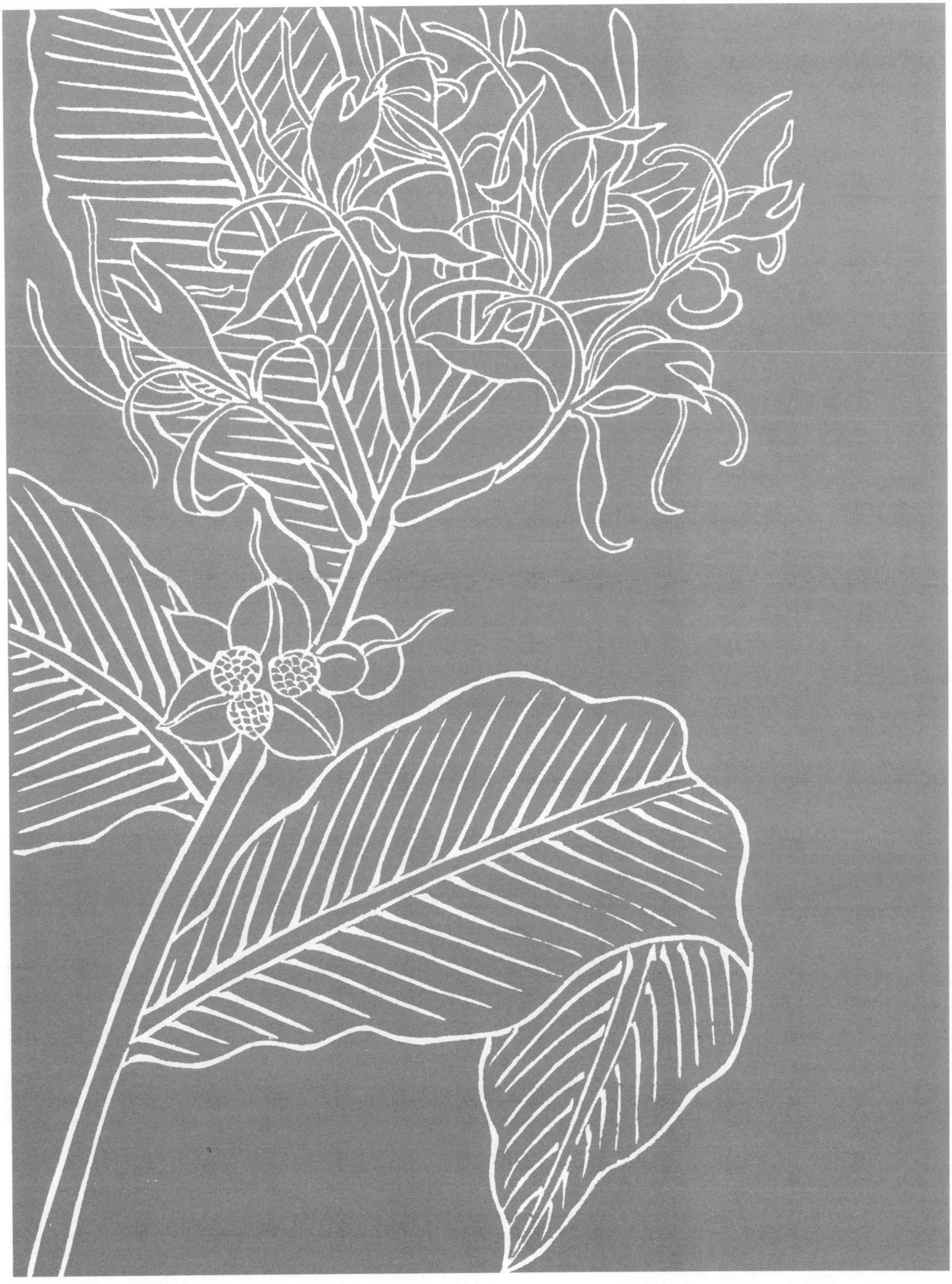

清炎解毒用药

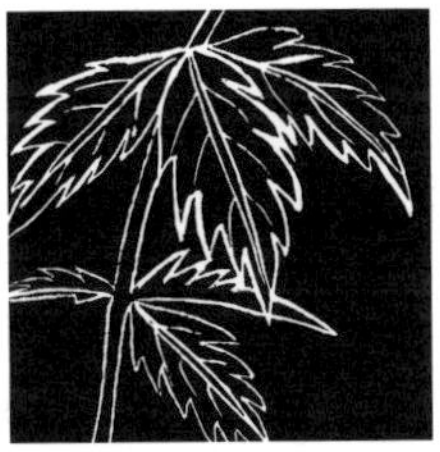

Remedies for Infection, Toxicosis and Parasitosis

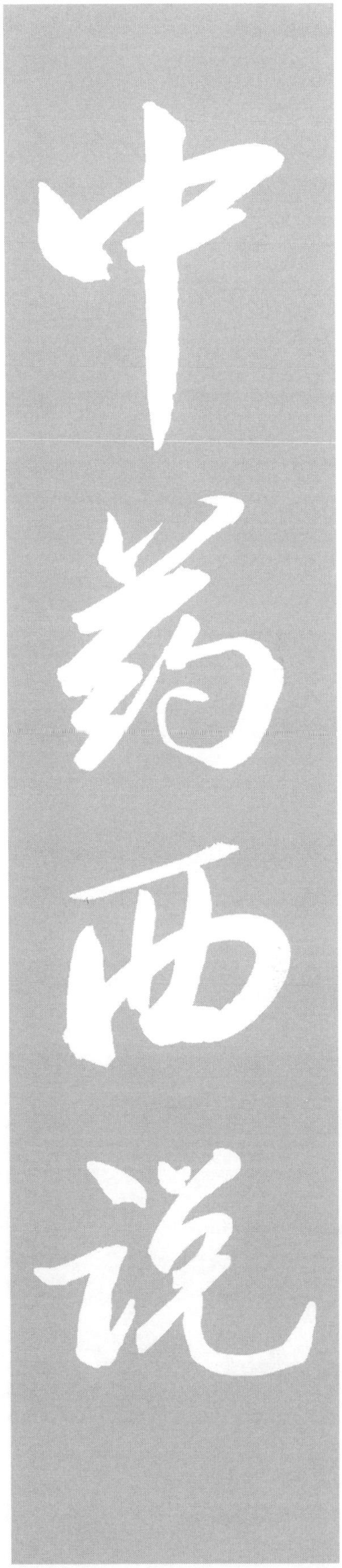

Herbal remedies that treat infection and toxicosis have served humankind since prehistory and continue to be used for these purposes the world over. Medicinal plants that stimulate immune functions, reduce infection and inflammation, reduce fever, clear toxins and enhance lymphatic drainage have been an integral part of the health care system of the Far East for millenniums.

More specifically, Asian medicine has at its disposal some of the most powerful botanical *antimicrobial* and *antiparasitic* agents known. These deal both remedially and preventively with infection and proliferation of various microorganisms, including bacteria, viruses, spirochetes, mycoses (funguses), protozoa, amoebas and helminths (worms). In addition, *resolvent detoxicant* remedies comprehensively address various forms of toxicosis—the excessive generation and/or retention of endogenous and exogenous toxins. By mainly addressing microbial and metabolic forms of toxicosis, these *detoxicants* are especially effective at treating eczema and tumors.

Remedies in this section are divided into three basic types: those that treat infection, those that treat toxicosis and those that treat parasitosis. The three remedy classes in this section consist of:

- ***broad-spectrum anti-infectives*** that treat infection involving fever and inflammation.
- ***resolvent detoxicants*** that address toxicosis accompanied by skin disorders and tumors.
- ***antiparasitics*** that clear internal and topical parasites.

The Remedies for Infection

Remedies in this section are used to treat infections with resulting fever and inflammation, conditions variously known in Chinese medicine as **wind heat, damp heat** and **fire toxin** or **toxic heat,** depending on the symptom picture presenting. These remedies are generally known as *broad-spectrum anti-infectives* because they counteract a wide variety of pathogenic microorganisms, especially bacteria, viruses and funguses. This they do in two ways: One, by stimulating immune functions and increasing defense response to pathogens; and second, by disinfecting locally at the site of infection. Because their *anti-infective* action consists, for the most part, of a combined systemic *immunostimulant* action and a local *antiseptic* one, their efficiency is very high in terminating infections.

Anti-infective remedies in this section are additionally strongly *antipyretic, anti-inflammatory* and *detoxicant.* That is to say, they reduce fever, inflammation and toxins—functions entirely appropriate and synergistic in promoting a resolution of infection. The multi-faceted action of these herbs results from a spontaneous and self-regulating synergism with the individual's own capacity to keep (potential) pathogens under control and maintain homeostasis. This occurs regardless of whether microorganismic dysbiosis (imbalance) is generated internally (endogenously), externally (exogenously), or by a combination of these two.

The infectious conditions treated by *anti-infective* remedies are essentially divided in Oriental medicine into **wind heat** and **damp heat** conditions. Both types of heat may additionally present **fire toxin,** which in particular refers to swollen, hot, discolored, painful and often pyogenic lesions accompanied by fever, such as acute laryngitis, furunculosis, abscesses, mastitis and stomatitis.

Wind heat denotes the onset of acute upper respiratory infections presenting fever and inflammation, such as laryngitis and sinusitis (for which the *cool diaphoretics* and *anti-inflammatories* of the Nose, Throat and Eyes section are also employed). With lower respiratory involvement, the syndrome is called **lung wind heat.**

Damp heat conditions are, for the most part, acute febrile bacterial infections. The essential features of **damp heat** are swelling due to exudates, redness from inflammation, and pain from tissue irritation. With **fire toxin** present there is also fetid, purulent discharge caused by irritation to the mucous membrane. The actual site of the infection will determine the specific type of damp heat syndrome generated, which is named accordingly. Thus, **intestines damp heat** consists of urgent, frequent loose stool, sometimes blood in the stool and burning passing of stool, along with fever. This is found in cases of acute enteritis and bacterial and amoebic dysentery. The keynote symptoms of **bladder damp heat,** on the other hand, are urgent, frequent, painful urination, cloudy urine, fever, thirst and dry mouth; they clearly signal urinary tract infections. In the bronchi, infections such as acute bronchitis or pneumonia may result in syndromes such as **lung phlegm heat** (with a productive cough present), **lung heat dryness** (with no cough present).

How do these natural *anti-infectives* work? In traditional energetic terms, they possess intensely bitter, astringent, cold, dry and sinking (downward moving) effective qualities that are known to clear heat, i.e., reduce fever and inflammation, and dry damp, i.e., stop discharge—producing a net disinfectant action. This is why, from the vitalistic perspective of the four essential herb actions—*restoring, relaxing, stimulating, sedating*—*anti-infective* remedies are considered *sedating* by nature. *Sedating* remedies in each body system address infection of that system, and under each system is found a full description of the infectious conditions they treat, together with their symptom pictures and Western diseases.

Some *anti-infectives* in this section are particularly effective *immune stimulants,* among them Andrographis Chuan Xin Lian (Heart-thread lotus leaf, common throughout South Asia) and Oldenlandia Bai Hua She She Cao (Snaketongue grass herb from Southeast Asia), the latter resembling Echinacea root in respect to this action. Others that are more widely and strongly *antiseptic* and entail *antiviral, antifungal* and *antiprotozoal* properties, include Coptis Huang Lian (Goldthread root from the Central China mountains) and Isatis Da Qing Ye (Woad leaf from South China).

Many *anti-infectives* contain flavonoid glycosides that give them their characteristic yellow color, another telltale sign of their *antimicrobial* nature. Biochemically, these plants contain such constituents as alkaloids, essential oils and glycosides, which are presumed responsible for their *anti-infective* and *immunostimulant* actions. Alkaloids are found in several plants in this section, notably in Coptis Huang Lian (Goldthread root), Berberis San Ke Zhen (the common three-needle barberry root) and Phellodendron Huang Bai (Siberian cork tree bark from Northeast Asia). Usnic acid contained in Usnea Song Luo (the common temperate Beard lichen thallus) is a strong *antibacterial* compound.

In modern times, *in vitro* (laboratory) and *in vivo* (clinical) studies both have shown that certain herbs are more effective against certain types of microorganisms than they are against others. Coptis Huang Lian (Goldthread root), for example, is known to be more effective with gram-negative bacilli than gram-positive ones, and more effective with influenza viruses than with others. Likewise, among the remedies that kill parasites, there are some that are more efficacious at killing and expelling intestinal worms, some that excel at ridding the body of blood flukes, others that will counteract malaria, and so on.

It is important to remember that, unlike synthetic antibiotic drugs, plant *anti-infectives* work with the organism's own defense functions, not against them. By acting in conjunction with the individual's life force rather than overriding it, they avoid the familiar side effects associated with antibiotics, such as weakened intestinal microflora and diminished immune functioning. Ultimately, their ease of use makes them superior to synthetic antibiotics, life-saving though these can sometimes be. It is known that antibiotics progressively weaken the organism as they carry out their "search and destroy" mission with mechanical disregard for the organism's own defense efforts. Besides, in working in cooperation with the organism rather than in spite of it, botanical *anti-infectives* also preserve the beneficial microorganisms that are needed to maintain the integrity of a person's eubiosis, or optimal balance of beneficial microorganisms.

Broad-spectrum anti-infectives are used in one of two ways: preventively or curatively. First, they can prevent contagion during an acute epidemic caused by an exogenous pathogen, such as influenza. They should be taken as soon as a person feels an infection coming on. At the onset of an infection, the immune system can mount a more effective defense, and the chances of a speedy resolution are much higher. Second, they can cure an infection that is already established.

Anti-infective remedies should not be taken, as they sometimes mistakenly are, for the purpose of strengthening immune functions in times of relative good health. They do not have the endocrine depth of action that *immune enhancers* alone possess, a type of action necessary for building general, nonspecific resistance. When taken over time, *immune enhancers* can prevent the occurrence of infections by reinforcing the ground of the individual on endocrine, nervous and humoral levels. In a predisposed environment, infection can ultimately only be prevented from flaring up by strengthening immune functions, balancing the intestinal flora and regulating the overall ecology of beneficial microorganisms (see Holmes 1989).

It should be emphasized that certain posological (dosage) protocols need to be adhered to for *anti-infectives* to work best. First, higher-than-normal dosages are the rule for unfolding *antimicrobial* action in these plants. Up to 60 g of a dried herb or herb combination may be needed for a single dose, repeated four or more times throughout the day. In tincture form, the equivalent dose would be one teaspoon of tincture.

Second, with acute infections, the herb, formula or tincture should be repeated several times throughout the day; in severe cases, one dose should be taken every hour. Thousands of years of experience, corroborated by scientific tests, also show that maximum *antimicrobial* results are achieved by judicious herb combining, rather than by administering a single remedy alone. In the phenomenon of herb synergy, taking two or more plants together potentiates—or increases—their individual actions, resulting in a greater, more powerful effect.

The Remedies for Toxicosis

Toxins are not solely generated from exogenous pathogens. They can accumulate internally from inadequately processed or excessively produced wastes, resulting in **microbial** and **metabolic** forms of **toxicosis.** The interstitial fluid environment and the connective tissue are normally bathed in such endogenous toxins. When a critical level of toxin saturation is reached, infection as we know it may arise. In the case of **microbial toxicosis,** external microorganisms are then more likely to trigger an infection lying dormant in the ground of internal systemic dysbiosis. In the case of **metabolic toxicosis,** symptoms such as malaise, fatigue, headaches, skin rashes, muscle and joint aches, fetid urine and stool, and tumors are liable to appear.

Skin conditions present a very clear example of the two endogenous forms of toxicosis. When acute, inflammatory, allergic and pruritic, and when presenting **wind heat** (e.g., atopic dermatitis), they arise from **microbial toxicosis.** Skin disorders that are chronic and cold, and when presenting **wind cold** (e.g., eczema, psoriasis) arise from **metabolic toxicosis.**

Clearly, although Chinese medicine does not have a concept equivalent to toxicosis as such, it certainly does define the results of toxicosis along the parameters of the vitalistic terms wind, damp, heat and cold.

Remedies in this section are called *resolvent detoxicants* because they promote endogenous toxins to be adequately processed and eliminated and, in the same action, resultant symptoms to be resolved. Frequently used general *detoxicants* include Taraxacum Pu Gong Ying (Mongolian dandelion root and herb from temperate Asia) and Viola Zi Hua Di Ding (the common temperate Asian violet root and herb).

The physiological effect of *resolvent detoxicants* can further be broken down into more specific actions, such as *lymphatic decongestant* (reducing lymphatic stasis and lymph gland swelling), *detumescent* (reducing swelling) and *anti-inflammatory* (reducing inflammation). *Resolvent detoxicants* commonly used for dermatitis include Sophora Ku Shen (Yellow pagoda tree root, from the Central Chinese shrub), Smilax Tu Fu Ling (Glabrous greenbrier root, the climber from Central China related to sarsaparilla), Lithospermum Zi Cao (Purple groomwell root from Northeast China) and Dictammus Bai Xian Pi (Dittany root bark from Mid China).

Those botanicals frequently occurring in formulas for cancers of various types include Solanum Long Kui (the Eurasian Winter cherry herb), Oldenlandia Bai Hua She She Cao (Snaketongue grass herb) and Scutellaria Ban Zhi Lian (Barbed skullcap root). It must be remembered, however, that excellent *antitumoral* remedies are found throughout the Materia Medica, not in this section alone.

A large variety of chemical compounds have been observed to be active in *detoxicant* botanicals. Foremost among them are saponins (in Smilax Tu Fu Ling and Solanum Long Kui, for example), flavonoids (in Scutellaria Ban Zhi Lian, Sophora Ku Shen and Viola Zi Hua Di Ding) and alkaloids (in Solanum Long Kui and Sophora Ku Shen). Like their companion *anti-infectives, detoxicants* in vitalistic pharmacology are considered cold in quality with stimulating, dissolving and astringing secondary qualities.

Many remedies in this section can be used to treat both acute infectious conditions and chronic toxicosic conditions presenting eczema or tumors. They include the commonly employed Lonicera Jin Yin Hua (Japanese honeysuckle flower, the aggressive twining vine from temperate East Asia also found on North America's east coast) and Forsythia Lian Qiao (Forsythia valve, another common sprawling lowland shrub). However, the majority of herbs have a primary therapeutic emphasis that determines their most common usage.

The Remedies for Parasitosis

Parasitic infestation also has been managed since time immemorial by Oriental plant remedies. Although most *antiparasitic* herbs will treat a variety of parasitic conditions, including worms (helminths), protozoa and rickettsiae, all have specific applications that produce optimal results. Cucurbita Nan Gua Zi (the common temperate Red squash seed), Areca Bing Lang (Betel nut from the Asian palm tree) and Torreya Fei Zi (Torreya seed from the East China tree) are the mildest, multi-purpose *anthelmintics.* They mainly treat intestinal parasites or worms, and are ideal for children's conditions. They are all, incidentally, especially effective for tapeworm (taeniasis). Quisqualis Shi Jun Zi (Rangoon creeper fruit from the Southeast Asian climbing vine), Melia Ku Lian Pi (Bead tree root bark from South China) and Melia Chuan Lian Zi (Sichuan bead tree berry from the deciduous Sichuanese tree) work best for roundworm (ascariasis).

Then there are those remedies that are more widely *antiparasitic* as well as specifically *anthelmintic,* among them Brucea Ya Dan Zi (Brucea berry from the southern Chinese shrub) and Dichroa Chang Shan (Feverflower root from Central China's valleys). Some are particularly effective in malaria, like both these and Artemisia Huang Hua Hao (the temperate Eurasian Annual wormwood herb), while the first two will also most effectively terminate amoebic conditions.

Because some of these remedies contain compounds that produce cumulative toxicity when taken every day, care should be taken with respect to dosage, administration and number of days ingested. The directions and cautions given at the end of each herb presentation should be read carefully by anyone using them, including when taken in patent remedy (e.g., pill, extract, etc.) form.

➤ DISPEL WIND HEAT AND DETOXIFY FIRE TOXIN

Broad-spectrum anti-infectives: immunostimulants, antivirals, antibacterials, antifungals, antipyretics, anti-inflammatories

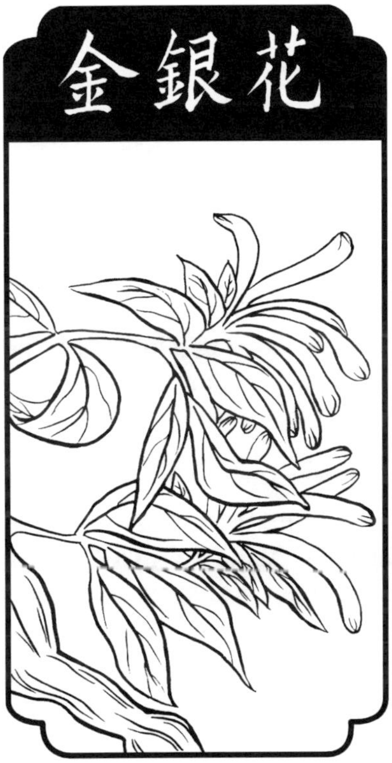

Lonicera Jin Yin Hua

Japanese Honeysuckle Flower

Botanical source: *Lonicera japonica* Thunberg and spp. (Caprifoliaceae)
Pharmaceutical name: Flos Lonicerae
Chinese names: Jin Yin Hua, Ren Dong Hua, (Shan) Yin Hua, Shuang Hua (Mand); Gam Ngan Fa, Yan Dung Fa (Cant)
Other names: Woodbine, "Gold silver flower", "Enduring winter flower"; Kinginka, Nindo (Jap)
Habit: Perennial twining shrub or vine from temperate East Asia, especially Shandong and Henan; grows in hilly forest outskirts, woods and ravines; also cultivated throughout China; flowers in early summer with aromatic white and later golden yellow, slender axillary flowers.
Part used: the flower bud and small flower

Therapeutic category: mild remedy with minimal chronic toxicity
Constituents: chlorogenic and isochlorogenic acids, saponins, flavonoid luteolin, inositol, tannins, essential oil (incl. linalool, ethyl palmitate)
Effective qualities: sweet, astringent, cold, dry
stimulating, astringing, dissolving
Tropism: respiratory, digestive, lymphatic systems
Lung, Stomach, Large Intestine channels; Warmth, Air bodies

Actions and Indications

broad-spectrum anti-infective: immunostimulant, antiviral, antibacterial, antifungal: acute infections (incl. common cold, influenza, herpes, HIV, enteritis, bacillary dysentery with melena, pneumonia, infected wounds, fungal/yeast infections, erysipelas, leptospirosis, scabies); esp. *Staphylococcus, Streptococcus*; many gram-negative bacilli
leukocytogenic: leukopenia
detoxicant, anti-inflammatory: microbial toxicosis with acute pyogenic local infections with heat, swelling and pain (incl. laryngitis, conjunctivitis, tonsillitis, lymphadenitis, mastitis, hepatitis; boils, carbuncles, abscesses)
lymphatic decongestant, dissolvent: swollen glands, fibrocystic breasts
antilipemic: hypercholesterolemia, atherosclerosis
antitumoral, interferon inducent: cancer (esp. mammary, lymphatic)
antipyretic: fever (esp. infectious)
hypotensive, diuretic: hypertension
uterine stimulant, abortive: miscarriage
astringent, detergent, vulnerary: skin ulcers, corneal ulcer, cervical erosion

Symptom Pictures

external wind heat with **fire toxin:** sore throat, swollen glands, red eyes, fever, fear of wind, headache
intestines damp heat: burning, difficult passing of stool, diarrhea with blood, abdominal pain, thirst, fever
microbial toxicosis with **fire toxin:** malaise, boils, skin rashes, frequent infections

Preparation

Use: The flower Lonicera Jin Yin Hua is prepared by a short decoction or used in tincture form. Topical washes, etc., can be made for surface conditions, especially ulcers.

Dosage: Decoction: 10-60 g
Tincture: 2-5 ml

Caution: Forbidden in diarrhea due to cold deficiency of the intestines, in sores with clear exudate due to low immunity, in chronic cold ulcers and during pregnancy.

Notes

The fragrant flower of the Japanese honeysuckle vine is a major *detoxicant* and *immune modulating* remedy. Its efficacity in resolving acute infections is due, among other components, to its content in chlorogenic acids and the monoterpenol linalool. Japanese honeysuckle is especially appropriate when fever, inflammation and purulence prevail. These manifestations are collectively known as "fire toxin" in Chinese medicine, and can be described as often arising from a deeper terrain condition of preinfectious microbial toxicosis, i.e., a proliferation and injurious pleomorphic deterioration of normally beneficial symbiotic microbes. As a *resolvent* to this systemic dysbiosis, therefore, Japanese honeysuckle (as many others in this section) will relieve external and internal signs of heat, i.e., both early and advanced stages of febrile or inflammatory infection. The remedy's *lymph decongestant* action is just a part of its overall *detoxicant* and *resolvent* effect.

Note also this remedy's tropism for the breast: fibrocystic conditions and breast cancer are among the conditions that have responded well to it.

This Japanese species of honeysuckle (*Lonicera japonica*) should not be confused with a less-used species, *Lonicera confusa,* properly known as **Tu Yin Hua** (Mand.) or **To Gan Fa** (Cant). The "confused honeysuckle" is mainly used for clearing fire toxin and local heat (e.g., boils, dermatitis, dysentery, etc.), and to that extent is interchangeable with the Japanese species.

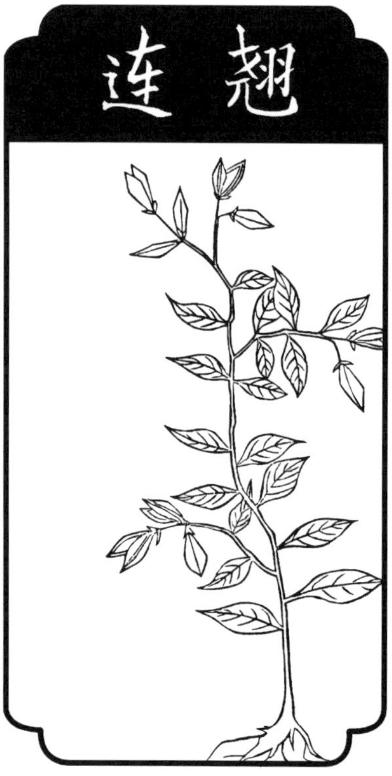

Forsythia Lian Qiao

Forsythia Valve

Botanical source: *Forsythia suspensa* (Thunb.) Vahl, *F. viridissima, F. koreana* (Oleaceae)
Pharmaceutical name: Fructus Forsythiae
Chinese names: Lian Qiao, Er Cao, San Lian (Mand); Lin Kiu (Cant)
Other names: Golden bells, Weeping forsythia; Rengyo (Jap)
Habit: Deciduous sprawling temperate shrub from North and Central China; found in sunny, warm, damp, low-lying areas and commonly cultivated; blooms in spring with shining yellow axillary flowers.
Part used: the immature, green fruit valve (capsule) with its seeds

---

Therapeutic category: mild remedy with minimal chronic toxicity
Constituents: essential oil, triterpenoid saponins (incl. phillyrin), forsythol, forsythiaside, pinoresinol glucosides, arctiin, forsythine, oleanolic/ursolic/betulinic acids, sterols, matairesinoids, alkaloids, flavonoids (incl. rutin), coumarins, lignan
Effective qualities: bitter, a bit pungent and astringent, cold
stimulating, dissolving, astringing, thickening
Tropism: respiratory, urinary, lymphatic, epidermal systems
Heart, Liver, Gallbladder, Lung, Triple Warmer channels

Actions and Indications

broad-spectrum anti-infective: immunotimulant, antiviral, antibacterial, antifungal, phagocyte stimulant: acute respiratory, urinary, skin infections, (incl. common cold, influenza, measles, nephritis, pyelitis, cystitis; dermatitis, ringworm); gram-positive and gram-negative bacilli (incl. *Staphylococcus aureus, Diplococcus pneumoniae, Shigella* spp., *Pasteurella pestis, Mycobacterium tuberculosis, Salmonella typhi/paratyphi, Eschericia coli*)

antiparasitic: tinea, scabies, pinworms [oxyuriasis]), giardiasis, malaria

detoxicant, anti-inflammatory, dermatropic: microbial toxicosis with acute pyogenic local infections with heat and swelling (incl. laryngitis, pharyngitis, lymphangitis, nephritis; boils, carbuncles, abscesses, acute and chronic dermatitis)

lymphatic decongestant, dissolvent: lymphadenitis, lymph gland TB, scrofula

antipyretic, diuretic: fevers (incl. eruptive fevers)

detergent, vulnerary: ulcers, wounds

hemostatic, coagulant: hemorrhage (incl. retinal)

laxative, emmenagogue

cardiotonic

antiemetic: vomiting in all conditions

Miscellaneous: deafness

Symptom Pictures

external wind heat with **fire toxin:** fever, slight chills, sore throat, swollen glands

microbial toxicosis with **fire toxin:** malaise, skin rashes, boils, urinary irritation, poor immunity

Preparation

Use: The fruit valve of Forsythia Lian Qiao is decocted or used in tincture form. Topical preparations such as swabs, compresses and gargles are also made with it.

Dosage: Infusion: 10-30 g
Tincture: 2-5 ml

Caution: Forbidden in diarrhea due to deficiency cold of the intestines, in sores with clear exudate due to low immunity, and in carbuncles that have already ulcerated.

Notes

Like Japanese honeysuckle flower with which it is often combined, Forsythia valve is a cold *detoxicant* remedy. Specifically, its broad-spectrum *anti-infective, immune stimulant* and *anti-inflammatory* actions are ideal for addressing microbial toxicosis presenting acute inflammatory and infectious forms of pathology. With purulence and lymphatic stasis present, this fire toxin removing herb is especially appropriate.

The bitter-cold Forsythia valve also excells in resolving acute or long-term skin conditions in particular—whether due to toxicosis, lymphatic stasis, inflammation, fungal infection or other causes. Its *antiparasitic* action completes the profile of a remedy that addresses some of the more long-term fruits of systemic (not just intestinal) dysbiosis.

Forsythia valve is reminiscent of Marigold flower (*Calendula officinalis*) in Western phytotherapy, yet somewhat *cooler* and overall more *draining*. As with Marigold, an impressive, broad range of components has been found active in this remedy, including active flavonoids, saponins, lignans and pinoresinol glucosides (Hikino 1990).

This remedy's reliable *antiemetic* effect operates by inhibiting the vomiting reflex originating in the medulla.

Forsythia root, Lian Qiao Gen (Mand.) or **Lin Kiu Gan** (Cant.), is reputed as an *antipyretic, hepatic* and *circulatory stimulant remedy.*

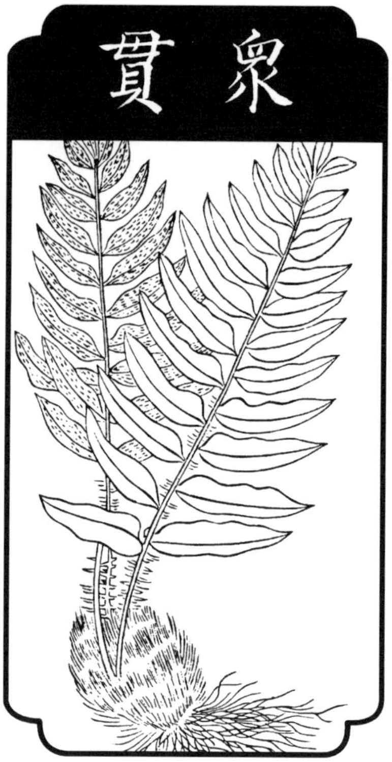

Dryopteris Guan Zhong

Shield Fern Root

Botanical source: *Dryopteris crassirhizoma* Nakai (Polypodiaceae) and *Osmunda japonica* Thunberg (Osmundaceae)
Pharmaceutical name: Rhizoma Dryopteris
Chinese names: Guan Zhong (Mand); Gwun Jung (Cant); *Dryopt.:* Mian Ma Guan Zhong, Dong Bei Guan Zhong; *Osm.:* Zi Qi Guan Zhong (Mand)
Other names: Wood fern, "Link masses"; *Osm.:* Flowering fern; Kanju, Tohokukanju (Jap)
Habit: *Dryopt.:* Perennial East Asian fern growing along ditches and roads and in rock crevices in damp, shady places.
Osm.: Perennial East Asian fern growing in very acidic soil; found in woods, by creek and streamsides and on slopes.
Part used: the rhizome and leaf stalk base

Therapeutic category: medium-strength remedy with some chronic toxicity
Constituents: *Dryopteris:* filicic/filicinic/flavaspidic acids, filicin, traces albaspidin and dryocrassin, filmarone, aspidin, paraspidin, aspidinol, deaspidin, fernene, pterosterone, tannin, essential oil, resin
Osmunda: ponasterone A, ecdysterone, ecdysone
Effective qualities: bitter, astringent, cool, dry
astringing, thickening, sinking, stabilizing
Tropism: digestive, respiratory, reproductive systems
Liver, Stomach, Spleen channels
Fluid, Warmth bodies

Actions and Indications

broad-spectrum anti-infective: antiviral, antibacterial: acute and chronic respiratory, intestinal, and systemic infections (incl. viral influenza, common cold, dysentery, epidemic meningitis, measles, viral pneumonia, acute infectious hepatitis, scarlet fever, typhoid; chronic bronchitis); esp. many strains of *Myxovirus influenzae, Shigella dysentericae, Salmonella typhi, Escherichia coli, Pseudomonas aeruginosa, Proteus vulgaris*
antiparasitic, anthelmintic: parasites, incl. tapeworm (taeniasis), hookworm (ancylostomiasis), pinworm (enterobiasis), roundworm (ascariasis), trichuriasis, giardiasis, trichomoniasis, schistosomiasis, filariasis
detoxicant, anti-inflammatory, analgesic: microbial toxicosis with boils, sores, furuncles (incl. from infection)
antipyretic: fever (esp. with macular eruptions)
coagulant hemostatic: hemorrhage (incl. uterine bleeding, postpartum bleeding, coughing up and vomiting blood, blood in stool)
astringent: dysentery, enteritis
uterine stimulant, parturient, abortive: uterine dystocia, miscarriage, placental retention
estrogenic
water purifying

Symptom Pictures

external wind heat/cold with **fire toxin:** sneezing, aches and pains, feverishness

intestines damp heat: burning, difficult passing of stool, diarrhea with blood, fever, abdominal pain, thirst

Preparation

Use: The root Dryopteris Guan Zhong is decocted or used in tincture form. The powder may be used in capsules or pill form.

Dosage: Decoction: 6-16 g
Pill, capsule: 0.6-1 g
Tincture: 0.4-1 ml (8-25 drops)

Caution: Contraindicated for pregnant women, children and weak people; also forbidden in peptic ulcers and organic disease in general. Dosages should not be exeeded because of Dryopteris Guan Zhong's medium-strength nature. Usage should be limited to one or two doses. Fatty foods should not be taken 6 hours before or after taking this remedy, as this increases absorption and hence toxicity. Signs of toxicity include indigestion, nausea, vomiting, diarrhea and visual disturbances.

Notes

Although Shield fern root is famed for both its *antiparasitic* and *antiviral* effects, today this remedy is definitely considered to possess a wider *anti-infective* action. Highly effective with a broad range of influenza and other viruses, the botanical also acts rapidly on many gram-negative bacillary conditions. Microbial toxicosis and parasitosis arising from intestinal dysbiosis are the two ground conditions that it addresses. The filicic acid content makes it *vermicidal* for tapeworms.

Shield fern root is also much used in veterinary medicine, e.g., for swine ascariasis, earthworms and leeches, and for bovine liver, flat and broad sucker flukes.

Shield fern root is closely related to the Western *Dryopteris filix mas*, **Male fern,** which is also used in China. However, Shield fern is preferred over Male fern as it is considerably less toxic.

Numerous plants are sourced for the remedy Guan Zhong. They include: *Osmunda japonica* Thunberg (Japanese flowering fern), *Lunathyrium crostichoides* (Sw.) Ching, also known as **E Mei Jue Guan Zhong;** *Matteuccia stuthiopteris* (L.) Todaro (Ostrich-feather fern), also called **Jia Guo Jue Guan Zhong** and **Xiao Yue Guan Zhong;** *Blechnum orientale* L. or **Wu Mao Jue Guan Zhong** or **Dong Fang Wu Mao Jue Ye** (Oriental hammock fern); *Brainia insignis* (Hook.) J. Sm. or **Su Tie Jue Guan Zhong;** *Woodwardia japonica* (L.f.) Sm. or **Gou Ji Guan Zhong** or **Da Ye Guan Zhong** (Japanese chain fern); *Cyrtomium fortunei* J. Sm. or **Hun Ji Tou.**

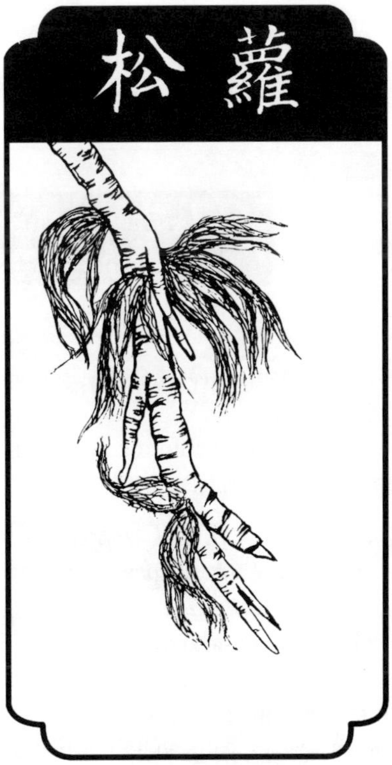

Usnea Song Luo

Beard Lichen Thallus

Botanical source: *Usnea diffracta* Vain. or *U. longissima* Ach. (Usneaceae)
Pharmaceutical name: Thallus Usneae
Chinese names: Song Luo, Hai Feng Teng (Mand) Chung Lo (Cant)
Other names: Old man's beard, Witch's broom; Saruogase (Jap)
Habit: Gray-green colored lichen growing in pantemperate woods and forests on the trunks and branches of coniferous trees; grows in tufts as well as longer, beard-like strands.
Part used: the mycelia or thallus

Therapeutic category: mild remedy with minimal chronic toxicity
Constituents: bitter substance usnic acid up to 5%, barbatic, diffractaic and evernic acids, polysaccharides, mucilage
Effective qualities: sweet, a bit bitter, cool
stimulating, relaxing
Tropism: respiratory, digestive, reproductive, immune, lymphatic systems
Lung, Liver channels
Air, Warmth bodies

Actions and Indications

broad-spectrum anti-infective: immunostimulant, antibacterial: respiratory, intestinal urinary infections (incl. common cold, influenza, sinusitis, pharyngitis, gastroenteritis, pleurisy, pneumonia, lung and lymph TB; typhus, vaginitis, gonorrhea, impetigo, cystitis, urethritis); esp. gram-positive bacilli and cocci (incl. *Streptococcus, Mycobacterium tuberculosis*)

antiparasitic, antiprotozoal, antifungal: trichomoniasis, schistosomiasis, giardiasis, ringworm, candidiasis

detoxicant, anti-inflammatory: microbial toxicosis, conjunctivitis, boils, carbuncles, burns

antipyretic, diuretic: fevers in general

analgesic: headache

vulnerary, antiseptic: wounds (incl. suppurative wounds); cervical erosion, cracked nipples

bronchodilator, expectorant, antitussive: acute and chronic bronchitis with coughing, asthma

Symptom Pictures

external wind heat/cold: headache, aches and pains, sneezing, sore throat, feverishness, nasal congestion

lung phlegm heat with **Qi constraint:** coughing, expectoration of thick yellow sputum, wheezing

Preparation

Use: The whole thallus Usnea Song Luo is infused in cold water for 6 hours or used in tincture form. Topical washes, compresses, douches, vaginal sponges, etc., are also prepared with it. Gargles are excellent for throat infections.

Dosage: Cold water infusion: 10-30 g
Tincture: 2-4ml

Caution: None.

Notes

Named for its beard-like growth on forest trees, all species of Beard lichen have a long history of use by the Chinese, European and Native American peoples. Beard lichen is more than just a good *anti-infective* remedy for bronchitis and lung tuberculosis: Its twin *immunostimulant* and *bacterio/fungostatic* actions, due to the polysaccharides and usnic acid content respectively, prevent and clear a wide variety of infections.

Because of its *anti-inflammatory, antipyretic* and *analgesic* actions, Beard lichen is particularly suited to resolving wind heat onsets of upper respiratory infections displaying feverishness and pain. Its *antifungal* action makes it ideal for treating dysbiotic terrain evolving into candidiasis.

Allium Da Suan
Garlic Bulb

大蒜

Botanical source: *Allium sativum* L. (Liliaceae)
Chinese names: Da Suan (Mand); Daai San (Cant)
Category: mild remedy with minimal chronic toxicity
Constituents: allicin, garlicin, allistatine, essential oil, glucokinins, ferments, cholin, silicic acid, trace elements and vitamins
Effective qualities: pungent, sweet, hot, dry; stimulating, decongesting, dispersing
Tropism: digestive, circulatory, cardiovascular, respiratory systems; Lung, Stomach, Spleen, Large Intestine

Actions: *Broad-spectrum anti-infective (imunostimulant, antibacterial, antiviral, antifungal, antiparasitic [antiamoebic], antivenomous), diaphoretic, vulnerary, analgesic, stimulant expectorant, circulatory stimulant, coronary decongestant, digestive stimulant, draining diuretic, anticoagulant, resolvent, antitumoral*

Indications: Bacterial and viral epidemics, onset of infections: flu, common cold, infections with damp heat (incl. enteritis, dysentery), diphtheria, typhus, encephalitis, bronchitis, laryngitis; early stage of boils, skin and lung TB, food poisoning with diarrhea; fungal infections (incl. tinea, ringworm, candidiasis); amoebic infestation (incl. amoebic dysentery); parasitic infestation (incl. pinworm, hookworm, scalp ringworm, giardiasis, scabies, gangrene); insect bites, chronic wounds and ulcers (incl. varicose); microbial and metabolic toxicosis; myalgia, earache, chronic bronchitis, emphysema; chronically cold extremities and chills, fatigue; coronary disease, angina pectoris, cardiac asthma; dyspepsia, intestinal dysbiosis with flatulence, abdominal pain and swelling; water retention; thrombosis, phlebitis, arterio- and atherosclerosis, liver sclerosis, benign and cancerous tumors.

Dosage: In acute infections: 1-2 freshly crushed cloves (8-20 g) eaten immediately.

In chronic conditions: lower end of the above dose. Garlic bulb may be infused but should never be decocted.

Tincture: 0.5-2 ml (12-50 drops)

Caution: Do not use in Yin, fluids and Blood (metabolic) deficiency conditions; in premature ejaculation, spermatorrhea and tendency to spontaneous bleeding; during pregnancy and lactation.

Broad-spectrum anti-infectives: immunostimulants, antivirals, antibacterials, antifungals, antipyretics, anti-inflammatories

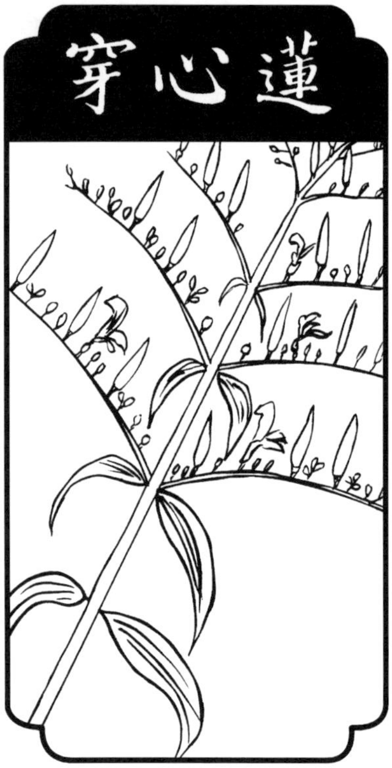

Andrographis Chuan Xin Lian

Heart-Thread Lotus Leaf *

Botanical source: *Andrographis paniculata* (Burman f.) Nees (Acanthaceae)
Pharmaceutical name: Folium Andrographis
Chinese names: Chuan Xin Lian, Yi Jian Xi, Lan He Lian (Mand); Chyun Sam Ling (Cant)
Other names: Creat, Halviva, Kariyat, Green chiretta; Senshinren (Jap)
Habit: Annual or perennial cultivated herb; also grows wild in thickets throughout South Asia; in summer and autumn cymes of small white terminal and axillary flowers appear.
Part used: the leaf

Therapeutic category: mild remedy with minimal chronic toxicity
Constituents: lactones, flavonoids, aldehydes, ketones, alkanes, andrographan, andrographolide, hydroxyandrographolide, andrographon, andrographosterin, panicolide, methylwithtin, apigenindimethyl ether, polysaccharides PA and PB (galacturonic acid, galactose, arabinose, rhamnose)
Effective qualities: very bitter, astringent, cold, dry
astringing, stimulating, sinking
Tropism: intestinal, respiratory, hepatobiliary, immune systems
Large Intestine, Lung, Liver channels
Warmth body

Actions and Indications

broad-spectrum anti-infective: immunostimulant, antibacterial, antiviral: acute hepatobiliary, respiratory, intestinal, urinary and systemic infections (incl. acute bacterial dysentery, gastroenteritis, hepatitis, cholecystitis, tonsillitis, influenza, viral pneumonia, pelvic inflammatory disease, HIV infection, urethritis, pyelonephritis; epidemics); esp. *Staphylococcus aureus, Pseudomonas aeruginosa, Proteus vulgaris, Shigella dysentericae, Escherichia coli*
antipyretic: fever, esp. with the above
anti-inflammatory, detoxicant, antivenomous: microbial toxicosis with laryngitis, sores, infected wounds, furunculosis, pustular dermatitis, pulmonary abscess, snakebite
vulnerary: infected wounds
expectorant: respiratory infections, cough with purulent sputum; pneumonia
uterine stimulant, parturient, abortive: miscarriage, prolonged pregnancy, retained placenta
anthelmintic: intestinal parasites

Symptom Pictures

intestines damp heat: burning, difficult passing of stool, diarrhea with blood, fever, abdominal pain, thirst
lung phlegm heat: coughing, expectoration of thick yellow-green sputum
gallbladder heat: sharp right subcostal pains, nausea, fatigue

Preparation

Use: The leaf Andrographis Chuan Xin Lian requires a very short decoction or a long infusion; alternately it may be used in tincture form. Very small doses may be taken as a *bitter digestive* before meals to stimulate digestion.

Dosage: Short decoction: 10-20 g
Tincture: 2-5 ml

Caution: Forbidden in deficiency cold intestinal conditions.

Notes

In light of repeated clinical trials, Heart-thread lotus leaf cultivated in the plains of Shanghai has emerged as one of China's foremost *immune stimulating anti-infective* remedies for a large variety of bacterial, viral and parasitic infections. The leaf's bitter, astringent, cold and dry nature indicates its most suitable applications to be acute conditions presenting fever, inflammation and purulence.

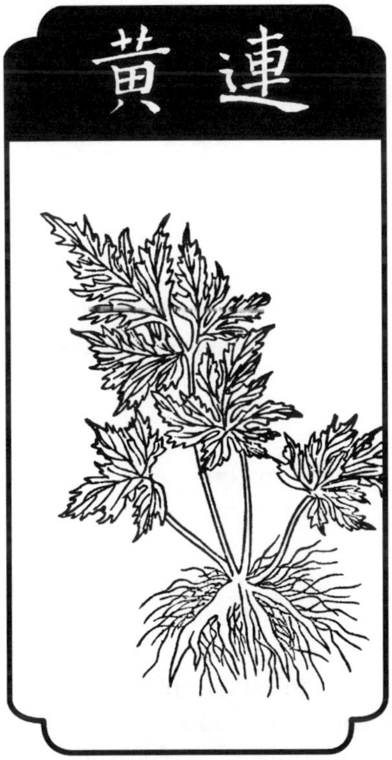

Coptis Huang Lian

Goldthread Root

Botanical source: *Coptis chinensis* Franchet, *C. omeiensis* (Chen) C.Y. Cheng, *C. teetoides* C.Y. Cheng, *C. deltoidea* C.Y.Cheng and spp. (Ranunculaceae)
Pharmaceutical name: Rhizoma Coptis
Chinese names: Huang Lian, Chuan Lian, Wei Lian, Ya Lian, Yun Lian (Mand); Wong Lin, Chyun Wong Lin (Cant)
Other names: Oren (Jap)
Habit: Perennial stemless herb growing in damp, tree-shaded locales in the Central China mountains, especially in Sichuan, Hubei and Yunnan; blooms in spring with cymes of small whitish green terminal flowers.
Part used: the rhizome

Therapeutic category: mild remedy with minimal chronic toxicity
Constituents: alkaloids (incl. berberine 5-8%, coptisine, worenine, palmatine, columbamine, jatrorrhizine, magnoflorine, epiberberine), obakunone, obakulactone, lumicaerulic and ferulic acid, trace minerals (incl. selenium)
Effective qualities: very bitter, astringent, cold, dry
astringing, relaxing, calming, stimulating, sinking
Tropism: digestive, cardiovascular, immune systems
Liver, Gallbladder, Stomach, Large Intestine, Heart channels

Actions and Indications

broad-spectrum anti-infective: immunostimulant, antibacterial, antiviral, broad-spectrum antifungal, antiprotozoal: acute intestinal, respiratory, biliary, gynecological infections (incl. bacillary and amoebic dysentery, cholera, acute gastroenteritis, giardiasis, Crohn's disease [esp. with bleeding]; typhoid fever, flu, whooping cough, lung TB, scarlet fever, diphtheria, pelvic inflammatory disease, trichomoniasis, yeast infections, candidiasis, scarlet fever, brucellosis), fungal skin conditions; esp. *Staphylococcus, Streptococcus, Vibrio cholerae, Bacillus anthracis, Bacillus dysentericae*, gram-negative bacilli

interferon inducent

antipyretic: high fever (esp. with thirst)

anti-inflammatory, detoxicant: toxicosis with acute conjunctivitis and blepharitis, otitis media, tonsillitis, ulcerative colitis, inflammatory bowel disease, cervicitis, vaginitis, glossitis, stomatitis, periodontitis; burns, boils, furuncles, abscesses

hemostatic, astringent: nosebleed, hematuria, hemafecia, hemoptysis, epistaxis; ulcers (all types), canker sores, non-suppurative sores, hemorrhoids
nervous sedative/relaxant, vasorelaxant hypotensive: febrile irritability and agitation; hypertension
biliary and gastric stimulant, choleretic: biliary and gastric dyspepsia, acute and chronic cholecystitis, gastritis, anorexia
intestinal stimulant: constipation
Miscellaneous: leukemia

Symptom Pictures

intestines damp heat: burning, difficult passing of stool, diarrhea with blood, fever, abdominal pain, thirst

stomach damp heat / gallbladder and stomach Qi stagnation: nausea, epigastric pain and bloating, sour regurgitation, vomiting, bad breath, diarrhea or constipation

gallbladder heat: sharp right subcostal pains, nausea, fatigue

Pericardium fire with **nerve excess:** irritability, delirium, insomnia, high fever, coma, bleeding

Preparation

Use: The root Coptis Huang Lian is either decocted or used in tincture form. A wash or swab can be made for eye, skin and middle ear infections and for anal fissures. Vaginal sponges and douches apply in all forms of vaginitis (fungal/ parasitic/bacterial).

Dosage: Decoction: 2-8 g
Tincture: 0.25-3 ml

Smaller doses should be used for stomach damp heat syndrome, larger ones for all other types of hot conditions.

Caution: Contraindicated in the following conditions: Yin deficiency, vomiting from stomach cold, and diarrhea from digestive deficiency and cold. Coptis Huang Lian should never be used on its own continuously, as its cold astringency will eventually impair digestive functions and injure the intestinal microflora.

Notes

Being one of the most cold-natured botanical remedies in the Oriental materia medica, Goldthread root is most commonly used in formulas addressing high fever conditions—when heat needs clearing quickly. In terms of the germ theory it shares with the other bitter, astringent, cold, dry remedies in this section powerful wide-spectrum *antimicrobial* properties. Goldthread is an especially broad-spectrum *antifungal* remedy, hence ideal for fungal terrain in general. Its excellent *astringent* and *anti-inflammatory* actions combine with its *antibacterial* and *antiprotozoal* effect for one of the best botanicals in the treatment of intestinal infections with bleeding present—as in various inflammatory bowel disorders, peptic ulcers and so on.

Like Scutellaria Huang Qin, Goldthread is superlative in chronic forms of cholecystitis and may also be used in small doses as a *biliary stimulant* for digestive distress arising from a stagnation of gallbladder and stomach Qi. Its reliable *astringent hemostatic* action is applied mainly to passive bleeding, including bleeding from ulcers and hemorrhoids.

The best grade of Goldthread is reputed to come from the mountain forests of the mid-western province Sichuan, and is therefore called **Chuan Lian** (Mand.) or **Chyun (Wong) Lin** (Cant.).

Two North American remedies stand out as very similar to this remedy: the indigenous **Goldthread root,** *Coptis teeta* Wall., and **Goldenseal root,** *Hydrastis canadensis.* The latter also belongs to the buttercup family (Ranunculaceae). The latter remedy shares all of Goldthread's properties except for the *hypotensive* action and also shares at least one of its components, the alkaloid berberine.

The root of *Coptis japonica* Makino, **Japanese goldthread,** indigenous to Japan, is sometimes used as a less expensive substitute for *Coptis chinesis.* It contains the alkaloids coptisine, worenine and berberine, and is considered inferior to the original product. The dose is 4-14 g

黄芩

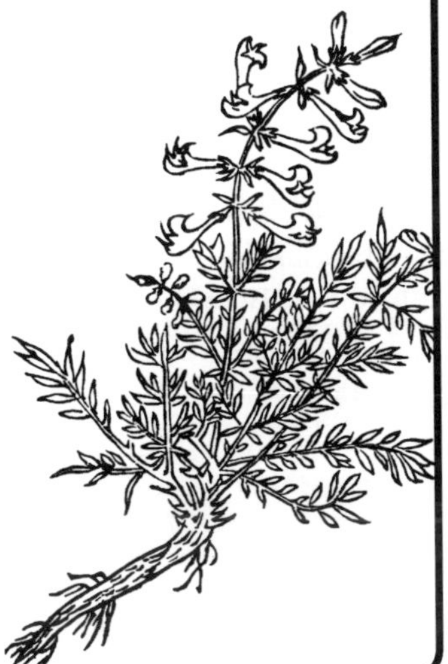

Scutellaria Huang Qin

Baikal Skullcap Root

Botanical source: *Scutellaria baicalensis* Georgi (syn. *B. macrantha* Fischer), *S. amoena* C.H. Wright, *S. viscidula* Bunge (Labiatae)
Pharmaceutical name: Radix Scutellariae
Chinese names: Huang Qin (Mand); Wong Sam, Wong Kam (Cant)
Other names: "Yellow *qin*"; Ogon (Jap)
Habit: Spreading perennial hardy herb from north China's mountain regions, Inner Mongolia and eastern Russia; found on exposed slopes and along roadsides; blooms in spring with racemes of magenta and violet flowers.
Part used: the root

Therapeutic category: mild herb with minimal chronic toxicity
Constituents: alkaloids (incl. baicalein, baicalin), flavonoids (incl. wogonin, wogonoside, oroxylin, skullcap flavonoids I and II, chrysin, various methoxy- and hydroxy-flavones), phytosterols (sitosterol, campestrol), koganebanin, scutellarin, benzoic acid, trace minerals (incl. copper, zinc, manganese)
Effective qualities: bitter, astringent, cold, dry
relaxing, stimulating, astringing, stabilizing, sinking
Tropism: digestive, respiratory, vascular, urogenital, immune systems
Gallbladder, Small Intestine, Large Intestine, Heart, Lung channels
Warmth, Air bodies

Actions and Indications

broad-spectrum anti-infective: immunostimulant, antibacterial, antifungal, antiviral: acute respiratory, intestinal, hepatobiliary, urinary, epidermal infections (incl. rhinitis, pneumonia, bronchitis, bacterial enteritis, dysentery, flu, HIV, adenovirus, rhinovirus, pelvic inflammatory disease, cystitis; yeast infections, fungal skin infections); esp. *Staphylococcus, Streptococcus hemolyticus*; many gram-positive and gram-negative bacilli

detoxicant, anti-inflammatory, astringent: microbial toxicosis, inflammatory bowel disease (incl. ulcerative colitis, Crohn's disease), vaginitis, conjunctivitis, mastitis, otitis, boils, furuncles, acute dermatitis, burns

hemostatic: nosebleed, coughing up blood, blood in stool or urine, excessive menstrual or uterine bleeding

hepatobiliary sedative/stimulant: choleretic, cholagogue, antilipemic: liver congestion, hepatitis (all types), cholecystitis, cholangitis, acute jaundice, biliary and hepatic dyspepsia, poor fats digestion, hyperlipidemia

nervous sedative, hypotensive: unrest, irritability, insomnia; hypertension

immune regulator, antiallergic, bronchodilator: immediate allergies (incl. rhinitis, asthma, otitis media); cytotoxic allergies (incl.food allergies), allergic edema and inflammation

relaxant diuretic: dysuria, strangury

fetal relaxant, antiabortive: fetal distress, threatened miscarriage

interferon inducent

Symptom Pictures

liver and gallbladder damp heat with **Liver Yang rising:** irritability, feeling stressed, headache, right subcostal pain, bitter taste in mouth, jaundice

gallbladder heat: sharp right subcostal pains, nausea, fatigue

lung phlegm heat: coughing, expectoration of thick yellow-green sputum

intestines damp heat: burning, difficult passing of stool, diarrhea with blood, fever, abdominal pain, thirst

lung Qi constraint: coughing fits, wheezing, allergies

bladder damp heat: burning, dribbling, urgent or ineffective urination, dark yellow urine

Preparation

Use: The root Scutellaria Huang Qin is decocted or used in tincture form. Washes, douches, sponges, etc. are also made.

Dosage: Decoction: 6-18 g
Tincture: 2-4 ml

Caution: Forbidden in diarrhea from intestines cold, fetal unrest from cold in the uterus, and deficiency lung heat.

Notes

The bitter, drying and very cooling Baikal skullcap root is noted for its wide-ranging *anti-infective, anti-inflammatory* and *antiallergic* actions. These are traditionally applied in the damp heat types of symptom pictures above—acute conditions for the most part.

For contemporary health concerns, the remedy should also specifically be seen as a comprehensive agent for the liver and gallbladder (including fat metabolism) and a remedy for various hypersensitivity/allergic conditions (including true food allergies). Baikal skullcap turns out to be important for treating hyperlipidemia as well as intestinal dysbiosis, microbial toxicosis and the many resultant forms of hypersensitivity, inflammatory and infectious pathology.

The North American **Skullcap herb,** *Scutellaria lateriflora,* has but few actions in common with the Baikal skullcap, and in herbal practice is used quite differently.

大青葉

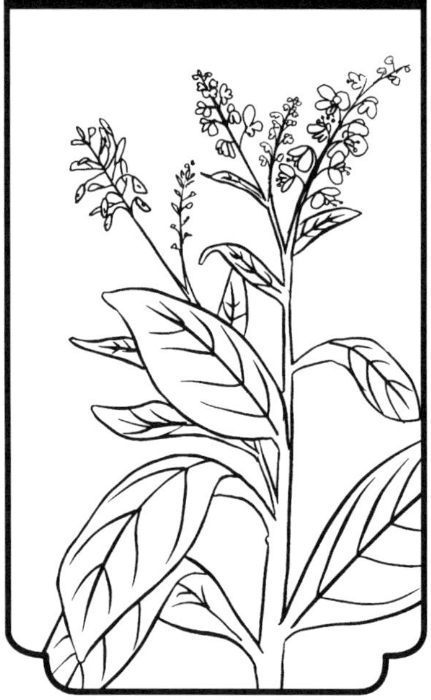

Isatis Da Qing Ye

Woad Leaf

Botanical source: *Isatis tinctoria* L. or *I. indigota* Fortune (Cruciferae), *Baphicacanthus cusia* (Nees) Bremekamp (syn. *Strobilanthes cusia* [Nees] O. Kuntze) (Acanthaceae), *Clerodendron cyrtophyllum* Turczaninow (Verbenaceae), *Polygonum tinctorium* Aiton (Polygonaceae)
Pharmaceutical name: Folium Isatis
Chinese names: Da Qing Ye (Mand); Daai Ching Yip (Cant)
Other names: "Big green leaf"; Taiseiyo (Jap)
Habit: Erect Eurasian and American herb growing in South China's wild areas, and on roadsides and hillsides; racemes of orange flowers bloom in spring.
Part used: the leaf

Therapeutic category: mild herb with minimal chronic toxicity
Constituents: isatan B, indican, glucobrassicin, glucobrassicinsulfonate, indigotin
Effective qualities: bitter, astringent, cold, dry
astringing, sinking
Tropism: respiratory, digestive, urinary, immune systems
Lung, Heart, Stomach, Large Intestine channels
Warmth, Fluid bodies

Actions and Indications

broad-spectrum anti-infective: immunostimulant, antibacterial, antiviral, antiamoebic: acute respiratory, intestinal, urinary infections (incl. flu, epidemic fevers, pneumonia, measles, mumps, encephalitis B, infectious hepatitis, mononucleosis, acute gastroenteritis, bacillary and amoebic dysentery; viral meningitis, HIV); esp. *Staphylococcus, Streptococcus, Neisseria* spp, many gram-positive and gram-negative bacilli

antipyretic: fevers (incl. rheumatic fever)

detoxicant, anti-inflammatory, detumescent, dermatropic, interferon inducent: microbial toxicosis, skin eruptions, dermatitis, boils, abscesses (esp. in throat and lungs); erysipelas, mumps, parotitis, pharyngitis

Symptom Pictures

lung phlegm heat: coughing, production of thick yellow-green sputum, swollen sore throat

intestines damp heat: burning, difficult passing of stool, diarrhea with blood, fever, abdominal pain, thirst

stomach damp heat: nausea, epigastric pain and bloating, sour regurgitation, bad breath, diarrhea or constipation, vomiting

Preparation

Use: The leaf Isatis Da Qing Ye is infused, decocted or used in tincture form.

Dosage: Infusion and decoction: 10-20 g
Tincture: 2-5 ml

Caution: Not to be used with intestinal cold deficiency.

Notes

Isatis leaf is a strong *antimicrobial* herb for acute febrile, pyogenic and epidemic conditions, especially for acute bronchial infections with heat. Its *antiviral* action frequently employed in formulations treating mumps, influenza and encephalitis makes it distinctive.

As seen above, there are four plants commonly used as source for the remedy Isatis Da Qing Ye: first, the leaf of *Isatis indigotica,* also called **Song Lan;** second, the leaf and root of *Clerodendron cyrtophyllum,* properly known as **Da Qing Gen,** green-white Clerodendron; third, the leaf of *Baphicacanthus cusia,* properly called **Ma Lan Ye,** Assam indigo; fourth, the whole plant of *Polygonum tinctorium,* **Lan Shi (Liao Lan),** Chinese indigo. Note that **Ma Lan Ye** itself is sometimes sourced from various species of *Strobilanthes,* such as *S. divaricatus, S. penstemonoides,* etc.

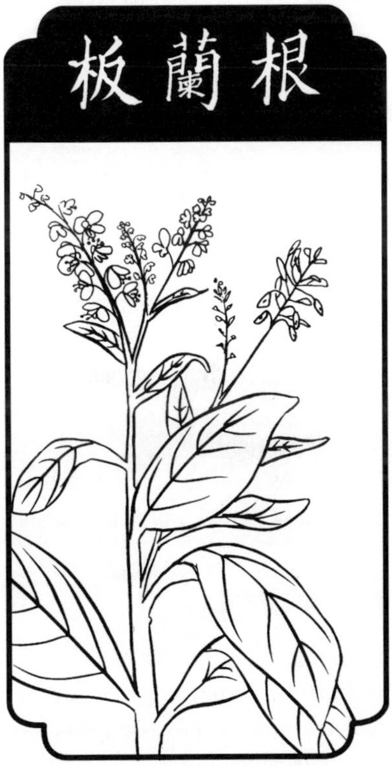

Isatis Ban Lan Gen

Woad Root

Botanical source: *Isatis tinctoria* L,. *I. indigotica* Fort. (Cruciferae), *Baphicacanthus cusia* (Nees) Bremekamp (syn. *Strobilanthes cusia* [Nees] O. Kuntze) (Acanthaceae)
Pharmaceutical name: Rhizoma et Radix Isatis seu Baphicacanthi
Chinese names: Ban Lan Gen (Mand); Baan Laam Gan (Cant)
Other names: Dyer's woad; Banrankon (Jap)
Habit: Erect Eurasian and American herb growing in wild areas, on roadsides and hillsides; racemes of orange flowers bloom in spring.
Part used: the rhizome and root

Therapeutic category: mild remedy with minimal chronic toxicity
Constituents: indoxyl glycoside, isatan, isatan B, quercetin, kaempferol, kinetin, resin, saccharides (stachyose, manneotetrose, lupeose)
Effective qualities: bitter, astringent, cold, dry
astringing, sinking
Tropism: respiratory, digestive systems
Liver, Stomach, Lung, Heart channels; Warmth body

Actions and Indications

broad-spectrum anti-infective: antibacterial, antiviral: acute hepatobiliary, repiratory, gastrointestinal infections (incl. hepatitis, chickenpox, enteritis, influenza, encephalitis B, mumps; pneumonia [all types], viral skin conditions, e.g. herpes zoster, herpes simplex, verruca plana); esp. *Staphylococcus, Streptococcus, Diplococcus pneumoniae, Hemophilus influenzae, Eschericia coli, Salmonella typhi, Shigella dysentericae, Neissera meningitis*

antipyretic: fevers due to infection
detoxicant, anti-inflammatory: microbial toxicosis, pharyngitis, laryngitis, parotitis, mumps, acute conjunctivitis, stomatitis, cerebrospinal meningitis, skin eruptions (incl. erysipelas, macula, papula)
antitumoral: bening and cancerous tumors, chronic leukemia
leukocytogenic: low WBC count (leukopenia)

Symptom Pictures

liver and gallbladder damp heat: jaundice, feverishness, right subcostal pain, thirst, nausea, fatigue

stomach damp heat / gallbladder and stomach Qi stagnation: nausea, epigastric pain and bloating, sour regurgitation, bad breath, diarrhea or constipation, vomiting

lung phlegm heat: coughing, expectoration of thick yellow-green sputum

Preparation

Use: The root Isatis Ban Lan Gen is decocted or used in tincture form both internally and externally.
Dosage: Decoction: 15-30 g
Tincture: 2-5 ml
Caution: Forbidden for weak people and in cases of deficiency cold in the intestines.

Notes

The strong, broad-spectrum *anti-infective* properties of this dye plant are used especially for treating acute liver, lung, throat and skin conditions, including those of viral origin. Many syndromes of the damp heat and fire toxin variety will therefore respond to it.

In South China, **Assam indigo root,** of *Baphicacanthus cusia,* is used for Isatis Ban Lan Gen. However, although similarly used, Assam indigo root is properly called **Ma Lan Gen** or **Nan Ban Lan** (Southern Ban Lan). In Taiwan, the root of *Indigofera suffruticosa* is normally used.

黄柏

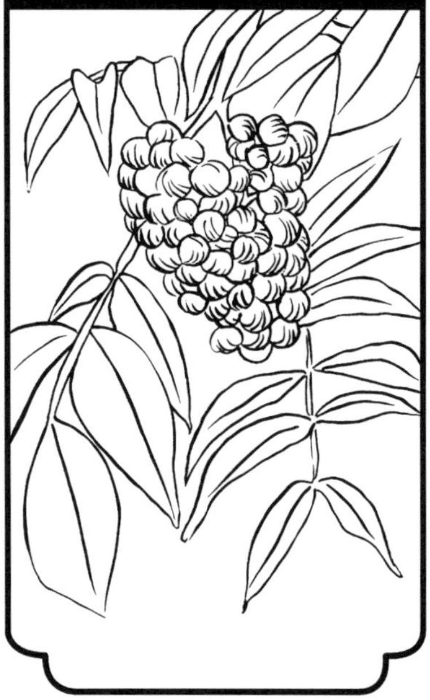

Phellodendron Huang Bai

Siberian Cork Tree Bark

Pharmaceutical name: Cortex Phellodendri
Botanical source: *Phellodendron amurense* Ruprecht or *P. chinense* Schneid (Rutaceae)
Chinese names: Huang Bai, Huang Bo, Chuan Bai (Mand); Wong Paak, Chyun Paak (Cant)
Other names: Amur cork tree, "Yellow fir"; Obaku (Jap)
Habit: Deciduous mountain tree from Northeast Asia, Sichuan and Guizhou, Siberia and Japan; blooms in summer with hairy panicles of yellow-green flowers.
Part used: the bark

Therapeutic category: mild remedy with minimal chronic toxicity
Constituents: alkloids (incl. berberine, jatrorrhizine, magnoflorine, phellodendrine, candicine, menisperine), sitosterol, campesterol, dehydrostigmasterol, triterpenes (incl. obacunobene, obakulactone, dictamnolide, lumicaeruleic and obakunonic acid), tannins
Effective qualities: very bitter, astringent, cold, dry
astringing, relaxing, sinking
Tropism: urogenital, digestive, nervous, cardiovascular systems
Kidney, Bladder, Large Intestine channels; Warmth, Air bodies

Actions and Indications

broad-spectrum anti-infective: antibacterial, antiprotozoal, broad-spectrum antifungal: acute urinary, genital, intestinal and skin infections with discharge (incl. cystitis, vaginitis, cervicitis, trichomoniasis, candidiasis, moniliasis, giardiasis, leucorrhea, gonorrhea; gastroenteritis, dysentery; meningitis, dermatitis, dermatomycoses); esp. *Shigella* spp, many gram-positive and gram-negative bacilli

anti-inflammatory, detoxicant, antilipemic: microbial toxicosis, acute conjunctivitis, dermatitis, otitis, peri-auricular eczema, inflammatory bowel disease, boils, sores, hemorrhoids, abscesses; scalds, burns; hyperlipidemia

antipyretic: low-grade fevers

biliary and pancreatic stimulant, cholagogue: biliary and pancreatic dyspepsia, jaundice

neurocardiac sedative, hypotensive: unrest, agitation, palpitations, pain in general; hypertension

genital sedative/astringent: sexual overstimulation, seminal incontinence, spermatorrhea; hemorrhoids with anal fistula

diuretic, spasmolytic: strangury, dysuria

Symptom Pictures

genitourinary damp heat: thick, yellow, purulent vaginal discharges, difficult/painful/ineffective urination

intestines damp heat: burning, difficult passing of stool, diarrhea with blood, abdominal pain, thirst, fever

stomach damp heat / gallbladder and stomach Qi stagnation: nausea, epigastric pain and bloating, sour regurgitation, bad breath, diarrhea or constipation, vomiting

Yin deficiency with **Kidney fire / Heart and Kidney Yin deficiency:** unrest, feeling stressed, palpitations, afternoon hot spells, night sweats, nocturnal emissions

Preparation

Use: The tree bark Phellodendron Huang Bai is decocted or used in tincture form. Washes, swabs, douches, vainal sponges, etc., can be applied to inflammatory skin, eye and genital conditions, and burns with or without discharge.

Dosage: Decoction: 3-12 g
Tincture: 2-4 ml

Caution: Forbidden in digestive deficiency and cold of any kind.

Notes

On the face of it, Siberian cork tree bark is much like the other bitter, astringent, dry, cold botanicals in this section employed for their *anti-infective* actions. However, this remedy alone is distinguished by its ability to clear heat arising from Yin deficiency conditions in particular. Being *relaxant* to the cardiovascular and reproductive systems (and *astringent* to the latter), Siberian cork tree is ideal for addressing such deficiency heat symptoms as hot spells and low-grade fevers. Cork tree bark is comparable to the bark of a Western tree, the willow, for treating Heart and Kidney Yin deficiency syndromes.

Because of its excellent *antifungal, anti-inflammatory* and *biliary/pancreatic stimulant* actions combined, Siberian cork tree today is also an excellent remedy for a range of intestinal dysbiosis and microbial toxicosis conditions. These include infectious and inflammatory conditions such as food allergies, candidiasis, yeast infections in general, giardiasis and acute skin and middle ear infections. This remedy's *antifungal* action is particularly wide, addressing chronic digestive and skin infections arising from fungal terrain. Inflammatory bowel disorders such as ulcerative colitis will also benefit partly for the same reason, and partly because of its *astringent* effect. With discharge present, regardless of type, Siberian cork tree again scores over many other bitter-cold *anti-infectives* as it dries these out with its astringency.

Berberis San Ke Zhen
Three-Needle Barberry Root

三棵针

Botanical source: *Berberis sargentiana* Schneider or *B. wilsonae* Hemslow or *B. vernae* Schneider and spp. (Berberidaceae)
Chinese names: San Ke Zhen, Tu Huang Lian, Ci Huang Lian (Mand); Saam Gwo Jam (Cant)
Category: mild remedy with minimal chronic toxicity
Constituents: alkaloids (incl. berberine 0.5-5.7%, palmatine, jatrorrhizine, berbamine, columbamine, oxyacanthine, isotetrandrine, magnoflorine)
Effective qualities: bitter, astringent, cold, dry; astringing, relaxing, sinking
Tropism: digestive, respiratory systems; Large Intestine, Stomach, Liver, Lung channels

Actions: *Broad-spectrum anti-infective (immunostimulant, antibacterial, antifungal, antiviral, leukocytogenic), antipyretic, anti-inflammatory, detoxicant, detumescent; detergent, analgesic, vulnerary; hepatobiliary and gastric stimulant, cholagogue; hypotensive, pituitary-adrenocortical stimulant.*
Indications: Acute intestinal, hepatobiliary, respiratory infections with damp heat (incl. bacillary dysentery, enteritis, bronchitis, candidiasis, vaginitis, influenza, dermatitis); esp. *Staphylococcus aureus, Streptococci, Shigella dysentericae, Proteus vulgaris, Pseudomonas aeruginosa, Escherichia coli, Leptospira*; gram-positive cocci; low WBC count (leukopenia) from radiotherapy, chemotherapy, tumors, benzene, uranium, aspirin, chloramphenicol, etc.; fevers, inflammations (incl. cholecystitis, gastritis, conjunctivitis, laryngitis, stomatitis, tonsillitis); burns, boils, abscesses, injuries; liver congestion, jaundice, anorexia, fatigue, gastritis, essential hypertension; silicosis.
Dosage: Decoction: 10-20 g
Tincture: 2-5 ml

As with the Western Barberry root bark, small doses of this remedy may be used as a bitter *digestive stimulant.*
Caution: Forbidden in deficiency cold of the intestines.
Notes: Although a wide variety of *Berberis* species are used in mainland China for the remedy San Ke Zhen, all contain the same basic cluster of alkaloids—though in varying amounts—as well as a few additional alkaloids unique to each. These ensure the same *antimicrobial, anti-inflammatory, antipyretic, detoxicant* and *immune-stimulating* effects here as in Coptis Huang Lian root and Goldenseal root.

Senecio Qian Li Guang
Climbing Ragwort Herb

千里光

Botanical source: *Senecio scandens* Buchanan-Hamilton (Compositae)
Chinese names: Qian Li Guang, Qian Li Ji, Jiu Li Guang, Jiu Li Ming (Mand); Chin Lei Gwong (Cant)
Other names: German ivy; Taikingiku, Yukimigiku (Jap)
Habit: Perennial herb from south China with a preference for thickets in damp, shady and hilly locales; bright yellow capitate flowers open in autumn.
Category: medium-strength remedy with chronic toxicity
Constituents: flavoxanthin, chrysanthemaxanthin, phenolic acid (incl. hydroxyphenylacetic/salicilic/vanillic/pyromucic acid, hydroquinone, senecionine, seneciphylline)
Effective qualities: bitter, astringent, cold; astringing, sinking
Tropism: digestive, respiratory systems; Liver, Lung, Large Intestine channels

Actions: *Broad-spectrum anti-infective (antibacterial, antiviral), antipyretic, resolvent detoxicant, dermatropic, anti-inflammatory, antivenomous, astringent, antipruritic, vision enhancer*
Indications: Acute intestinal, respiratory, gynecological infections with damp heat, with or without fever (incl. tonsillitis, bronchitis, enteritis, bacillary dysentery, trichomonas vaginalis; leptospirosis; malaria, epidemic influenza, septicemia, scarlet fever); intestines damp heat, lung phlegm heat and genitourinary damp heat syndromes; esp. *Staphylococcus aureus, Shigella sonnei* and *boydii, Salmonella typhi/paratyphi/sarcinae;* gram-positive and gram-

negative bacilli; microbial toxicosis with acute appendicitis, conjunctivitis, lymphangitis; boils, sores, furunculosis, abscesses; dermatitis, eczema, pruritus; insect and animal bites; diarrhea; poor eyesight.

Dosage: Decoction or long infusion: 15-30 g
Tincture: 2-4 ml

Local washes, compresses, eyewashes, etc. are also excellent.

Caution: Avoid using this remedy for over four weeks at full dose as it does contain slight cumulative toxicity due to the alkaloid senecionine.

Notes: Predictably for a *Senecio,* this is an excellent wide-spectrum *antimicrobial* remedy. Its principal use is for acute febrile infections, i.e., damp heat and fire toxin conditions. Topical applications with trichomonas vaginalis over a 12-24 hour period have also achieved good results.

Isatis Qing Dai
Woad Leaf and Stem Pigment

青黛

Botanical source: *Isatis tinctoria* L. or *I. indigotica* Fortune (Cruciferae) and *Baphicacanthus cusia* (Nees) Bremekamp (Acanthaceae) and *Indigofera suffruticosa* Miller (Leguminosae) and *Polygonum tinctorium* Aiton (Polygonaceae)
Chinese names: Qing Dai (Mand); Ching Doi (Cant)
Category: mild remedy with minimal chronic toxicity
Constituents: indican, indirubin
Effective qualities: bitter, salty, cold, dry; calming, relaxing
Tropism: respiratory, epidermal, digestive systems; Lung, Liver, Stomach channels

Actions: *Broad-spectrum antibacterial, anti-inflammatory, antipyretic, nervous sedative, spasmolytic, hemostatic, detoxicant, anti-inflammatory, detumescent.*

Indications: Febrile and inflammatory conditions with hemorrhage (esp. nosebleed and hemoptysis), acute bronchitis (lung heat) with cough, enteritis; infantile febrile agitation or seizures; intestinal parasites.

Topically for mouth and throat inflammation, middle ear infection (otitis), macula, papula, erysipelas, thrush, parotitis, mumps, boils, swellings, tumors, bruises and stings; chronic granulocytic leukemia.

Dosage: Decoction: 1.5-3 g
Tincture: 0.2-1 ml

Mouthwashes, gargles and a range of external preparations are also prepared.

Caution: None.

Note: This remedy is the pigment of woad's powdered leaf and stem. Recent research has shown indirubin, one of Qing Dai's chemical constituents, to have an *antitumoral* effect. Both the remedy and its extract indirubin have been used very successfully for this action.

Picrorrhiza Hu Huang Lian
Picrorrhiza Root

胡黃連

Botanical source: *Picrorrhiza kurroa* Royle ex Benth., *P. scriphulariaeflora* Pennell (Scrophulariaceae)
Chinese names: Hu Huang Lian (M); Wu Wong Lin (C)
Category: mild remedy with minimal chronic toxicity
Constituents: alkaloid berberine, kutkin, mannitol, vannillic acid, apocynin, kutkiol, kutkisterol
Effective qualities: bitter, cold, dry; astringing, relaxing, sinking
Tropism: digestive systems; Liver, Large Intestine, Stomach channels

Actions: *Antibacterial, antifungal, antipyretic, cholagogue*

Indications: Acute infectious damp heat conditions, incl. dysentery with bloody stool, urinary tract infections; febrile infections in general, remittent low-grade fevers, malaria, jaundice, boils, conjunctivitis, hemorrhoids, infantile seizures, childhood malnutrition.

Dosage: Decoction: 2-8 g
Tincture: 1-4 ml
Caution: Use carefully in digestive weakness.

Pyrola Lu Xian Cao

鹿銜草

Asian Wintergreen Root and Herb

Botanical source: *Pyrola rotundifolia* L. subsp. *chinensis* H. Andres (Pyrolaceae)
Chinese names: Lu Xian Cao, Lu Ti Cao, Lu Han Cao (Mand); Lok Heun Chou, Lok Ham Chou (Cant)
Category: mild remedy with minimal chronic toxicity
Constituents: methylhydroquinone (luticaosu), gallic and ursolic acid, ursone, quinone chimaphilin, arbutin, ericolin, tannins, bitters, essential oil, sucrose, invertase, renifolin, emulsin
Effective qualities: bitter, sweet, dry, warm; calming, restoring, relaxing
Tropism: respiratory, digestive, musculoskeletal, cardiovascular, reproductive systems; Lung, Liver, Heart channels

Actions: *Broad-spectrum anti-infective (antibacterial), musculoskeletal restorative, antirheumatic, hemostatic, hypotensive, coronary restorative, detoxicant, contraceptive*
Indications: Respiratory, intestinal, bronchial and urinary infections with damp heat; liver abscess; cough, lung TB, hemoptysis from internal injury, uterine bleeding; rheumatic myalgia, lumbar pain, general weakness; hypertension, angina; insect and animal bites; contraception.
Dosage: Decoction: 10-30 g
Tincture: 2-5 ml
Caution: None.

Polygonum Huo Tan Mu

火炭母

Chinese Smartweed Herb

Botanical source: *Polygonum chinense* L. (Polygonaceae)
Chinese names: Huo Tan Mu (Cao), San Qi (Mand); Fuk Tan Mou (Cant)
Category: mild remedy with minimal chronic toxicity
Constituents: flavonoid glycosides
Effective qualities: sour, pungent, cool; calming
Tropism: digestive, respiratory, cardiovascular, reproductive systems; Spleen, Lung, Liver channels

Actions: *Broad-spectrum anti-infective (antifungal, antibacterial), detoxicant, anti-inflammatory, detumescent, astringent, antidiarrheal, antivenomous*
Indications: Fungal and bacterial intestinal, hepatic and reproductive infections with damp heat, incl. intestinal dysbiosis with dyspepsia, enteritis, candidiasis (local, systemic), fungal vaginitis with leucorrhea, hepatitis, dermatitis; bacterial infections with toxic heat (incl. bloody dysentery, pharyngitis, tonsillitis, diptheria, whooping cough, mastitis, abscesses, furunculosis, impetigo); snake and insect bites; corneal opacity; traumatic injuries, vesicular/suppurative sores and eczema.
Dosage: Decoction: 15-30 g (twice this amount for the fresh herb)
Tincture: 3-6 ml

Topical applications can also be prepared as required, including poultice (crush the fresh large leaves), compress, vaginal sponge, pessary and douche.
Caution: None.
Notes: Chinese smartweed or knotweed is a highly effective *antifungal* remedy for altering fungal terrain in general, as well as in the treatment of damp candida-like conditions both systemic and local.

REMEDIES TO REDUCE TOXICOSIS AND RESOLVE ECZEMA AND TUMORS

Resolvent detoxicants: lymphatic decongestants, antitumorals, detumescents

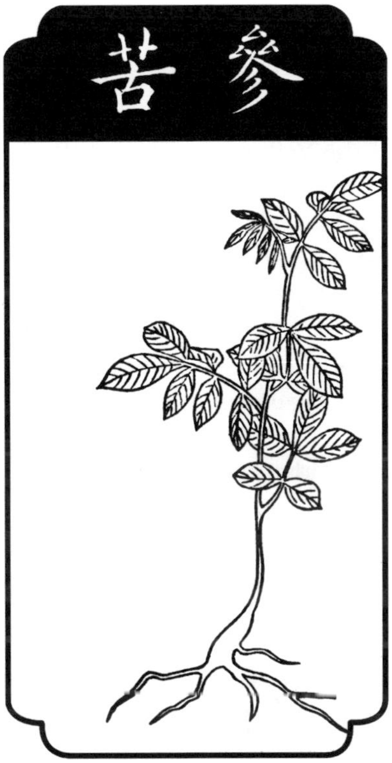

Sophora Ku Shen

Yellow Pagoda Tree Root

Botanical source: *Sophora flavescens* Aiton (Leguminosae)
Pharmaceutical name: Radix Sophorae flavescentis
Chinese names: Ku Shen, Ye Huai, Shui Hai, Di Huai (Mand); Fu Sam (Cant)
Other names: Yellow sophora, "Bitter ginseng"; Kujin (Jap)
Habit: Deciduous woody shrub from Central China, growing on grassland and sunny hillsides; blooms in early summer with racemes of etiolated yellow axillary/terminal flowers.
Part used: the root

Therapeutic category: mild remedy with minimal chronic toxicity
Constituents: 8 alkaloids (matrine, oxymatrine, hydroxymatrine, sophoranol, methylcytisine, baptifoline, sophocarpine, anagyrine), sophoridin, flavonoids
Effective qualities: very bitter, astringent, very cold, dry
calming, astringing, relaxing
Tropism: digestive, urogenital, circulatory, epidermal systems
Liver, Kidney, Stomach, Large Intestine, Small Intestine, Dai channels
Warmth, Fluid bodies

Actions and Indications

resolvent detoxicant, dermatropic, anti-inflammatory: microbial toxicosis with chronic skin lesions/ dermatitis (esp. with pruritus, weeping and bleeding); impetigo, urticaria, psoriasis (incl. purulent, pruritic); atopic/allergic eczema, sores, boils, burns
antitumoral, interferon-inducent: cancer (esp. cervical, rectal, dermal)
broad-spectrum anti-infective: immunostimulant (lymphocyte stimulant), antibacterial, antifungal: genital/intestinal infections (incl. enteritis, dysentery, candidiasis, syphilis); fungal skin infections, yeast infections
antiparasitic, antiprotozoal: intestinal parasites, scabies, trichomoniasis, giardiasis, leprosy
genital astringent, antipruritic: genital and other pruritus, leucorrhea, vaginitis with discharges
hepatic, diuretic, liver-protective: jaundice, liver congestiom, edema, dysuria
cardiac relaxant, hypotensive: neurocardiac syndrome with arrhythmia, hypertension
analgesic, astringent: diarrhea, abdominal pain
bronchodilator, expectorant: bronchial asthma, chronic bronchitis
immune regulator, antiallergic: immune stress with immediate allergies (incl. atopic dermatitis, urticaria, angioedema, bronchial asthma, rhinitis)
radiation-protective, leukocytogenic: radiation damage, leukopenia

Symptom Pictures

microbial toxicosis with **skin wind/damp/heat:** red, itching skin rashes, sores, headaches, food allergies
intestines damp heat: burning, difficult passing of stool, diarrhea with blood, abdominal pain, thirst, fever
genitourinary damp heat: genital itching, vaginal discharges with purulence, unrest
fluid congestion with **heat:** water retention, thirst, feverishness, painful dribbling urination
heart Qi constraint: palpitations, irregular heartbeat, stress, unrest

Preparation

Use: The root Sophora Ku Shen should be decocted or used in tincture form. A wash or compress is also made for external/skin conditions, as well as douches and vaginal sponges for various genital infections and discharges

Dosage: Decoction: 4-15 g
Tincture: 1-4 ml

Caution: Forbidden in indigestion due to cold. Avoid using in deficient and cold conditions in general.

Notes

The typically yellow and intensely bitter, cold, dry-natured root of the Yellow pagoda tree from Henan is traditionally used for infectious damp heat and fire toxin conditions involving the skin, genital and digestive organs. Nowadays, where this brilliant remedy really shines is in those pathologies arising from microbial toxicosis. Yellow pagoda tree covers them virtually all: allergic, inflammatory, infectious and tumoral. Immediate allergies such as atopic dermatitis and bronchial asthma (Qiu and Wu 1986) presenting acute inflammation and irritation is one example. Not only microbial, but the derived fungal and parasitic forms of pleomorphic proliferation can also be reduced with its use, including candidiasis, fungal skin infections and a range of parasites.

With the definition and extraction of Yellow pagoda tree's alkaloids came an extension of its field of applications. The plant's alkaloids have been shown to produce a *relaxant* effect on the organs of the rhythmic zone, the heart and lungs. Cardiac arrhythmia of various types—including premature beats and sinus tachycardia—responds particularly well to this remedy (Ding 1987). In energetic terms, the syndrome implicated is Qi constraint affecting the heart.

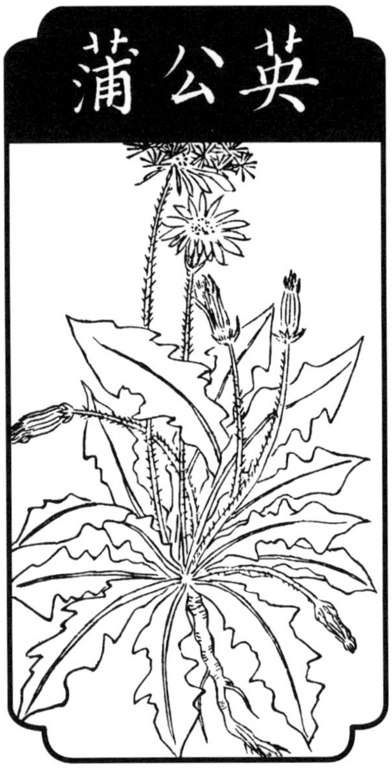

Taraxacum Pu Gong Ying

Mongolian Dandelion Root and Herb *

Botanical source: *Taraxacum mongolicum* Handel-Mazzetti and spp. (Compositae)
Pharmaceutical name: Radix et herba Taraxaci
Chinese names: Pu Gong Ying, Huang Hua Di Ding, Gong Ying (Mand); Pou Gung Ying (Cant)
Other names: Asian dandelion; Hokoei (Jap)
Habit: Perennial herb found in temperate Asian grasslands, on hillsides and roadsides; bright yellow terminal capitate flowers bloom in spring.
Part used: the whole plant

Therapeutic category: mild remedy with minimal chronic toxicity
Constituents: bitter glycosides, sitosterol, taraxerol, tannins, cholin, saponin, inulin, minerals and trace minerals, carotinoids, resin, levulose, essential oil, silicic and citric acid
Effective qualities: bitter, a bit salty and sweet, cool, dry
stimulating, decongesting, restoring, softening dissolving, sinking
Tropism: hepatobiliary, urinary, venous, lymphatic systems
Liver, Gallbladder, Stomach channels; Fluid, Warmth, Air bodies

Actions and Indications

resolvent detoxicant, dermatropic: metabolic toxicosis with chronic arthritic, rheumatic, eczematic, gouty conditions (incl. hyperuricemia), hypercholesterolemia; nephritis; microbial toxicosis with pyogenic infections (incl. firm boils, carbuncles, abscesses, appendicitis, lymphangitis, non-suppurative sores)

connective tissue restorative: connective tissue weakness or degeneration
resolvent antilithic: hard deposits, e.g. hepatic cirrhosis, arteriosclerosis, biliary/urinary stones; weight gain, cellulite
lymphatic decongestant: lymphadenitis
immunostimulant anti-infective (phagocyte stimulant), anti-inflammatory: acute infections (incl. cholecystitis, tonsillitis, pharyngitis, early acute mastitis, appendicitis, pelvic inflammatory disease, urinary tract infection, chronic gastritis, osteomyelitis)
antiviral: herpes simplex
venous decongestant: varicose veins, hemorrhoids
choleretic, laxative: liver congestion with lethargy, dyspepsia, jaundice, constipation
draining diuretic: generalized edema
liver/metabolic restorative, liver protective: hepatic and metabolic deficiency conditions; chronic hepatitis, anemia, gylcogen storage disorders, autotoxicosis, infection proneness
hypoglycemiant: hyperglycemia, diabetes (supportive)
galactagogue: insufficient breast milk

Symptom Pictures

metabolic toxicosis: malaise, headaches, muscle aches, joint pains, skin rashes

microbial toxicosis with **fire toxin:** sore throat, swollen glands, boils, headache, fever

liver and gallbladder Qi stagnation: general congestion better with exercise, epigastric pain with eating, constipation, right subcostal distension and tenderness

liver fire: right subcostal pain and distension, congested face, red swollen eyes

liver fluid congestion: generalized water retention, fatigue

venous blood stagnation: varicose veins, hemorrhoids, tired legs

liver and pancreas Yin deficiency: low motivation, fatigue, frequent infections, underweight

Preparation

Use: The root and herb Taraxacum Pu Gong Ying is decocted or used in tincture form. External preparations are also applied to boils, sores, etc.

Dosage: Decoction: 10-25 g
Tincture: 2-4 ml

Smaller doses are more *stimulating* and *restoring,* while larger ones are more *heat-clearing* and *draining.*

Caution: This herb may occasionally cause some heartburn, nausea, abdominal discomfort or loose stool.

Notes

Many different dandelion species, including the Western *T. officinalis,* are used in China as sources for this remedy. Not surprisingly, contemporary Chinese research on this plant has confirmed and enlarged many of the findings familiar to us in the West.

From the clinical and historical point of view, the actions and uses of Mongolian dandelion root and herb clearly indicate a *draining, detoxicant* remedy. Unlike most other remedies in this section, however, this remedy addresses both metabolic and microbial forms of toxicosis. Its *metabolic detoxicant* action serves numerous chronic and degenerative conditions involving weakened connective tissue. Its *microbial detoxicant,* i.e., *anti-infective,* action—together with immune stimulation, lymph activation and diuresis—targets both acute and chronic forms of infections, especially those presenting swollen tissues such as glands, boils, etc.

Mongolian dandelion's tropism for the liver and pancreas (like that of the Western dandelion) is intrinsic to its action on metabolism in general. The remedy is both a *stimulant* to liver Yang functions (*liver decongestant, choleretic*) and a *restorative* to liver Yin functions (*liver restorative/protective*). On the other hand, its use for such syndromes as liver fire (in both traditional Chinese and Greek medicine) is based on its final *heat-clearing* and *diuretic* effect. These various actions are traditionally corroborated by its bitter, salty and sweet taste qualities.

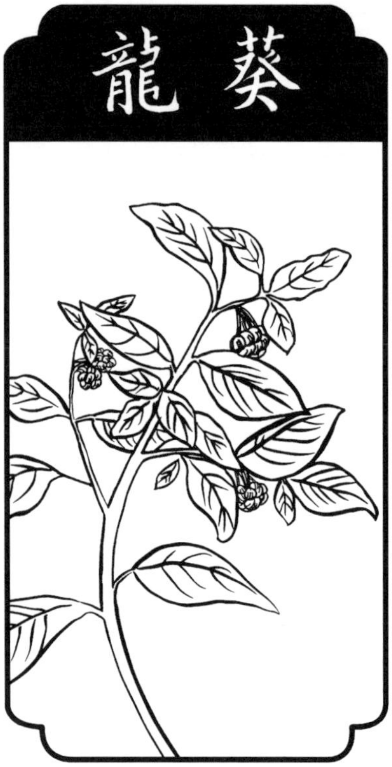

Solanum Long Kui

Winter Cherry Herb

Botanical source: *Solanum nigrum* L. (Solanaceae)
Pharmaceutical name: Herba Solani nigri
Chinese names: Long Kui, Ye Hai Jiao, Tian Qie Zi (Mand); Lung Kwai (Cant)
Other names: Black/Garden nightshade, Morel; Inuhozuki (Jap)
Habit: Annual Eurasian herb found in damp soil in wild places, roadsides, field borders and gardens; racemes of small white blossoms flower in summer.
Part used: the herb

Therapeutic category: medium-strength remedy with some chronic toxicity
Constituents: glycoalkaloids (incl. solanine, solasonine, solamatgine, atropine), saponins
Effective qualities: bitter, a bit sweet, cold, dry
stimulating, relaxing, dissolving, astringing
Tropism: respiratory, urinary, cardiovascular, epidermal systems
Lung, Bladder channels
Air, Warmth bodies

Actions and Indications

resolvent detoxicant, dermatropic: toxicosis with eczema (pruritic), dermatitis, urticaria, impetigo; carbuncles
broad-spectrum anti-infective, antipyretic, anti-inflammatory, antivenomous: febrile infections (incl. urinary infections, acute nephritis, mastitis, laryngitis); fungal/yeast infections, vaginitis with pruritus; poisonous snakebite
antitumoral: cancer (incl. cervical, dermal)
astringent, antipruritic, mucostatic: genital and other pruritus, vaginitis; severe leucorrhea
diuretic, hypotensive: cystitis, dysuria; hypertension
stimulant expectorant, antitussive: chronic bronchitis with coughing, wheezing; whooping cough
analgesic

Symptom Pictures

microbial/metabolic toxicosis with **skin damp/heat:** skin rashes/itching, headaches, fungal/yeast infections
lung phlegm damp: coughing, wheezing, expectoration of white sputum

Preparation

Use: The herb Solanum Long Kui is decocted or used in tincture form. Topical applications (including washes, douches, etc.) can be made for eczema, skin and vaginal itching, etc. The fruit and the fresh herb are more toxic than the dried, as they contain more of the alkaloid solanine, and should be given only at the lowest dosage.
Dosage: Decoction: 3-10 g
Tincture: 1-3 ml
Caution: Not for continuous use as the herb has some cumulative toxicity. Contraindicated during pregnancy and breastfeeding.

Notes

Winter cherry herb was used in traditional Greek medicine in the same way as in Chinese medicine. The bitter-cold herb has superior *detoxicant* and *skin cleansing* effects, and has demonstrated an ability to reverse a wide variety of carcinomas.

Winter cherry herb is also a highly effective *expectorant* in cases of chronic bronchitis.

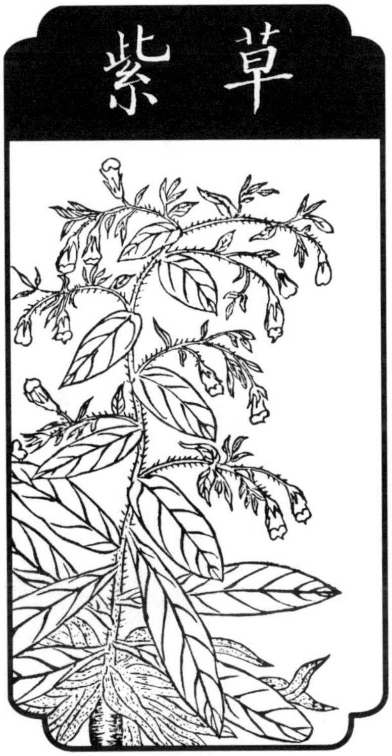

Lithospermum Zi Cao

Purple Groomwell Root

Botanical source: *Lithospermum erythrorhizon* Siebold et Zuccarini; also *Arnebia euchroma* (Royle) Johnston (syn. *Macrotomia euchroma* [Royle] Pauls), *A. guttata* Bunge, *Onosma paniculatum* Bureau et Franchet, *O. hookeri* (Boraginaceae)
Pharmaceutical name: Radix Lithospermi seu Arnebiae seu Macrotomiae
Chinese names: Zi Cao, Zi Dan, Zi Gen, Hong Tiao Zi Cao (M); Ji Chou (C)
Other names: Chinese stoneseed, "Purple weed"; Shikon (Jap)
Habit: Hairy perennial herb from Northeast China and Japan, growing on sunny hillsides; white racemes of terminal flowers appear during spring.
Part used: the root

Therapeutic category: mild remedy with minimal chronic toxicity
Constituents: naphthoquinones (incl. shikonin, ectylshikonin, acetylshikonin, isobutylshikonin, dimethylacryloshikonin, hydroxyisovalerylshikonin, teracrylshikonin), allantoin, alkannan, bornesitol, valeric/isovaleric acid, calcium, mucilage
Effective qualities: sweet, salty, bitter, cold, moist
stimulating, softening, astringing
Tropism: hormonal, digestive, epidermal systems
Pericardium, Heart, Liver, Ren channels; Fluid, Warmth bodies

Actions and Indications

resolvent detoxicant, dermatropic, anti-inflammatory: metabolic and microbial toxicosis with skin rashes, eczema, dermatitis, boils, burns, frostbite, cervicitis, vaginitis, pityriasis rosea
astringent, antipruritic, vulnerary: vaginal and other pruritus, ulcers, wounds
antitumoral: tumors, cancer (incl. liver, skin)
antibacterial, antiviral, immunostimulant (phagocyte stimulant): infections (incl. HIV, vaginitis, flu)
rash-promoting, diuretic: measles with little or no rashes, smallpox, chickenpox
demulcent laxative: constipation, hard dry stool
estrogen inhibitor: excess estrogen conditions
contraceptive, pituitary gonadotropic inhibitor

Preparation

Use: The root Lithospermum Zi Cao is decocted, tinctured and used topically in swabs, salves, douches, etc.
Dosage: Decoction: 4-20 g
Tincture: 1-4 ml
Caution: Forbidden in measles if the rash has already appeared.

Notes

A *cool demulcent* in the Borage family, Purple groomwell root is a purple dye plant entirely similar in function to the European stoneseed and the various Alkanets. Indeed, we may apply here Culpeper's words for the latter: "As gallant a remedy to drive out the smallpox and measles as any." Fire toxin, skin rashes and itching are Purple groomwell root's particular indications.

Like other varieties of *Lithospermum,* such as *L. officinale* and the Indian *L. ruderale,* Purple groomwell root will prevent conception when given long enough for its effects to accumulate. This result is obtained by an inhibiting action on pituitary gonadotropic hormones, thereby reducing ovulation.

土茯苓

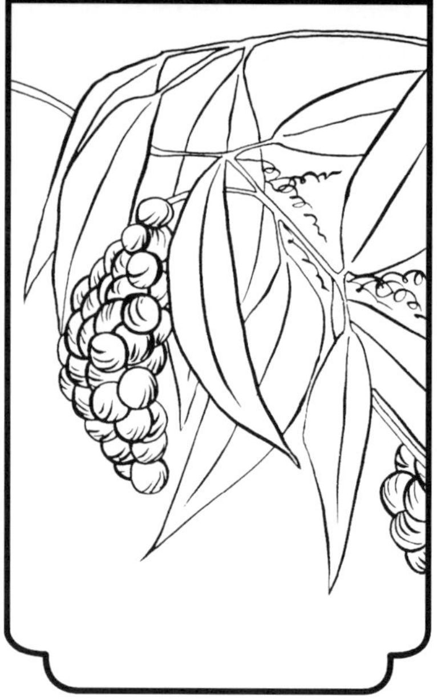

Smilax Tu Fu Ling

Glabrous Greenbrier Root *

Botanical source: *Smilax glabra* Roxburgh (Liliaceae)
Pharmaceutical name: Rhizoma Smilacis glabrae
Chinese names: Tu Fu Ling, Zi Ju Ling, Leng Fen Tuan, Xian Yi Liang (Mand); Tou Fuk Ling (Cant)
Other names: China root, "Native hoelen," "Immortals' leftover food"; Dobukuryo (Jap)
Habit: Climbing mountain shrub from mideast China, growing in thickets in valleys and uplands; umbels of pale yellow blossoms bloom in early summer.
Part used: the rhizome

Therapeutic category: mild remedy with minimal chronic toxicity
Constituents: saponins (incl. smilacin, beta-sitosterol, stigmasterol), tannins, resin, starch, glucoside
Effective qualities: sweet, bland, cool
restoring, dissolving
Tropism: musculoskeletal, hepatobiliary, urinary, dermal systems
Liver, Stomach, Kidney channels; Warmth, Fluid bodies

Actions and Indications

resolvent detoxicant, dermatropic: metabolic and heavy metal toxicosis with eczema, chronic suppurative dermatoses, psoriasis, syphilis; furunculosis, skin ulcers, boils, abscesses (incl. lymphatic); mercury/silver poisoning
lymphatic decongestant, dissolvent, progesteronic: lymphadenitis, fibrocystic breasts; progesterone deficiency
antitumoral: cancer (incl. skin, lymphatic)
analgesic, anti-inflammatory: acute rheumatoid arthritis, lymph gland pain, gout
diuretic, anti-inflammatory: dysuria, albuminuria, chyluria, nephritis, cystitis, jaundice, hepatitis A
anastative digestive: dyspepsia, diarrhea, malabsorption, weight loss
antileptospiral

Symptom Pictures

metabolic toxicosis with **skin damp heat:** skin rashes, boils, skin ulcers, headaches

metabolic toxicosis with **damp heat obstruction:** hot, painful, swollen, stiff joints

bladder damp: turbid white urine, difficult urination

Preparation

Use: The root Smilax Tu Fu Ling is decocted or used in tincture form.
Dosage: Decoction: 15-30 g
Tincture: 2-4 ml
Caution: Use with care in Liver and Kidney Yin deficiency syndromes. Never drink this remedy with black tea containing tannin.

Notes

Closely related to Jamaica sarsaparilla, *Smilax officinalis,* is the climber Glabrous greenbrier from China's eastern highlands. Containing saponins (some steroidal), the faintly sweet–tasting rhizome is successfully used for eczema and other toxicosis conditions because of its deep *detoxicant* action on metabolic waste accumulations. The remedy is reported to be 90% effective for primary syphilis, reduces heavy metal toxicosis and is active in leptospiral infections. Prescriptions treating acute, painful arthritic conditions also frequently contain Glabrous greenbrier.

白花蛇舌草

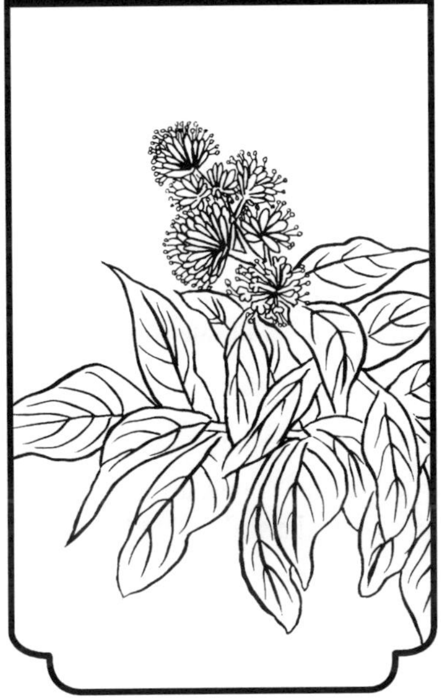

Oldenlandia Bai Hua She She Cao

Snaketongue Grass Herb *

Botanical source: *Oldenlandia diffusa* (Willd.) Roxburgh, syn. *Hedyotis diffusa* Willdenow (Rubiaceae)
Pharmaceutical name: Herba Oldenlandiae
Chinese names: Bai Hua She She Cao, She She Cao, She Zhen Cao (Mand); Baak Fa Se Sit Chou (Cant)
Other names: "White pattern snake tongue weed"; Byakkajazetsuso (Jap)
Habit: Thin, delicate annual spreading herb from (sub)tropical Asia; grows on hillsides, in damp grasslands, gardens, field borders and water ditches; small, white single or paired axillary flowers bloom in late summer.
Part used: the herb

Therapeutic category: mild remedy with minimal chronic toxicity
Constituents: hentriacontane, stigmasterol, sitosterol, ursolic and oleanolic acid, coumaric acid, flavonoids
Effective qualities: a bit sweet and bitter, cool, dry
calming, restoring, stimulating
Tropism: digestive, reproductive, urinary, immune systems
Liver, Stomach, Large Intestine channels; Warmth body

Actions and Indications

resolvant detoxicant, anti-inflammatory, antivenomous: metabolic and microbial toxicosis with acute local pyogenic infections (incl. deep boils, carbuncles, furuncles, intestinal abscess); sores, ulcers, laryngitis, appendicitis, pelvic inflammatory disease, snakebites
antitumoral: cancer (incl. of cervix, esophagus, stomach, intestines, liver, skin, lymph); acute leukemia (all types)
anti-infective, immunostimulant, antipyretic: infections (incl. urinary tract infections [cystitis, urethritis], pneumonia, bronchitis, lymphadenitis, hepatitis, enteritis, septicemia), radiotherapy; fever, heatstroke
anticontusion, vulnerary, analgesic: sprains, strains, contusions, fractures
diuretic: oliguria, anuria, edema
hepatic stimulant: jaundice, hepatomegaly, depression
adrenocortical restorative
antispermatogenic

Preparation

Use: The herb Oldenlandia Bai Hua She She Cao is infused, briefly decocted or prepared in tincture form. Topical preparations are also made for boils, snakebites, etc. The remedy is *antivenomous* to a variety of snakebites.
Dosage: Infusion and Decoction: 20-60 g
Tincture: 2-5 ml
Caution: Use with caution during pregnancy.

Notes

Frequently used in treating a wide variety of infections, the remedy Snaketongue grass has now become one of the main components of formulas treating acute appendicitis (considered a type of fire toxin). The herb's effectiveness in combating infection lies in its ability to control microbial and metabolic toxicosis on one hand, and modulate immune functions on the other. It has shown to increase lymphocyte phagocytosis and stimulate reticuloendothelial functioning (Chang and But 1987). Snake-tongue grass' *antitumoral* activity is inconsistent, however. In clinical practice, best results have been obtained when it is combined with other *antitumoral* remedies.

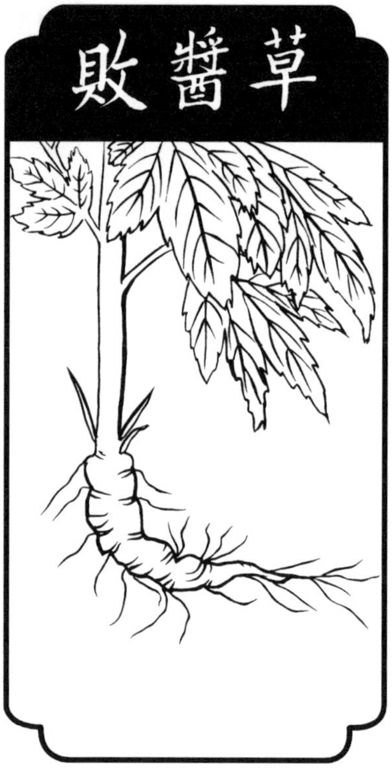

Patrinia Bai Jiang Cao

Patrinia Herb and Root

Botanical source: *Patrinia scabiosaefolia* Fischer or *P. villosa* Jussieu (Valerianaceae)
Pharmaceutical name: Herba et rhizoma Patriniae
Chinese names: Bai Jiang Cao, Bai Jiang, Ku Zhai Gong (Mand); Baai Jeung Chou (Cant)
Other names: "Spoilt soy"; Haishoso (Jap)
Habit: Perennial mountain herb from Central China; grows in grasslands, waste ground, by forest borders and roadsides; flowers in late summer with small umbels of terminal yellow or white blossoms.
Part used: the herb and/or rhizome

Therapeutic category: mild remedy with minimal chronic toxicity
Constituents: *P. scab.:* patrinoside yielding oleanolic acid, scabioside, essential oil (incl. patrinine, isopatrinine), isopentanoic acid, sitosterol, hederagenin
P. vill.: sinigrin, morroniside, loganin, villoside
Effective qualities: pungent, a bit bitter, cool
relaxing, calming, dissolving
Tropism: digestive, lymphatic, nervous systems
Liver, Stomach, Large Intestine channels; Warmth, Air bodies

Actions and Indications

resolvent detoxicant, anti-inflammatory: toxicosis with acute pyogenic local infections (incl. boils, sores, internal or external abscesses [incl. liver abscess], suppurative tonsillitis, acute appendicitis, lymphangitis)
lymphatic decongestant, detumescent: lymphadenitis
antitumoral: tumors, cancer (esp. skin)
antibacterial: enteritis, dysentery, cholecystitis, pneumonia; eczema, endometritis
antiparasitic: parasitic skin infections
antiviral: herpes simplex, influenza
antipyretic: eruptive fevers (e.g. measles)
nervous sedative: unrest, insomnia, dizziness; neurosis
analgesic: abdominal or chest pain, postpartum and postoperative pain, dysmenorrhea
liver protective: hepatitis

Symptom Pictures

microbial/metabolic toxicosis: chronic or recurring boils, skin rashes, malaise

Qi constraint with **nerve excess (Liver Yang rising):** insomnia, stress, dizziness, irritability, palpitations

Preparation

Use: The herb and root Patrinia Bai Jiang Cao are briefly decocted or used in tincture form. The herb may also be infused. Local swabs, fomentations, etc. are excellent for topical use, especially for mumps.
Dosage: Infusion and decoction: 10-30 g
Tincture: 2-5 ml
Caution: Forbidden in weak digestion.

Notes

This fragrant, white-flowered herb was traditionally used in formulas to clear internal and surface infections. The *nervous sedative* and *liver protective* actions of Patrinia herb and root, however, have been put to use only recently. Research has evinced *sedative* activity twice the strength of its Western relative, Valerian root (Chang and But 1987). This strongly suggests use in syndromes of rising Liver Yang. Patrinia also exerts a *liver protective* action that is presumed to operate via its oleanolic acid content. As of printing date, however, both this and its *antitumoral* actions require more definitive investigation.

In South China and Taiwan, *Thlaspi arvense* L. (pennycress) is the botanical source of the remedy Bai Jiang Cao. This remedy is more accurately called **Nan Bai Jiang,** "Southern Bai Jiang."

Polygonum Hu Zhang

Japanese Knotweed Root and Leaf

虎杖

Botanical source: *Polygonum cuspidatum* Siebold et Zuccharini (Polygonaceae)
Chinese names: Hu Zhang, Ban Zhang, Chuan Jin Long, Tu Da Huang, Yin Yang Lian (Mand); Fu Jeung (Cant)
Other names: Bushy knotweed
Habit: Perennial herb from Central China found in dank, cool, shady spots along streams and in woods.
Category: mild remedy with minimal chronic toxicity

Constituents: *root:* anthraquinones (incl. emodin, chrysophanol, rheic acid, physcion, polygonin), hydroxyanthraquinones, polydatin, resveratrol, piceid, polysaccharides, condensed tannins
leaf: quercetin, isoquercetin, reynoutrin, vitamin C
Effective qualities: bitter, sour, astringent, cold, dry; sinking, stimulating, astringing
Tropism: digestive, urinary, reproductive, respiratory, immune systems; Lung, Liver, Gallbladder channels

ACTIONS: *Detoxicant, antibacterial, antiviral, immunostimulant (phagocyte and leukocyte stimulant), antivenomous, anti-inflammatory, antipyretic, analgesic, vulnerary, detumescent, liver decongestant, laxative, diuretic, uterine stimulant, parturient, expectorant, antitussive, capillary stimulant, antilipemic*

INDICATIONS: Toxicosis (metabolic, microbial) with acute abscesses, boils, appendicitis, eczema, snakebites; burns, traumatic injuries, swelling of unknown origin; bronchitis, pneumonia, cough, pleurisy; influenza, leukopenia; acute hepatitis, jaundice, cholecystitis, dysentery, enteritis, constipation; urinary tract infection, acute nephritis, anuria; dysmenorrhea, amenorrhea, stalled labor, retained placenta; rheumatoid arthritis; bleeding hemorrhoids, anal fissure.

Dosage: Decoction: 8-26 g
Tincture: 2-4 ml

Caution: Contraindicated during pregnancy.

NOTES: Supported by recent research, Japanese knotweed is a very wide-ranging botanical for acute fire toxin/pyogenic conditions, more systemic forms of toxicosis and infections as well as gynecological, urinary and hepatic disorders.

In North America, the plant was once introduced from Asia as an ornamental, and now exists as a weed along roadsides, fields and watse areas.

Dictamnus Bai Xian Pi

Asian Dittany Root Bark

白鲜皮

Botanical source: *Dictamnus dasycarpus* Turczaninow (Rutaceae)
Chinese names: Bai Xian Pi (M); Baak Sin Pei (C)
Other names: "White fresh bark"; Hakusenpi (Jap)
Habit: Perennial temperate herb from mid China, growing in hilly forested country; pale red five-petaled flowers appear in spring.
Category: mild remedy with minimal chronic toxicity

Constituents: choline, dictamnine, limonin, obacunone, fraxinellone, obaculactone, dictamnolactone, obacunonic acid, phytosterol, trigonelline, fagarin, dasycarpamin
Efective qualities: bitter, salty, astringent, cold, dry; calming, stimulating, sinking
Tropism: epidermal, cardiac, reproductive systems; Spleen, Stomach, Bladder, Small Intestine channels

ACTIONS: *Resolvent detoxicant, dermatropic, anti-inflammatory, antipruritic, broad-spectrum antifungal, antibacterial, hepatic, cardiac stimulant, uterine stimulant, analgesic, antipyretic*
INDICATIONS: Toxicosis with chronic eczema, dermatitis (esp. with pruritus); impetigo, boils, scabies, German measles (rubella), all fungal skin conditions (tinea); jaundice, arthralgia
Dosage: Decoction: 6-16 g
Tincture: 2-4 ml
Topical applications for skin conditions are made with this remedy.
Caution: Use cautiously in deficiency cold conditions with Qi deficiency; forbidden in pregnancy.
NOTES: The skin is the focus of Asian dittany root bark's multifaceted *detoxicant, antipruritic* and *antifungal* actions. They are effective in conditions ranging from eczema due to chronic toxicosis, to acute, itchy, red skin rashes.

Viola Zi Hua Di Ding
Asian Violet Root and Herb

紫花地丁

Botanical source: *Viola yedoensis* Makino or *V. japonica* Langsdorf (Violaceae)
Chinese names: Zi Hua Di Ding, Di Ding (Mand); Ji Fa Dei Ding (Cant)
Other names: "Purple flower earth nail"; Shikajicho (Jap)
Habit: Perennial temperate East Asian herb growing on hillsides and damp places; magenta terminal flowers bloom in spring.
Category: mild remedy with minimal chronic toxicity
Constituents: cerotic acid, flavonoids, alkaloids
Effective qualities: pungent, bitter, a bit astringent, cold; astringing, dissolving, calming
Tropism: hepatobiliary, lymphatic, epidermal systems; Liver, Heart channels

ACTIONS: *Resolvent detoxicant, anti-infective, anti-inflammatory, lymphatic decongestant, detumescent, vulnerary, interferon inducent, leukocytogenic, hepatic*
INDICATIONS: Toxicosis with acute local pyogenic infections with heat, redness and swelling; conjunctivitis, laryngitis, otitis media, lymphangitis; abscesses (esp. of head, back, breast, intestines); boils, furuncles, mumps, suppurative osteomyelitis, erysipelas; lymphadenitis; sores, wounds; lung TB, HIV infection; acute icteric hepatitis, jaundice; leukopenia.
Dosage: Decoction: 10-30 g
Tincture: 2-5 ml
Caution: Contraindicated in deficiency cold conditions.
NOTES: The remedy Asian violet root and herb is commonly found in *detoxicant, heat-clearing* and *detumescent* formulas of many types. In this respect the focus is different from the violet types used in the West, although similar to other East Asian violet varieties such as *Viola diffusa*, Di Bai Cao, *Viola japonica*, Li Tou Cao, *Viola patrinii*, Hua To Cao, and *Viola inconspicua.*

Tinospora Jin Guo Lan
Tinospora Tuber

金果榄

Botanical source: *Tinospora sagittata* Gagnepain or *T. capillipes* Gagnepain (Menispermaceae)
Chinese names: Jin Guo Lan, Qing Niu Dan, Jiu Niu Dan (Mand); Gam Gwo Laam (Cant)
Category: mild remedy with minimal chronic toxicity
Constituents: alkaloids (incl. columbin)
Habit: Perennial twining vine from Mid and South China, growing in dank, shady places in woods or thickets; panicles of small white blossoms open in summer.
Effective qualities: bitter, cold, dry; dissolving, calming
Tropism: epidermal, respiratory, digestive, lymphatic systems; Lung, Stomach channels

ACTIONS: *Resolvent detoxicant, anti-inflammatory, detumescent, lymphatic decongestant, anti-infective, antipyretic, antitussive, hemostatic, antivenomous*

INDICATIONS: Toxicosis with boils, carbuncles, furuncles; infected wounds; acute laryngitis, sore throat, tonsillitis, stomatitis, parotitis, mastitis; swollen lymphangitis, lymphadenitis (incl. tubercular); acute gastroenteritis, bacillary dysentery, abdominal pain; insect and snake bites.

Dosage: Decoction: 4-10 g.
Tincture: 1-3 ml

Topical preparations are also made for insect bites, wounds and boils especially.

Caution: Use cautiously with digestive deficiency present.

Wikstroemia Liao Ge Wang 了哥王

Wikstroemia Root

Botanical source: *Wickstroemia indica* (L.) C.A. Meyer (Thymelaeaceae)

Chinese names: Liao Ge Wang (Gen), Jiu Xin Cao, Nan Ling Zhao Hua, Pu Yin Gen (Mand); Liu Go Wong (Cant)

Habit: Deciduous shrub primarily from the southern province Guangdong, found on hillsides, roadsides and around villages; racemes of small yellow-green blossoms open in summer.

Category: medium-strength remedy with chronic toxicity

Constituents: daphnoretin, glycoside wikstroemin, tricin, saponins (incl. nortrachelogenin, arctigenin, kaempferolglucopyranoside)

Effective qualities: bitter, cold, dry; calming, decongesting

Tropism: epidermal, lymphatic, respiratory systems; Liver, Lung channels

ACTIONS: *Resolvent detoxicant, anti-inflammatory, lymphatic decongestant, detumescent, antivenomous, antifungal, antiparasitic, vulnerary, antipyretic, diuretic*

INDICATIONS: Acute pyodermias, incl. boils, abscesses; acute mastitis, lymphangitis (esp. cervical), acute lymphadenitis, mumps, cellulitis, parotitis; pneumonia, whooping cough, bronchial asthma; insect stings, snakebites, fungal scalp infections; intestinal parasites; traumatic injury with swelling and contusion; edema.

Dosage: Long decoction: 6-12 g. Decoct for 5 hours or more to decrease its toxicity.
Tincture: 1-4 ml

Swabs, compresses, liniments, etc., are often prepared for topical use.

Caution: Do not use continuously at the maximum dosage. Signs of cumulative toxicity include diarrhea and vomiting. Forbidden during pregnancy and breastfeeding.

NOTES: Wickstroemia root is a very effective remedy from South China for fire toxin conditions and traumatic injuries.

Wikstroemia leaf and **stem** are specifically used for cancer treatment.

Ampelopsis Bai Lian 白蔹

Japanese Peppervine Root

Botanical source: *Ampelopsis japonica* (Thunb.) Makino (Vitaceae)

Chinese names: Bai Lian, Qi Zi Mei (Mand); Baak Lim (Cant)

Habit: Perennial herb from montane temperate China and Japan; yellow flower cymes bloom in summer.

Category: mild remedy with minimal chronic toxicity

Constituents: myricetin

Effective qualities: sweet, a bit pungent, bitter and astringent, neutral; astringing, dissolving, restoring

Tropism: epidermal, vascular, lymphatic systems; Heart, Stomach, Liver channels

Actions: *Detoxicant, anti-inflammatory, detumescent, vulnerary, analgesic, astringent, mucostatic, expectorant, antifungal, antibacterial*

Indications: Boils, carbuncles, lymphadenitis, weeping and suppurative sores/lesions, sloughing ulcers, wounds, dermatitis, acne; burns, scalds, frostbite; bleeding hemorrhoids, leucorrhea; syphilis, lymph gland TB; fungal infections.

Dosage: Decoction: 10-16 g
Tincture: 1-3 ml

In addition to internal use, topical applications for all of the indicated conditions are frequently prepared.

Caution: In digestive deficiency with chills.

Polygonum Quan Shen
Bistort Root

拳参

Botanical source: *Polygonum bistorta* L. (Polygonaceae)
Chinese names: Quan Shen, Cao He Che, Zhong Lou, Zi Shen (Mand); Kyun Sam (Cant)
Category: mild remedy with minimal chronic toxicity
Constituents: tannin, gallic acid, phlobaphene, phloroglucinol, methylanthraquinone, flavonoid
Effective qualities: bitter, astringent, cold; dissolving, astringing, decongesting, stimulating
Tropism: epidermal, urinary , reproductive systems; Liver, Spleen channels

Actions: *Detoxicant, antivenomous, anti-inflammatory, astringent, hemostatic, draining diuretic, laxative, emmenagogue, spasmolytic*

Indications: Toxicosis with boils, abscesses, sore throat; enteritis, snakebites; leucorrhea, tumors, the early stage of cancer; wounds, hemorrhage; water retention, constipation, amenorrhea.

Dosage: Decoction: 10-18 g
Tincture: 2-5 ml

Caution: This remedy is best used for severe infections.

Notes: Also known as alpine knotweed or snakeweed, this remedy is used for similar indications in Western herbal medicine.

Smilax Jin Gang Teng
China Root

金刚藤

Botanical source: *Smilax china* L. (Lilliaceae)
Chinese names: Jin Gang Teng, Ba Qia, Ba Ji, Gou Gu Zi (Mand); Gam Gong Tang (Cant)
Habit: Perennial climbing shrub from temperate China, growing on hillsides; umbels of small viridian blossoms open in summer.
Category: mild remedy with minimal chronic toxicity
Constituents: steroidal saponins (sarsasapogenin, diosgenin), cinchonin, resin, tannins
Effective qualities: sweet, neutral; dissolving, decongesting, calming
Tropism: epidermal, musculoskeletal, urinary systems; Spleen, Liver channels

Actions: *Resolvent detoxicant, antitumoral, anti-inflammatory, analgesic, anti-infective, diuretic*

Indications: Metabolic toxicosis with eczema, psoriasis, boils, abscesses, gout, rheumatism; cancer (esp. gastric, esophageal, rectal, breast, cervical and nasopharyngeal); acute, painful arthritis and rheumatism; traumatic injury; enteritis, dysentery, urinary tract infection, syphilis; diabetes, chyluria.

Dosage: Decoction: 30-60 g
Tincture: 2-5 ml

Very high doses are used for treating cancer.

Caution: None.

Echinops Lou Lu

Globe Thistle Root

漏芦

Botanical source: *Echinops latifolius* Tausch or *E. gmelinii* Turczaninov (Compositae)
Chinese names: Lou Lu (Mand); Lok Lu (Cant)
Category: mild remedy with minimal chronic toxicity
Constituents: echinopsine, ehinorine, echinine, essential oil
Effective qualities: bitter, salty, cold; dissolving, calming
Tropism: epidermal, cardiovascular, digestive systems; Large Intestine, Stomach channels

Actions: *Resolvent detoxicant, anti-inflammatory, antitumoral, galactagogue, hypotensive*
Indications: Toxicosis with boils, abscesses; acute mastitis, breast swelling and pain; hemorrhoids; early stage sores and ulcers; contusions, gout; tumors; insufficient breast milk.
Dosage: Decoction: 4-14 g
Tincture: 1-4 ml
Caution: Forbidden during pregnancy and in weak people or Qi deficiency conditions.
Notes: The root of *Rhaponticum uniflorum* (L.) De Candolle, **Swiss centaury,** is used interchangeably with the Globe thistle root as botanical source for the remedy Lou Lu.

Scutellaria Ban Zhi Lian

Barbed Skullcap Root and Herb

半枝蓮

Botanical source: *Scutellaria barbata* Don or *S. rivularis* (Labiatae)
Chinese names: Ban Zhi Lian (Mand); Bun Ji Lin (Cant)
Category: mild remedy with minimal chronic toxicity
Constituents: alkaloids
Effective qualities: a bit bitter, astringent, cold, dry; calming, decongesting
Tropism: digestive, respiratory, immune systems; Liver, Lung, Stomach channels

Actions: *Resolvent detoxicant, antitumoral, broad-spectrum anti-infective, anti-inflammatory, antipyretic, hepatobiliary decongestant, diuretic, antivenomous, detumescent, analgesic*
Indications: Toxicosis with tumors, incl. cancer (many types); boils, laryngitis, lung abscess; damp heat febrile infections, influenza, schistosomiasis; hepatitis, cirrhosis, edema with dysuria.
Topically for boils, pyodermas, snakebites and traumatic injury.
Dosage: Decoction: 10-60 g
Tincture: 2-5 ml
External applications are also prepared.
Caution: None.
Notes: Barbed skullcap root and herb is one of the most frequent components of *anticancer* formulas of all types in mainland China. However, it may be more useful for symptom relief rather than cure of cancer.

Solanum Bai Ying

Climbing Nightshade Herb

白英

Botanical source: *Solanum lyratum* Thunberg (Solanaceae)
Chinese names: Bai Ying, Gu Cai, Bai Cao, Bai Mao Teng (Mand); Baak Ying (Cant)
Habit: Perennial trailing vine from temperate China; blooms in summer with cymes of white flowers.
Category: mild remedy with minimal chronic toxicity
Constituents: alkaloids
Effective qualities: a bit bitter, cool, dry; dissolving, calming
Tropism: hepatobiliary, reproductive, urinary systems; Liver, Stomach channels

Actions: *Resolvent detoxicant, antitumoral, anti-inflammatory, mucostatic, hemostatic*
Indications: Toxicosis with boils, abscesses; tumors, cancer (many types, incl. of liver, stomach, esophagus, lung, bladder); hepatitis, cholecystitis, liver cirrhosis, thyroid enlargement; leucorrhea, menorrhagia, lumbar pain.
Dosage: Decoction: 16-30 g
Tincture: 2-5 ml
Caution: None.
Notes: This remedy is a frequent ingredient in *anticancer* formulas in China and Taiwan.

Selaginella Shi Shang Bai
Spikemoss Herb

石上柏

Botanical source: *Selaginella doederleinii* Hieron (Selaginellaceae)
Chinese names: Shi Shang Bai, Pa Bai, Sheng Ye Chuan Bai, Da Ye Cai (Mand); Sek Song Paak (Cant)
Category: mild remedy with minimal chronic toxicity
Effective qualities: sweet, pungent, neutral; dissolving, calming
Constituents: alkaloids, saponins, phytosterols
Tropism: respiratory, digetive, urinary systems; Lung, Spleen, Bladder channels

Actions: *Resolvent detoxicant, antitumoral, anti-inflammatory, anti-infective, hepatic, hemostatic*
Indications: Toxicosis with boils, sore throat, cough; cancer (incl. of lung, nasopharynx, esophagus, chorion [chorioepithelioma, choriocarcinoma], liver, skin); bronchitis, pneumonia, tonsillitis; chronic hepatitis with jaundice, cholecystitis, ascites, cirrhosis; acute cystitis.
Dosage: Decoction: 15-30 g
Tincture: 2-5 ml
For cancer treatment, high doses of up to 100 g of the herb decocted for three or four hours are used.
Caution: None.

Momordica Mu Bie Zi
Cochin Bitter Melon Seed

木鱉子

Botanical source: *Momordica cochinchinensis* (Lour.) Sprengel (Cucurbitaceae)
Chinese names: Mu Bie Zi, Tu Mu Bi, Mu Bi, Mu Bie Gua (Mand); Muk Bit Ji (Cant)
Habit: Large perennial climbing vine from Southeast Asia and India, found in open woods, thickets and on hillsides; also cultivated; yellow flowers open in summer.
Category: medium-strength remedy with some chronic toxicity
Constituents: gypsogenin, momordic/eleostearic/pipecolic/oleanolic/trychosanic acid, phytosterol, mycose
Effective qualities: bitter, a bit sweet, warm; dissolving
Tropism: epidermal, digestive, lymphatic systems; Liver, Lung, Spleen, Stomach channels

Actions: *Resolvent detoxicant, detumescent, lymphatic decongestant, antitumoral, anti-inflammatory, anthelmintic, digestant, vulnerary*
Indications: Toxicosis with boils, sores, lymphangitis, lymphadenitis, hemangioma, psoriasis, scrofula, mastitis; tumors, malignant ulcers; intestinal parasites in infants, enteritis, dysentery, ringworm, mumps; hemorrhoids, sebaceous cysts, freckles, moles; swelling and pain from injury, contusion, fracture, lumbar/hemorrhoidal/anal pain.
Dosage: Decoction: 1-1.5 g
Tincture: 0.1-0.25 ml
Topical applications are much used, using the powder, swab, paste or compress.
Caution: Not for continuous use because of medium-strength status. Forbidden during pregnancy and in weak people.

Paris Qi Ye Yi Zhi Hua

Paris Root

七叶一枝花

Botanical source: *Paris polyphylla* Smith, *P. formosana* Hayata and var., *P. chinensis* Franchet (Liliaceae)
Chinese names: Qi Ye Yi Zhi Hua, Zao Xiu, Chong Lou, Qi Ye Lian (Mand); Chat Yip Yat Ji Fa, Sat Yau (Cant)
Category: medium-strength remedy with chronic toxicity
Constituents: steroidal saponins (diosgenin, alpha-paristyphin, dioscin), amino acids
Effective qualities: bitter, cool; dissolving, calming, relaxing
Tropism: epidermal, nervous systems; Bladder, Lung channels

Actions: *Resolvent detoxicant, anti-inflammatory, detumescent, antitumoral, antipyretic, spasmolytic, anticonvulsant, antitussive, nervous sedative, analgesic*

Indications: Toxicosis with boils, abscesses, ulcers, sore throat, fever, tumors (incl. cancer); encephalitis, meningitis (incl. tuberculous), typhoid; allergic asthma, spasmodic cough; seizures (esp. febrile, with spasms, infantile); snake and insect bites.

Dosage: Decoction: 5-10 g. For cancer treatment, 15-30 g is used.
Tincture: 1-3 ml

Caution: Not for continuous use because of its medium-strength status. Toxic signs include nausea, vomiting, headache and seizures.

Notes: This remedy is derived from the rhizome of the above-listed species of *Paris* in the lily family.

Camptotheca Xi Shu

Happy Tree Root Bark

喜树

Botanical source: *Camptotheca acuminata* Decne. (Nyssaceae)
Chinese names: Xi Shu, Han Lian (Mand); Sei Sat (Cant)
Category: medium-strength remedy with chronic toxicity
Constituents: quinoline alkaloids (incl. camptothecine, hydroxy/methoxy/deoxy-camptothecine, venoterpine, trimethylellagic acid)
Effective qualities: bitter, cool; calming, dissolving
Tropism: digestive, epidermal, urinary, immune systems; Lung, Spleen channels

Actions: *Antitumoral, immunosuppressant, antiviral, abortive, dermatropic*

Indications: Tumors (incl. cancer: gastric, intestinal, rectal, urinary; lymphatic, ovarian); leukemia, leukosis (incl. lymphatic, myeloid); psoriasis, dermatitis, pityriasis rosea, neurodermatitis.

Dosage: Decoction: 8-16g
Tincture: 1-3 ml

Caution: Do not use long-term or exceed doses because of cumulative toxicity. Toxic effects include nausea, vomiting, diarrhea, gastric bleeding, hairloss and blood in urine. Forbidden in pregnancy and lactation.

Notes: In China the extracted and synthesized alkaloids from this remedy are also used.

Happy tree fruit is used in the same way as the root bark at a dose of 4-10 g. If the whole **root** and **branch** are used, the dosage is 15-35 g.

Crotalaria Ye Bai He
Thin-Leaf Rattlebox Herb

野百合

Botanical source: *Crotalaria sessiliflora* L. (Leguminosae)
Chinese names: Ye Bai He, Nong Ji Li, Yang Shi Dan, Hua Gu Cao, Long Ju Li (Mand); Ye Baak Hap (Cant)
Part used: the herb, including the seeds
Habit: Annual pilose herb from Mid and South China, found on sunny hillsides, roadsides and in grass thickets; purple flower spikes open in September.
Category: medium-strength remedy with some chronic toxicity
Constituents: pyrrolizidine alkaloids (incl. monocrotalines I and II, senecionine)
Effective qualities: sweet, bland, warm; softening, dissolving
Tropism: epidermal, digestive, immune, nervous systems; Lung, Liver channels

Actions: *Resolvent detoxicant, anti-inflammatory, antitumoral, dissolvent, diuretic, antidotal, antivenomous*
Indications: Toxicosis with boils, sores; tumors, cancer (incl. of skin, cervix, rectum, penis, stomach, lung, breast, esophagus, liver, blood); food poisoning, mushroom/mineral/pesticide/cigarette poisoning (incl. arsenic, DDT, hexachlorobenzene); dysentery; bones stuck in throat; deafness, tinnitus, dizziness; infantile malnutrition.
Dosage: Decoction: 10-16 g
Tincture: 1-3 ml
Up to 30 g of the decoction is traditionally used in severe cases.
Skin cancer is treated with topical as well as internal preparations of this remedy.
Caution: This remedy is not for long-term internal use because of its medium-strength status, achieved through its content in pyrrolizidine alkaloids. Signs of toxicity include appetite loss and abdominal bloating.
Notes: This remedy has achieved prominence in treating a variety of cancers. Although some modern researchers feel that the dosage should be lower because of Crotalaria's cumulative toxicity, the doses given here are the ones traditionally, empirically found effective for the above condi-tions (especially for concerous conditions). In any case, truly long-term treatment is not desirable.

Lycoris Shi Suan
Red Spiderlily Corm

石蒜

Botanical source: *Lycoris radiata* (L'Her.) Herbert (Amaryllidaceae)
Chinese names: Shi Suan, Lao Ya Suan, Wu Suan (Mand); Sek Syun (Cant); "Stone garlic"
Habit: Perennial mountain herb from China and Japan growing in shady, wooded areas; umbels of large scarlet flowers open in summer.
Category: medium-strength remedy with some chronic toxicity
Constituents: alkaloids (incl. lycorine, lycoramine, lycoreine, galanthamine, dihydro- and pseudolycorine, tazettine, pluvine, norpluviine, squamigerine, vittatine)
Effective qualities: pungent, sweet, warm; dissolving, calming
Tropism: epidermal, nervous, respiratory, urinary systems; Bladder, Lung channels

Actions: *Resolvent detoxicant, detumescent, anti-inflammatory, antitumoral, antiparasitic, expectorant, emetic, uricosuric diuretic*
Indications: Toxicosis with sores, virulent boils, furuncles, abscesses, deep-rooted ulcers; acute laryngitis with swallowing difficulty; tumors, cancer; lymph gland TB; scabies; infantile neurodermatitis.
Dosage: Decoction: 1.5 g
Tincture: 0.1-0.25 ml
Caution: Use only under supervision. This medium-strength remedy is not for long-term use because of its cumulative toxicity. Doses must not be exceeded.

Cantharis Ban Mao

Cantharides

斑毛

Zoological source: *Mylabris phalerata* Pallas and spp., *Cantharis vesicatoria* De Geer and spp. (Meloidae/Coleoptera)
Chinese names: Ban Mao (Mand); Ban Mou (Cant)
Other names: Spanish fly, Chinese blister beetle; Hanmyo (Jap)
Part used: the whole animal
Category: strong remedy with acute toxicity

Constituents: cantharidin 1-1.2%, fats 12%, formic acid, wax, pigments
Effective qualities: pungent, cold, dry; stimulating, decongesting, relaxing, dissolving, softening, sinking
Tropism: immune, lymphatic, reproductive, digestive systems; Large Intestine, Small Intestine, Liver, Kidney channels

ACTIONS: *Resolvent detoxicant, antithrombotic, detumescent, antitumoral, antifungal, antiviral, leukocyte stimulant, urogenital mucostatic, diuretic urinary relaxant, uterine stimulant, abortive, reproductive stimulant/restorative, estrogenic*
INDICATIONS: Toxicosis with boils, furunculosis, lymphangitis, ulcers, non-suppurative sores, psoriasis; immobile palpable lumps, lymphadenitis and TB; tumors (incl. hepatic cancer, thyroid tumor); fungal skin conditions, viral conditions (incl. viral hepatitis, rabies); chemotherapy with decreased WBC count, chronic leucorrhea, spermatorrhea, enuresis, gonorrhea, bladder irritation; urgent, painful urination (dysuria), neurogenic bladder, strangury, amenorrhea, miscarriage; frigidity, impotence, hypoplastic and atonic sterility; allergic rhinitis.

In plaster form as external *counterirritant* and *vesicant:*

ACTIONS: *anti-inflammatory, analgesic, spasmolytic, dissolving, breaking up; nervous and circulatory stimulant; attractive*
INDICATIONS: Meningitis, encephalitis, myelitis, spondylitis, multiple sclerosis, spasms, epilepsy, headache, migraine, neuralgia (incl. sciatica), arthralgia, gout, otitis media, laryngitis, pleuritis, pneumonia, bronchial asthma, lung TB, angina pectoris, pericarditis, cholecystitis, pelvic inflammatory disease, thrombophlebitis, typhoid; psychosis, catatonia, paralysis, stroke; frigidity, impotence, sterility, chronic amenorrhea.

PREPARATION

Use: Cantharis Ban Mao is dry toasted or fried, or alkali processed, and then decocted or tinctured. Recent research shows the alkali-processing method to produce least toxicity. The same is true if the entire insect is used, rather than just the trunk (without head, feet and wings attached).

Because of its toxicity, Cantharis Ban Mao can only be safely taken internally if the dosage and administration protocols (see below) are followed to the letter. It is also found in compound pills. External preparations are far more common, however, and include washes and compresses for infectious and pyogenic (fire toxin) conditions such as fungal skin conditions, carbuncles, ulcers, etc. A plaster is also prepared or available for vesicant, or blistering, therapy. See Caution and Notes below.

Dosage: Decoction: 0.03-0.09 g

Tincture: 5-15 drops (10 drops is the average dose) taken for one week, discontinued for a week, then taken again and discontinued again for one week, etc. According to Aschner (1986), it is best to start with 5 drops and increase by 1 drop daily to reach the optimal dose, while watching for signs of toxicity (see below). Should these appear, stop immediately for a week, then restart and stay at the lower dose.

Caution: Do not use this remedy without professional supervision. Dosages must not be exceeded because of the strong nature of this remedy, a consequence of its kidney-irritating constituent cantharidin. Intake must be strictly limited to a week at a time, followed by a week's break. Cantharides is forbidden during pregnancy and for weak people, and is to be used cautiously with diabetics. Signs of toxicity include mouth-burning, thirst, vomiting, diarrhea, abdominal and urinary pain, and frequent urination. Toxicity should be counteracted with plenty of green tea (e.g., bancha) and a *gastrointestinal demulcent* such as Licorice root, Marshmallow root, Codonopsis Dang Shen or Dendrobium Shi Hu.

When used topically, Cantharides causes erythema and blistering, but only mild pain, and its blisters heal rapidly. The remedy should never be used on any broken skin or mucus membrane surface as it may then cause permanent damage.

Notes

Cantharides occupies a unique place in the pharmacopeia of both Asia and the West. Although infrequently used internally because of its acute and cumulative toxicity, it nevertheless is a significant remedy for treating severe conditions such as carcinomas, viral and fungal infections, leucocyte deficiency and reproductive deficiencies including sterility and impotence. Various Cantharides derivatives, such as sodium cantharidinate, often injected, are also used in Chinese hospitals, especially for their *antineoplastic* effect (Chang and But 1987).

Turning to the external applications of Cantharides, we find consistent useage in all major medical systems past and present. As a topical treatment, Cantharides was a mainstay of traditional Greek medicine in Europe up to the early 1800s, while until this century Chinese medicine used it in a more conservative way.

Making use of its *stimulant* nature, traditional Greek medicine applies Cantharides as a plaster for the express purpose of *vesicant* therapy. This is a derivative technique designed to draw blood and Qi to the area of irritation and away from the locale of pain and inflammation. As a topical *counterirritant vesicant,* the Cantharides plaster is unsurpassed in the variety of its applications, and is historically the most effective, widely used and important counterirritant known. Its historical origins are obscure, but Greek doctors in Alexandria and the near East, such as Aretaios and Oribasos in the first century A.D., are kown to have used Cantharides in this way. In the Renaissance, physicians applied it with great success from the time of Paracelsus to the time of Fyens, Sydenham, Baglivi and Tissot.

Cantharides is indicated in external conditions presenting pain, inflammation, stuck Blood and Qi/energy, being essentially *analgesic, spasmolytic, "Blood-vitalizing," dissolving.* With painful arthritis, neuralgia and rheumatism, i.e., wind/damp/cold obstruction conditions, Cantharides plaster is said to be the most effective topical treatment of all (Aschner 1968). The conditions listed for it above further divide into ear, throat, lung, heart, biliary, reproductive, musculoskeletal, mental and nervous conditions.

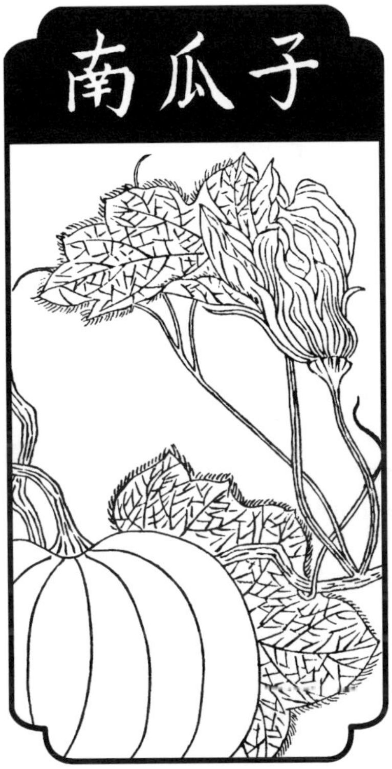

Cucurbita Nan Gua Zi

Red Squash Seed

Botanical source: *Cucurbita moschata* Duchesne (Cucurbitaceae)
Pharmaceutical name: Semen Cucurbitae moschatae
Chinese names: Nan Gua Zi (Mand); Naam Gwa Ji (Cant)
Other names: Winter squash, "Southern melon"; Nankashi (Jap)
Habit: Common annual temperate vine; yellow single axillary flowers appear in midsummer.
Part used: the seed and husk

Therapeutic category: mild remedy with minimal chronic toxicity
Constituents: glycerrhetin, linoleic and palmitic acid, urease, stearin, amino acid curcurbitine, fixed oil, vitamins B1 and 2
Effective qualities: sweet, warm, moist
calming
Tropism: digestive, urinary, respiratory, endocrine systems
Liver, Large Intestine channels
Fluid body

Actions and Indications

antiparasitic: anthelmintic; analgesic: tapeworm, roundworm, abdominal pain due to parasites; early stage of schistosomiasis
detumescent: postpartum peripheral edema with swelling
antitussive: whooping cough
galactagogue: insufficient lactation

Preparation

Use: The seed Cucurbita Nan Gua Zi may be decocted or powdered and eaten fresh, plain or toasted. Suppositories can also be prepared for tapeworms. Thirty day courses are standard for treating parasites.
Dosage: All forms: 30-60 g
Caution: This remedy may occasionally cause dizziness, nausea, vomiting, diarrhea and loss of appetite.

Notes

Red squash seed is most efficacious in tapeworm and the early stage of schistosoma. For this purpose this gentle yet effective *anthelmintic* is often combined with Betel nut (Areca Bing lang). Based on pharmacological research, the amino acid curcurbitine is thought to account for Red squash seed's ability to kill blood flukes (schistosoma).

The red squash, or winter squash, should not be confused with the pumpkin, *Cucurbita maxima,* whose seed is used mainly for prostate hyperplasia.

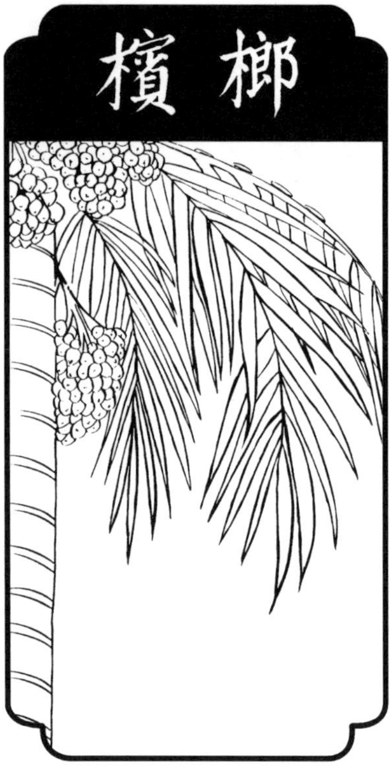

Areca Bing Lang

Betel Nut

Botanical source: *Areca catechu* L. (Arecaceae)
Pharmaceutical name: Semen Arecae
Chinese names: Bing Lang, Jian Lang (Mand); Ban Long (Cant)
Other names: Areca nut, Pinang; Binroji (Jap)
Habitat: Solitary palm tree found throughout the Asian (sub)tropics, including South China, Taiwan, Thailand, Malaysia and India.
Part used: the ripe seed

Therapeutic category: mild remedy with minimal chronic toxicity
Constituents: alkaloids (incl. arecoline, arecaidine, guvacine, guvacoline, arecolidine, homoarecoline), condensed tannins 15%, resin, catechin, starch, areca red pigment, fixed oil (palmitic/oleic/stearic/caprylic/lauric/myristic acids)
Effective qualities: pungent, bitter, astringent, warm
stimulating, decongesting, astringing
Tropism: digestive, urinary systems
Spleen, Stomach, Large Intestine channels
Air, Fluid bodies

Actions and Indications

antiparasitic: anthelmintic, vermicidal, antiviral: intestinal parasites; esp. tapeworm, pinworm, roundworm; taeniasis, fasciolopsiasis, ancylostomiasis, ascariasis, schistosomiasis (blood flukes), trichuriasis, malaria, influenza
digestive stimulant, carminative, enzymatic digestant: intestinal dyspepsia
astringent, spasmolytic: diarrhea, dysentery with tenesmus
draining diuretic: edema (esp. of lower limbs), dysuria
emmenagogue: scanty or absent menses
antifungal: fungal skin conditions
interferon inducent
Miscellaneous: beriberi; glaucoma (topically)

Symptom Picture

food stagnation: indigestion with mild abdominal pain, flatulence, distension, diarrhea or constipation

Preparation

Use: The nut Areca Bing Lang is decocted or used in tincture form. The raw nut only should be used, as it can be up to 50% higher in alkaloid content than the processed nut. The decoction should be drunk cold, as it may cause vomiting when taken warm. Eyedrops for treating glaucoma are also prepared.

Dosage: Decoction: 6-14 g. High doses of between 60-120 g are used for tapeworm if the remedy is taken alone.
Tincture: 2-4 ml

Caution: Use with caution in people with tendency to organ prolapse. Do not overdose, as this may cause salivation, nausea, vomiting, dizziness or nervousness.

Notes

Betel nut is a commonly used *wide-spectrum anthelmintic* remedy from the southern provinces. The remedy works by paralyzing and eliminating parasites, and is most effective for tapeworm and other intestinal worms. The cholinergic alkaloid arecoline is not only deemed *vermicidal,* but also has shown to stimulate salivation, peristalsis and enzyme secretion. Clinically, the optimum use of this botanical is when food stagnation and intestinal parasites present together.

使君子

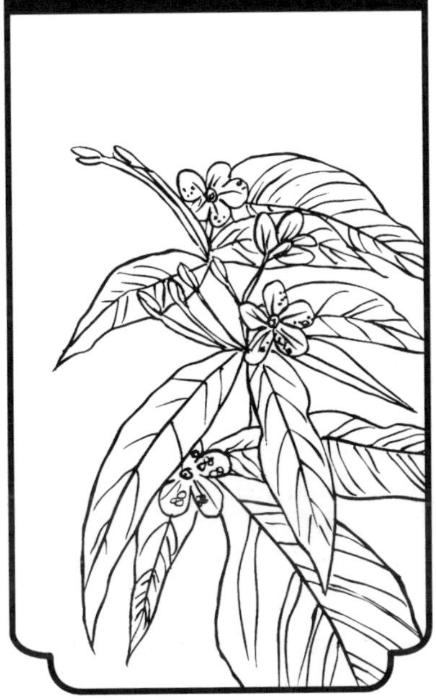

Quisqualis Shi Jun Zi

Rangoon Creeper Nut

Botanical source: *Quisqualis indica* L. (Combretaceae)
Pharmaceutical name: Fructus Quisqualis
Chinese names: Shi Jun Zi (Mand); Si Gwan Ji (Cant)
Other names: Shikunshi (Jap)
Habit: Woody climbing vine from the forests and mountains of South China, Southeast Asia and India; cymes of carmine terminal flowers bloom in summer.
Part used: the fruit with seed kernel

Therapeutic category: medium-strength remedy with some chronic toxicity
Constituents: potassium quisqualate, quisqualic acid, fixed oil 0-27% (incl. myristic/oleic/palmitic/stearic/linoleic acid), trigonelline, pyridine, resin
Effective qualities: sweet, warm, moist
restoring, stimulating
Tropism: digestive, urogenital systems
Spleen, Stomach channels
Fluid body

Actions and Indications

antiparasitic: anthelmintic, ascaricidal: intestinal parasites, esp. roundworm (ascariasis) with abdominal pain; tapeworm (taeniasis), pinworm/threadworm (oxyuriasis); tapeworm (taeniasis); parasitic skin conditions, intestinal trichomoniasis, enterobiasis
antifungal: fungal skin conditions (incl. tinea), yeast infections
gastric stimulant, carminative: gastric dyspepsia, infantile malnutrition, marasmus, anorexia
Miscellaneous*:* leucorrhea

Symptom Picture

stomach Qi stagnation: weakness, appetite loss, indigestion, abdominal pain and distension

Preparation

Use: The nut Quisqualis Shi Jun Zi is decocted or used in tincture form. Washes, compresses, douches (etc.) may be made using either. Roasting the fruits beforehand seems to decrease any side effects (see below). The roasted ripe seeds are given in diarrhea and fever.
Dosage: Decoction: 6-12 g
Tincture: 2-4 ml
Caution: This remedy may provoke nausea, hiccups and vomiting, especially in the higher dosage, and should not be taken continuously for more than two weeks. Do not drink tea before or after taking this remedy as it may increase these side effects.

Notes

The dark brown, ribbed nut of the Rangoon creeper is named after the physician Guo Shi-jun who, in the fourteenth century, made extensive use of the remedy's *antiparasitic* and *ascaricidal* properties in his pediatrics practice. In children, marasmus, abdominal swelling and pain due to worms are the keynote symptoms of Rangoon creeper nut. This *broad-spectrum anthelmintic* is also particularly suited to weak constitutions.

The key *anthelmintic* component of this *stimulant* remedy appears to be quisqualic acid.

苦楝皮

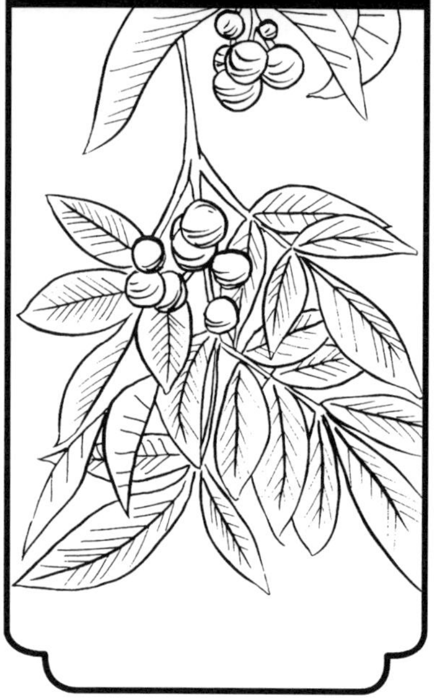

Melia Ku Lian Pi

Bead Tree Root Bark

Botanical source: *Melia azedarach* L. or *M. toosendan* Siebold et Zuccarini (Meliaceae)
Pharmaceutical name: Cortex radicis Meliae
Chinese names: Ku Lian Pi, Ku Lian Gen Pi (Mand); Fu Lin Pei (Cant)
Other names: Persian lilac, Chinaberry, Umbrella tree; Kurenkonpi (Jap)
Habit: Tall deciduous tree from South and Central China, growing wild by roadsides and waste places; also cultivated; blooms in summer with panicled terminal/axillary purple flowers.
Part used: the root bark; also the bark and leaf

Therapeutic category: medium-strength remedy with some chronic toxicity
Constituents: *M. azed.:* alkaloid margosine, tannin, resin
M. toos.: toosendanin, margoside, resin tannin, triacontane, sitosterol, triterpene kulinone, kulolactone, meliantriol, nimbolin A and B, fraxinellone, gedunin, glucose
Effective qualities: bitter, astrigent, cold, dry, restoring, astringing
Tropism: digestive, reproductive, epidermal systems
Liver, Spleen, Stomach channels
Air body

Actions and Indications

antiparasitic: anthelmintic, ascaricidal: roundworms (ascariasis); threadworms (oxyuriasis), tapeworms (taeniasis), hookworms (ancylostomiasis), trichmoniasis with vaginitis; trichuriasis, scabies, rubella, erysipelas, sores, leprosy
antifungal: ringworm (tinea), yeast infections
dermatropic: weeping/vesicular eczema, urticaria

Preparation

Use: The root bark Melia Ku Lian Pi is decocted or used in tincture form. The latter is the more effective for topical application for the indicated skin and gynecological conditions. The remedy is also used powdered and mixed with vinegar.

Dosage: Decoction: 6-20 g
Tincture: 2-4 ml

Caution: Contraindicated in liver disease, and to be used cautiously in weak digestion and weak constitutions. Prolonged intake of this medium-strength remedy is forbidden. Signs of intoxication include vomiting, dizziness, abdominal pain and numb extremities.

Notes

So named because its seeds are used for fashioning ornamental and rosary beads, the deciduous bead tree from the East Asian tropics also furnishes in its root bark a *broad-spectrum antiparasitic* remedy. The reliably *anthelmintic* compound is toosendanin, one of the most effective for ascariasis known.

Bead tree stem bark can be also used as an *anthelmintic,* but is somewhat less effective than the root bark. The tree's less used long, serrated leaves, fragrant lilac flowers, golden yellow drupes and seeds are each also used for various ailments.

Brucea Ya Dan Zi

鴉膽子

Brucea Berry

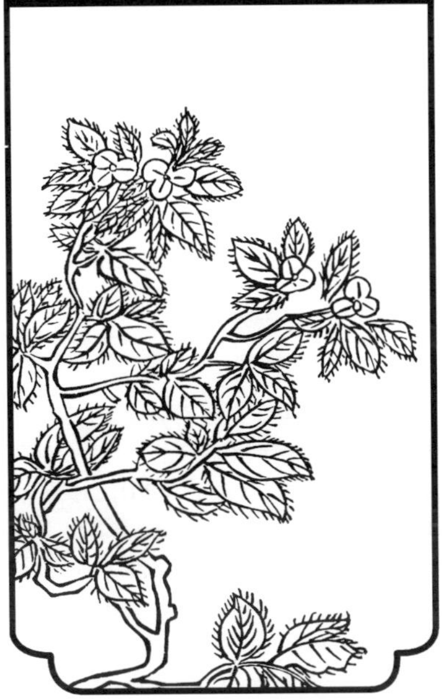

Botanical source: *Brucea javanica* (L.) Merrill (Simarubaceae)
Pharmaceutical name: Fructus Bruceae
Chinese names: Ya Dan Zi, Ku Shen Zi (Mand); Nga Daan Ji (Cant)
Other names: Java brucea, Kosam, "Crow gallbladder seed"; Atanshi (Jap)
Habit: Shrub or small tree from South China, Sumatra and India, growing on slopes, roadside shrubland and near villages; flowers in June with minute purple blossom clusters forming axillary panicles.
Part used: the ripe fruit

Therapeutic category: medium-strength remedy with high chronic toxicity
Constituents: bitters (incl. brusatol, bruceolide, bruceines), quassinoid glycosides (incl. bruceosides A and B, bruceantin, bruceantinol, yadaziosides, bruceantarin, dehydrobruceine A and B), glycosides (yatanoside, kosamine, brucealin), alkaloids (incl. yatanine, brucamarine), chrysophanol, chrysophanein, fixed oil (incl. oleic/ stearic linolic acids), phenol brucenol, bruceolic acid, ethyl gallate, emodin, vanillic acid
Effective qualities: very bitter, cold, dry
restoring
Tropism: digestive, circulatory systems
Large Intestine, Gallbladder channels; Warmth, Fluid bodies

Actions and Indications

antiparasitic: anthelmintic, vermicidal: hookworm, pinworm, tapeworm, nematodes; ancylostomiasis, schistosomiasis, paramecium
antiprotozoal: antiamoebic, antimalarial: protozoa infestation, amoebic conditions (incl. dysentery), giardiasis, trichomoniasis, malaria (all types)
antidysenteric, anti-inflammatory, detoxicant: chronic diarrhea, dysentery, hemorrhoids
antipyretic, nervous sedative: low fevers, malaria
antitumoral: tumors (incl. cancer, esp. of breasts, cervix, lung, stomach, skin)
necrotizing (locally): warts, corns, papilloma, keloids, verruca, condyloma, skin cancer

Symptom Picture

intestines damp cold: chronic diarrhea, alternating soft and hard stool, fatigue

Preparation

Use: The berry Brucea Ya Dan Zi is taken in decoction, tincture, or else is eaten unprocessed, either wrapped in a longan fruit or ground and put into capsules. Topical preparations like compresses are also made for tumors, wens, corns and parasitic conditions. The extracted fatty oil may also be applied for topical/local conditions.

Dosage: Decoction for internal use: 0.5-2 g, i.e., 7-20 berries. 10-15 berries are generally used for malaria, 10-30 berries for amoebic dysentery.
Tincture: 0.8-0.2 ml, i.e. 5-20 drops

Caution: Brucea berry is contraindicated during pregnancy and nursing, and in young children. It should also be used cautiously in gastrointestinal bleeding and liver and kidney disease. Brucea berry should generally be used very carefully because its toxicity is rapidly cumulative. Use should always be discontinued after a 7- to 10-day course.

Being a local irritant, Brucea berry frequently causes mild side-effects such as nausea, vomiting, abdominal discomfort or pain, diarrhea, dizziness and fatigue. However, no fatal overdose of this remedy has been recorded in China in the last two-hundred years (Chang and But 1987).

NOTES

A highly effective *broad-spectrum antiparasitic* remedy, Brucea berry is valued throughout Asia for treating stubborn intestinal parasites, malaria and amoebic dysentery. In addition, the berry is especially useful for chronic and recurring enteritis and dysentery.

The quassinoids and bitter compound brusatol have shown good *antitumoral* activity in a variety of cancers. Topical preaparations are also made for skin cancer and other skin conditions (see Preparation).

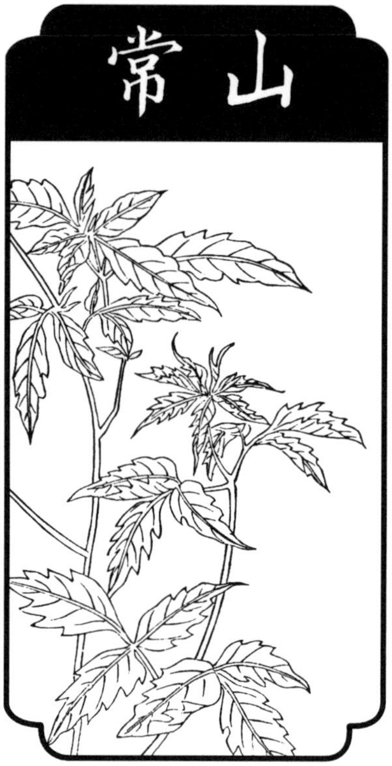

Dichroa Chang Shan

Feverflower Root

Botanical source: *Dichroa febrifuga* Loureiro (Saxifragaceae)
Pharmaceutical name: Radix Dichroae
Chinese names: Chang Shan, Shou Qi, Shu Qi, Hen Shan (Mand); Seung San (Cant)
Other names: Chinese quinine, "Eternal mountain"; Aseru, Basak; Josan (J)
Habit: Deciduous semi-shrub from Central China's mountain valleys; also Java, Philippines, Himalayas; found along streams, on slopes and in open woods; umbels of light blue terminal/axillary flowers appear in autumn.
Part used: the root; also the leaf and young twig

Therapeutic category: medium-strength remedy with some chronic toxicity
Constituents: alkaloids (incl. alpha/beta/gamma dichroine [febrifugine], dichroidine, changrolin [quinazoline]), umbelliferone, trimethylamine
Effective qualities: bitter, pungent, cool, dry
stimulating, relaxing
Tropism: cardiovascular, respiratory, digestive systems
Liver, Gallbladder, Lung channels; Warmth, Air bodies

ACTIONS AND INDICATIONS

antiparasitic, antiprotozoal (antimalarial, antiamoebic): malaria (all types), giardiasis, amoebiasis, trichomoniasis, food poisoning
antipyretic: fevers in general (incl. intermittent/remittent fever)
cardiac relaxant, hypotensive: hypertension, arrhythmia, tachycardia, fibrillation, premature beats
expectorant: bronchitis with productive cough
diuretic
emetic
antitumoral: cancer

SYMPTOM PICTURE

heart Qi constraint (Liver Yang rising): dizziness, ringing in ears, headache, irregular or fast heart beats

PREPARATION

Use: The root Dichroa Chang Shan is decocted or used in tincture form. It can also be used as an *emetic* to cause therapeutic vomiting (see Holmes 1989). The *emetic* effect can be counteracted by stir-frying the sliced root in ginger juice or white wine, or by combining it with *antiemetics* such as Pinellia Ban Xia, Agastache Huo Xiang, Citrus Chen Pi (Ripe tangerine rind) or Peppermint herb. Topical applications include swabs, douches and vaginal sponges.
Dosage: Decoction: 5-10 g
Tincture: 2-3 ml

Caution: Forbidden in pregnancy and nursing, and in senile debility. Because of its alpha-dichroine content, Dichroa Chang Shan is a medium-strength remedy with cumulative toxicity. It should be discontinued after a two-week period. It may also cause nausea and vomiting in some people at any time. However, this reaction decreases with every day of intake. Note that in Taiwan, the root of *Hydrangea chinensis* is the normal source of this remedy.

Notes

The name "Chang Shan" derives from the original discovery of this plant, supposedly by a feverish Buddhist monk, on Chang Shan, Mount Eternity. As its English name suggests, Feverflower root is a reliable *antipyretic* remedy, and is perfect when parasitic infestation is involved. The cluster of dichroine alkaloids also ensures a reliable remedy for malaria—a time-tested as well as scientifically proven usage.

The recently discovered excellent *cardiorelaxant* action of Feverflower root (which has been traced down to its alkaloidal derivative changrolin), has in recent years shown remarkable results in hypertension and other cardiac conditions (Ding 1987). In terms of vitalistic medicine this effect points tothe treatment of constrained Qi affecting the heart.

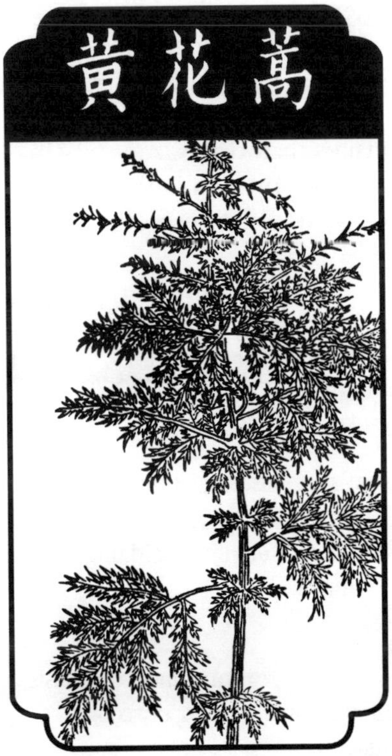

Artemisia Huang Hua Hao

Annual Wormwood Herb

Botanical source: *Artemisia annua* L. (Compositae)
Pharmaceutical name: Herba Artemisiae annnuae
Chinese names: Huang Hua Hao, Qing Hao (Mand); Wong Fa Hou (Cant)
Other names: Sweet Annie; "Yellow flowered wormwood"; Kusoninjin, Hosobaninjin (Jap)
Habit: Aromatic annual herb from temperate China, Siberia and Eurasia, growing on sunny hillsides, streamsides, roadsides and disturbed soil; yellow, tube-shaped capitulate flowers appear in August through October.
Part used: the herb

Therapeutic category: mild remedy with minimal chronic toxicity
Constituents: essential oil 0.9% (incl. terpenoid esters, ketone thujone, camphor, 1,8 cineol, linalool, monoterpenes [caryophyllene, myrcene]), sesquiterpene lactone arteannuin (artemisinin, qinghaosu) with peroxide group, dihydroarteannuic acid, qinhaosu A and B, scopolin, scopoletin, flavonoids (incl. chrysophlenetin, cirsilineol), methoxylated flavones (incl. casticin)
Effective qualities: bitter, cold, dry
relaxing, astringing, diluting, sinking
Tropism: digestive, hepatic, epidermal systems
Liver, Gallbladder channels; Warmth body

Actions and Indications

antiparasitic, antiprotozoal: schistosomiasis, giardiasis, trichomoniasis, malaria, scabies
anti-infective: antibacterial, antifungal: intestinal dysbiosis, chronic dysentery, food poisoning, candidiasis
detoxicant, antipruritic, vulnerary: abscesses, pruritus, urticaria, dermatitis, malignant ulcers, sores
antipyretic: fevers (esp. from food poisoning); low-grade fever with night sweats, heat syndrome, heatstroke
immunoregulator: autoimmune and immunodeficiency disorders (incl. lupus erythematosus)
anticoagulant: cerebral thrombosis
radiation-protective: radiation damage
insect repellent

PREPARATION

Use: The herb Artemisia Huang Hua Hao is briefly decocted, infused or taken in tincture form. External preparations are used for pruritic and eczematous skin conditions, and as *insect repellant*. Extracts of several of its constituents, notably arteannuin, have also been used for their *antiparasitic* action.

Dosage: Short decoction and infusion: 3-12 g
Tincture: 2-4 ml

Caution: None.

NOTES

This yellow flowered variety of *Artemisia,* although also traditionally called Qing Hao, today is more properly named Huang Hua Hao to distinguish it from *Artemisia apiacea,* Celery wormwood, also called Qing Hao.

Like other *Artemisia* varieties, Annual wormwood herb is a good *detoxicant, anti-infective* and *antipyretic.* In particular, the remedy is needed when intestinal dysbiosis and microbial toxicosis tend to cause hypersensitivity disorders on one hand and parasites on the other. Autoimmune conditions especially have responded to it, although the herb seems to act as an *immune regulator* in the truest sense, rather than an *immune-suppressant.* Because it contains such a broad range of constituents, it should also be investigated for potential *antiallergic* activity.

Blood parasites and protozoa is the parasitic terrain that requires Annual wormwood. Blood flukes, malaria (including the drug-resistant falciparum malarias) and giardiasis respond well to it. The plant contains the lactone arteannuin, the flavone casticin and the ketone thujone which together often act more quickly in destroying asexual parasites than drugs. Any possible relapse associated with the use of this remedy will usually be prevented by combining the herb with an *immune stimulant* such as Astragalus root, Echinacea root, Marigold flower, etc.

Torreya Fei Zi

Japanese Torreya Nut

榧子

Botanical source: *Torreya grandis* Fortune or *T. nucifera* Siebold et Zuccarini (Taxaceae)
Chinese names: Fei Zi (Mand); Fei Ji (Cant); Kaya
Category: mild remedy with minimal chronic toxicity
Constituents: gliadine, palmitic/oxalic/linoleic/stearic/oleic acid, tannin, sterol, lipids
Effective qualities: sweet, astringent, neutral, moist; softening
Tropism: digestive, respiratory systems; Lung, Large Intestine, Stomach channels

ACTIONS: *Anthelmintic, analgesic, demulcent laxative, antitussive*

INDICATIONS: Intestinal parasites with pain and marasmus: tapeworm (taeniasis), hookworm (ancylostomiasis), pinworm (oxyuriasis), roundworm (ascariasis); constipation from hemorrhoids; infantile malnutrition; dry cough.

Dosage: Decoction and powder: 10-25 g (10 to 20 seeds). Lightly toast the seeds first.
Tincture: 2-5 ml

Caution: None.

Mylitta Lei Wan

Thunder Ball Fungus

雷丸

Botanical source: *Mylitta lapidescens* Hortorum (syn. *Omphalia lapidescens* Schroeter) (Polyporaceae)
Chinese names: Lei Wan, Lei Yuan (Mand); Lai Yan (Cant)
Habit: Underground fungus from North China growing around the roots of bamboo.
Category: medium-strength remedy with chronic toxicity
Constituents: hydrolytic protease (mylittine) 3%
Effective qualities: bitter, cold
Tropism: digestive system; Stomach, Large Intestine ch.

ACTIONS: *Anthelmintic, vermicidal, antiprotozoal (antitrichomonal), antitumoral*
INDICATIONS: Intestinal parasites with marasmus; tapeworm (taeniasis); hookworm (ancylostomiasis), pinworm (oxyuriasis), roundworm (ascariasis), trichomoniasis.
Dosage: Powder and pill: 4-10 g
Caution: Use with caution with digestive deficiency present. Do not decoct, as temperature destroys the active enzyme mylittine. Because of its medium-strength status, this remedy is not for continuous high dosage use.
NOTES: Most effective of all for tapeworms, Thunder ball fungus operates by directly destroying them.

Carpesium He Shi
Starwort Fruit or Seed

鹤虱

Botanical source: *Carpesium abrotanoides* L. (Compositae)
Chinese names: He Shi, Tian Ming Jing (Mand); Ho Chi (Cant); "Stork flea"
Habit: Erect herb from China, Japan and North Vietnam.
Category: medium-strength remedy with some chronic toxicity
Constituents: coleic acid, stigmasterol, carpesialactone, carabrine, valine
Effective qualities: bitter, pungent, neutral; stimulating, calming
Tropism: digestive system; Spleen, Stomach, Liver ch.

ACTIONS: *Anthelmintic, analgesic*
INDICATIONS: Tapeworms (taeniasis), pinworms (oxyuriasis) roundworms (ascariasis); abdominal pain from intestinal parasites.
Dosage: Powder and pill: 6-12 g
Caution: Belonging to the medium-strength category, Carpesium He Shi should not be taken continuously on its own. Also watch for passing signs of dizziness, ringing in ears and abdominal pain.

Agrimonia He Cao Ya
Furry Agrimony Winter Bud

鹤草芽

Botanical source: *Agrimonia pilosa* Ledebour (Rosaceae)
Chinese names: He Cao Ya, Xian He Cao Gan Ya (Mand); Ho Chou Nga (Cant)
Category: medium-strength remedy with chronic toxicity
Constituents: hydroxycinnamic esters, isocoumarin glycoside, phenol agrimophol, nonacosane, sitosterol, pseudoaspidin, agrimol B, ellagic acid glycoside, agrimonolide, taxifolin, tormentic and ellagic acid
Effective qualities: bitter, cool
Tropism: digestive system; Spleen channel

ACTIONS: *Anthelmintic, antiprotozoal*
INDICATIONS: Parasitic conditions, incl. tapeworms, roundworms, bladder worms, schistosoma, giardiasis, trichomoniasis, malaria.
Dosage: Decoction: 6-12 g
Tincture: 2-4 ml

In Chinese clinics the extracted active constituent, the phenol agrimophol, is also given on its own.
Caution: Watch for side-effects of nausea and vomiting. Not for continuous high dosage use.

Aloe Lu Hui

Aloe Resin

芦荟

Botanical source: *Aloe vera* L. var. *chinensis* (Haw.) Berg (Liliaceae)
Chinese names: Lu Hui (Mand); Lou Wei (Cant)
Habit: (Sub)tropical succulent from Africa, the West Indies, the Mediterranean and India.
Category: mild remedy with minimal chronic toxicity

Constituents: glycosides, aloe-emodin, resin 16-36%, mucopolysaccharides, formic acids, glucose, electrolytes, trace minerals
Effective qualities: bitter, cool
Tropism: digestive, nervous systems; Liver, Stomach, Large Intestine channels

Actions: *Anthelmintic, antifungal, antiseptic, vulnerary, anti-inflammatory, antitumoral, nervous sedative, anticonvulsant, uterine stimulant, emmenagogue, purgative laxative*
Indications: Intestinal parasites, fungal/yeast infections (topically), caries, sores, burns; cancer (e.g. acute monocytic leukemia); headache, dizziness, unrest, infantile seizures (incl. epileptic); obstinate amenorrhea, constipation; fever from malnutrition; whooping cough.
Dosage: Decoction, powder or pill: 1.5-4 g
Tincture: 0.2-1 ml
Whole leaf decoction: 10-15 g

Topical preparations, including douches, vaginal sponges and enemas are prepared in addition to internal use.
Caution: Forbidden during pregnancy, in weak digestion, pelvic congestion, hemorrhoids and uterine bleeding.
Notes: This remedy is prepared from the dried leaf exterior of the aloe plant, yielding a resinous juice which is then dried. Most species of aloe contain this resin.

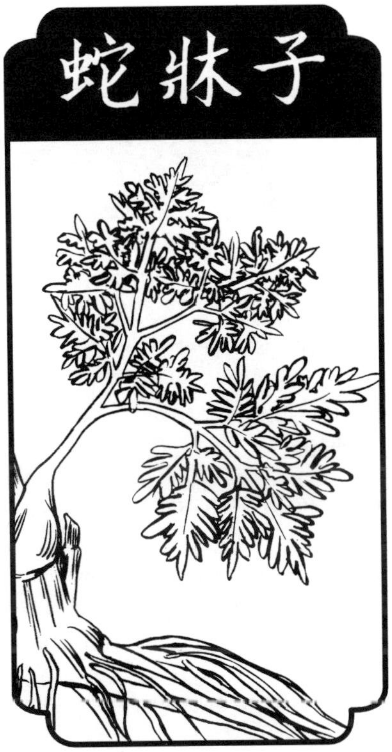

Cnidium She Chuang Zi

Cnidium Seed

Botanical source: *Cnidium monnieri* Cuss., *C formosanum* Yabe (Umbelliferae)
Pharmaceutical name: Fructus Cnidii
Chinese names: She Chuang Zi, She Su (Mand); Se Chong Ji (Cant)
Other names: "Snake bed seed"; Jashoshi (Jap)
Habit: Perennial temperate herb from Central and North China, Vietnam and Siberia, growing in river valleys along fields and ditches; lateral/terminal compound umbels of small white blossoms flower during summer and autumn.
Part used: the fruit (with the seeds)

Therapeutic category: mild remedy with minimal chronic toxicity
Constituents: essential oil 1.3% (incl. pinene, camphene, bornyl isovalerate, isovalerate, isoborneol, terpineol), osthol, coumarins (incl. columbianetin, cnidimine [edultin], cnidiadin, isopimpinelline, archangelicin, columbianetin, calumbianadin, dihydroroselol, xanthotoxin, imperatorine, alloimperatorine, xanthoxol), trace elements
Effective qualities: pungent, bitter, warm, dry
astringing, restoring, relaxing
Tropism: urogenital, digestive, epidermal systems
Kidney, Spleen, Dai channels; Warmth body

Actions and Indications

antiparasitic: antifungal, antiprotozoal: scabies, tinea (ringworm), yeast infections with vaginitis (incl. candidiasis, moniliasis); trichomoniasis, ascariasis, giardiasis
antiviral, interferon inducent: influenza, common cold
aphrodosiac, estrogenic, androgenic: infertility, impotence, sexual disinterest, frigidity
spasmolytic, analgesic: dyspepsia, abdominal and rheumatic pain, dysmenorrhea, strangury
bronchodilator: bronchial asthma, bronchitis
urinary astringent: incontinence with enuresis, pollakiuria
astringent, mucostatic, antipruritic (topical): leucorrhea, trichomonal vaginitis, eczema (esp. vesicular, scrotal); genital and other pruritus
vulnerary, anesthetic (topical): sores, injuries
Miscellaneous: uterine displacement

Preparation

Use: The fruit Cnidium She Chuang Zi is decocted or used in tincture form. It is both used internally and prepared for external use in douches, vaginal sponges, swabs, washes, salves or powders for the above genital and skin conditions.
Dosage: Decoction: 4-14 g
Tincture: 2-4 ml
Caution: Contraindicated in acute urogenital infections with discharge, and in Yin deficiency heat.
Note: In Hong Kong and Taiwan the species *Cnidium formosanum* is normally used.

Notes

Cnidium seed is a reliable topical remedy traditionally reserved for itchy, weeping skin conditions and pruritic vaginitis. However, the seed's general *antiparasitic, antiviral* and *gonadotropic* actions are also significant, and are much employed at the present day. Possessing a *relaxant* effect, the extracted coumarins are sometimes used for treating asthma and bronchitis.

Hibiscus Mu Jin Pi

Rose of Sharon Root Bark

木槿皮

Botanical source: *Hibiscus syriacus* L. (Malvaceae)
Chinese names: Mu Jin Pi, Mu Jing Hua (Mand); Mut Gan Pei (Cant)
Habit: Deciduous shrub from South China, Japan and Taiwan, mostly cultivated; pale pink or lilac single flowers open in fall.

Category: mild remedy with minimal chronic toxicity
Constituents: saponin, saponaretin, vitexin
Effective qualities: sweet, astringent, cool, dry; astringing, restoring
Tropism: epidermal, respiratory, digestive systems; Large Intestine, Lung channels

Actions: *Broad-spectrum antifungal, antibacterial, vermifuge, insecticidal, antipruritic, astringent, anti-infective, anti-inflammatory, hemostatic, mucostatic, diuretic*

Indications: Topically for fungal skin infections (esp. from dermatophytes, incl. tinea, favus), yeast infections, vaginitis with pruritus, eczema (esp. scrotal), squamous conditions, erythrasma, pruritus, hemorrhoids.

Internally for intestinal parasites (ascariasis, amoebiasis, giardiasis); diarrhea, enteritis, dysentery with bloody stool, gas and dizziness; intestines damp heat syndrome; leucorrhea.

Dosage: Decoction: 6-14 g
Tincture: 2-4 ml

External applications are routine for the above skin conditions, using the tincture or paste (the powdered root bark mixed with vinegar is best).

Caution: None.

Notes: Rose of Sharon root bark is a specific for dermatophytosis and a good general remedy for skin infections.

Rose of Sharon flower, Mu Jin Hua (Mand.) or **Mut Gan Fa** (Cant.) is given internally for dysentery, leucorrhea and bleeding hemorrhoids, and externally for boils. Dose: 10-30 g.

Kochia Di Fu Zi

Kochia seed

地肤子

Botanical source: *Kochia scoparia* (L.) Schrader (Chenopodiaceae)
Chinese names: Di Fu Zi (Mand); Dei Fu Ji (Cant)
Other names: Broom/Summer cypress, "Earth skin seed"

Category: mild remedy with minimal chronic toxicity
Constituents: triterpenoid saponins, alklaoids, vitamin A
Effective qualities: sweet, bitter, cold; calming
Tropism: epidermal, urinary, reproductive systems; Bladder, Kidney channels

Actions: *Broad-spectrum antifungal, antibacterial, dermatropic detoxicant, antipruritic, diuretic* (mild)

Indications: Topically and internally for fungal skin infections (incl. tinea), pruritus, eczema, scabies, ulcers; yeast infections with vaginitis, discharge and itching, dysuria, acute urinary tract infection, nephritis.

Dosage: Decoction: 4-14 g
Tincture: 2-4 ml

This remedy is for both internal and topical use.

Caution: Use only in damp heat conditions, such as those above.

Lithargyrum Mi Tuo Seng

Litharge

密佗僧

Geological source: *Lithargyrum*
Chinese names: Mi Tuo Seng (M); Muk Toi Sang (C)
Source: Mid China, Sichuan, Yunnan
Category: medium-strength remedy with chronic toxicity

Constituents: lead oxide, impurities silica and iron
Effective qualities: salty, pungent, neutral; astringing
Tropism: epidermal, digestive systems; Liver, Large Intestine channels

Actions: *Antifungal, detumescent, hemostatic*
Indications: Topically for fungal skin conditions (tinea), vaginitis, yeast infections, scabies; chronic draining ulcers and sores, pyodermia, swollen bleeding hemorrhoids, leukoderma, underarm odor.

Internally for chronic dysentery with blood, infantile seizures.

Dosage: The powder and paste are applied topically. Facial ointiments containing Litharge were prepared for skin blemishes.

Powder and pill for internal use: 1-3 g

Caution: Being medium-strength, do not use this remedy continuously internally. Contraindicated in weak people.
Notes: Litharge, or lead monoxide is a by-product of the smelting of the mineral galena for its silver and lead content.

Realgar Xiong Huang

Realgar

雄黄

Geological source: *Realgar*
Chinese names: Xiong Huang, Xiong Jing (M); Song Wong (C); "Male yellow," "Cinnabar mountain soul"
Other names: Red arsenic
Source: Central China, Sichuan, Yunnan
Category: mild remedy with minimal chronic toxicity

Constituents: arsenic di/trisulfide, traces calcium, iron, chloride, antimony
Effective qualities: pungent, bitter, warm; stimulating
Tropism: epidermal, digestive systems; Liver, Large Intestine channels

Actions: *Antiparasitic, antifungal, anthelmintic, antibacterial, detoxicant, antipruritic*
Indications: Topically for scabies, ringworm, lice, tinea and other fungal skin conditions, vaginitis; yeast infections, trichomoniasis, neurodermatitis, abscesses, boils, pyodermia, skin ulcers, pruritus; insect/snake bites.

Internally for roundworm (ascariasis) with marasmus, blood flukes (schistosomiasis); chronic malaria, giardiasis

Dosage: Powder: 0.2-0.4 g for swabs, compresses, etc., as well as internal use.
The mineral remedy should never be heated as it oxidizes and becomes highly toxic. Use directly in powder form only.
Caution: Contraindicated in pregnancy and with Blood/metabolic deficiency conditions.
Notes: Realgar was one of the main minerals used in mediaeval Daoist alchemy. It was believed to possess the ability to transform copper into gold. Realgar was the emblem of the color yellow in the preparation of longevity elixirs.

Polistes Lu Feng Fang

Hornet Nest

露蜂房

Zoological source: *Polistes mandarinus* Saussure and spp. and *Parapolybia varia* Fabricius
Chinese names: Lu Feng Fang, Feng Fang (Mand); Lou Fun Fong (Cant)
Source: Primarily South China

Part used: the hornet or wasp nest
Category: medium-strength remedy with chronic toxicity
Constituents: resin, beeswax, minerals, amino acids
Effective qualities: sweet, neutral; calming
Tropism: epidermal systems; Lung, Liver, Stomach ch.

Actions: *Antiparasitic, antifungal, antipruritic, dermatropic, vulnerary, analgesic, detoxicant, coagulant, antitumoral, anticonvulsant, antitussive, diuretic*
Indications: Scabies, tinea, vaginitis, yeast infections, urticaria, eczema, pruritus, simple sores, boils, carbuncles, pyodermia; toothache, gum swelling and pain, arthralgia, myalgia; gastric/cervical cancer; seizures, chronic cough.
Dosage: Decoction: 3-8 g

Swabs, salves, compresses, douches, etc. are also applied for topical conditions.

A warm gargle is used for toothache and gum pain and swelling.

Caution: Do not use continuously internally, nor overstep the dosage of this medium-strength remedy. Contraindicated in Qi or Blood (metabolic) deficiency and for sores that have already burst.

Sulphur Liu Huang
Sulphur

硫黃

Geological source: *Sulphurum*
Chinese names: Liu Huang, Shi Liu Huang (Mand); Lau Wong (Cant); "Sulphur yellow"
Source: Central and South China, Taiwan
Category: medium-strength remedy with chronic toxicity

Constituents: sulphur, impurities selenium, tellurium
Effective qualities: sour, pungent, hot; softening, stimulating
Tropism: epidermal, digestive, respiratory systems; Kidney, Spleen, Pericardium channels

Actions: *Antiparasitic, antifungal, detoxicant, vulnerary, antipruritic, laxative, reproductive and adrenal restorative*
Indications: Topically for tinea, scabies, vaginitis with pruritus; sicosis; cold boils (e.g. carbuncles), pyodermia, festering sores with pruritus, chronic ulcers.

Internally for Yang deficiency with cold symptoms, incl. impotence, asthma, urinary frequency, constipation; lumbar and knee weakness, pain or coldness.

Dosage: Decoction of the powder: 1.5-6 g for topical (compress, swab, etc.) and internal use.

Sulphur is usually processed with tofu for internal use.

Caution: This mineral remedy is contraindicated during pregnancy, and in Yin deficiency and empty heat conditions. Do not take internally continuously because of its medium-strength status.
Notes: Not only doctors, but also alchemists, cosmetics manufacturers and painters made extensive use of sulphur in the past. The mineral was an essential ingredient in Daoist cinnabar pills, for example. Dioskurides' *On Therapeutic Substances*, a basic textbook of Greek medicine, also lists detailed medical applications for sulphur.

Hydnocarpus Da Feng Zi
Chaulmoogra Seed

大楓子

Botanical source: *Hydnocarpus anthelmintica* Pierre (Flacourtiaceae)
Chinese names: Da Feng Zi (Mand); Daai Fun Ji (Cant)
Category: medium-strength remedy with chronic toxicity

Constituents: 15-56% oil with fatty acids (hydnocarpic/chaulmoogric/oleic/gorlic/palmitic)
Effective qualities: pungent, hot; stimulating
Tropism: epidermal, digestive systems; Spleen, Liver, Kidney channels

Actions: *Antiparasitic, antifungal, antibacterial, antiputrefacient, antiseptic*
Indications: Topically for scabies, trichomoniasis, tinea, yeast infection, vaginitis; leprosy, elephantiasis, syphilis, smallpox, dermatitis, burns, scalds; rheumatism; esp. *Mycobacterium leprae* and *M. tuberculosis.*
Dosage: Decoction: 0.3-0.9 g for external use only in swabs, washes, compresses, vaginal sponges, etc.
Caution: None.
Notes: Used throughout tropical Asia, this remedy is also called **Krabao oil tree seed.**

Alumen Ming Fan
Alum

明矾

Geological source: *Alumen*
Chinese names: Ming Fan, Bai Fan (M); Ming Faan (C)
Source: Central and East China
Category: medium-strength remedy with chronic toxicity

Constituents: aluminum potassium sulfate
Effective qualities: sour, astringent, cold
Tropism: digestive, vascular systems; Lung, Spleen, Stomach, Large Intestine channels

Actions: *Antiparasitic, antifungal, anti-infective, astringent, amti-inflammatory, hemostatic, styptic, antipruritic, detumescent, mucolytic expectorant, anticonvulsant, nervous sedative*

Indications: Topically for scabies, tinea, trichomoniasis, yeast infections, vaginitis, pruritus; streptococcal and diphtherial infections; chronic diarrhea, nosebleed, blood in stool, uterine bleeding, bleeding hemorrhoids, bleeding gums; swollen, painful eyes, gums and throat; middle ear infection; bleeding traumatic injuries, leucorrhea, weeping eczema, cough with difficult expectoration, seizures with delirium (wind phlegm syndrome).

Dosage: Powder: 0.6-3 g

Use this mineral remedy topically in a 5-10% dilution for most conditions (e.g. wash, swab, compress, vaginal sponge, douche, gargle).

Caution: Because of its medium-strength status, use Alum with caution internally, and then never for prolonged periods of time. Signs of toxicity include diarrhea, vomiting and ulceration.

Notes: Also known as Potash alum, the mineral was also commonly used as an industrial mineral in the past, especially by leather-workers, papermakers and dyers (as a mordent). Although North-west China produced some alum, the highest quality was imported from Qoco in Central Asia.

Calomelas Qing Fen
Calomel

轻粉

Geological source: *Calomelas*
Chinese names: Qing Fen, Shui Yin Fen (Mand); Ching Fan (Cant)
Source: Central China, Yunnan
Category: strong remedy with acute toxicity

Constituents: mercurous chloride, calcium sulphate, trace iron
Effective qualities: pungent, cold
Tropism: epidermal urinary system; Kidney, Bladder channels

Actions: *Antiparasitic, antifungal, draining diuretic, purgative laxative*

Indications: Topically for scabies, syphilitic chancres, fungal skin infections, neurogenic dermatitis (incl. shingles).

Internally for edema, anuria, constipation.

Dosage: Powder or paste for topical use
Powder for internal use: 0.1-0.2 g

Caution: Because it is in the strong category, the mineral remedy Calomel is best kept for external use only. The main sign of toxicity is acute nephritis.

Notes: Calomel purified by careful sublimation is called **Fen Shuang** or **Shui Yin Shuang.**

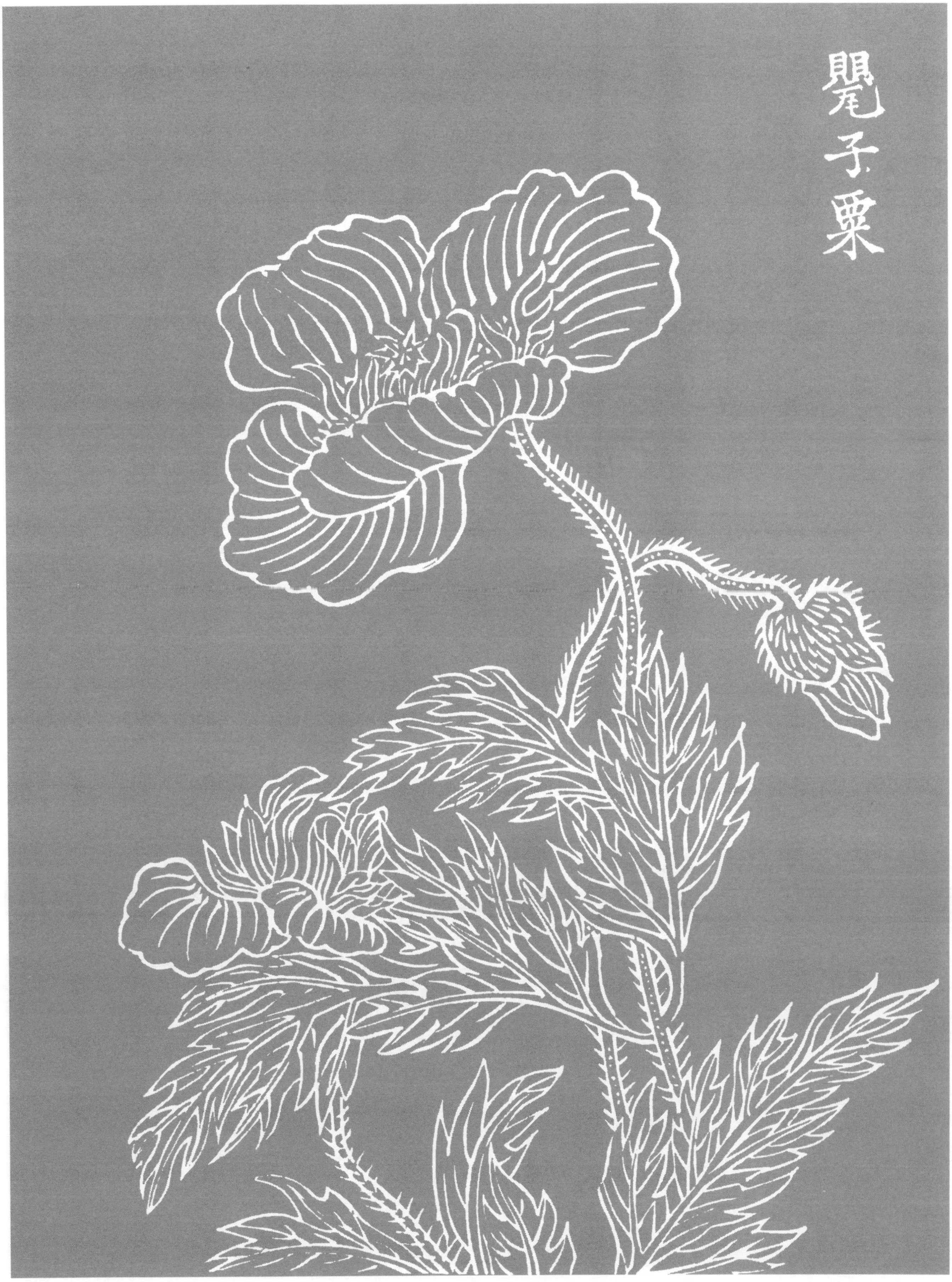
罌子粟

组织创伤用药

Remedies for Tissue Trauma

There are a few Oriental remedies traditionally used mainly for treating tissue trauma. They possess properties that heal tissue and relieve pain and swelling, respectively called *vulnerary, analgesic* and *detumescent*.

In traditional textbooks the action of many *vulnerary* and *analgesic* remedies is described as arising from their "Blood vitalizing" property. In traditional Oriental pathology pain, especially sharp, stabbing pain, is held to be caused by "Blood stasis." Indeed, numerous *analgesic* and *spasmolytic* herbs that treat such painful conditions as dysmenorrhea, arthralgia and myalgia, are defined as "Blood activators" that "disperse" or "break up congealed Blood." Outstanding cases in point are Corydalis Yan Hu Suo (Chinese corydalis root), an effective *central nervous sedative* and *pain-reliever;* Prunus Tao Ren (Peach kernel), a *uterine spasmolytic* and *analgesic* for menstrual pain; Milettia Ji Xue Teng (Milettia root and vine), a *nervous relaxant, sedative* and *analgesic* that treats menstrual, neuralgic, rheumatic and arthritic pain; and Zedoaria E Zhu (Zedoary root), a systemic *nervous relaxant* and *analgesic* for abdominal, uterine and tissue trauma pain.

Clearly, however, the main pathway for the *analgesic* action of these remedies is a neural one, not a blood-connected or even humoral one. For this reason, it is important to understand the traditional term "vitalizing Blood," not in a literal sense, but simply as a concept from traditional Oriental medicine for explaining pain of a sharp, colicky nature. In the case of tissue trauma, pain arises from tissue necrosis, not ecchymosis. Although ecchymosis and hematoma often accompany certain injuries, they are by-products of injury, not primary factors.

The Remedies for Tissue Repair

Vulnerary, analgesic and *detumescent* remedies deal with conditions such as soft tissue injury (called *jin shang,* "sinew damage," e.g., sprains, strains, contusions), open trauma wounds (e.g., cuts, abrasions, crush wounds) and fractures and dislocations. To the extent that their action works on the tissue trauma, it also includes relief of the symptoms that accompany such injury, including pain, red or purple discoloration and swelling from edema or hematoma.

Throughout the treatment of tissue trauma in its various stages, these remedies are given both by topical application and internally by decoction. In addition, massage therapy, acupuncture, bone-setting and exercise are frequent accompaniments to herbal treatment, as the condition requires. Topical preparations, which are fairly easily available and ready to use, include liniments, salves, soft and hard plasters and compresses. Some preparations are based on a water decoction and require steam-soaking the affected part. Herbal formulas for internal use, like the topical preparations, are also available in patent remedy or some other pre-packaged form.

For the most part, the recipes of the compound topical and internal preparations are fully or almost fully disclosed. The highly effective liquid liniment for soft tissue injury, Zheng Gu Shui (literally "bone-regulating water"), for example, which is produced in the South China province Guangxi, contains Panax San Qi, Croton Ba Dou and Cassia Rou Gui among its eight ingredients. Textbooks also describe the functions and uses of various preparations according to the different types of tissue injury and their particular stage of progress. For each formula the texts usually also detail the actions of the ingredients on the tissues in the conditions they are used for.

However, there are many preparations that to this day remain undisclosed proprietary formulas. This is because they originate in martial arts lineages where the treatment of *die da sun shang*—literally "injury from falls and blows"—has evolved over many centuries into a fine art. While in many of these compound formulations it is possible to accurately guess at some of the ingredients, their exact composition and proportion of ingredients still remain the secret of the inheritors and teachers of those lineages. A well-known case in point is the Yunnan Bai Yao formula, available as a patent remedy. This famous formula is given in tissue trauma of most types, especially with bleeding present. The main ingredient is known to be Panax San Qi (Pseudoginseng root), while the other ingredients can only be guessed at. Yunnan province, where this remedy is produced, is extremely rich and diverse in its flora!

The most valued of *vulnerary* remedies without question is Pseudoginseng root from South China, Panax San Qi in the ginseng family, the Araliaceae. One of its many names is Jin Bu Huan, or "Gold no recompense," as it is peerless in treating traumatic injuries with pain, discoloration, swelling and bleeding. Another important *vulnerary* remedy is the root of an evergreen fern, Drynaria Gu Sui Bu. Its literal translation, "bone-knit," is, interestingly, the same as that of the traditional name for the Western herb, Comfrey, *Symphytum officinalis.* This "bone-mender" is mainly taken internally but is also applied externally for sprains, strains and fractures. Frankincense and Myrrh, both types of gummy oleoresins which long ago were incorporated into Chinese medicine from ancient Egyptian, Greek and Ayurvedic medicine, are also frequent ingredients in compound remedies for tissue trauma.

Three natural minerals are also among the remedies often used topically for tissue injury: Pyritum Zi Ran Tong (Pyrite from the South); Ophicalcitum Hua Rui Shi (Dolomite, a compact limestone from northern and coastal China) and Calamina Lu Gan Shi (Calamine, also known as Smithsonite).

Many other significant herbs for tissue trauma are found in other sections of this book, notably Bletilla Bai Ji (the montane Amethyst orchid root), Oldenlandia Bai Hua She She Cao (Snaketongue grass herb from tropical Asia), Wikstroemia Liao Ge Wang (Wikstroemia root from South China) and Dipsacus Xu Duan (Japanese teasel root) However, it must be remembered that, because of the diversity of the flora and the sheer size of the Chinese mainland, there are numerous herbal remedies which, although superlative in their tissue healing and pain relieving actions, are used only regionally rather than nationally. Space limitations make it impossible to present them here.

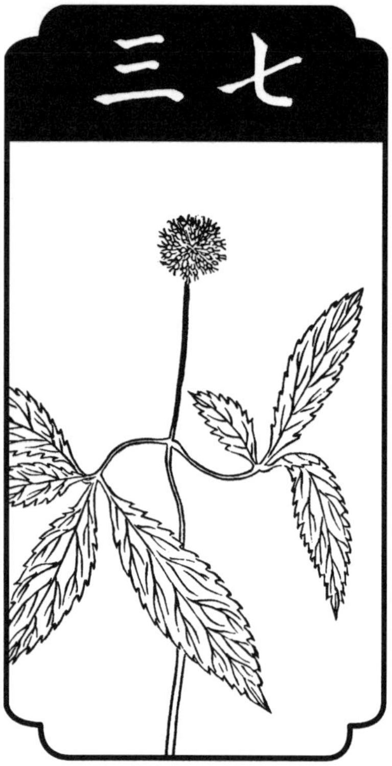

Panax San Qi

Pseudoginseng Root

Botanical source: *Panax notoginseng* (Burk.) F.H. Chen, syn. *P. pseudoginseng* Wall. (Araliaceae)
Pharmaceutical name: Radix Panacis notoginsengis
Chinese names: San Qi, Tian Qi, Shan Qi, Jin Bu Huan (Mand); Saam Chat, Tin Chat (Cant)
Other names: "Three/Seven"; Sanshichi (Jap)
Habit: Perennial mountain herb from South China, especially Yunnan and Guangxi, growing wild and under cultivation in forested hilly regions; prefers moderately warm, damp, shady conditions with black loamy soil; terminal umbels of five-petaled red flowers appear in summer.
Part used: the root

Therapeutic category: mild remedy with minimal chronic toxicity
Constituents: triterpenoid saponins 12% (arasaponins A and B, panaxatriol saponins [ginsenosides], sanchinosides A and B [dammaranes]), flavonoids, pectic polysaccharides, sterols beta-sitosterol/daucosterol, alkaloids, essential oil (incl. methoxyethylbenzene, phenylethanal, nonanoic acid), guaiene, isoallylbenzene, octadecane, methyl palmitate, dencichine
Effective qualities: sweet, astringent, bitter, warm, dry
astringing, thickening, restoring, relaxing
Tropism: cardiovascular, digestive, urinary, immune systems
Liver, Stomach, Yang Wei channels; Warmth, Fluid bodies

Actions and Indications

vulnerary, detergent, anti-inflammatory, detumescent: wounds, injuries, fractures, sprains, strains (esp. with pain, discoloration, swelling)
analgesic, anticontusion: pain of trauma; postpartum, abdominal, chest pain
hemostatic, coagulant, styptic: internal and external bleeding (incl. hematemesis, epistaxis, melena, hematuria, hemorrhage due to trauma or passive); hematoma; metrorrhagia
adaptogenic: fatigue, chronic stress, low vitality, weight loss
vasodilator, hypotensive: hypertension, coronary deficiency/disease, angina pectoris, thrombocytopenic purpura, arrhythmia
hepatic restorative, diuretic: chronic hepatitis
hypoglycemiant
immunostimulant anti-infective: antibacterial, antifungal, antiviral

Symptom Picture

heart blood and Qi stagnation: chest tightness or pain, palpitations, fatigue

Preparation

Use: The root Panax San Qi is taken decocted, powdered or tinctured. All preparations are also used externally in washes, liniments, compresses, etc. Hematuria, i.e., blood in the urine, is traditionally treated with the charred root.

Dosage: Decoction: 2-8 g
Powder: 1-3 g
Tincture: 1-4 ml
Caution: Contraindicated during pregnancy. Use with caution in Blood (metabolic) deficiency conditions.

Notes

Cultivated in the Southern provinces Guangxi and Yunnan, Pseudoginseng root is the most highly valued botanical in Asian medicine for tissue trauma. The root very effectively relieves pain, bleeding, inflammation and contusion all at once, and has long been a standard by which the performance of all other tissue trauma remedies is judged.

Recent research reveals additional values in this remedy. First, its polysaccharides have shown activity with immune stimulation via the reticuloendothelial system, indicating application for infections in general, not just infected wounds. Second, Pseudoginseng root is now used for its *vasodilatant* action in treating coronary blood deficiency leading to angina. The *cardiovascular relaxant* action of Pseudoginseng root is to be expected from its very high saponin content: Saponins have a rejuvenating effect on red blood cells and plasma—a fact that helps account for the remedy's traditional status as a "magic root for life preservation." One of its other popular names, Jin Bu Huan, meaning "gold no recompense," also attests to the stellar reputation past and present of this ginseng variety.

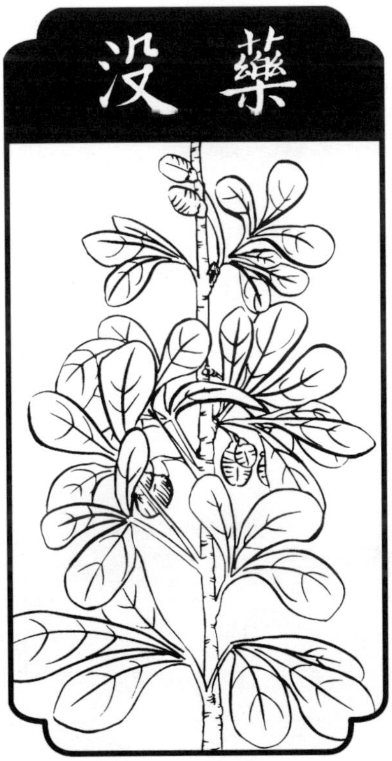

Commiphora Mo Yao

Myrrh Resin

Botanical source: *Commiphora myrrha* L. (Burseraceae)
Pharmaceutical name: Resina Commiphorae
Chinese names: Mo Yao (Mand); Mut Yeuk (Cant)
Other names: Motsuyaku (Jap)
Habit: Perennial shrub or small tree from tropical West Asia and East Africa; small flowers blossom in summer.
Part used: the oleo-gum-resin

Therapeutic category: mild remedy with minimal chronic toxicity
Constituents: essential oil (incl. limonene, pinene, dipentene, heerabolene, octadiene, farnesene, cinnamic aldehyde, eugenol, cresol, methoxyphenyl ether, benzofuranoacetate), resin (incl. commiphoric acid, commiphorinic acid, heerabomyrrhol), gums, salts, sulfates, oxydase, xyloe, galactose
Effective qualities: bitter, a bit pungent, warm, dry
restoring, astringing, stimulating, decongesting
Tropism: digestive, respiratory, urogenital, circulatory systems
Liver, Lung, Ren channels; Air, Fluid, Warmth bodies

Actions and Indications

vulnerary, detergent (topically only): chronic sores, ulcers, wounds (esp. with swelling or putrefaction); ulcerated throat, voice loss
analgesic, anticontusion: pain of trauma; chest, abdominal and menstrual pain
astringent, mucostatic: diarrhea, leucorrhea, loose gums
antifungal, antibacterial, anti-inflammatory: fungal conditions of all types; mouth, gum, throat, vaginal, lung infections with inflammation; putrefactive conditions
detumescent: boils, carbuncles, abscesses

circulatory stimulant: cold extremities, fatigue, weakness
stimulant expectorant: bronchitis (esp. chronic)
uterine stimulant, oxytocic parturient: amenorrhea, dysmenorrhea; stalled labor, hypotonic uterine dystocia, postpartum placental retention
digestive stimulant, carminative: indigestion, appetite loss
antitumoral

Symptom Pictures

uterus Qi stagnation with cold: difficult, painful or stopped menses, cold extremities, fatigue

lung phlegm cold: expectoration of copious sputum, coughing, wheezing, fatigue, chilliness

intestines mucous damp (Spleen damp): gurgling distended abdomen, diarrhea, appetite loss, indigestion

Preparation

Use: The resin Commiphora Mo Yao is decocted or used in essential oil or tincture form. It is often used topically or used in preparations such as compresses and plasters along with other herbs. Mouthwashes, gargles and douches are used for infections of the mucosa. As an *oxytocic parturient*, Myrrh will stimulate more effective labor contractions.

Dosage: Decoction: 3-12 g
Essential oil: 2 drops in a gel cap with some olive oil
Tincture: 1-3 ml

Caution: Forbidden during pregnancy and in heavy uterine bleeding.

Notes

Like Frankincense, Myrrh resin also spans traditional Western and Oriental herbal medicine, having been introduced to China by Arabic traders in the seventh century. In the West the remedy is given for chronic cold catarrhal conditions, both infectious and non-infectious, as in the respiratory and digestive syndromes presented. Recognizing its value in topical preparations and first-aid trauma medicine, Chinese doctors use Myrrh mainly for acute tissue trauma presenting pain and swelling, or for chronic sores, ulcers and non-healing or putrifying wounds.

乳香

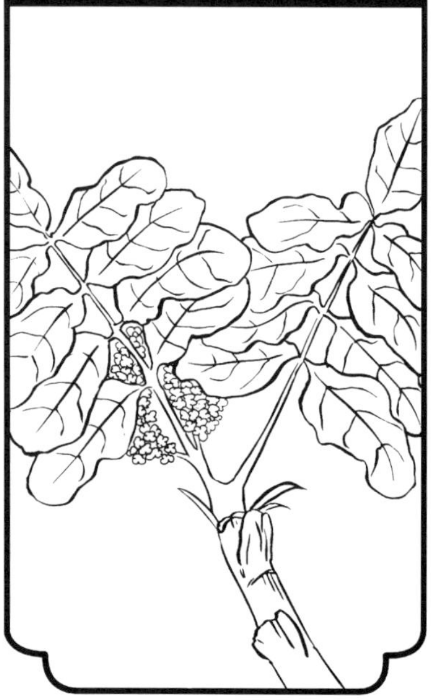

Boswellia Ru Xiang

Frankincense Resin

Botanical source: *Boswellia carterii* Birdw. and spp. (Burseraceae)
Pharmaceutical name: Resina Boswelliae
Chinese names: Ru Xiang, Xun Lu Xiang (Mand); Yu Heung (Cant)
Other names: Olibanum, "Milk aromatic"; Nyuko (Jap)
Habit: Perennial subtropical shrub from the desert Middle East; blooms with racemes of small, pale yellow flowers.
Part used: the oleo-gum-resin

Therapeutic category: mild remedy with minimal chronic toxicity
Constituents: resin (boswellic acids), arabic acid, essential oil (incl. pinene, phellandrene, dipentene, limonene), gum, olibanoresene, bassorin
Effective qualities: pungent and bitter, warm, dry
restoring, astringing, solidifying, stimulating, relaxing
Tropism: respiratory, reproductive, muscular, digestive systems
Heart, Liver, Spleen, Chong, Ren channels
Warmth, Air, Fluid bodies

Actions and Indications

vulnerary, detergent: non-suppurating sores, ulcers, wounds, swollen gums
analgesic, anti-inflammatory: pain of trauma, arthritis, rheumatism, menstruation; mouth, throat, chest, epigastric and abdominal pain
hemostatic, styptic: uterine, lung or traumatic bleeding
urogenital astringent, mucostatic: leucorrhea, spermatorrhea, mucoid diarrhea
antiseptic: respiratory and urogenital infections
detumescent: boils, carbuncles, abscesses, scrofula
muscular relaxant: stiffness and spasms of joints
uterine stimulant, emmenagogue: amenorrhea
stimulant expectorant: bronchitis, lung TB
immunostimulant: immune deficiency disorders
antidepressant: nervous depression

Symptom Pictures

wind damp obstruction: painful, stiff joints of hands and feet

uterus Qi stagnation: painful menses, stopped menses, heavy menstrual bleeding

lung phlegm damp: coughing, wheezing, production of copious white sputum, chest pain and tightness

Preparation

Use: The resin Boswellia Ru Xiang is decocted or used in essential oil or tincture form. This important topical remedy is often prepared into a variety of ointments, compresses, plasters, etc., together with other ingredients The essential oil of Frankincense is also used as an inhalant for catarrhal head colds, and in douches for leucorrhea.

Dosage: Decoction: 3-10 g
Essential oil: 2 drops in a gel cap with some olive oil
Tincture: 1-4 ml

Caution: Although forbidden during the main part of pregnancy, Frankincense resin may be used as a gentle *uterine stimulant* to prepare for childbirth, thereby ensuring a smooth birth. The remedy may be taken once a day beginning one or two weeks before the due date.

Notes

An exudate from the bark of a small, hardy desert tree in Saudi Arabia, Somaliland and Western India, Frankincense is one of the several *xiang* or "aromatics" used in Chinese medicine. The resin was and is used in Egyptian, Greek, Hebrew, Ayurvedic and Chinese medicine, in addition to being burned as a costly ceremonial incense for its sweet-woody, balsamic fragrance.

There is a difference between the traditional Western/Middle-Eastern uses of Frankincense, and the Oriental applications. Traditional Greek medicine uses Frankincense more systemically for catarrhal/mucousy/damp cold/excess *kapha* conditions involving the head, digestive and urogenital organs. As a systemic remedy, Frankincense excells at relieving chronic discharges of different kinds with its dry, astringent, solidifying qualities. Frankincense's pungent-warm *stimulant* effect, on the other hand, is directed mainly at the uterus and bronchi, promoting uterine contractions on one hand, and expectoration on the other. In the same vein, contemporary French usage of Frankincense essential oil includes the treatment of nervous depression and immune deficiency conditions.

Chinese medicine applies the resin mainly in first-aid formulas for various types of pain, as well as to stop bleeding. Traumatic, menstrual, arthritic and rheumatic pain are the main types addressed. *Analgesic, anti-inflammatory* and gently *hemostatic* actions work here in concert.

骨碎補

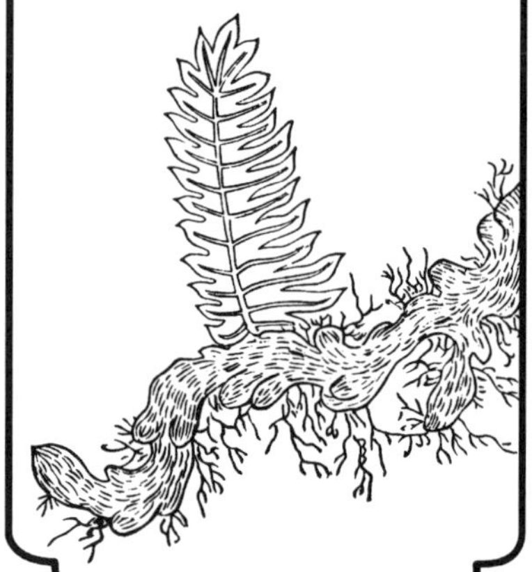

Drynaria Gu Sui Bu

Boneknit Root *

Botanical source: *Drynaria fortunei* (Kunze) J. Small or *D. baronii* (Christ) Diels or *D. propinqua* (Wall.) J. Small; also *Davallia divaricata* Blume and *Pseudodrynaria coronans* (Wall.) Ching and *Phymatodes lucida* (Roxb.) Ching (Polypodiaceae)
Pharmaceutical name: Rhizoma Drynariae
Chinese names: Gu Sui Bu, Gu Cui Bu, Hou Jiang, Mao Jiang (Mand); Gwat Seui Bou (Cant)
Other names: Oakleaf fern, "Broken bone-mender"; Kotsusaiho (Jap)
Habit: Perennial evergreen epiphytic fern from temperate East Asia; grows on tree trunks and branches, and rocky cliff faces.
Part used: the rhizome

Therapeutic category: mild remedy with minimal chronic toxicity
Constituents: naringin, glucose, starch
Effective qualities: bitter, astringent, warm, dry
restoring, astringing, solidifying
Tropism: musculoskeletal, urinary, digestive systems;
Kidney, Liver channels
Fluid body

Actions and Indications

vulnerary: traumatic injury from falls, fractures, strains, sprains (esp. involving ligaments and simple fractures)
analgesic, anticontusion: pain of trauma, contusions; lumbar pain, arthralgia, myalgia, toothache from cold; rheumatoid arthritis
astringent: bleeding gums
musculoskeletal restorative: weak back, legs and knees
intestinal astringent: chronic diarrhea, infantile marasmus
hair stimulant (topical): hair loss

Symptom Picture

musculoskeletal deficiency (Liver and Kidney depletion): weakness of lower back and knees, backache, joint pain

Preparation

Use: The root Drynaria Gu Sui Bu is decocted or used in tincture form. The remedy is also used topically for injuries and hair loss. Internal use is most important for a complete tissue-healing effect.
Dosage: Decoction: 6-16 g
Tincture: 2-5 ml
Caution: Use cautiously in Yin deficiency conditions.

Notes

Gu Sui Bu literally means "shattered bone mender," reminiscent of Comfrey's traditional name, "Consolida," which refers to the same function. Derived from species of *Drynaria* ferns, Boneknit root especially helps ligaments heal, but unlike its Western counterpart has received only scanty biochemical research. Like Comfrey, however, Boneknit root is more than a first-aid remedy. It is additionally considered *restorative* and *analgesic* to the whole musculoskeletal system.

More experimentation and research is clearly needed into the variety of East Asian botanical genera and species of epiphytic ferns that furnish this remedy (see also the Cross-indexes).

血竭

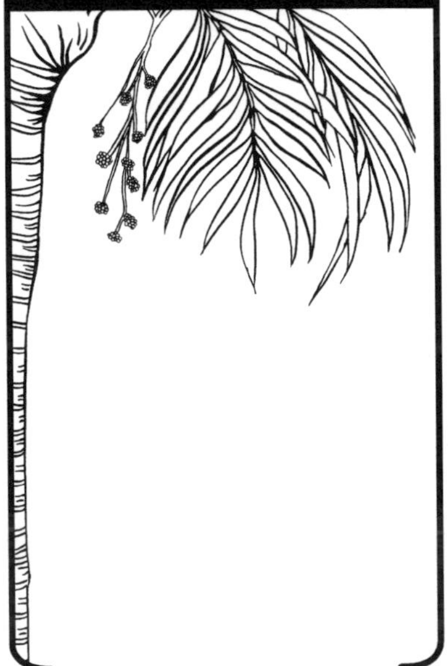

Daemonorops Xue Jie

Dragon's-Blood Resin

Botanical source: *Daemonorops draco* Blume (syn. *Calamus draco* Willdenow) (Arecaceae)
Pharmaceutical name: Resina Daemonoropsis (Sanguis Draco)
Chinese names: Xue Jie, Qi Lin Jie (Mand); Hyut Kit (Cant)
Other names: "Blood exhausted"; Kekketsu (Jap)
Habit: Perennial evergreen climbing rattan palm from (sub)tropical East Asia (incl. Guangdong and Taiwan); blooms with pale yellow helmet-shaped flowers forming spadix patterns.
Part used: the red fruit resin

Therapeutic category: mild remedy with minimal chronic toxicity
Constituents: dacroresinotannol (benzoic and benzoyl acetic esters), dracoalban 2.5%, yellow dracoresene, phlobaphene, abietic acid, cinnamic acid, red pigments dracocarmin and anthocyanidin, dracorubin
Effective qualities: sweet, salty and astringent, neutral, dry
astringing, restoring
Tropism: vascular system
Liver, Heart channels; Fluid, Air bodies

Actions and Indications

vulnerary, detergent, analgesic: traumatic injuries (incl. wounds, contusions, sprains, fractures); chronic ulcers, cancerous sores
hemostatic, coagulant, styptic: hemorrhage, traumatic bleeding, dysentery, diarrhea
antitumoral: uterine cancer
antifungal

Preparation

Use: The resin Daemonorops Xue Jie is powdered and used both internally and externally. Applied topically, its *detergent* action prevents ulcerous and cancerous decay as well as bleeding.
Dosage: Decoction: 0.3-0.6 g
Tincture: 0.2-0.5 ml
Caution: Forbidden during pregnancy and in bleeding due to deficiency heat conditions.

Notes

A common *tissue-repairing* remedy in Southeast Asia, Dragon's-blood resin is most often found in formulas for traumatic injury with pain and bleeding. Preventing ulcerous or cancerous decay is another of its special indications.

Cissampelos Xi Sheng Teng

錫生藤

Ice Vine Root

Botanical source: *Cissampelos pareira* L. (Menispermaceae)
Chinese name: Xi Sheng Teng (M); Sak Sang Tang (C)
Habitat: Small woody climber from the Asian tropics.
Category: mild remedy with minimal chronic toxicity
Constituents: alkaloids (incl. cissamparine, bebeerine, cissamine, hayatidine, hayatine, isochondrodendrine, methylcurine, menismine, pareirine), quercitol, sterols
Effective qualities: bitter, a bit sweet, warm; restoring
Tropism: musculoskeletal/nervous systems; Liver, Lung ch.

ACTIONS: *Analgesic, vulnerary, hemostatic, muscle relaxant, diuretic, emmenagogue, bronchodilator*
INDICATIONS: Contusions, sprains, strains, wounds, traumatic hemorrhage; rheumatic myalgia, lumbar pain; muscle spasms, asthma, heart disease.
Dosage: Decoction: 6-16 g
Tincture: 2-4 ml
Caution: None.

Dalbergia Jiang Xiang 降香
Asian Rosewood

Botanical source: *Dalbergia odorifera* T. Chen (Fabaceae)
Chinese names: Jiang Xiang, Jiang Zhen Xiang (Mand); Geung Heung (Cant)
Category: mild remedy with minimal chronic toxicity

Constituents: dalbergin, nordalbergin, methyldalbergin, dalbergenone, dalbergichromine
Effective qualities: pungent, warm, dry; astringing, solidifying, calming
Tropism: vascular, digestive s.; Liver, Spleen, Stomach ch.

ACTIONS: *Vulnerary, hemostatic, analgesic*
INDICATIONS: Sprains, strains, fractures; bleeding from internal or external trauma; spasmodic abdominal, epigastric or chest pain.
Dosage: Decoction: 6-10 g
Powder: 1.5-3 g
Tincture: 1-4 ml
Caution: None.

Eupolyphaga Tu Bie Chong 土鳖虫
Cockroach

Zoological source: *Eupolyphaga sinensis* Walker (Corydiidae)
Chinese names: Tu Bie Chong, Zhe Chong, Di Bi Chong (Mand)

Category: mild remedy with minimal chronic toxicity
Effective qualities: salty, cold; calming, stimulating
Tropism: reproductive, musculoskeletal systems; Liver, Spleen channels

ACTIONS: *Vulnerary, detumescent, analgesic, emmenagogue*
INDICATIONS: Contusions, sprains, strains, lacerations, fractures, lumbar pain, mouth sores; abdominal lumps, hypochondriac swelling and pain from liver or spleen enlargement.; amenorrhea
Dosage: Decoction: 3-6 g
Caution: During pregnancy.

Hirudo Shui Zhi 水蛭
Leech

Botanical source: *Hirudo nipponia* Whitman and *Whitmania pigra* or *W. acranulata*
Chinese names: Shui Zhi, Zhi Chang (Mand); Seui Jik (Cant)
Category: medium-strength remedy with chronic toxicity

Constituents: hirudin, heparin
Effective qualities: salty, bitter, neutral; calming, relaxing
Tropism: nervous, epidermal, reproductive, cardiovascular systems; Liver, Bladder channels

Actions: *Analgesic, detumescent, anti-inflammatory, spasmolytic, emmenagogue, vasodilator, diuretic*
Indications: Tissue trauma with swelling and pain; abdominal lumps; amenorrhea.
Dosage: Decoction: 1-3 g
Caution: Do not use this medium-strength remedy long-term. Forbidden in pregnancy and Qi or Blood (metabolic) deficiency conditions.

Pyritum Zi Ran Tong
Pyrite

自然铜

Geological source: *Pyritum*
Chinese names: Zi Ran Tong, Ran Tong, Shi Sui Chien (Mand); Ji Wan Tong (Cant); "Natural copper"
Source: Sichuan, Yunnan, Guangdong, Jiangsu provinces
Category: mild remedy with minimal chronic toxicity
Constituents: ferrous disulfide, copper, nickel, arsenic
Effective qualities: pungent, bitter, neutral; astrin-ging
Tropism: epidermal systems; Liver, Kidney channels

Actions: *Vulnerary, analgesic, detumescent*
Indications: Fractures, traumatic injuries with swelling and pain; endemic goiter.
Dosage: Decoction, powder and pill: 3-10 g
When part of a formula, this mineral should first be cooked alone for 30 minutes.
Caution: Forbidden in Yin deficiency and Blood (metabolic) deficiency conditions with empty heat.

Ophicalcitum Hua Rui Shi
Dolomite

花蕊石

Geological source: *Ophicalcitum*
Chinese names: Hua Rui Shi, Shi E (Mand); Fa Yuk Sek (Cant); "Flower stamen stone," Limestone
Category: mild remedy with minimal chronic toxicity
Constituents: calcium and magnesium carbonate
Effective qualities: sour, astringent, neutral; astrin-ging, relaxing
Tropism: epidermal, respiratory systems; Liver channel

Actions: *Vulnerary, thrombolytic, hemostatic*
Indications: Topically for traumatic injuries with ecchymosis, with or without bleeding.
Internally for coughing and vomiting of blood.
Dosage: The powdered mineral is applied topically for traumatic injuries.
Decoction and powder: 3-10 g
Caution: Forbidden during pregnancy.

Calamina Lu Gan Shi
Calamine

炉甘石

Geological source: *Calamina, Smithsonitum*
Chinese names: Lu Gan Shi, Lu Xian Sheng (Mand)
Category: strong remedy with acute toxicity
Constituents: zinc carbonate, calcium/magnesium/ferric manganese oxide, sodium
Effective qualities: sweet, neutral; astringing
Tropism: epidermal, optic systems; Liver, Spleen, Stomach, Lung channels

Actions: *Vulnerary, cicatrisant, anti-inflammatory, antiseptic*
Indications: Topically for chronic indolent wounds, ulcers, open sores with pus drainage; eczema; eye inflammation, pterygium, nebula, corneal opacity.
Dosage: Powder: 6-30 g for external use only. The powder of the calcined mineral is mixed with water before applying.
Caution: Not for internal use.
Notes: This mineral is also known as Smithsonite (native zinc carbonate).

PART THREE

Cross Indexes, Glossaries & Charts

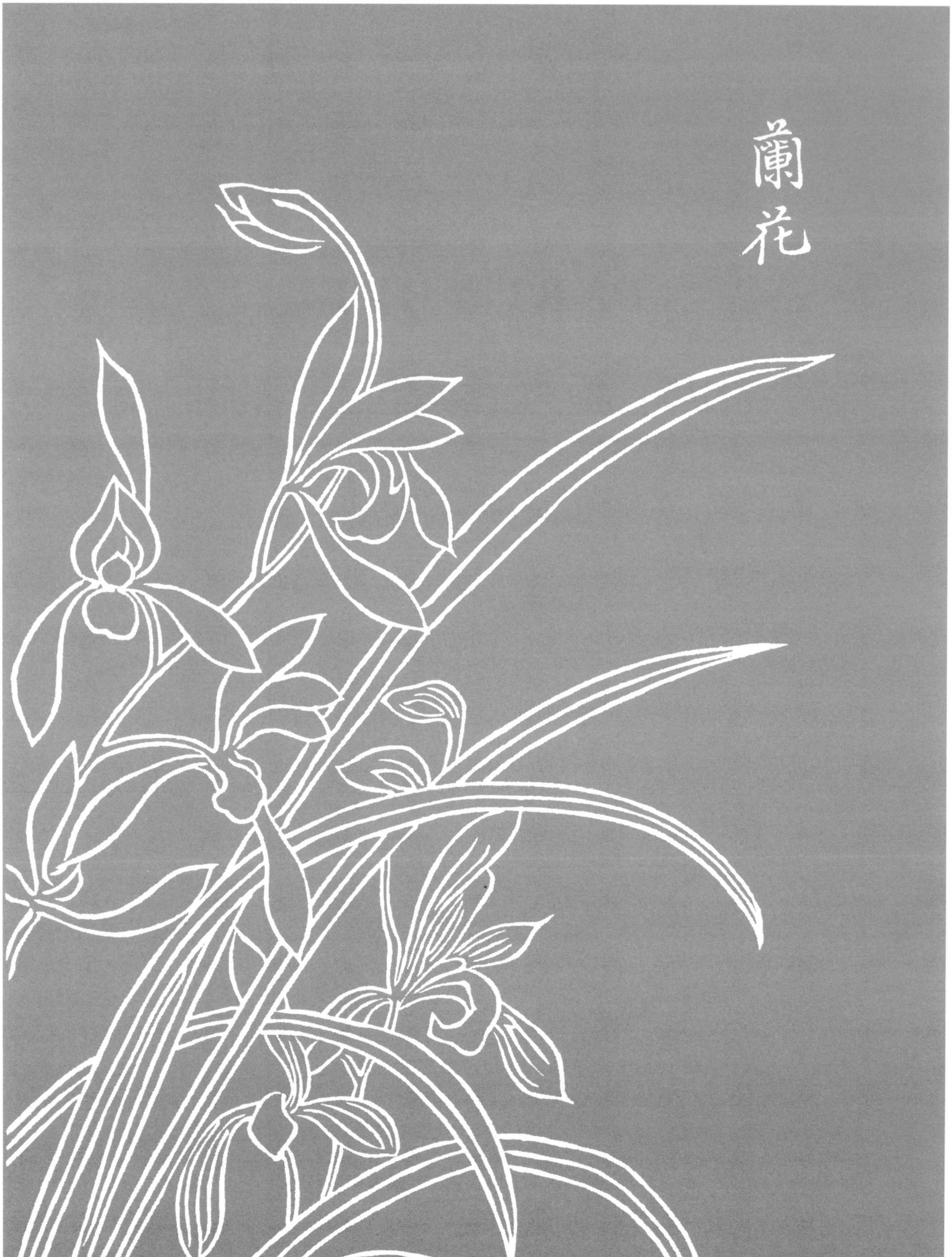
蘭花

Cross Index of Scientific Remedy Names

SCIENTIFIC	PHARMACEUTICAL	CANTONESE	MANDARIN	JAPANESE	ENGLISH
	Massa fermentata	Shen Qu	Sam Chau	Shinkiku	Medicated leaven
	Massa fermentata	Shen Qu Cha	Sam Chau Cha		Medicated leaven tea
	Pulvus fumi carbonisati	Bai Cao Shuang	Baak Chou Sheung		Boiler or chimney soot
	Terra flava usta, Bolus usta	Fu Long Gan	Fuk Lung Gon	Bukuryukan	Wood stove clay
Abrus precatorius, A. cantoniensis	Herba Abri	Ji Gu Cao	Gai Gwat Chou		Licorice bean herb
Abrus precatorius, A. cantoniensis	Radix Abri	Xiang Si Zi Gen	Seung Si Ji Gan		Licorice bean root
Abutilon indicum	Herba Abutilonis indici	Mo Pan Cao, Mi Lan Cao	Mo Bun Chou		Country mallow herb
Abutilon theophrastii	Semen Abutili theophrasti	Qing Ma (Zi)	King Ma (Ji)		China jute seed
Acacia catechu	Pasta Acaciae seu Uncariae	Er Cha	Yi Cha	Asenyaku	Catechu paste
Acalypha australis	Herba Acalyphae	Tie Xian (Cai)	Tit Yin		Annual copperleaf herb
Acanthopanax gracilistylus	Cortex radicis Acanthopanacis gracilistylus	Wu Jia Pi, Xi Zhu Wu Jia	Ng Ga Pei, Sai Chu Ng Ga		Five additions root bark
Acanthopanax gracilistylus, A. spinosus, A. sessiliflorus and spp	Cortex radicis Acanthopanacis	Wu Jia Pi	Ng Ga Pei	Gokahi	Five additions root bark
Acanthopanax trifoliatus	Cortex radicis Acanthopanacis trifoliati	Wu Jia Pi, Bai Le	Ng Ga Pei, Baak Lak		Three-leaf acanthopanax root bark
Acanthus ilicifolius	Radix Acanthi ilicifolii	Lao Shu Le	Lou Syu Laak		Holly-leaf acanthus root
Achyranthes aspera	Radix Achyranthis asperae	Wei Niu Xi, Ju Niu Xi, Dou Kou Cao	Wai Ngau Sat, Dou Kau Chou		Rough oxknee root
Achyranthes bidentata	Radix Achyranthis	Niu Xi, Huai Niu Xi	Ngau Sat, Wai Ngau Sat	Goshitsu	White oxknee Root
Achyranthes longifolia	Radix Achyranthis longae	Tu Niu Xi	Tou Ngau Sat		Long-leaf oxknee root
Acipenser sinensis, Miichthys spp	Colla piscis	Yu Biao Jiao	Yu Biu Gaau		Fish airbladder
Aconitum brachypodum and spp	Radix Aconiti brachypodi	Xue Shang Yi Zhi Yao	Syu Seung Yat Ji Hou		Brachypode aconite root
Aconitum carmichaeli	Radix Aconiti carmichaeli	Chuan Wu Wu Tou	Chyun Wu, Wu Tau	Uzu	Prepared Sichuan aconite root tuber
Aconitum carmichaeli	Radix lateralis Aconiti carmichaeli praeparatae	Fu Zi	Fu Ji	Bushi	Prepared Sichuan aconite root
Aconitum chinense, A. kusnezoffii and spp	Radix Aconiti chinensis	Cao Wu, Bei Wu Tou	Chou Wu, Mai Wu Tau	So-u	Prepared wild aconite root tuber

SCIENTIFIC	PHARMACEUTICAL	CANTONESE	MANDARIN	JAPANESE	ENGLISH
Aconitum coreanum	Rhizoma Aconiti coreani	Bai Fu Zi, Guan Bai Fu	Baak Fu Ji, Gwan Baak Fu Ji		Prepared Korean aconite root
Acorus calamus	Rhizoma Acori calami	Shui Chang Pu, Bai Chang Pu	Seui Cheung Pou, Baak Cheung Pou	Shobu	Sweetflag root
Acorus gramineus	Rhizoma Acori graminei	Shi Chang Pu	Sek Cheung Pou		Rock sweetflag root
Acorus tatarinowii	Rhizoma Acori tatarinowii	Jie Chang Pu	Jik Cheung Pou		Tatarinow's sweetflag root
Acronychia laurifolia	Lignum Acronychiae	Sha Tang Mu, Jiang Xiang	Sa Tong Muk		Acronychia heartwood
Actinidia chinensis	Fructus Actinidiae chinensis	Mi Hou Tao, Teng Li	Nei Hau Tou		Kiwi fruit
Actinidia chinensis	Fructus Actinidiae chinensis	Teng Li Gen	Tang Li Gan		Kiwi root
Actinidia polygama	Galla fructi Actinidiae	Mu Tian Lian	Muk Tin Lin	Mokutenryo	Actinidia gall
Actinolitum	Actinolitum	Yang Qi Shi	Yeung Hei Sek		Actinolite
Actinostemma lobata	Folium at semen Actinostemmae	He Zi Cao	Hap Ji Chou		Actinostemma leaf and seed
Adenophora stricta, A. capillaris, A. tetraphylla and spp	Radix Adenophorae strictae	Nan Sha Shen	Naam Sa Sam	Nanshajin	Upright ladybell root
Adenophora trachelioides	Radix Adenophorae trachelioidis	Gan Jie Geng	Gam Gaat Gan, Ai Ji Sam		Sweet ladybell root
Adenophora trachelioides, A. remotifolia	Radix Adenophorae trachelioidis	Ji Ni	Chai Ni		Common harebell root
Adenosma glutinosum	Herba Adenosmae glutinosi	Mao She Xiang	Mou Se Heung		Adenosma herb
Adenostemma lavenia	Herba Adenostemmae	Ma Zhi Hu, Feng Qi Cao	Ma Ji Wu, Fung Hei Chou		Adenostemma herb
Adina rubella	Flos Adinae	Shui Yang Mei	Seui Yeung Mui		Red modelwood flower
Adonis amurensis	Herba Adonis	Fu Shou Cao	Fuk Sau Chou		Amur adonis herb
Aeginetia indica	Herba Aeginetiae	Guan Zhen Huang, Ye Gu	Gwon Jam Wong, Ye Gu		Aeginetia herb
Aesculus wilsonii, A. chinensis	Fructrus Aesculi	Suo Luo Zi	So Lo Ji		Chinese horse chestnut
Agastache rugosa	Herba Agastachis	Huo Xiang	Fok Heung	Kakko	Rugose giant hyssop herb
Agate	Agate	Ma Nao			Agate
Agave americana	Folium Agavis americanae	Jin Bian Long She Lan	Gam Bin Lung Sit Laan		Agave leaf
Agkistrodon acutus and *Bungarus multicinctus*	Agkistrodon seu Bungarus	Bai Hua She	Baak Fa Se	Hakkada	Multibanded krait
Agkistrodon halys	Agkistrodon	Fan Bi	Faan Bei		Viper
Agrimonia pilosa var. *japonica*	Gemma Agrimoniae pilosae	He Cao Ya	Hok Chou Nga		Furry agrimony winter bud
Agrimonia pilosa var. *japonica*	Herba Agrimoniae pilosae	Xian He Cao	Sin Hok Chou	Senkakuso	Furry agrimony herb
Ailanthus altissima	Fructus Ailanthi	Feng Yen Cao	Fung Ngaan Chou		Tree of heaven fruit

SCIENTIFIC	PHARMACEUTICAL	CANTONESE	MANDARIN	JAPANESE	ENGLISH
Ailanthus altissima	Cortex Ailanthi	Chun (Bai) Pi	Chan (Baak) Pei		Tree of heaven bark
Ailanthus altissima	Cortex radicis Ailanthi	Chun Gen Pi	Chan Gan Pei		Tree of heaven root bark
Ajuga decumbens	Herba Ajugae	Bai Mao Xia Ku Cao, Jing Gu Cao	Baak Mou Ha Fu Chou, Gan Gwat Chou		Bugleweed herb
Akebia quinata	Fructus Akebiae	Ba Yue Zha, Yu Zhi Zi	Baat Yut Jaat, Yu Ji Ji		Akebia fruit
Akebia quinata, A. trifoliata	Caulis Akebiae	Mu Tong, Bai Mu Tong	Baak Muk Tong	Mokutsu	Akebia stem
Alangium chinense	Radix Alangii	Ba Jiao Feng	Baat Gok Fung		Alangium root
Albizzia julibrissin, A. lebbak and spp	Cortex Albizziae	He Huan Pi	Hap Fun Pei	Gokanhi	Mimosa bark
Albizzia julibrissin, A. lebbek and spp	Flos Albizziae	He Huan Hua	Hap Fun Fa	Gokanka	Mimosa flower
Aleurites fordii	Semen Aleuritis	You Tong Zi	Yau Tung Ji		Tung seed
Alisma orientalis	Rhizoma Alismae	Ze Xie	Jaak Se	Takusha	Water plantain root
Allium fistulosum	Bulbus Allii fistulosi	Cong Bai	Chung Baak		Fresh scallion bulb
Allium fistulosum	Semen Allii fistulosi	Cong Zi	Chung Ji	Sohaku	Scallion seed
Allium macrostemon	Bulbus Allii macrostemonis	Xie Bai	Se Baak	Gaihaku	Chinese chive bulb
Allium sativum	Bulbus Allii sativi	Da Suan	Daai Syun	Taisan	Garlic bulb
Allium tuberosum	Semen Alii tuberosi	Jiu Cai Zi	Gau Choi Ji	Kyushi	Asian leek seed
Alocasia odora	Rhizoma Alocasiae	Guang Lang Du, Hai Yu	Hoi Wu		Alocasia root
Aloe vera var. *chinensis*	Resina Aloidis	Lu Hui	Lou Wui		Aloe resin
Alpinia galanga	Radix Alpiniae galangae	Da Liang Jiang	Daai Leung Geung		Greater galangal root
Alpinia galanga	Fructus Alpiniae Galangae	Hong Dou Kou	Hung Dau Kau		Greater galangal berry
Alpinia katsumadai	Semen Alpiniae katsumadis	Cao Dou Kou	Chou Dau Kau	Sozuku	Katsumada's galangal seed
Alpinia officinarum	Rhizoma Alpiniae officinari	Gao Liang Jiang	Gou Leung Geung	Koryokyo	Galangal root
Alpinia oxyphylla	Fructus Alpiniae oxyphyllae	Yi Zhi Ren	Yik Ji Yan	Yakuchinin	Sharp-leaf galangal berry
Alpinia zerumbet	Fructus Alpiniae zerumbetsis	Da Cao Kou	Daai Chou Kau		Beautiful galangal berry
Alternanthera philoxeroides	Herba Alternantherae	Kong Xiu Lian Zi Cao	Hung Sam Lin Ji Chou		Alligator Alternanthera herb
Alumen	Alumen praeparatum	Ku Fan	Gu Faan		Prepared alum
Alumen	Alumen	Ming Fan	Ming Faan	Myoban	Alum
Amomum cardamomum	Flos Amomi cardamomi	(Bai) Dou Kou Hua	(Baak) Dau Kau Fa	Byakuzu-kuka	Cluster cardamom flower
Amomum cardamomum	Fructus Amomi cardamomi	Bai Dou Kou	Baak Dau Kau	Byakuzuku	Cluster cardamom pod
Amomum longiligulare	Fructus Amomi longiligularis	Sha Ren, Hai Nan Sha Ren	Sai Yan, Hoi Naam Sa Yan		Hainan cardamom pod

SCIENTIFIC	PHARMACEUTICAL	CANTONESE	MANDARIN	JAPANESE	ENGLISH
Amomum tsao-ko	Fructus Amomi tsao-konis	Cao Guo (Ren)	Chou Gwat (Yan)	Soka	Cochin cardamom fruit
Amomum villosum	Fructus Amomi villosi	Sha Ren, (Yang) Chun Sha Ren	Sa Yan, (Yeung) Chyun Sa Yan	Sanin	Wild cardamom pod (fruit)
Amomum villosum	Flos Amomi villosi	Sha Ren Hua, (Yang) Chun Sha Hua	Sa Yan Fa, (Yeung) Chyun Sa Fa	Saninka	Wild cardamom flower
Amomum villosum	Pericarpium Amomi villosi	Sha Ren Ke	Sa Yan Hok		Wild cardamom shell
Amomum villosum	Semen Amomi villosi	Guang Sha Ren	Gwong Sa Yan		Wild cardamom seed
Amomum xanthioides	Fructus Amomi xanthioidis	Sha Ren, Suo Sha Mi	Sa Yan, Suk Sa Mat		Cocklebur cardamom pod
Amorphophallus rivieri, A. sinensis, A. knojac	Rhizoma Amorphophalli	Ju Ruo	Geui Yeuk		Amorpho-phallus root
Ampelopsis brevipedunculata	Radix et folium Ampelopsis brevipedunculatae	She Pu Tao, Shan Pu Tao	Se Pou Tou, Saan Pou Tou		Snake grape root and leaf
Ampelopsis japonica	Radix Ampelopsis	Bai Lian	Baak Lim	Byakuran	Japanese peppervine root
Amyda sinensis, Trionix sinensis	Carapax Amydae seu Trionis	Bie Jia	Bit Gaap	Bekko	Asian soft-shell turtle shell
Anagallis arvensis	Herba Anagallis	Jian Feng Hong	Gin Fung Hung		Scarlet pimpernel herb
Andrographis paniculata	Folium Andrographis	Chuan Xin Lian	Chyun Sam Lin	Senshinren	Heart-thread lotus leaf
Androsaca umbellata	Herba Androsacae	Dian Di Mei			Androsaca herb
Anemarrhena asphodeloides	Radix Anemarrhenae	Zhi Mu	Ji Mou	Chimo	Know mother root
Anemone altaica	Rhizoma Anemoni altaicae	Jiu Jie Chang Pu	Gau Jit Cheung Pou	Arutai ginrenkon	Altai anemone root
Anemone hupehensis	Herba Anemonis hupehensis	Da Po Wan Hua Hua	Da Po Wun Fa Fa		Hubei anemone herb
Anemone raddeana	Rhizoma Anemonis raddeanae	Liang Tou Jian	Leung Tau Jim		Anemone root
Angelica acutiloba	Radix Angelicae acutilobae	Dang Gui	Dong Gwai		Dong quai root
Angelica dahurica, A. anomala, A. taiwaniana	Radix Angelicae dahuricae	Bai Zhi	Baak Ji	Byakushi	White angelica Root
Angelica pubescens, A. laxiflora and spp	Radix Angelicae pubescentis	Du Huo	Duk Wut	Dokkatsu	Hairy angelica Root
Angelica sinensis	Radix Angelicae sinensis	Dang Gui	Dong Gwai	Toki	Dong quai root
Angelica sinensis, A. acutiloba	Caput Angelicae sinensis	Dang Gui Tou	Dong Gwai Tou	Tokito	Dong quai head
Angelica sinensis, A. acutiloba	Extremas radicis Angelicae sinensis	Dang Gui Wei	Dong Gwai Mai	Tokio	Dong quai tail
Anisodus tanguticus	Redix seu semen Anisodi	Zang Qie	Jong Ke		Anisodus root or seed

SCIENTIFIC	PHARMACEUTICAL	CANTONESE	MANDARIN	JAPANESE	ENGLISH
Apis cerana and spp	Cera flava	Feng La	Fung Laap		Beeswax
Apis cerana and spp	Mel	Feng Mi	Fung Mat		Honey
Apocynum lancifolium, A. venetum, A. hendersonii	Radix et herba Apocyni	Luo Bu Ma	Lo Bou Ma		Dogbane root and herb
Aquilaria agallocha, A. sinensis	Lignum Aquilariae	Chen Xiang	Cham Heung	Jinko	Aloeswood
Arachis hypogaea	Pericarpium Arachis	Hua Sheng Pi	Fa Sang Pei	Kashohi	Peanut skin
Aralia chinensis	Radix Araliae chinensis	Song Mu Bai Pi	Sung Muk Baak Pei		Chinese aralia root
Aralia cordata	Radix Araliae cordatae	Tu Dang Gui	Tou Dong Gwai		Heart-leaf aralia root
Aralia elata, A. elata var. *suninermis*	Cortex Araliae elatate	Ci Lao Ya Pi	Chu Lou Nga	Taranoki	Aralia bark
Arca inflata and spp	Concha Arcae	Wa Leng Zi	Nga Ling Ji	Garyoshi	Cockle shell
Arctium lappa	Fructus Arctii	Niu Bang Zi	Ngau Pong Ji	Goboshi	Burdock seed
Ardisia crenata, A. bicolor	Radix Ardisiae crenatae	Da Lo San, Zhu Sha Gen	Jyu Sa Gan	Shushakon	Coralberry root
Ardisia crispa	Herba Ardisiae crispae	Bai Liang Jin	Baak Leung Gam		Crisp ardisia herb
Ardisia gigantifolia	Rhizoma Ardisiae gigantifoliae	Zou Ma Tai	Jau Ma Toi		Ardisia root
Ardisia japonica	Radix et herba Ardisiae japonicae	Zi Jin Niu, Jin Niu Cao	Ji Gam Ngau		Marlberry root and herb
Areca catechu, A. dicksonii	Semen Arecae catechu	Bing Lang	Ban Long	Binroji	Betel nut
Areca catechu, A. dicksonii	Flos Arecae catechu	Bing Lang Hua	Ban Long Fa	Binroka	Betel nut flower
Areca catechu, A. dicksonii	Pericarpium Arecae	Da Fu Pi	Daai Fuk Pei	Daifukuhi	Betel husk
Arisaema consanguineum, A. amurense and spp	Pulvis Arisaemae cum felle Bovis	Dan Nan Xing	Daam Naam Sing	Tannansho	Powdered dragon arum corm with ox bile
Arisaema consanguineum, A. amurense and spp	Rhizoma Arisaemae preparatae	Tian Nan Xing, Zhi Nan Xing	Tin Naam Sing, Jek Naam Sing		Prepared dragon arum corm
Aristolochia contorta, A. debilis	Fructus Aristolochiae	Ma Dou Ling	Ma Dau Ling	Batorei	Green birthwort capsule
Aristolochia contorta, A. debilis	Radix Aristolochiae	Qing Mu Xiang, Ma Dou Ling Gen	Ching Muk Heung	Seimokko	Green birthwort root
Aristolochia contorta, A. debilis	Caulis Aristolochiae	Tian Xian Teng	Tin Sin Tang	Tensendo	Green birthwort stem
Aristolochia fangchi, A. westlandii	Radix Aristolochiae fangchis	Fang Ji, Guang Fang Ji	Fong Gei, Gwong Fong Gei		Fangchi birthwort root
Aristolochia manshuriensis, A. moupinensis	Caulis Aristolochiae manshuriensis	Guan Mu Tong	Gwaan Muk Tung		Manchurian birthwort stem
Aristolochia mollissima	Herba Aristolochiae mollissimae	Xun Gu Feng, Mian Mao Ma Dou Ling	Cham Gwat Fung, Min Mou Ma Dou Ling		Soft birthwort herb

SCIENTIFIC	PHARMACEUTICAL	CANTONESE	MANDARIN	JAPANESE	ENGLISH
Aristolochia moupiensis	Radix seu caulis Aristolochiae moupiensis	Huai Tong	Waai Tung		Birthwort root or stem
Armadillidium vulgare, Porcellio scaber	Armadillidium	Shu Fu	Syu Fu		Wood louse
Armillaria mellea	Sclerotium Armillariae	Mi Huan Jun			Honey mushroom
Arnebia euchroma, A. guttata	Radix Arnebiae	Zi Cao, Xin Jiang Zi Cao	Ji Chou, San Geung Ji Chou	Shikon	Arnebia root
Arsenicum album	Arsenolitum	Pi Shi, Xin Shi			White arsenic
Artemisia annua	Herba Artemisiae annuae	Huang Hua Hao Qing Hao	Wong Fa Hou, Ching Hou		Annual wormwood herb
Artemisia anomala	Herba Artemisiae anomalae	Liu Ji Niu	Lau Gei Nou	Ryukido	Anomalous wormwood herb
Artemisia apiacea	Herba Artemisiae apiaceae	Qing Hao	Ching Hou	Seiko	Celery wormwood herb
Artemisia argyi	Folium Artemisiae argyi	Ai Ye	Ngaai Yang, Ngaai Yip	Gaiyo	Asian mugwort leaf
Artemisia capillaris, A. scoparia	Herba Artemisiae capillaris	Yin Chen (Hao), Mian Yin Chen	Yan Chan (Hou), Min Yan Chan	Inchinko	Downy wormwood herb
Artemisia keiskeana	Fructus Artemisiae keiskeanae	An Lu Zi	Am Leui Ji		Keiskeana mugwort seed
Artemisia scoparia	Herba Artemisiae scopariae	Bei Yin Chen	Bak Yan Chan		Northern wormwood herb
Asarum forbesii	Rhizoma Asari forbesii	Du Heng	Dou Hang		Forbes' wild ginger root
Asarum heterotropoides	Herba Asari heterotropoidis	Xi Xin, Bei Xi Xin	Bak Sai San		Northern wild ginger root
Asarum maximum	Herba Asari maximi	Ta Hua Xi Xin	Daai Fa Sai San		Large flower wild ginger herb
Asarum sieboldii	Herba Asari sieboldii	Xi Xin, Hua Xi Xin	Wa Sai San		Siebold's wild ginger herb
Asarum sieboldii, A. heterotropoides **and spp**	Radix et herba Asari	Xi Xin	Sai San	Saishin	Asian wild ginger root and herb
Asparagus cochinchinensis	Rhizoma Asparagi cochinchinensis	Tian (Men) Dong	Tin (Mun) Dung	Tenmondo	Shiny asparagus root
Asparagus officinalis	Rhizoma Asparagi officinalis	Shi Diao Bai	Sek Diu Baak		Asparagus root
Aspongopus	Aspongopus	Jiu Xiang Chong	Gau Heung Chung		Stinkbug
Aster indicus **and spp**	Herba Asteris indici	Ma Lan	Ma Laan		Indian aster herb
Aster tataricus	Radix Asteris tatarici	Zi Wan	Ji Yun	Shion	Tartary aster root
Astilbe chinensis	Rhizoma Astilbis	Luo Xin Fu	Lok San Fu		Astilbe root
Astragalus membranaceus, A. mongholicus **and spp**	Radix Astragali	Huang Qi	Wong Kei, Paak Kei	Ogi	Astragalus root
Astragalus complanatus **and spp**	Semen Astragali complanati	Sha Yuan Zi, Sha Yuan Ji Li	Sa Yun Ji, Sa Yun Jek Lai	Saenshi, Toshitsuri	Flat milkvetch seed
Atalantia buxifolia	Radix Atalantiae	Dong Feng Ju Gen	Dung Fung Gwat Gan	Tofukitsu	Atalantia root

SCIENTIFIC	PHARMACEUTICAL	CANTONESE	MANDARIN	JAPANESE	ENGLISH
Atractylodes japonica	Rhizoma Atractylodis japonicae	Cang Zhu, Guan Cang Zhu	Chong Seut, Gwan Chong Seut		Japanese black Atractylodes root
Atractylodes lancea, A. sinensis **and spp**	Rhizoma Atractylodis lanceae	Cang Zhu, Mao Cang Zhu	Chong Seut, Mau Chong Seut	Sojutsu	Black atractylodes root
Atractylodes macrocephala	Rhizoma Atractylodis macrocephalae	Bai Zhu	Baak Seut	Byakujutsu	White atractylodes root
Auricularia auricula	Sclerotium Auriculariae	Mu Er	Muk Yi	Kikurage	Wood ear mushroom
Aurum	Folium Auri	Jin Bo	Gam Bok		Gold foil
Averrhoa carambola	Fructus Averrhoae	Yang Tao	Yeung Tou		Carambola fruit
Averrhoa carambola	Flos Averrhoae	Yang Tao Hua	Yeung Tou Fa		Carambola flower
Baphicacanthus cusia	Radix Baphicacanthi	Ma Lan Gen	Ma Laam Gan	Banrankon	Assam indigo root
Baphicacanthus cusia	Folium Baphicacanthi	Ma Lan Ye	Ma Laam Yip	Banranyo	Assam indigo leaf
Bauhinia championi	Caulis bauhiniae championi	Jiu Long Teng, Wu Teng	Gaau Lung Tang, Lung Sou Tang		Bauhinia stem
Bauhinia paraglauca	Herba Bauhiniae paraglaucae	Hu Die Cao			Green bauhinia herb
Bauhinia variegata	Cortex Bauhiniae variegatae	Lao Bai Hua Pi	Lou Baak Fa Pei		Orchid tree bark
Begonia crassirostris	Herba Begoniae crassirostris	Hong Ban Bian Lian	Hung Bun Bin Lin		Begonia herb
Begonia fimbristipula	Herba Begoniae fimbristipulae	Zi Bei Tian Kuei, Hong Tian Kui	Ji Mai Tin Kwai, Hung Tin Kwai		Begonia herb
Belamcanda chinensis	Herba Belamcandae	She Gan Miao	Se Gon Miu		Leopard flower herb
Belamcanda chinensis	Rhizoma Belamcandae	She Gan	Se Gon	Yakan	Leopard flower root
Benincasa hispida	Epicarpium Benincasae	Dong Gua Pi	Dung Gwa Pei	Tokahi	Waxgourd fruit rind
Benincasa hispida	Semen Benincasae	Dong Gua Ren	Dong Gwa Yan	Tokanin	Waxgourd seed
Berberis sargentiana, B. wilsonae, B. vernae **and spp**	Radix Berberis sargentianae	San Ke Zhen	Saam Gwo Jam		Three-needle barberry root
Berberis thunbergii	Lignum Berberis thunbergii	Xiao Nie	Siu Maak	Megi	Barberry wood
Berchemia lineata	Radix Berchemiae	Tie Bao Jin	Tit Bau Gam		Supplejack root
Betula platyphylla	Cortex Betulae	Hua Mu Pi	Wa Muk Pei		Asian birch bark
Bidens bipinnata	Herba Bidentis bipinnatae	Gui Zhen Cao	Gwai Jam Chou		Beggartick herb
Bidens pilosa **var.** ***minor*** **and spp**	Herba Bidentis pilosae	Xian Feng Cao	Heun Fung Chou		Hairy beggartick herb
Biota orientalis	Semen Biotae orientalis	Bai Zi Ren	(Baak) Ji Yan	Hakushinin	Oriental arborvitae berry
Biota orientalis	Cacumen Biotae orientalis	Ce Bai Ye	Jak Paak Yip	Sokuhakuyo	Oriental arborvitae tip

SCIENTIFIC	PHARMACEUTICAL	CANTONESE	MANDARIN	JAPANESE	ENGLISH
Blechnum orientale	Rhizoma Blechni	Guan Zhong, Wu Mao Jue Guan Zhong, Dong Fang Wu Mao Jue Ye	Gwun Jung, Dung Fong Wu Mou Kyut Yip	Kanju	Oriental hammock fern root
Bletilla striata	Rhizoma Bletillae	Bai Ji	Baak Gap	Byakukyu	Amethyst orchid root
Blumea balsamifera	Herba Blumeae balsamiferae	Ai Na Xiang, Da Feng Cao	Ngaai Naap Heung	Daifuso	Camphor plant
Bodens pilosa	Herba Bidentis pilosae	San Ye Gui Zhen Cao	Sam Yip Gwai Jam Chou		
Boehmeria nivea	Radix Boehmeriae	Zhu Ma Gen	Chyu Ma Gan		Ramie root
Bombyx mori	Excrementum Bombicis	Can Sha	Chaam Sa	Sansha	Silkworm dropping
Bombyx mori	Periostracum Bombycis	Ma Ming Dui	Ma Ming Teui		Silkworm slough
Bombyx mori artificially infected with *Beauveria bassiana*	Bombyx beauveriatus	Jiang Yong	Geung Yung		Silkworm larva
Bombyx mori infected with *Beauveria bassiana*	Bombyx beauveriatus	Jiang Can	Geung Chaam		Silkworm larva
Borax	Borax	Peng Sha	Pang Sa	Hosha	Borax
Borax	Borax	Shu Peng Sha	Syu Pang Sa		Roasted borax
Bos taurus domesticus, Bubalis bubalis	Corium Bovis	Niu Pi	Ngau Pei		Ox hide
Bos taurus domesticus, Bubalis bubalis	Vesica fellae Bovis	Niu Dan	Ngau Daam	Gyutan	Ox gallbladder
Bos taurus domesticus, Bubalis bubalis	Calculus Bovis	Niu Huang	Ngau Wong	Goo	Ox gallstone
Boswellia carterii and spp	Resina Boswelliae	Ru Xiang	Yu Heung	Nyuko	Frankincense resin
Breynia fruticosa	Cacumen Breyniae	Hei Mian Ye	Haak Min Yip		Breynia tip
Broussonetia papyrifera	Fructus Broussonetiae	Chu Shi Zi	Chyu Sat Ji		Paper mulberry fruit
Brucea javanica	Fructus Bruceae	Ya Dan Zi	Nga Daan Ji	Atanshi	Brucea berry
Bubalus bubalis	Cornu Bubali	Shui Niu Jiao	Seui Ngau Gok		Water buffalo horn
Buchnera cruciata	Herba Buchnerae	Gui Yu Jian	Gwai Yu Jin		Cruciate bluehart herb
Buddleia asiatica	Radix Buddleiae asiaticae	Bai Pu Jiang	Baak Pou Geung		Asian Buddleia root
Buddleia lindleyana	Radix Buddleiae lindleyanae	Qi Li Xiang	Chat Lei Heung		Buddleia root
Buddleia officinalis	Flos Buddleiae	Mi Meng Hua	Mat Mung Fa	Mitsumoka	Buddleia flower and bud
Bufo gargarizans, B. melanostictus	Secretio Bufonis	Chan Su	Sim Sou	Senjo	Toad venom
Bupleurum scorzonerifolium	Radix Bupleuri scorzonerifolii	Chai Hu, Xia Ye Chai Hu	Chaai Wu, Hap Yip Chaai Wu		Thin-leaf buplever root
Bupleurum chinense, B. falcatum, B. longiradiatum and spp	Radix Bupleuri	Chai Hu	Chaai Wu	Saiko	Asian buplever root
Buthus Martensi	Buthus	Quan Xie	Chyun Kit	Zenkatsu	Scorpion

SCIENTIFIC	PHARMACEUTICAL	CANTONESE	MANDARIN	JAPANESE	ENGLISH
Caesalpinia minax	Semen Caesalpiniae minacis	Ku Shi Lian (Zi)	Fu Sek Lin (Ji)		Caesalpinia seed
Caesalpinia sappan	Lignum Caesalpiniae	Su Mu	Sou Muk	Soboku	Sappanwood
Cajanus cajan	Semen Cajani	Mu Dou Zi	Muk Dau Ji		Pigeon pea seed
Calamina, Smithsonitum	Calamina, Smithsonitum	Lu Gan Shi	Lou Gam Sek	Rokanseki	Calamine
Calcaria	Calcaria	Chen Shi Hui	Chan Sek Wei		Calcium hydroxide
Calcitum	Calcitum	Han Shui Shi, Fang Jie Shi	Hon Seui Sek	Kansuiseki	Calcite
Callicarpa macrophylla	Folium Callicarpae macrophyllae	Zi Zhu Ye, Ta Ye Zi Zhu	Ji Jyu Yip, Daai Yip Ji Jyu		Large-leaf Callicarpa leaf
Callicarpa pedunculata	Folium Callicarpae pedunculatae	Zi Zhu Ye	Ji Jyu Yip	Jijuso	Callicarpa leaf
Callorhinus ursinus, Phoca vitulina	Testes et penis Callorhini seu Phocae	Hai Gou Shen	Hoi Gau Sam	Kaikujin	Seal genitals
Calomelas	Calomelas	Qing Fen	Ching Fan	Keifun	Calomel
Calophyllum inophyllum	Resina Calophylli	Hu Tong Lei	Ng Tung Leui		Foraha resin
Camellia japonica	Flos Camelliae japonicae	Shan Cha Hua	Saan Cha Fa		Common camellia flower
Camellia sinensis	Folium Camelliae sinensis	Cha Ye	Cha Yip	Fujucha, Chayo	Tea leaf
Campanumoea javanica	Radix Campanumoeae	Tu Dang Shen	Tou Dong Sam		Java bellflower root
Campsis grandiflora	Radix Campsis grandiflorae	Ling Xiao Gen	Ling Siu Gan	Ryoshoka	Asian trumpetcree-per root
Campsis grandiflora	Flos Campsis grandiflorae	Ling Xiao Hua	Ling Siu Fa		Asian trumpetcree-per flower
Campsis radicans	Flos Campsis radicantis	Ling Xiao Hua, Mei Jou Ling Xiao	Ling Siu Fa, Mei Jau Ling Siu		Common trumpetcree-per flower
Camptotheca acuminata	Cortex radicis Camptothecae	Xi Shu	Hei Syu		Happy tree root bark
Camptotheca acuminata	Fructus Camptothecae	Xi Shu Guo	Hei Syu Gwo		Happy tree seed
Canarium album	Fructus Canarii	Gan Lan, Jing Guo	Gaam Laam		Asian olive fruit
Canavalia gladiata, C. ensiformis	Semen Canavaliae	Dao Dou	Dou Dau		Swordbean seed
Canis	Testes et penis canis	Guang Gou Shen	Gwong Gau Sam	Kujin	Male dog genitals
Canna indica	Rhizoma Cannae	Mei Ren Jiao (Gen)	Mei Yan Jiu (Gan)	Dandoku	Canna lily root
Cannabis sativa	Semen Cannabis	Huo Ma Ren	Fo Ma Yan	Mashinin	Cannabis seed
Cantharis vesicatoria	Cantharis	Ban Mao	Ban Mou	Hanmyo	Cantharides
Capparis masaikai	Semen Capparis	Ma Bin Lang	Ma Ban Long	Kuttokei	Capparis berry
Capsella bursa-pastoris	Herba Capsellae	Ji Cai	Chai Choi	Seisai	Shepherd's purse herb
Caragana sinica and spp	Flos Caraganae	Jin Que Hua	Gam Jeuk Fa		Caragana flower

SCIENTIFIC	PHARMACEUTICAL	CANTONESE	MANDARIN	JAPANESE	ENGLISH
Caragana sinica, C. microphylla and spp	Radix Caraganae	Jin Ji Er	Gam Jik Yi		Caragana root
Carpesium abrotanoides	Fructus seu semen Carpesii	He Shi	Hok Sat	Kakushitsu	Starwort fuit or seed
Carpesium abrotanoides	Herba Carpesii	Tian Ming Jing	Tin Ming Jing		Starwort herb
Carthamus tinctorius	Flos Carthami tinctorii	Hong Hua	Hung Fa	Koka	Safflower
Cassia alata	Folium Cassiae alatae	Dui Ye Dou Ye	Deui Yip Dau Yip		Ringworm bush leaf
Cassia occidentalis	Semen Cassiae occidentalis	Wang Jiang Nan Zi	Mong Gong Naam	Banshashi	Coffee senna seed
Cassia tora, C. obtusifolia and spp	Semen Cassiae torae	Jue Ming Zi, Cao Jue Ming	Kyut Ming Ji, Chou Kyut Ming	Ketsumeishi	Sickle senna seed
Castanea mollissima	Fructus Castaneae	Li Zi, Feng Li Gu	Leut Ji	Furitsukaku	Chinese chestnut
Catalpa bungei	Cortex Catalpae	Zi Bai Pi, Qiu Mu Pi	San Baak Pei, Chau Muk Pei		Catalpa bark
Catalpa ovata	Fructus Catalpae	Zhi Shi	San Sat	Kisasage	Catalpa fruit
Catharanthus roseus	Radix et herba Catharanthi	Chang Chun Hua	Cheung Cheun Fa		Madagascar periwinkle root and herb
Catharsius molossus, Xylotrupes dichotomus	Catharsius seu Xylotrupes	Jiang Lan Chong	Jeung Long Chung		Dung beetle
Cayratia japonica	Herba Cayratiae	Wu Lian Mei	Wu Lin Mui		Cayratia herb
Cedrela sinensis	Cortex radicis Cedrelae	Chun Gen Bai Pi	Jung Gan Baak Pei		Cedrela root bark
Celosia argentea	Semen Celosiae argenteae	Qing Xiang Zi	Ching Seung Ji	Seisoshi	Silver quail-grass seed
Celosia cristata	Herba Celosiae cristatae	Ji Guan Hua	Gai Gun Fa		Cock'scomb herb
Centella asiatica	Folium Centellae	Ji Xue Cao, Peng Da Wan	Jik Syut Chou, Pang Daai Yan		Gotu kola leaf
Centipeda minima	Herba Centipedae	E Bu Shi Cao	Ngo Bat Sik Chou	Sekikozui, Gabusho-kuso	Centipeda herb
Cephalanoplos segetum	Radix et herba Cephalanoplis	Xiao Ji	Siu Gai		Field thistle herb and root
Cephalotaxus fortunei	Ramulus et folium Cephalotaxi	San Jian Shan	Saam Jim Chaam		Yew twig and leaf
Cephalotaxus sinensis	Ramulus et folium Cephalotaxi sinensis	Tu Xiang Fei	Tou Heung Fei		Plum yew twig and leaf
Cercis chinensis	Cortex Cercis	Zi Jing Pi	Ji Ging Pei		Chinese redbud bark
Cerussa	Cerussa	Qian Fen	Yun Fan		Cerusite
Cervus nippon and spp	Testes et penis Cervi	Hua Lu Shen	Fa Luk Sam		Male deer genitals
Cervus nippon and spp	Cornu Cervi	Lu Jiao	Luk Gok	Rokkaku	Mature deer antler
Cervus nippon and spp	Colla cornu Cervi	Lu Jiao Jiao	Luk Gok Gaau	Rokkakukyo	Mature deer antler glue
Cervus nippon and spp	Cornu Cervi degelatinatum	Lu Jiao Shuang, Rong Mo	Luk Gok Shuen	Rokkakuso	Mature deer antler powder
Cervus nippon and spp	Cornu cervi parvum	Lu Rong, Rong Tou, Nen Lu Rong	Luk Yan	Rokujo	Velvet deer antler

SCIENTIFIC	PHARMACEUTICAL	CANTONESE	MANDARIN	JAPANESE	ENGLISH
Cervus nippon and spp	Cauda Cervi	Lu Wei Ba	Luk Mei Ba		Mature deer tail
Chaenomeles lagenaria	Fructus Chaenomelis lagenariae	Mu Gua, Chuan Mu Gua	Muk Gwa, Chyun Muk Gwa	Mokka	Chinese quince fruit
Chaenomeles sinensis	Fructus Chaenomelis sinensis	Mu Gua, Ming Za	Muk Gwa		Chinese quince fruit
Chaenomeles speciosa	Fructus Chaenomelis speciosae	Mu Gua, Tie Geng Hai Tang	Muk Gwa, Tip Gang Hoi Teng		Flowering quince fruit
Chalcanthitum	Chalcanthitum	Dan Fan, Shi Dan	Daan Faan	Tanban	Crystallized blue vitriol
Changium smyrnioides	Radix Changii	Ming Dang Shen	Ming Dong Sam	Mintojin	Bright changium root
Chelidonium majus var. ***asiaticum***	Herba Chelidonii	Bai Qu Cai	Baak Wat Choi	Hakkutusai	Asian celandine herb
Chenopodium ambrosioides	Herba Chenopodii ambrosioidis	Tu Jing Jie	Tou Ging Gai		Wormseed herb
Chimonanthus praecox	Flos Chimonanthi	La Mei Hua	Laap Mui Fa	Sakubaika	Wintersweet flower
Chinemys reevesii	Gelatinum carapaxis Chinemis	Gui Ban Jiao	Gwai Baan Gaau		Tortoise shell gel
Chinemys reevesii	Plastrum Chinemis	Gui Ban	Gwai Baan	Kiban	Tortoise shell
Chloranthus serratus	Radix Chloranthi	Ji Ji	Kap Gei		Serrate-leaf chloranthus
Chloris	Chloris	Jin Meng Shi	Gam Mein Sek		Mica schist
Chloris	Chloris	Qing Meng Shi	Ching Mein Sek		Chlorite schist
Chrysanthemum indicum	Flos Chrysanthemi indici	Ye Ju Hua	Gam Guk Fa, Ye Guk Fa	Nogikuka	Wild chrysanthe-mum flower
Chrysanthemum x ***morifolium***	Flos Chrysanthemi	Ju Hua, Gan Ju Hua	Guk Fa		Chrysanthe-mum flower
Chrysomyia megacephala and spp	Larva Chrysomyiae	Wu Gu Chong	Ng Guk Chung		Maggot
Cibotium barometz	Rhizoma Cibotii	Gou Ji	Gau Jek	Kuseki	Dogspine root
Cimicifuga dahurica	Radix Cimicifugae dahuricae	Sheng Ma, Xing An Sheng Ma	Sing Ma, Hing On Sing Ma	Shoma	Dahurian rising hemp root
Cimicifuga foetida	Radix Cimicifugae foetidae	Sheng Ma	Sing Ma	Shoma	Rising hemp root
Cimicifuga heracleifolia	Radix Cimicifugae heracleifoliae	Sheng Ma, Ta San Ye Sheng Ma	Sing Ma, Da Sam Yip Sing Ma	Shoma	Heraclean rising hemp root
Cinchona succiruba and spp	Cortex Cinchonae	Jin Ji Le, Jin Ji Na Pi	Gam Gai Laak		Cinchona bark
Cinnabarum	Cinnabarum	Zhu Sha	Ju Sa	Shusha	Cinnabar
Cinnamomum camphora	Lignum Cinnamomi camphorae	Zhang Mu	Jeung Muk		Camphor wood
Cinnamomum camphora	Camphora	Zhang Nao	Jeung Naau	Shono	Camphor flake
Cinnamomum cassia	Cortex intimum Cinnamomi cassiae	Rou Gui Xin	Yuk Gwai San		Cassia cinnamon inner bark
Cinnamomum cassia	Ramulus Cinnamomi cassiae	Gui Zhi , Rou Gui Zhi	Gwai Ji	Keishi	Cassia cinnamon twig

SCIENTIFIC	PHARMACEUTICAL	CANTONESE	MANDARIN	JAPANESE	ENGLISH
Cinnamomum cassia	Cortex Cinnamomi cassiae	Rou Gui (Pi)	Yuk Gwai (Pei)	Nikkei	Cassia Cinnamon bark
Cinnamomum japonicum, C. zeylanicum, C. obtusifolium	Cortex Cinnamomi japonici	Gui Pi	Gwai Pei		Cinnamon bark
Cinnamomum zeylanicum	Cortex Cinnamomi zeylanici	Rou Gui, Xi Lan Rou Gui	Yuk Gwai, Sek Laan Yuk Gwai		Ceylon cinnamon bark
Cirsium japonicum	Herba Cirsii japonici	Da Ji	Daai Gai	Taikei	Japanese thistle herb
Cissampelos pareira	Radix Cissampeli	Xi Sheng Teng	Sak Sang Tang		Ice vine root
Cissus pteroclada	Caulis Cissi	Kuan Jin Teng	Gwan Gam Tang		Cissus stem
Cistanche salsa and spp	Herba Cistanchis	Rou Cong Rong	Yuk Chung Yung	Nikujuyo	Fleshy broomrape herb
Citrullus vulgaris	Fructus Citrulli	Xi Gua	Sai Gwa	Seika	Watermelon fruit
Citrullus vulgaris	Pericarpium Citrulli	Xi Gua Pi	Sai Pa Pei		Watermelon rind
Citrus aurantium var. *amara*	Fructus Citri aurantii amarae	Zhi Ke, Zhi Qiao, Dai Dai Hua Zhi Qiao	Ji Hok, Doi Doi Fa Ji Hok	Kikoku	Ripe bitter orange fruit
Citrus aurantium, C. wilsonii	Fructus Citri aurantii immaturi	Zhi Shi	Ji Sat	Kijitsu	Unripe bitter orange fruit
Citrus grandis	Folium Citri grandi immaturi	You Ye	Yau Yip		Pomelo leaf
Citrus grandis	Pericarpium Citri grandi immaturi	You Pi (Ju Hong), Hua Ju Hong	Yau Pei (Gwat Hung), Fa Gwat Hung		Pomelo rind
Citrus grandis	Semen Citri grandi immaturi	You He	Yau Hat		Pomelo seed
Citrus grandis and spp	Flos Citri grandi	Ju Hong Hua	Gwat Heung Fa		Citrus flower
Citrus grandis and spp	Exocarpium rubrum Citri	Ju Hong (Pi), Hua Ju Pi	Gwat Heung (Pei), Fa Gwat Pei		Red citrus outer rind
Citrus grandis and spp	Fructus Citri grandi immaturi	Ju Hong Zhu	Gwat Heung		Unripe citrus fruit
Citrus medica var. *sarcodactylis*	Fructus Citri medicae	Fo Shou (Gan)	Fut Sau (Gam)		Finger lemon fruit
Citrus medica var. *sarctodactylus*	Flos Citri sarctodactylis	Fo Shou (Gan) Hua	Fut Sao Fa	Bushukan	Finger lemon flower
Citrus medica, C. wilsonii	Pericarpium Citri medicae	Xiang Yuan Pi, Gou Yuan Pi	Heung Yun Pei, Gau Yun Pei		Citron rind
Citrus medica, C. wilsonii	Fructus Citri medicae	Xiang Yuan, Gou Yuan	Heung Yun		Citron fruit
Citrus reticulata, C. tangerina, C. erythrosa	Pericarpium Citri reticulatae	Chen Pi, Ju Pi	Chan Pei, Gwat Pei	Chimpi	Ripe tangerine rind
Citrus reticulata, C. tangerina, C. erythrosa	Semen Citri reticulatae	Ju He	Gwat Hat		Tangerine seed
Citrus reticulata, C. tangerina, C. erythrosa	Pericarpium Citri reticulatae viride	Qing Pi	Ching Pei	Johi	Unripe tangerine rind
Citrus sinensis	Fructus Citri sinensis	Tian Chen	Tim Chaang		Sweet orange fruit

SCIENTIFIC	PHARMACEUTICAL	CANTONESE	MANDARIN	JAPANESE	ENGLISH
Citrus spp	Fasciculus vascularis Citri, Endocarpium Citri	Ju Luo, Ju Bai	Gwat Lok		Citrus fibre
Citrus spp	Folium Aurantium	Ju Ye	Gwat Yip		Citrus leaf
Clausenia lansium	Folium Clauseniae	Huang Pi Ye	Wong Pei Yip		Wampi leaf
Clausenia lansium	Pericarpium Clauseniae	Huang Pi Guo	Wong Pei Gwo		Wampi fruit
Clausenia lansium	Semen Clauseniae	Huang Pi He	Wong Pei Ho		Wampi seed
Cleistocalyx operculatus	Gemma Cleistocalycis	Shui Weng Hua	Seui Yung Fa		Cleistolcalyx bud
Clematis chinensis, C. hexapetala and spp	Radix Clematis chinensis	Wei Ling Xian	Wai Ling Sin	Ireisen	Chinese clematis root
Clematis florida	Herba Clematis floridae	Tie Xian Lian	Ti Chik Lin		Flowering clematis herb
Clematis hexapetala	Radix Clematis hexapetalae	Wei Ling Xian, Mian Tuan Tie Xian Lian	Wai Ling Sin, Min Tyun Ti Chik Lin		Six-petal clematis root
Clematis montana, C. armandii	Caulis Clematis montanae	Chuan Mu Tong	Chyun Muk Tong		Mountain clematis stem
Clerodendranthus spicatus	Herba Clerodendranthi	Mao Xu Cao	Maau Sao Chou		Orthosiphon herb
Clerodendron bungei	Folium Clerodendronis bungeis	Chou Mu Dan	Chau Maau Daan		Bung's Clerodendron leaf
Clerodendron cyrtophyllum	Folium Clerodendronis cyrtophylli	Da Qing Ye	Daai Cheng Yip		Green-white clerodendron leaf
Clerodendron inerme	Folium Clerodendronis inermis	Shui Hu Man	Seui Wu Mun		Glorybower leaf
Clerodendron paniculatum	Radix Clerodendronis paniculati	Bai Long Chuan Gen	Baak Lung Chyun Gan		Panicled clerodendron root
Clerodendron trichotomum	Folium Clerodendronis trichotomi	Chou Wu Tong (Ye)	Chau Ng Tung (Yip)		Forked glorybower leaf
Clinopodium confine	Herba Clinopodii	Jian Dao Cao	Jin Dou Chou		Clinopodium herb
Cnidium monnieri	Fructus Cnidii	She Chuang Zi	Se Chong Ji	Jashoshi	Cnidium seed
Cocculus trilobus	Radix Cocculi	Mu Fang Ji	Muk Fong Gei		Three-leaf cocculus root
Codonopsis lanceolata	Radix Codonopsis lanceolatae	Yang Ju, Shi Ye Shen	Yang Guk, Sei Yip Sam	Yonyu, Shiyojin	Goat's-tit bellflower root
Codonopsis pilosula, C. tangshen, C. nervosa	Radix Codonopsis	Dang Shen	Fong Dong Sam	Tojin	Downy bellflower root
Codonopsis subglobosa	Radix Codonopsis subglobosae	Dang Shen, Qiu Hua Dang Shen	Dong Sam, Kau Fa Dong Sam		Subglobular bellflower root
Codonopsis tangshen	Radix Codonopsis tangshenis	Dang Shen, Chuan Dang Shen	Chyun Dong Sam		Sichuan bellflower root
Coix lachryma-jobi var. *Ma-yuen*	Semen Coicis preparatae	Shu Yi Ren	Suk Yi Mai		Dry-fried Job's-tears seed

SCIENTIFIC	PHARMACEUTICAL	CANTONESE	MANDARIN	JAPANESE	ENGLISH
Coix lachryma-jobi var. *Ma-yuen*	Radix Coicis	Yi Yi Gen	Yi Yi Gan		Job's-tears root
Coix lachryma-jobi var. *Ma-yuen*	Semen Coicis	Yi Yi Ren	San Yi Mai, Yi Yi Yan	Yokuinin	Job's-tears seed
Colocasia esculenta	Radix Colocasiae	Yu Tou Gen	Wu Tau Gan		Taro root
Commelina benghalensis	Herba Commelinae	Tang Shi Song	Tong Sek Chung		Bengal dayflower herb
Commelina communis	Herba Commelinae	Ya Zhi Cao	Ngaap Jek Chou		Common dayflower herb
Commiphora myrrha	Resina Commiphorae	Mo Yao	Mut Yeuk	Motsuyaku	Myrrh resin
Coniogramme japonica	Herba Coniogrammis	Huo Xue Lian	Fo Hyut Lin		Bamboo fern herb
Coptis chinensis, C. omeiensis and spp	Rhizoma Coptis	Huang Lian, Chuan Lian	Wong Lin, Chyun Wong Lin	Oren	Goldthread root
Cordyceps scotianus and host *Cryptotympana atrata* and spp	Sclerotium Cordycepsis scotianus	Chan Hua, Jin Chan Hua	Sim Fa, Gam Sim Fa		Cicada fungus
Cordyceps sinensis and host larvae *Hepialus armoricanus* or *Holotrichia koraiensis*	Sclerotium Cordycepsis	Dong Chong Xia Cao	Dung Chung Ha Chou	Tochukaso	Chinese caterpillar mushroom
Coriandrum sativum	Herba Coriandri	Hu Sui	Wu Sai		Coriander herb
Coriandrum sativum	Fructus Coriandri	Yan Sui Zi	Yun Sai Ji		Coriander seed
Coriaria sinica	Folium Coriariae	Ma Sang Ye	Ma Song Yip		Coriaria leaf
*Coriolus versicolor (*syn. *Trametes versicolor)*	Sclerotium Corioli versicolori	Yun Zhi	Wan Ji		Turkey tail mushroom
Cornus officinalis	Fructus Corni	Shan Zhu Yu, Shan Yu Rou	San Jyu Yu, San Yu Yuk	Sanshuyu	Japanese dogwood berry
Corydalis ambigua var. *amurensis*	Rhizoma Corydalis ambiguae	Yan Hu Suo, Dong Bei Yan Hu Suo	Yin Wu Sok, Dung Bak Yin Wu Sok		Amur corydalis corm
Corydalis decumbens	Herba Corydalis decumbensis	Xia Tian Wu	Ha Tin Mou		Decumbent corydalis herb
Corydalis turtschaninovii	Rhizoma Corydalis	Yan Hu Suo, Chi Ban Yan Hu Suo	Yin Wu Sok, Chi Faan Yin Wu Sok	Engosaku	Dentate-leaf corydalis corm
Corydalis yanhusuo	Rizoma Corydalis yanhusuoidis	Yan Hu Suo, Yuan Hu	Yin Wu Sok, Yun Wu	Engosaku	Asian corydalis corm
Crataegus cuneata	Fructus Crataegus cuneatae	Ye Shan Zha	Ye Saan Ja		Wild hawthorn berry
Crataegus pinnatifida, C. cuneata and spp	Fructus Crataegi	Shan Zha (Rou)	Saan Ja (Yuk)	Sanzashi	Asian hawthorn berry
Crataegus pinnatifida, C. cuneata and spp	Fructus Crataegi carbonisatus	Shan Zha Tan	Saan Ja Tan		Charred Asian hawthorn berry
Cratoxylon ligustrinum	Folium Cratoxyli	Huang Niu Cha	Wong Ngau Cha		Cratoxylon leaf

SCIENTIFIC	PHARMACEUTICAL	CANTONESE	MANDARIN	JAPANESE	ENGLISH
Cremastra variabilis	Rhizoma et radix Cremastrae	Shan Ci Gu	Saan Chi Gu		Cremastra corm
Crocus sativus	Stigma Croci	Xi Hong Hua, Fan Hong Hua	Fun Hung Fa	Bankoka	Saffron stigma
Crossostephium chinense	Herba Crossostephii	Fu Rong	Fu Yung		Crossosteph-ium herb
Crotalaria assamica	Semen seu herba Crotalariae assamicae	Da Zhu Shi Dou, Zi Xiao Rong	Daai Ju Si Dau		Assam crotalaria seed or herb
Crotalaria sessiliflora	Herba Crotalariae	Ye Bai He	Ye Baak Hap		Thin-leaf rattlebox herb
Croton crassifolius	Radix Crotonis crassifolii	Ji Gu Xiang	Gai Gwat Heung		Thick-leaf croton root
Croton tiglium	Semen Crotonis	Ba Dou	Ba Dau		Croton seed
Cryptotympana atrata and spp	Periostracum Cryptotympanae	Chan Tui	Sim Teui, Sim Tyut	Sentai	Cicada slough
Cuccubala baccifer	Radix Cuccubalae bacciferis	Bai Niu Xi	Baak Ngao Sat		White oxknee root
Cucumis melo	Caulis Cucumis	Tian Gua Di	Tim Gwa Dai	Katei	Young cantaloupe stalk
Cucumis melo	Semen Cucumis	Tian Gua Zi	Tim Gwa Ji		Cantaloupe seed
Cucurbita moschata	Semen Cucurbitae	Nan Gua Zi	Naam Gwa Ji	Nankashi	Red squash seed
Cudrania cochinchinensis	Radix Cudraniae cochinchinensis	Chuan Po Shi	Chyun Po Sek		Cochin cudrania root
Cudrania tricuspidata	Lignum Cudraniae tricuspidatae	Da Ding Huang, Zhe Mu	Je Muk		Cudrania heartwood
Curculigo orchioides	Rhizoma Curculigonis	Xian Mao	Sin Maau	Sembo	Golden eye-grass root
Curcuma kwangsiensis	Rhizoma Curcumae kwangsiensis	E Zhu, Guang Xi Er Zhu	Ngo Seut, Gwong Sai Ngo Seut		Guangxi turmeric root
Curcuma longa, C. aromatica	Tuber Curcumae	Yu Jin	Yuk Gam	Ukon	Turmeric tuber
Curcuma longa. C. aromatica	Rhizoma Curcumae	Jiang Huang	Geung Wong	Kyoo	Turmeric root
Curcuma zedoaria, C. aeruginosa and spp	Rhizoma Curcumae zedoariae	E Zhu, Peng Er Zhu	Ngo Seut, Fung Ngo Seut	Gajutsu	Zedoary root
Cuscuta chinensis, C. japonica	Semen Cuscutae	Tu Si Zi	Tou Si Ji	Toshishi	Asian dodder seed
Cyathea spinulosa	Rhizoma Cyatheae	Guan Zhong	Gwun Jung		Cyathea root
Cyathula officinalis,. C. officinalis	Radix Cyathulae	Chuan Niu Xi	Chyun Ngau Sat		Hookweed root
Cycas revoluta	Semen Cycadis	Su Tie Zi	Sou Tit Ji		Sago palm seed
Cycas revoluta	Folium Cycadis	Tie Shu	Tit Syu		Sago palm leaf
Cyclina sinensis	Concha Cyclinae	Hai Ge Ke, Ke Li	Hoi Gap Hok	Kaigokaku	Clam shell
Cymbidium ensifolium	Radix Cymbidii	Jian Lan Gen	Gin Laan Gan		Cymbidium orchid root
Cymbidium ensifolium	Herba et radix Cymbidii	Jian Lan Hua	Gin Laan Fa		Cymbidium orchid herb and root
Cymbidium ensifolium	Folium Cymbidii	Jian Lan Ye	Gin Laan Yip		Cymbidium orchid leaf
Cymbopogon citratus	Herba Cymbopogonis	Xiang Mao	Heung Maau		Lemongrass herb

SCIENTIFIC	PHARMACEUTICAL	CANTONESE	MANDARIN	JAPANESE	ENGLISH
Cymbopogon distans	Herba Cymbopogonis distansis	Yun Xiang Cao	Yun Heung Chou		Distant lemongrass herb
Cynanchum atratum, C. versicolor	Radix Cynanchi atrati	Bai Wei	Baak Mei	Byakubi	Swallow-wort root
Cynanchum auriculatum	Radix Cynanchi auriculati	Bai Shou Wu, Niu Pi Xiao	Baak Sau Wu, Ngau Pei Siu		Auricle dogbane root
Cynanchum paniculatum	Radix et herba Cynanchi paniculati	Xu Chang Qing, Liao Diao Zhu	Cheui Cheung Hing		Panicled dogbane root and herb
Cynanchum stauntoni, C. glaucescens	Radix et rhizoma Cynanchi stauntoni	Bai Qian	Baak Chin	Byakuzen	Prime white root
Cynomorium songaricum	Herba Cynomorii	Suo Yang	Soi Yeung	Sayo	Lock yang stem
Cyperus rotundus	Rhizoma Cyperi	Xiang Fu	Heung Fu	Kobushi	Purple nutsedge root
Cypraea moneta, C. macula and spp	Concha Cypraeae	Bei Zi	Chan Bu Chi		Cowrie shell
Cyprinus carpio	Cyprinus	Li Yu	Lei Yu		Carp
Cypripedium formosanum	Herba Cypripedii	Yi Dian Hong	Yut Dim Hung		Formosa lady' slipper herb
Cyrtomium fortunei	Rhizoma Cyrtomi	Guan Zhong, Hun Ji Tou,	Gwun Jung, Fan Gai Tau		Boss fern root
Daemonorops draco	Resina Daemonoropsis (Sanguis draconis)	Xue Jie	Hyut Kit	Kekketsu	Dragon's-blood resin
Daemonorops margaritae	Radix Daemonoropsis	Huang Teng Gen	Wong Tang Gan		Daemonorops root
Dalbergia hupeana	Folium Dalbergiae hupeanae	Tan Gen	Taan Gan		Hupei rosewood
Dalbergia odorifera	Lignum Dalbergiae odoriferae	Jiang Xiang	Geung Heung		Asian rosewood
Daphne genkwa	Flos Daphnis genkwae	Yuan Hua	Yun Fa	Genka	Lilac daphne flower
Daphne giraldii, D. tangutica, D. retusa	Cortex Daphnis giraldii	Zu Shi Ma	Jou Si Ma		Giraldi's daphne bark
Daphne odora	Flos Daphnis odorae	Rui Xiang Hua	Seui Heung Fa		Mezerum flower
Datura metel	Flos Daturae	Yang Jin Hua	Yeung Gam Fa		Jimsonweed flower
Daucus carota	Fructus Dauci	Nan He Zao	Naam Hok Sat		Wild carrot seed
Davallia divaricata	Rhizoma Davalliae	Gu Sui Bu	Gwat Seui Bou	Kotsusaiho	Boneknit root
Dendrobium chrysanthum	Herba Dendrobii chrysanthi	Shi Hu, Shu Hua Shi Hu	Sek Wu, Chuk Fa Shi Hu		Stonebushel stem
Dendrobium fimbriatum	Herba Dendrobii fimbriati	Shi Hu, Ma Bian Shi Hu	Sek Wu, Ma Bin Sek Wu		Stonebushel stem
Dendrobium loddigesii	Herba Dendrobii loddigesii	Shi Hu, Wan Cao Shi Hu	Sek Wu, Waan Chou Sek Wu		Stonebushel stem
Dendrobium moniliforme	Caulis Dendrobii miniliformis	Xi Jing Shi Hu, Xiao Wan Chai	Sai Ging Sek Wu		Stonebushel stem
Dendrobium nobile	Herba Dendrobii nobilis	Shi Hu, Jin Sha Shi Hu	Sek Wu, Gam Ja Sek Wu		Stonebushel stem
Dendrobium nobile, D. linawianum, D. officinale and spp	Herba Dendrobii	Shi Hu	Sek Wu	Sekkoku	Stonebushel stem
Dendrobium officinalis	Herba Dendrobii officinalis	Shi Hu, Tie Pi Shi Hu	Sek Wu, Tit Pei Sek Wu		Stonebushel stem

SCIENTIFIC	PHARMACEUTICAL	CANTONESE	MANDARIN	JAPANESE	ENGLISH
Descurainia sophia	Semen Descurainiae	Ting Li Zi	Ting Lai Ji	Teirekishi	Tansy mustard seed
Desmodium pseudotriquetrum D. triquetrum	Herba Desmodii pseudotriquetrii	Long Shi Huang	Lung Sek Wong		Bottlegourd herb
Desmodium sinnatum	Herba Desmodii sinnati	Guo Lu Huang, Nian Ren Hua	Lim Yan Fa		Sinnate desmodium herb
Desmodium styracifolium	Herba Desmodii	Guang Dong (Jin) Qian Cao	Gwong Dung (Gam) Chin Chou	Kinsenso	Coin-leaf desmodium herb
Desmodium umbellatum	Flos Desmodii umbellati	Gu Su Hua	Gu Sou Fa		Umbel desmodium flower
Dianthus chinensis	Herba Dianthi chinensis	Qu Mai, Shi Zhu	Geui Mak, Sek Juk		Chinese pink herb
Dianthus superbus, D. chinensis	Herba Dianthi	Qu Mai	Geui Mak	Kubaku	Proud pink herb
Dichondra repens	Herba Dichondrae	Ma Di Jin	Ma Dei Jing	Kinsenso	Dichondra herb
Dichroa febrifuga	Radix Dichroae	Chang Shan	Seung Saan	Joszan	Feverflower root
Dichroa febrifuga	Folium Dichroae	Shu Qi	Suk Chat	Shokushitsu	Feverflower leaf
Dictamnus dasycarpus	Cortex radicis Dictamni	Bai Xian Pi	Baak Sin Pei	Hakusempi	Asian dittany root bark
Dioscorea bulbifera	Rhizoma Dioscoreae bulbiferae	Huang Yao Zi	Wong Yeuk Ji	Oyakushi	Potato yam tuber
Dioscorea cirrhosa	Rhizoma Dioscoreae cirrhosae	Shu Liang	Syu Leung		Dyer's yam root
Dioscorea hypoglauca	Rhizoma Dioscoreae hypoglaucae	Bi Xie, Fen Bi Xie, Bei Xie	Bei Gaai, Fan Bei Gaai	Hikai	Long yam root
Dioscorea japonica	Rhizoma Dioscoreae japonicae	Feng Che Er	Fung Che Yi		Japanese yam root
Dioscorea nipponica	Rhizoma Dioscoreae nipponicae	Chuan Shan Long	Chyun Saan Lung		Nippon yam root
Dioscorea opposita, D. batatas	Rhizoma Dioscoreae oppositae	Shan Yao Shu Yu	Wai Saan, Saan Yeuk	Sanyaku	Mountain yam root
Dioscorea septemloba	Rhizoma Dioscoreae septemlobae	Bi Xie, Mian Bi Xie	Bei Gaai, Min Bei Gaai		Seven-lobe yam root
Dioscorea zingiberensis	Rhizoma Dioscoreae zingiberis	Dun Ye Shu Yu	Teun Yip Syu Yu		Shield-leaf yam root
Diospyros kaki	Saccharum Diospyris	Shi Bing Shuang	Chi Beng Sheung		Persimmon frost
Diospyros kaki	Calyx Diospyri	Shi Di	Chi Dai	Shitei	Persimmon calyx
Diospyros kaki	Fructus Diospyri	Shi Shuang Bing	Chi Shuen Bing		Persimmon frosted fruit
Diospyros kaki	Folium Diospyri	Shi Ye	Chi Yip		Persimmon leaf
Dipsacus asperoides	Radix Dipsaci asperoides	Xu Duan, Chuan Duan	Juk Dyun, Chyun Dyun		Sichuan teasel root
Dipsacus chinensis and spp	Fructus Dipsaci	Ju Sheng Zi	Geui Sing Ji		Chinese teasel fruit

SCIENTIFIC	PHARMACEUTICAL	CANTONESE	MANDARIN	JAPANESE	ENGLISH
Dipsacus japonica	Radix Dipsaci japonicae	Xu Duan	Juk Dyun	Zokudan	Japanese teasel root
Dolichos lablab	Radix Dolichoris	Rou Dou Gen	Yuk Dau Gan		Hyacinth bean root
Dolichos lablab	Semen Dolichis	Bai Bian Dou	Baak Bin Dau	Hakuhenzu	Hyacinth bean
Dolichos lablab	Gemma Dolichis	Bian Dou Hua	Bin Dau Fa	Henzuka	Hyacinth bean bud
Dolichos lablab	Testa Dolichoris	Bian Dou Yi	Bin Dau Yi		Hyacinth bean capsule
Dolomiaea berardioidea	Radix Dolomiaea berardioidea	Hou Ye Chuan Mu Xiang	Hau Yip Chyun Muk Heung		Thick-leaf Dolomiaea root
Dolomiaea souliei	Radix Dolomiaeae souliei	Chuan Mu Xiang	Chyun Muk Heung		Sichuan Dolomiaea root
Drosera burmanni	Herba Droserae	Jin Di Luo	Gam Dei Lo		Sundew herb
Drynaria fortunei and spp	Rhizoma Drynariae	Gu Sui Bu	Gwat Seui Bou	Kotsusaiho	Boneknit root
Dryobalanops camphora	Borneolum	Bing Pian	Bing Pin	Ryuno	Borneo camphor
Dryopteris crassirhizoma	Rhizoma Dryopteris	Guan Zhong, Mian Ma Guan Zhong	Gwun Jung, Min Ma Gwun Jung	Tohoku-kanju	Shield fern root
Duchesnea indica	Herba Duchesneae	She Mei	Se Mui		Mock strawberry herb
Dysosma pleiantha	Rhizoma Dysosmae pleianthae	Ba Jiao Lian	Baat Gok Lin		Pleianth dysosma root
Dysosma versipellis	Rhizoma Dysosmae versipellis	Gui Jiu	Gwai Kau		Common dysosma root
Echinops latifolius, E. gmelinii	Radix Echinopsis	Lou Lu	Lau Lou		Globe thistle root
Eclipta prostata, E. alba	Herba Ecliptae	Han Lian Cao, Mo Han Lian	Hon Lin Chou	Kanrenso	Field lotus herb
Edgeworthiae chrysantha	Flos Edgeworthiae chrysanthae	Jie Xiang Hua, Meng Hua	Git Heung Fa, Mung Fa		Oriental paperbush flower
Eleagnus oldhamii	Radix Eleagni oldhamii	Yi Wu Gen	Yi Ng Gan		Oldham's eleagnus root
Eleagnus pungens	Folium Eleagni pungensis	Hu Tui (Zi) Ye	Wu Teui (Ji) Yip		Thorny eleagnus leaf
Elephantopus scaber	Herba Elephantopi	Di Dan Tou, Ku Di Dan, Tu Gong Ying	Fu Dei Daam		Rough elephant's foot herb
Elephe taeniurus and spp, *Dinodon rufozonatum*	Periostracum/Exuviae Elephis	She Tui (Pi)	Se Teui (Pei)	Dataihi	Snakeskin slough
Eleutherococcus senticosus	Radix seu cortex radicis Eleutherococci senticosi	Ci Wu Jia (Gen Pi)	Chi Ng Ga (Gan Pei)		Eleuthero ginseng root
Elsholtzia splendens, E. stauntonii	Herba Elsholtziae	Xiang Ru (Cao)	Heung Yu (Chou)	Koju	Aromatic madder herb
Emilia sonchifolia	Herba Emiliae	Yang Ti Cao	Yeung Tai Chou		Red tasselflower herb
Ephedra sinica	Herba Ephedrae	Ma Huang	Ma Wong	Mao	Ephedra stem
Ephedra sinica	Radix Ephedrae	Ma Huang Gen	Ma Wong Gan	Maokon	Ephedra root

SCIENTIFIC	PHARMACEUTICAL	CANTONESE	MANDARIN	JAPANESE	ENGLISH
Ephemerantha fimbriata	Herba Ephemeranthae	Shi Hu	Sek Hap	Sekkoku	Ephemerantha stem
Epimedium saggitatum, E. macranthum and spp	Folium Epimedii	Yin Yang Huo, Xian Ling Pi	Yam Yeung Fok, Sin Ling Pei	Inyokaku	Horny goat weed leaf
Equisetum hiemale	Herba Equiseti hiemalis	Mu Zei	Muuk Chaak	Mokuzoku	Horsetail herb
Equisetum ramosissimum	Herba Equiseti ramosissimi	Bi Tong Cao	Bat Tung Chou		Ramose horsetail herb
Equus asinus and spp	Gelatinum corii Equi asini	E Jiao	O Gaau	Akyo	Ass hide glue
Equus caballos	Calculus Equi	Ma Bao	Ma Bou		Horse bezoar
Eretmochelys imbricata	Plastrum Eretmochelis	Dai Mao	Doi Mou	Taimai	Hawksbill turtle shell
Ericerus pela	Ericerus	Chong Bai La	Chung Baak Laap		Ericerus worm
Erinaceaus europoeus, Hemichianum dauricus	Corium Erinacei	Ci Wei Pi	Chi Wai Pei		Hedgehog hide
Eriobotrya japonica	Fructus Eriobotryae	Pi Pa	Pei Pa		Loquat fruit
Eriobotrya japonica	Folium Eriobotryae	Pi Pa Ye	Pei Pa Yip	Biwayo	Loquat leaf
Eriocaulon buergerianum, E. sieboldianum	Herba Eriocaulonis	Gu Jing Cao	Guk Jing Chou	Kokuseiso	Pipewort herb
Eriocaulon buergerianum, E. sieboldianum	Fructus Eriocaulonis	Gu Jing Zi	Guk Jing Ji		Pipewort seed
Eriocheir sinensis, E. japonicus	Eriocheir	Jin Xie	Jeun Haai	Zukani	Tianjin crab
Erodium stephaniarum, Geranium spp	Herba Erodii seu Geranii	Lao Guan Cao	Lou Gwun Chou		Storksbill or cranesbill herb
Ervatamia divaricata, E. hainaensis	Herba Ervatamiae	Gou Ya Hua	Gaau Nga Fa		Crepe jasmine herb
Erycibes obtusifolia	Radix et caulis Erycibis	Ding Gong Teng	Ding Gung Tang		Erycibe root and stem
Erythrina variegata var. *orientalis*	Cortex Erythrinae	Hai Tong Pi	Hoi Tung Pei	Kaitohi	Asian coral tree bark
Eucalyptus globulus	Folium Eucalypti globuli	An Ye	Ngon Yip		Eucalyptus leaf
Eucommia ulmoides	Cortex Eucommiae	Du Zhong	Dou Jung	Tochu	Eucommia bark
Eucommia ulmoides	Folium Eucommiae	Du Zhong Ye	Dou Jung Yip		Eucommia leaf
Eugenia caryophyllata	Gemma Eugeniae	Ding Xiang	Ding Heung	Choko	Clove bud
Eulota peliomphala	Eulota	Gua Niu	Wo Ngau		Snail
Euonymus alata	Ramulus Eunymi alati	Gui Jian Yu	Gwai Jin Yu		Winged spindletree twig
Eupatorium fortunei	Herba Eupatorii fortunei	Pei Lan	Pui Laan	Haikan	Orchid-grass herb
Eupatorium lindleyanum	Herba Eupatorii lindleyani	Cheng Gan Sheng Ma	Ping Gon Sing Ma		Lindley's eupatorium herb

SCIENTIFIC	PHARMACEUTICAL	CANTONESE	MANDARIN	JAPANESE	ENGLISH
Eupatorium lindleyanum var. *tripartum*	Herba Eupatorii	Ye Ma Zhui, Jian Pei Lan	Ye Ma Jeui, Jim Pui Laan		Lindley's eupatorium herb
Euphorbia ebracteolata	Radix Euphorbiae ebracteolatae	Lang Du, Yue Xian Da Ji	Long Duk, Yu Sin Daai Gik		Bractless spurge root
Euphorbia fischeriana	Radix Euphorbiae fischerianae	Lang Du, Lang Du Da Ji	Long Duk, Long Duk Daai Gik		Fischer's spurge root
Euphorbia helioscopia	Herba Euphorbiaehelioscopiae	Ze Qi	Jaak Chat	Takushitsu	Sunspurge herb
Euphorbia humifusa	Herba Euphorbiae humifusae	Di Jin Cao	Dei Gam Chou		Wolf'smilk herb
Euphorbia kansui	Radix Euphorbiae kansui	Gan Sui	Gam Seui	Kansui	Sweet spurge root
Euphorbia lathyris	Semen Euphorbiae lathyris	Qian Jin Zi	Chin Gam Ji	Zokuzuishi	Caper spurge seed
Euphorbia milii	Herba Euphorbiae milii	Ci Peng Hua	Chi Fung Fa		Prickly spurge herb
Euphorbia nematocypha	Radix Euphorbiae nematocyphae	Lang Du, Da Lang Du	Long Duk, Daai Long Duk		Gigantic spurge root
Euphorbia pallasii, E. abracteolatae, E. fischerianae	Radix Euphorbiae pallasii seu ebracteolatae	(Bai) Lang Du	(Baak) Long Duk		White spurge root
Euphorbia pekinensis	Radix Euphorbiae pekinensis	Jing Da Ji	Ging Daai Gik	Taigeki	Peking spurge root
Euphorbia prolifera	Radix Euphorbiae proliferae	Lang Du, Ji Chang Lang Du	Long Duk, Gai Cheung Long Duk		Prolific spurge root
Euphoria longan	Semen Euphoriae	Long Yan He	Lung Ngaan Ho		Longan seed
Euphoria longan	Flos Euphoriae	Long Yan Hua	Lung Ngaan Fa		Longan flower
Euphoria longan	Arillus Euphoriae	Long Yan Rou	Lung Ngaan Yuk	Ryuganniku	Longan fruit pulp
Eupolyphaga sinensis	Eupolyphaga	Tu Bie Chong	Dei Bit Chung	Shachu	Cockroach
Euryale ferox	Semen Euryalis	Qian Shi	Him Sat	Kenjitsu	Foxnut
Evodia lepta	Radix Evodiae leptae	San Ya Ku (Gen)	Sam Nga Fu (Gan)		Bitter evodia root
Evodia rutaecarpa	Fructus Evodiae rutecarpae	Wu Zhu Yu	Ng Jyu Yu	Goshuyu	Evodia berry
Fagopyrum cymosum	Rhizoma Fagopyri	Jin Qiao Mai Gen	Gam Kiu Mak Gan		Buckwheat root
Ferrum	Pulvis ferri	Chen Sha	Chan Sa		Black iron oxide
Ferrum	Frusta Ferrum	Sheng Tie Luo	Sang Tit Lo		Iron filing/cinder
Ferrum	Pulvis ferri	Chen Sha	San Sa		Black ferric oxide
Ferula foetida	Resina Ferulae (Asafoetidae)	A Wei	A Ngai	Agi	Asafoetida resin
Ficus carica	Flos Fici	Wu Hua Guo	Wu Fa Gwat		Fig flower
Ficus microcarpa, F. retusa	Radix Fici microcarpae seu retusae	Lao Gong Xu, Rong Shu Xu	Lou Gung Chuk		Aerial fig root
Ficus pumila	Fructus Fici pumilae	Bi Li, Mu Man Tou	Bai La		Creeping fig fruit
Firmiana simplex	Semen Firmianae	Wu Tong Zi	Ng Tung Ji		Chinese parasol tree seed
Fissistigma glaucescens	Herba Fissistigmae	Wu Gu Teng	Wu Gwat Tang		Fissistigma herb

SCIENTIFIC	PHARMACEUTICAL	CANTONESE	MANDARIN	JAPANESE	ENGLISH
Fluoritum	Fluoritum	Zi Shi Ying	Ji Sek Ying		Purple fluorite
Foeniculum vulgare	Fructus Foeniculi	Xiao Hui Xiang	Siu Wui Heung	Shouikyo	Fennel seed
Fomes applanatus and host fruit *Euphoria longana*	Sclerotium Fomis	Long Yan Gu	Lung Ngan Gu		Longan fungus
Forsythia suspensa	Fructus Forsythiae	Lian Qiao	Lin Kiu	Rengyo	Forsythia valve
Fraxinus rhynchophyllae, F. bungeana, F. chinensis and spp	Cortex Fraxini	Qin Pi	Cheun Pei		Korean ash bark
Fritillaria cirrhosa	Bulbus Fritillariae cirrhosae	Chuan Bei Mu	Chyun Bui Mou	Senbaimo	Sichuan fritillary bulb
Fritillaria hupehensis	Bulbus Fritillariae hupehensis	Hu Bei Bei Mu	Wu Bak Bui Mou		Hubei fritillary bulb
Fritillaria pallidiflora	Bulbus Fritillariae pallidiflorae	Yi Bei Mu	Yi Bui Mou		Pale-flower fritillary bulb
Fritillaria puqiensis	Bulbus Fritillariae puqiensis	Hu Bei Bei Mu, Pu Qi Bei Mu	Wu Bak Bui Mou, Pou Kei Bui Mou		Puqi fritillary bulb
Fritillaria taipaiensis	Bulbus Fritillariae taipaiensis	Chuan Bei Mu, Tai Bai Bei Mu	Chyun Bui Mou, Taai Baak Bui Mou		Taipei fritillary bulb
Fritillaria thunbergii	Bulbus Fritillariae thunbergii	Zhe Bei Mu	Chit Bui Mou	Setsubaimo	Zhejiang fritillary bulb
Fritillaria tortifolia	Bulbus Fritillariae tortifoliae	Yi Bei Mu, Tuo Li Bei Mu	Yi Bui Mou, Tok Lei Bui Mou		Twist-leaf fritillary bulb
Fritillaria unibracteata	Bulbus Fritillariae unibracteatae	Chuan Bei Mu, An Zi Bei Mu	Chyun Bui Mou, Am Ji Bui Mou		Single-bract fritillary bulb
Fritillaria yuminensis	Bulbus Fritillariae yuminensis	Yi Bei Mu, Yu Min Bei Mu	Yi Bui Mou, Yu Man Bui Mou		Yumin fritillary bulb
Galium aparine	Herba Galii aparinis	Ba Xian Cao, Zhu Yang Yang	Baat Sin Chou		Cleavers herb
Gallus gallus domesticus	Endothelium corneum gigeriae Galli	Ji Nei Jin	Gai Na Gam	Keinaikin	Chicken gizzard lining
Gallus gallus domesticus	Membrana follicularis ovi	Feng Huang Yi			Chicken egg membrane
Gallus gallus domesticus	Vitellus Galli	Ji Zi Huang	Gai Ji Wong		Egg yolk
Ganoderma lucidum, G. sinense, G applanatum and spp	Sclerotium Ganodermae	Ling Zhi (Cao)	Ling Ji (Chou)	Reishi	Reishi mushroom
Garcinia morella	Resina Garciniae	Teng Huang	Tang Wong		Gamboge resin
Gardenia jasminoides	Fructus Gardeniae	Zhi Zi Shan Zhi Zi	Ji Ji, Saan Ji Ji	Sanshishi	Gardenia pod
Gastrodia elata	Rhizoma Gastrodiae	Tian Ma	Tin Ma	Temma	Celestial hemp corm
Gecko chinensis, G. japonicus and spp	Gecko chinensis	Shou Gong, Bi Hu	Sau Gung, Bik Fu		House lizard
Gecko gecko, G. verticilatus	Gecko	Ge Jie	Gap Gaai	Gokai	Toad-headed lizard
Gelsemium elegans	Radix Gelsemii	Gou Wen	Au Man		Chinese gelsemium

SCIENTIFIC	PHARMACEUTICAL	CANTONESE	MANDARIN	JAPANESE	ENGLISH
Gendarussa vulgaris	Herba Gendarussae	Bo Gu Dan	Bok Gwat Daam		Gendarussa herb
Gentiana macrophylla, G. tibetica, G. daburica and spp	Radix Gentianae macrophyllae	Qin Jiao	Cheun Gau	Jingyo	Large-leaf gentian root
Gentiana scabra, G. triflora, G. mansburica	Radix Gentianae scabrae	Long Dan Cao	Lung Daam Chou	Ryutan	Scabrous gentian root
Geranium wilfordii, G. thunbergii	Herba Geranii	Lao He Cao	Lou Hap Chou	Gennoshio-uko	Geranium herb
Ginkgo biloba	Fructus Ginkgoidis	Bai Guo, Yin Xing He	Baak Gwo, Ngan Hang Wat	Ginkyo	Ginkgo nut
Ginkgo biloba	Folium Ginkgoidis	Yin Xing Ye, Bai Guo Ye	Ngan Hang Yip, Baak Gwo Yip	Ginkyoyo	Ginkgo leaf
Glechoma hederacea, G. longituba	Herba Glechomae	Lian Qian Cao	Ling Chin Chou		Ground ivy herb
Gleditsia sinensis and spp	Spina Gleditsiae	Zao Jiao Ci	Jou Gok Chi	Sokakushi	Honeylocust spine
Gleditsia sinensis and spp	Fructus Gleditsiae	Zao Jiao, Zao Jia	Jou Gok, Jou Gaap	Sokaku	Honeylocust pod
Gleditsia sinensis and spp	Semen Gleditsiae	Zao Jiao Zi	Jou Gok Ji		Honeylocust fruit
Glehnia littoralis	Radix Glehniae	Bei Sha Shen	Mai Sa Sam	Shajin	Northern sandroot
Glossogyne tenuifolia	Herba Glossogyne	Shan Shen Zi	Saan Sam Jai		Thin-leaf glossgyne herb
Glycene max	Semen Glycinis germinati	Dou (Huang) Juan	Dau (Wong) Geun		Sprouting soybean
Glycine max	Semen Glycinis preparatum	Dan Dou Chi	Taam Dau Si	Tantoshi	Fermented soybean
Glycine max	Pericarpium Glycinis	Hei Dou Yi	Haak Dau Yi		Soybean husk
Glycirrhiza uralensis, G. glabra and spp	Radix Glycirrhizae	Gan Cao	Gam Chou	Kanzo	Ural licorice root
Glycirrhiza uralensis, G. glabra and spp	Radix Glycirrhizae preparatae	Zhi Gan Cao	Jek Gam Chou	Shakanzo	Honey-fried licorice root
Glycirrhiza uralensis, G. glabra and spp	Radix Glycirrhizae preparatae cum urina	Ren Zhong Huang	Yan Chung Wong		Urine-prepared licorice root
Glyptostrobus pensilis	Cacumen Glyptostrobi	Shui Song Mao	Seui Chung Ma		Chinese water pine tip
Gnaphalium affine	Herba Gnaphalii	Shu Qu Cao	Syu Guk Chou		Cudweed herb
Gomphrena globosa	Flos Gomphrenae	Qian Ri Hong	Jin Yat Hung		Globe amaranth flower
Gossampinus malabarica	Flos Gossampini	Mu Mian Hua	Muk Min Fa		Silk cotton tree flower
Gossypium hirsutum, G. herbaceum	Semen Gossypii	Mian Hua Zi	Min Fa Ji		Cotton seed
Gossypium hirsutum, G. herbaceum	Cortex radicis Gossypii	Mian Hua Gen	Min Fa Gan		Cotton root bark

SCIENTIFIC	PHARMACEUTICAL	CANTONESE	MANDARIN	JAPANESE	ENGLISH
Grifola frondosa	Sclerotium Grifolae frondosae			Maitake	Maitake, Hen of the woods mushroom
Gryllulus chinensis, G. mitratus, Gampsocleis buergeri	Gryllulus	Xi Shuai	Sik Seut		Cricket
Gymnema sylvestre and spp	Caulis et radix Gymnemae	Wu Xue Teng	Mou Heu Tang		Gymnema stem and root
Gymnocladus chinensis	Fructus Gymnocladi	Fei Zao Jia	Fei Jou Choi		Chinese gymnocladus berry
Gynostemma pentaphyllum	Herba Gynostemmae	Jiao Gu Lan	Gaan Gu Laam		Gynostemma herb
Gynura segetum	Folium Gynurae	San Qi Cao, Ju San Qi	Sam Chat Chou		Canton sanchi leaf
Gypsophyla oldhamiana	Radix Gypsophylae	Yin Chai Hu	Ngan Chaai Wu		Gypsophyla root
Gypsum fibrosum	Gypsum	Shi Gao	Sek Gou	Sekko	Gypsum
Gypsum fibrosum	Gypsum dehydratum	Shu Shi Gao	Chek Sek Gou		Dehydrated gypsum
Gypsum rubrum	Gypsum rubrum	Han Shui Shi, Hong Shi Gao	Hon Seui Sek, Hung Sek Gau		Red gypsum
Haematitum	Haematitum	Dai Zhe Shi	Doi Jyu Sek	Taishaseki	Hematite
Haliotis diversicolor, H. gigantea and spp	Concha Haliotis	Shi Jue Ming	Sek Kyut Ming	Sekketsumei	Abalone shell
Halitum	Halitum	Da Qing Yan	Daai Ching Yim		Rock salt
Halloysitum album	Halloysitum album	Bai Shi Zhi	Baak Sek Ji		White kaolin
Halloysitum rubrum	Halloysitum	Chi Shi Zhi	Chek Sek Chi	Shakusek-ishi	Red kaolin
Halloysitum rubrum	Halloysitum	Shu Chi Shi	Chek Sek Ji		Roasted red kaolin
Hedera nepalensis var. *sinensis*	Herba Hederae nepalensis	Chang Chun Teng	Seung Cheun Tang		Nepalese ivy leaf
Hedysarum polybotrys and spp	Radix Hedysari polybotris	Huang Qi, Hong Qi	Wong Kei		Hedysarum root
Heleocharis plantaginea	Herba Heleocharis	Bi Qi	But Chai	Bossai	Water chestnut herb
Helianthus annuus	Receptaculum Helianthi	Xian Ji Gui Hua Pan	Heung Yat Kwai Fa Bun		Sunflower receptacle
Helicteres angustifolia	Herba Helicteres	Shan Zhi Ma	Saan Ji Ma		Helicteres herb
Heliotropium indicum	Herba Heliotropi	Da Wei Yao, Er Gou Cao	Daai Mei Yiu		Heliotrope herb
Heliotropium indicum	Herba Heliotropi	Er Gou Cao	Yi Ngau Chou		Indian heliotrope herb
Helminthostachys zeylanica	Rhizoma Helminthostachys	Di Wu Song	Dei Ng Gung		Helmintho-stachys root
Hemerocallis fulva	Radix Hemerocallis	Xuan Cao (Gen)	Syun Chou Gan		Tawny day lily root
Hemerocallis fulva	Flos Hemerocallis	Xuan Cao Hua	Syun Chou Fa		Tawny day lily flower
Hemerocallis thunbergii	Rhizoma et radix Hemerocallis thunbergii	Li Lu	Lai Lou		Day lily root

SCIENTIFIC	PHARMACEUTICAL	CANTONESE	MANDARIN	JAPANESE	ENGLISH
Hemsleya amabilis, H. macrosperma and spp	Radix Hemsleyae	Xue Dan	Hat Daam		Hemsleya tuber
Heracleum candicans	Radix Heraclei candicantis	Du Huo	Duk Wut		White cow parsnip root
Hericium erinaceus	Sclerotium Hericii	Hou Gu			Hedgehog fungus
Hibiscus mutabilis	Folium Hibisci mutabilis	Fu Rong Ye	Fu Yung Yip		Cotton rose leaf
Hibiscus mutabilis	Flos Hibisci mutabili	Fu Rong Hua	Fu Yung Fa		Cotton rose flower
Hibiscus rosa-sinensis	Flos Hibisci rosa-sinensis	Fu Sang Hua	Fu Song Fa		Shoe flower
Hibiscus syriacus	Cortex radicis Hibisci syriacus	Mu Jin Pi	Mut Gan Pei		Rose of Sharon root bark
Hibiscus syriacus	Flos Hibisci syriaci	Mu Jin Hua	Mut Gan Fa		Rose of Sharon flower
Hippocampus kelloggi and spp	Hippocampus	Hai Ma	Hoi Ma	Kaiba	Sea horse
Hippophae rhamnoides	Fructus Hippophae	Sha Ji	Sa Jik		Sea buckthorn berry
Hirudo nipponia, Whitmania pigra and spp	Hirudo seu Whitmania	Shui Zhi	Seui Jik		Leech
Holarrhenia antidysenterica	Cortex Holarrheniae	Zhi Xie Mu Pi	Ji Se Muk Pei		Conessi bark
Holotrichia diomphalia	Holotrichia	Qi Cao	Chai Chou		June beetle grub (larva)
Homalomena occulta	Rhizoma Homalomenae	Qian Nian Jian	Chin Nin Gin	Sennenken	Homalomena root
Homo sapiens	Funis umbilici Hominis	Qi Dai	Chi Daai		Umbilical cord
Homo sapiens	Urina Hominis	Ren Niao	Yan Niu		Human urine
Homo sapiens	Sedimen urinae Hominis	Ren Zhong Bai, Qiu Shi Dan	Yan Jung Baak		Human urine sediment
Homo sapiens	Crinis carbonisatus Hominis	Xue Yu Tan	Hyut Yu Taan		Charred human hair
Homo sapiens	Placenta Hominis	Zi He Che	Ji Ho Je	Shikasha	Human placenta
Hordeum vulgare	Fructus germinatus Hordei	Mai Ya	San Man Nga	Bakuga	Sprouted barley grain
Hordeum vulgare	Saccharum Hordei	Yi Tang, Jiao Yi	Yi Tong		Barley malt sugar
Houttuynia cordata	Herba Houttuyniae	Yu Xing Cao	Yu Seng Chou	Juyakuso	Fishwort herb
Hovenia dulcis	Semen et fructus Hoveniae	Zhi Ju Zi	Ji Gwat Ji		Hovenia seed and fruit
Huechys sanguinea, H, philaemata	Huechys	Hong Niang Zi	Hung Leung Ji		Red cicada
Humulus lupulus	Flos Humuli lupuli	Pi Jiu Hua	Be Jau Fa		Hops flower
Humulus scandens	Herba Humuli scandentis	Lu Cao	Leut Chou		Climbing hops flower
Hydnocarpus anthelmintica, H. hainanensis	Semen Hydnocarpi	Da Feng Zi	Daai Fung Ji	Daifushi	Chaulmoogra seed
Hydragyrum	Hydragyrum	Shui Yin	Seui Yin		Mercury
Hydragyrum chloratum	Compositum Hydragyri chlorati	Bai Jiang Dan	Baak Geung Daan		Mercury chloride

SCIENTIFIC	PHARMACEUTICAL	CANTONESE	MANDARIN	JAPANESE	ENGLISH
Hydragyrum chloratum	Compositum Hydragyri oxydati crudi	San Xian Dan	Sam Gong Daan		Mercury oxide (crude)
Hydrangea macrophylla	Flos Hydrangeae	Ba Xian Hua	Baat Sin Fa		French hydrangea flower
Hydrangea serrata var. *thunbergii*	Folium Hydrangeae	Gan Cha	Gam Cha	Amatya, Dochouzan	Sweet tea leaf
Hydrocotyle sibthorpioides	Herba Hydrocotylis	Tian Hu Sui	Tin Wu Seui		Lawn (water) pennywort herb
Hylocereus undatus	Flos Hylocerei	Jian Hua, Ba Wang Hua	Gim Fa		Cereus flower
Hyoscyamus niger	Semen Hyoscyami	Tian Xian Zi	Tin Sin Ji		Black henbane seed
Hypericum ascyron	Herba Hyperici ascyronis	Hong Han Lian	Hung Hon Lin		St. John's wort
Hypericum chinense	Herba Hyperici Chinensis	Jin Si Tao			Chinese St. John's wort herb
Hypericum japonicum	Herba Hyperici japonici	Tian Ji Huang, Di Er Cao	Tin Jik Wong, Dei Yi Chou		Japanese St. John's wort herb
Hypericum sampsonii	Herba Hyperici sampsonii	Yuan Bao Cao	Yun Bou Chou		South China St. John's wort herb
Ilex asprella	Folium et radix Ilicis asprellae	Gang Mei (Gen), Wang Dian Jing	Gong Mui Gan, Maan Dim Gam		Rough holly leaf and root
Ilex chinensis	Folium Ilicis chinensis	Si Ji Qing, Dong Qing Ye	Sei Gwai Ching, Dung Ching Yip		Wintergreen holly leaf
Ilex cornuta	Folium Ilicis cornutae	Gou Gu Ye	Gau Gwat Yip		Cat thorn holly leaf
Ilex latifolia	Folium Ilicis latifoliae	Ku Ding Cha	Fu Ding Cha		Broadleaf holly leaf
Ilex pubescens	Radix Ilicis pubescentis	Mao Dong Qing	Mou Dung Ching	Motosei	Furry holly root
Ilex rotunda	Folium Ilicis rotundis	Jiu Bi Ying	Gau Bit Ying		Round-leaf holly leaf
Illicium verum	Fructus Illicii	Ba Jiao Hui Xiang	Baat Gok Wui Heung		Star anise fruit
Impatiens balsamina	Flos Impatiensis	Ji Xing Hua	Jek Chin Fa		Garden balsam flower
Impatiens balsamina	Semen Impatiensis	Ji Xing Zi	Jek Chin Ji	Kyuseishi	Garden balsam seed
Impatiens balsamina	Herba Impatientis	Tou Gu Cao	Tau Gwat Chou		Garden balsam herb
Imperata cylindrica var. *major*	Rhizoma Imperatae	Bai Mao Gen	Baak Maau Gan	Bokon	Woolly grass root
Imperata cylindrica var. *major*	Flos Imperatae	Bai Mao Hua	Baak Maau Fa		Woolly grass flower
Indigofera tinctoria	Folium Indigoferae	Mu Lan Ye	Muuk Laam Yip		Indigo leaf
Inula cappa	Herba Inulae cappae	Bai Niu Dan, Bai Mian Feng	Baak Ngau Daam		Goatear herb
Inula helenium	Radix Inula helenii	Tu Mu Xiang	Tou Muk Heung		Elecampane root

SCIENTIFIC	PHARMACEUTICAL	CANTONESE	MANDARIN	JAPANESE	ENGLISH
Inula japonica, I. brittanica, I. linariaefolia	Herba Inulae	Jin Fei Cao	Gam Fai Chou	Kinfutsuso	Elecampane herb
Inula japonica, I. brittanica, I. linariaefolia	Flos Inulae	Xuan Fu Hua	Syun Fuk Fa	Sembukuka	Elecampane flower
Inula racemosa	Radix Inulae racemosae	Tu Mu Xiang, Zong Zhuang Tu Mu Xiang	Tou Muk Heung, Chung Ching Tou Muk Heung		Racemose elecampane root
Iphigenia indica	Bulbus Iphigeniae	Shan Ci Gu	San Chi Gok		Iphigenia bulb
Ipomoea cairica	Herba Ipomoeae cairicae	Wu Zhao Long	Ng Jaau Lung		Cairo morning-glory herb
Iris pallasii var. *chinensis*	Semen Iris pallasii	Ma Lin Zi	Ma Leun Ji		North China iris seed
Iris tectorum	Rhizoma Iris tectoris	Yuan Wei	Yun Mei		Kite-tail iris root
Isatis indigotica	Folium Isatis indigoticae	Song Lan Ye	Song Laan Yip		Woad leaf
Isatis tinctoria	Folium Isatis tinctoriae	Da Qing Ye	Daai Ching Yip		Woad leaf
Isatis tinctoria and spp, *Baphicacanthus cusia, Indigofera suffruticosa, Polygonum tinctorium*	Indigo pulverata levis	Qing Dai	Ching Doi		Woad pigment
Isatis tinctoria, I. indigotica	Radix Isatis tinctoriae	Ban Lan Gen	Baan Laam Gan		Woad root
Isodon japonicus	Herba Isodonis	Ye Ming Cao	Yin Ming Chou	Enmeiso	Isodon herb
Ixeris denticulata	Herba Ixeris	Mu Dou Hui	Mou Tau Wui		Ixeris herb
Ixora chinensis	Radox Ixorae	Long Chuan Hua Gen	Lung Syun Fa Gan		Ixora root
Jasminum officinale var. *grandiflorum*	Flos Jasmini officinalis	Su Xin Hua	Sou Hing Fa		Jasmine flower
Jasminum sambac	Radix Jasmini sambacis	Mo Li Gen	Mut Lei Gan		Jasmine sambac root
Jasminum sambac	Flos Jasmini sambacis	Mo Li Hua	Mut Lei Fa		Jasmine sambac flower
Juglans regia	Semen Juglandis	Hu Tao Ren	Wu Tou Yan	Kotoniku	Walnut meat
Juglans regia	Folium Juglandis	Hu Tao Ye	Wu Tou Yip		Walnut leaf
Juglans regia	Ramulus Juglandis	Hu Tao Zhi	Wu Tou Ji		Walnut twig
Juncus effusus	Medulla Junci	Deng Xin Cao	Dang Sam Chou	Toshinso	Bulrush pith
Juncus effusus	Flos Junci	Deng Xin Hua	Ding Sam Fa		Bulrush flower
Jussiaea repens	Herba Jussiaeae	Kuo Tang She	Gwo Tong Se		Clove strip herb
Justicia procumbens	Herba Justiciae	Jue Chuang Cao, Shu Wei Huang	Jeuk Chong, Syu Mei Wong		Justicia herb
Kadsura longipedunculata	Radix Kadsurae longipedunculatae	Hong Mu Xiang	Hung Muk Heung		Long-stalk kadsura root
Kadsura coccinea	Caulis Kadsurae coccineae	Fan Tuan Teng	Faan Tyun Tang		Scarlet kadsura stem
Kadsura heteroclita	Caulis Kadsurae heteroclitae	Hai Feng Teng	Hoi Fung Tang		Heteroclite kadsura stem
Kadsura peltigera	Cortex Kadsurae peltigerae	Zi Jing Pi	Ji Ging Pei		Chinese redbud bark

SCIENTIFIC	PHARMACEUTICAL	CANTONESE	MANDARIN	JAPANESE	ENGLISH
Kaempferia galanga	Rhizoma Kaempferiae	Shan Nai, Sha Jiang	Saan Noi		Galanga root
Kalopanax septemlobus	Cortex Septemlobi	Chuan Tong Pi	Chyun Tung Pei		Kalopanax bark
Knoxia valerianoides	Radix Knoxiae	Hong Da Ji	Hung Daai Gik	Kogataigeki	Knoxia root
Kochia scoparia	Semen Kochiae	Di Fu Zi	Dei Fu Ji	Jibushi	Kochia seed
Kyllinga brevifolia	Herba Kyllingae	Shui Wu Gong	Seui Ng Gung		Kyllinga herb
Lagenaria siceraria	Fructus Lagenariae	Hu Lu Ke	Wu Lok Hok		Bottle gourd fruit
***Laminaria japonica* and spp**	Thallus Laminariae	Kun Bu	Gwan Bou	Kombu	Kelp seaweed
***Laminaria* spp**	Herba Laminariae	Hai Dai	Hoi Daai		Algae
Lantana camara	Herba Lantanae	Wu Se Mei	Ng Sik Mui		Wild sage herb
Lasiosphaera fenslii* and spp, *Calvatia lilacina, C. fenzlii, C. gigantea	Sclerotium Lasiosphaerae seu Calvatiae	Ma Bo	Ma But	Babotsu	Puffball mushroom
Ledebouriella divaricata, L. seseloides	Radix Ledebouriellae	Fang Feng	Fong Fung	Bofu	Wind-protector root
Lemna minor	Herba Lemnae	Fu Ping	Fau Ping		Duckweed herb
Lentinula edodes	Sclerotium Lentinulae	Xiang Gu	Heung Gu	Shiitake	Shiitake mushroom
***Leonorus heterophyllus* and spp**	Semen Leonori	Chong Wei Zi	Chong Wai Ji		Asian motherwort seed
***Leonorus heterophyllus, L. japonicus, L. sibiricus* and spp**	Herba Leonori	Yi Mu Cao, Chong Wei	Yik Mou Chou, Chong Wai	Yakumoso	Asian motherwort herb
Leontice robustum	Radix Leonticis	Hong Mao Qi	Hung Mou Chat		Leontice root
Lepidium apetalum, L. virginicum	Semen Lepidii	Ting Li Zi	Ting Lai Ji	Teirekishi	Wood whitlow grass seed
***Lepus* spp**	Excrementum Lepi	Wang Yue Sha	Mong Yut Sa		Rabbit dropping
Lespedeza cuneata	Herba Lespedezae	Ye Guan Men	Ye Gwaan Mun		Perennial lespedeza herb
Leucas mollissima	Herba Leuci	Bai Hua Zi Cao, Hu Yao Huang	Baak Fa Ji Chou, Fu Ngao Wong		Leucas herb
Ligusticum levisticum	Radix Ligustici levistici	Ou Dang Gui	Au Dong Gwai		Garden lovage root
Ligusticum sinense, L. jeholense	Radix Ligustici sinensis	Gao Ben	Gou Bun	Kohon	Chinese lovage root
Ligusticum walichii	Radix Ligustici walichii	Chuan Xiong, Xiong Qiong	Chyun Gung	Senkyu	Sichuan lovage root
Ligustrum japonicum, L. lucidum	Fructus Ligustri	Nu Zhen Zi	Neui Jing Ji	Joteishi	Glossy privet berry
Lilium brownii* var. *colchesteri	Flos Lilii	Bai He Hua	Baak Hap Fa		Brown's lily flower
Lilium brownii* var. *colchesteri	Radix Lilii	Bai He Gen	Baak Hap Gan		Brown's lily root

SCIENTIFIC	PHARMACEUTICAL	CANTONESE	MANDARIN	JAPANESE	ENGLISH
Lilium brownii var. *colchesteri*	Bulbus Lilii	Bai He	Baak Hap	Hyakugo	Brown's lily bulb
Lilium concolor	Bulbus Liliii concoloris	Shan Dan	Saan Daan		Japanese red star lily bulb
Lilium lancifolium	Bulbus Liliii lancifolii	Bai He, Juan Duan	Baak Hap, Gyun Daan		Lance-leaf lily bulb
Limax agrestic	Limax	Guo Yu	Gwat Kut		Slug
Limnophila sessiliflora	Herba Limnophilae	Shuang Liu Huang	Seung Lan Wong		Limnophila herb
Limonitum	Limonitum	Yu Liang Shi	Yu Leung Sek	Uyoryo	Clay ironstone
Lindera strychnifolia	Radix Linderae	Wu Yao, Tai Wu	Wu Yeuk, Toi Wu	Uyaku	Lindera root
Lindernia anagallis	Herba Linderniae	Ding Jing Cao	Ding Ging Chou		Lindernia herb
Linum usitatissimum	Semen Lini	Ya Ma Zi	A Ma Ji		Flax seed
Lippia nodiflora	Herba Lippiae	Peng Lai Cao, Ya She Huang	Fung Loi Chou, Ngaap Sit Wong		Frogfruit herb
Liquidambar orientalis	Resina Liquidambaris (Styrax liquidis)	Su He Xiang	Sou Hap Heung	Sogoko	Storax resin
Liquidambar taiwaniana	Resina Liquidambaris taiwaninanae	Bai Jiao Xiang	Baak Gaau Heung		Taiwan maple fruit resin
Liquidambar taiwaniana	Fructus Liquidambaris	Lu Lu Tong	Lou Lou Tung	Rorotsu	Taiwan maple fruit
Liriope platyphylla	Radix Liriopis platyphyllae	Mai Men Dong	Mak (Mun) Dung		Broad-leaf liriope root
Liriope spicata	Radix Liriopis spicatae	Mai (Men) Dong, Hu Bei Mai Men Dong	Mak (Mun) Dung, Wu Ba Mak Dung		Lance-leaf liriope root
Litchi chinensis	Semen Litchis	Li Zhi He	Lai Ji Ho		Lychee seed
Litchi chinensis	Pericarpium Litchis	Li Zhi Ke	Lai Ji Hok		Lychee rind
Lithargyrum	Lithagyrum	Mi Tuo Seng	Muk Toi Sang	Mitsudaso	Litharge
Lithospermum erythrorhizon	Radix Lithospermi	Zi Cao	Ji Chou	Shikon	Purple groomwell root
Lithospermum erythrorhizon	Flos Lithospermi	Zi Cao Rong	Ji Chou Yan		Purple groomwell flower
Litsea cubeba	Fructus Litseae	Bi Cheng Qie	Bat Ching Ke		Cubeb peppercorn
Litsea cubeba	Radix et caulis Litseae	Dou Chi Jiang	Dau Chek Geung	Toshikyo	Cubeb root and stem
Livistona chinensis	Semen Livistonae	Kui Shu Zi	Kwai Sat Ji		Fan palm seed
Lobelia chinensis	Herba et radix Lobeliae chinensis	Ban Bian Lian	Bau Bin Ling	Hanbanren	Rooting lobelia herb and root
Lonicera confusa	Flos Lonicerae confusae	Tu Yin Hua, Shan Yin Hua	Tou Ngan Fa		Wild honeysuckle flower
Lonicera japonica	Flos Lonicerae japonicae	Jin Yin Hua, Ren Dong Hua	Gam Ngan Fa Yan Dung Fa	Kinginka	Japanese honeysuckle flower
Lonicera japonica	Ramus et folium Lonicerae japonicae	Jin Yin Teng, Ren Dong Teng	Gam Ngan Tang, Yan Dung Tang		Japanese honeysuckle stem and leaf
Lopatherum gracile	Radix Lopatheri	Dan Zhu Gen	Daam Juk Gan		Bamboo grass root

SCIENTIFIC	PHARMACEUTICAL	CANTONESE	MANDARIN	JAPANESE	ENGLISH
Lopatherum gracile	Folium Lopatheri	Dan Zhu Ye	Daam Juk Yip	Tanchikuyo	Bamboo grass leaf
Loranthus parasiticus, L. yadorici and spp	Ramulus Loranthi	Sang Ji Sheng	Song Gei Sang	Sokisei	Asian mistletoe twig
Loropetalum chinense	Flos Loropetali	Ji Hua	Gai Fa		Strap flower
Loropetalum chinense	Cortex Loropetali	Ji Mu	Gai Muk		Strap flower bark
Ludwigia prostata	Herba Ludwigiae	Shui Ding Xiang	Seui Ding Heung		Water clove herb
Luffa cylindrica, L. acutangula	Pericarpium Luffae	Si Gua Pi	Si Gwa Pei		Luffa skin
Luffa cylindrica, L. acutangula	Fasciculus vascularis Luffae	Si Gua Luo	Si Gwa Lou	Shikaraku	Spongegourd
Lunathyrum vegetius, L. giraldii	Rhizoma Lunathyri	Guan Zhong	Gwun Jung		Lunathyrum fern root
Lutra lutra	Jecur Lutrae	Ta Gan	Taap Gon		Otter liver
Lycium chinense	Cortex radicis Lycii	Di Gu Pi	Dei Gwat Pei	Jikoppi	Wolfberry root bark
Lycium chinense, L. barbarum	Fructus Lycii	Gou Qi Zi	Gau Gei Ji, Gei Ji	Kukoshi	Wolfberry
Lycium chinense, L. barbarum	Folium Lycii chinensis	Gou Qi Ye	Gau Ji Yip		Wolfberry leaf
Lycopodium clavatum	Herba Lycopodi	Shen Jin Cao	Sam Gam Chou		Clubmoss herb
Lycopodium serratum and spp	Pollen Lycopodii	Qian Cang Ta, Pu Di Wu Gong, Guo Jiang Long, Yu Bai	Jin Jang Tap		Lycopodium pollen
Lycopodium serratum and *varieties*	Herba Lycopodii serrati	Jin Bu Huan	Gam Bat Wun		Serrated clubmoss
Lycopus lucidus	Rhizoma Lycopi lucidi	Di Sun	Dei Seun		Bright bugleweed root
Lycopus lucidus	Herba Lycopi	Ze Lan	Jaak Laan	Takuran	Bright bugleweed herb
Lycoris radiata	Rhizoma Lycoris	Shi Suan	Sek Syun		Red spiderlily corm
Lygodium japonicum	Spora Lygodii	Hai Jin Sha	Hoi Gam Sa	Kaikinsha	Japanese climbing fern spore
Lygodium japonicum	Herba Lygodii	Hai Jin Sha Teng	Hoi Gam Sa Tang	Kaikinshato	Japanese climbing fern herb
Lyonia ovafolia, L. neziki	Herba Lyoniae	Nan Zhu	Naam Juk		Lyonia herb
Lysimachia candida	Herba Lysimachiae candidae	Dan Tian Cao	Daan Tiu Chou		White lysimachia herb
Lysimachia capillipes	Rhizoma seu herba Lysimachiae capillipis	Man Shan Xiang	Mun Sam Heung		Lysimachia root or herb
Lysimachia christinae, L. hemsleyana	Herba Lysimachiae	Jin Qian Cao, Guo Lu Huang	Gam Chin Chou, Gwo Lou Wong	Kinsenso	Asian moneywort herb
Lysimachia congestiflora	Herba Lysimachiae congestiflorae	Xiao Guo Lu Huang	Siu Gwo Lou Wong		Full-flowered lysimachia

SCIENTIFIC	PHARMACEUTICAL	CANTONESE	MANDARIN	JAPANESE	ENGLISH
Lysimachia sikokiana	Herba Lysimachiae sikokianae	Ling Ling Xiang	Ling Ling Heung		Lysimachia herb
Lysionotus pauciflora	Herba Lysinoti	Shi Diao Lan	Sek Diu Laan		Lysionotus herb
Lythrum salicaria	Herba Lythri salicariae	Qian Cu Cai	Jin Wat Choi		Loosestrife herb
Macaca mulatta	Calculus Macacae	Hou Zao	Hau Jou	Koso	Macaque bezoar
Macaca mulatta	Gelatinum Macacae	Hou Jiao	Hao Gaau		Macaque gel
Macleaya cordata	Herba Macleayae	Bo Luo Hui	Bok Lok Wui		Plum poppy herb
Macrotomia euchroma	Radix Macrotomiae	Zi Cao	Ji Chou	Shikon	Macrotomia root
Mactra sulcataria	Concha Mactrae	Ge	Hok	Jiseki	Mactra shell
Magnetitum	Magnetitum	Ci Shi	Chi Sek		Magnetite
Magnolia liliflora, M. denudata, M. yulan and spp	Gemma Magnoliae	Xin Yi Hua	San Yi Fa	Shinika	Yulan magnolia bud
Magnolia officinalis, M. biloba, M. obovata	Cortex Magnoliae officinalis	Hou Po Chuan Po	Hau Pok, Chyun Pok	Koboku	Magnolia bark
Magnolia officinalis, M. biloba, M. obovata	Flos Magnoliae officinalis	Hou Po Hua	Hau Pok Fa	Koboka, Kobokuka	Magnolia flower
Mahonia bealei	Folium Mahoniae bealei	Shi Da Gong Lao Ye, Kuo Ye Shi Da Gong Lao Ye	Sap Daai Gung Lou Yip, Fut Yip Sap Daai Gung Lou Yip	Judaikoro	Leather-leaf mahonia leaf
Mahonia fortunei	Folium Mahoniae fortunei	Shi Da Gong Lao Ye, Xi Ye Shi Da Gong Lao Ye	Gung Lou Yip, Sai Yip Sap Daai Gung Lou Yip	Judaikoro	Mahonia leaf
Mahonia japonica	Radix Mahoniae japonicae	Shi Da Gong Lao Gen	Sap Daai Gung Lou Gan		Japanese mahonia root
Malachitum	Malachitum	Tong Lu	Tung Luk		Copper rust
Malva verticillata	Semen Malvae	Dong Kui Zi	Dung Kwai Ji		Musk mallow seed
Manganitum	Manganitum	Wu Ming Yi	Mon Ming Yi		Manganite
Mangifera indica	Semen Mangiferae	Mang Guo Zi	Man Gou Wat		Mango seed
Manis pentadactyla	Squama manis	Chuan Shan Jia	Chyun San Gaap	Senzanko	Pangolin scale
Marsdenia tenacissima	Herba Marsdeniae	Wu Gu Teng	Wu Gwat Tang		Marsdenia herb
Marsilea quaddrifolia	Folium Marsileae	Ping	Ping		European water clover leaf
Matteucia struthiopteris	Rhizoma Matteuciae	Guan Zhong, Jia Guo Jue Guan Zhong	Gwun Jung, Ying Gwo Kyut Gwun Jung		Ostrich-feather fern root
Melaleuca leucadendron	Folium Melaleucae leucadendronis	Bai Qian Ceng	Baak Chin Chang		Cajeput leaf
Melanteritum	Melanteritum	Zao Fan, Lu Fan	Jou Faan		Green vitriol
Melastoma candidum	Herba Melastomae candidae	Ye Mu Dan	Ye Maau Daan		Melastoma herb
Melia azedarach, M. toosendan	Cortex radicis Meliae	Ku Lian (Gen) Pi	Fu Lin (Gan) Pei	Kurenkombi	Bead tree root bark
Melia toosendan	Fructus Meliae toosendanis	Chuan Lian Zi	Chyun Lin Ji		Sichuan bead tree berry
Melodinus suaveolens	Fructus Melodini	Shan Chen, Qu Tou Ji	Saan Chaang		Melodinus fruit

SCIENTIFIC	PHARMACEUTICAL	CANTONESE	MANDARIN	JAPANESE	ENGLISH
Melothria heterophylla	Radix Melothriae heterolphyllae	Tu Bai Lian	Taou Baak Lin		Native peppervine root
Melothria mederospatana	Radix Melothriae mederospatanae	Diao Jin Zhong	Diu Gam Jung		Melothria root
Menispermum dauricum	Radix Menispermi	Bei Dou Gen	Pan Dau Gan		Siberian moonseed root
Mentha arvensis	Herba Menthae arvensis	Bo He	Bok Ho	Hakka	Asian fieldmint herb
Mentha spicata	Herba Menthae spicatae	Xiang Hua Cai, Liu Lan Xiang	Heung Fa Choi, Lou Laan Heung		Spearmint herb
Menyanthes trifoliata	Folium Menyanthis	Shui Cai Ye	Seui Choi Yip	Suisayo, Meisai	Bogbean leaf
Meretrix meretrix	Concha Metretris	Wen Ge	Man Gap		Asian venus clam shell
Mesona chinensis	Herba Mesonae	Xian Cao, Liang Fen Cao	Heun Chou, Leung Fan Chou		Jellywort herb
Metaplexis japonica	Herba Metaplexis	Guo Lu Huang, Luo Mo	Lo Mo		Metaplexis herb
Metaplexis japonica	Fructus Metaplexis	Tian Qiang Ke	Tin Cheung Hok		Metaplexis fruit
Mica, Chloritum	Mica, Chloritum	Meng Shi, Jin Meng Shi	Mung Sek, Ching Mung Sek		Mica, Chlorite schist
Michelia alba	Flos Micheliae	Bai Lan Hua	Baak Laan Fa		White champac flower
Microcos paniculata	Folium Microcotis	Bu Zha Ye	Bou Jai Yip		Microcos leaf
Microsorium hancockii, M. dilatatum	Herba Microsorii	Lu Ji Wei	Luk Gai Mei		Microsorium herb
Millettia dielsiana, M. reticulata, M. nitida	Radix et caulis Millettiae dielsianae	Ji Xue Teng	Gai Yut Tang	Keiketto	Millettia root and stem
Millettia philipinensis	Radix Millettiae philipinensis	Niu Da Li	Ngao Daai Lik		Millettia root
Millettia reticulata	Radix et caulis Millettiae reticulatae	Ji Xue Teng, Kun Ming Ji Xue Teng	Kwan Ming Gai Yut Tang		Millettia root and stem
Mimosa pudica	Herba mimosae pudicae	Han Xiu Cao	Ham Sau Chou		Mimosa herb
Minium	Minium	Qian Dan, Huang Dan	Chin Daan, Wong Daan	Entan	Red lead oxide
Mirabilitum	Mirabilitum	Mang Xiao	Mong Seu	Bosho	Mirabilite
Mirabilitum	Mirabilitum purum	Xuan Ming Fan	San Ming Fun	Bosho	Glauber's salt, Pure mirabilite
Miscanthus sinensis	Herba Miscanthi	Mang Jing	Mong Hong		Miscanthus herb
Mogera robusta and spp, *Scaptochirus moschatus*	Mogera carbonisatus	Yan Shu Shuang	Yim Syu Seung	Ensosu	Carbonized mogera
Moghania macrophylla, M. philippinensis	Radix Moghaniae	Yi Tiao Gen	Yat Tiu Gan		Moghania root

SCIENTIFIC	PHARMACEUTICAL	CANTONESE	MANDARIN	JAPANESE	ENGLISH
Momordica cochinchinensis	Semen Momordicae cochinchinensis	Mu Bie Zi	Muk Bit Ji	Mokubesshi	Cochin bitter melon seed
Momordica charantia	Fructus Momordicae charantiae	Ku Gua (Gan)	Fu Gwa (Gam)		Bitter melon fruit
Momordica grosvenori	Fructus Momordicae grosvenorii	Luo Han Guo	Lou Haan Kwo	Rakanka	Arhat fruit
Momordica grosvenori	Folium Momordicae grosvenorii	Luo Han Ye	Lou Haan Yip	Rakankayo	Arhat leaf
Morinda officinalis	Radix Morindae	Ba Ji Tian	Ba Gik Tin	Hagekiten	Morinda root
Morus alba	Cortex radicis Mori	Sang Bai Pi	Song Baak Pei	Sohakuhi	Mulberry root bark
Morus alba	Fructus Mori	Sang Shen (Zi)	Song Sam (Ji)	Sojin	Mulberry fruit
Morus alba	Folium Mori	Sang Ye	Song Yip	Soyo	Mulberry leaf
Morus alba	Ramulus Mori	Sang Zhi	Song Ji	Soshi	Mulberry twig
Moschus berezovskii and spp	Secretio Moschi	She Xiang	Se Heung	Jako	Musk
Mucuna birdwoodiana, M. sempervirens	Radix et caulis Mucunae	Ji Xue Teng, Chang Chun You Ma Teng	Gei Hat Tang, Seung Cheun Yao Ma Tang		Mucuna root and stem
Murraya paniculata	Ramulus et folium Murrayae	Jiu Li Xiang	Gau Lei Heung		Burma boxwood twig and leaf
Musa basjoo	Caudex Musae	Ba Jiao Gen	Ba Jiu Gan		Ryukyu banana root
Muscovitum	Muscovitum	Yun Mu Shi	Wan Mou Sek		Muscovite
Mussaenda pubescens, M. parviflora	Caulis et folium Mussaendae	Shan Gan Cao	Saan Gam Chou		Mountain licorice stem and leaf
Mylabris	Mylabris	Ban Mao	Ban Mou	Hanmyo	Asian cantharides
Mylitta lapidescens	Sclerotium Mylittae	Lei Wan	Leui Yun		Thunder ball fungus
Myrica rubra	Cortex Myricae rubrae	Yang Mei Pi	Yeung Miu Pei		Red bayberry bark
Myristica fragrans	Semen Myristicae	Rou Dou Kou	Yuk Dau Kau	Nikuzuku	Nutmeg seed
Mytilus crassitesta and spp	Mytilus	Dan Cai	Daam Choi		Mussel
Naemorrhedis	Cornu Naemorrhedis	Shan Yang Jiao	San Yeung Gok	Sanyokaku	Goat horn
Naja naja atra, Bungarus fasciatus, Elaphe radiata	Fel Najae seu Bungari seu Elaphis	She Dan	Se Daam		Viper gallbladder
Nandina domestica	Radix et caulis Nandinae	(Nan) Tian Zhu Gen	(Naam) Tin Juk Gan		Sacred bamboo root and stem
Nandina domestica	Folium Nandinae	(Nan) Tian Zhu Ye	(Naam) Tin Juk Yip		Sacred bamboo leaf
Nandina domestica	Fructus Nandinae	(Nan) Tian Zhu Zi	(Naam) Tin Juk Ji		Sacred bamboo fruit
Narcissus tazetta var. *chinensis*	Fructus Narcissi	Shui Xian Zi	Seui Sin Ji		Chinese sacred lily seed
Narcissus tazetta var. *chinensis*	Bulbus Narcissi	Shui Xian Gen	Seui Sin Gan		Chinese sacred lily bulb

SCIENTIFIC	PHARMACEUTICAL	CANTONESE	MANDARIN	JAPANESE	ENGLISH
Nardostachys jatamansi, N. chinensis	Radix Nardostachis	Gan Song	Gam Chung		Indian spikenard root
Nelumbo nucifera	Flos Nelumbinis	Bai Lian Hua	Baak Lin Fa		Lotus flower
Nelumbo nucifera	Folium Nelumbinis	He Ye, Lian Lie	Ho Yip	Kayo	Lotus leaf
Nelumbo nucifera	Receptaculum Nelumbinis	Lian Fang	Lin Fong	Renshin	Lotus receptacle
Nelumbo nucifera	Ramulus Nelumbinis	Lian Geng	Lin Gang		Lotus stem
Nelumbo nucifera	Plumula Nelumbinis	Lian Xin	Lin Sam		Lotus plumule
Nelumbo nucifera	Stamen Nelumbinis	Lian Xu	Lin Sou	Renshu	Lotus stamen
Nelumbo nucifera	Semen Nelumbinis	Lian Zi	Lin Ji	Renshi	Lotus seed
Nelumbo nucifera	Epicentrum seminis Nelumbinis	Lian Zi Xin	Lin Ji Sam		Lotus seed heart
Nelumbo nucifera	Rhizoma nodi Nelumbinis	Ou Jie	Ngau Jit		Lotus root node
Nepenthes mirabilis	Herba Nepenthis	Zhu Long Cao	Jyu Lung Chou		Pitcher plant herb
Nephelium lappaceum	Fructus Nephelii	Shao Zi	Siu Ji		Rambutan fruit
Nerium indicum	Folium Nerii	Jiao Zhu Tao Ye	Gap Juk Tou Yip		Indian oleander leaf
Nervilia fordii	Herba Nerviliae	Qing Tian Kui	Ching Tin Kwai		Nervilia herb
Niter	Niter	Xiao Shi	Siu Sek	Shoseki	Potassium nitrate
Notopterygium incisum, N. forbesii, N. francherii	Rhizoma et radix Notopterigii	Qiang Huo	Geung Wut	Kyokatsu	Notoptery-gium root
Nuphar japonicum, N. pumilum	Rhizoma Nupharis	Ping Peng Cao Gan	Ping Fung Chou Gan	Senkotu	Yellow pond lily root
Ocimum Basilicum	Fructus Ocimi	Guang Ming Zi	Gwong Ming Ji		Basil seed
Ocimum basilicum	Herba Ocimi	Jiu Ceng Ta, Luo Le	Lo Lak		Basil herb
Oenanthe javanica	Herba Oenanthis	Shui Qin	Seui Kan		Water dropwort
Oldenlandia diffusa	Herba Oldenlandiae	Bai Hua She She Cao	Baak Fa Se Sit Chou	Byakkaja-zesso	Snaketongue grass herb
Onosma paniculatum	Radix Onosmae	Zi Cao	Ji Chou		Onosma root
Ophicalcitum	Ophicalcitum	Hua Rui Shi	Fa Yeui Sek	Kazuiseki	Dolomite
Ophioglossum vulgatum	Herba Ophioglossi	Ping Er Xiao Cao	Ping Yi Siu Chou		Adder's tongue herb
Ophiopogon japonicus	Radix Ophiopogonis	Mai (Men) Dong	Mak (Mun) Dung	Bakumondo	Dwarf lilyturf root
Opuntia dillenii and spp	Rhizoma Opuntiae	Xian Ren Zhang	Sin Yan Jeung		Prickly pear root
Origanum vulgare	Herba Origani vulgaris	Tu Yin Chen, Tu Xiang Ru	Tou Gam Chan, Tou Heung Yu		Oregano herb
Orobanche caerulescens and spp	Herba Orobanchis	Lie Dang	Lit Dong		Orobanche herb
Orostachys fimbriatus	Herba Orostachis fimbriati	Wa Song	Nga Chung		Fimbriate orostachys herb

SCIENTIFIC	PHARMACEUTICAL	CANTONESE	MANDARIN	JAPANESE	ENGLISH
Orostachys japonica, O. fimbriatus	Herba Orostachis	Wa Song	Nga Chung		Hens-and-chickens herb
Oroxylum indicum	Semen Oroxyli	Mu Hu Die	Muk Wu Dip	Mokukocho	Oroxylum seed
Orpimentum	Orpimentum	Ci Huang, Xiong Huang	Chi Wong		Orpiment
Orthosiphon aristatus, O. grandiflorus	Herba Orthosiphonis	Mao Xu Kao, Hua Shi Cao	Maau Sou Chou, Fa Sek Chou		Orthosiphon herb
Oryza sativa	Saccharum Oryzae			Koi	Rice malt (syrup)
Oryza sativa	Fructus Oryzae	Nuo Mi	Lo Mai		Sweet rice
Oryza sativa	Fructus Oryzae germinatus	Gu Ya	Gu Nga	Kokuga	Sprouted rice grain
Oryza sativa	Fructus Oryzae	Jing Mi	Gang Mai		Rice grain
Oryza sativa	Radix Oryzae	Nuo Dao Gen (Xu)	No Du Gan	Jubeikon	Sweet rice root
Oryza sativa and *Monascus purpureus*	Fructus Oryzae fermentatus cum Monasco	Hong Qu Mi	Hung Ju Mai		Fermented rice with red yeast
Osbeckia chinensis	Herba Osbeckiae	Tian Xiang Lu, Jin Shi Lu	Tin Heung Lou		Chinese osbeckia herb
Osmanthus fragrans	Cortex ramuli Osmanthi	Gui Hua Pi	Gwai Fa Pei		Osmanthus twig bark
Osmunda japonica	Rhizoma Osmundae	Guan Zhong, Zi Qi Guan Zhong	Gwun Jung, Ji Kei Gwun Jung	Tohoku-kanju	Japanese flowering fern root
Ostrea gigas	Concha Ostreae calcinati	Duan Mu Li	Taan Mou Lai		Calcined oyster shell
Ostrea gigas and spp	Concha Ostreae	Mu Li	Mou Lai	Borei	Oyster shell
Oxalis corniculata	Herba Oxalis	Cu Jiang Cao	Chou Jeung Chou		Indian sorrel herb
Paederia scandens	Radix et caulis Paederiae	Ji Shi Teng	Gai Niu Tang	Hakumokeis hito	Chicken dung vine root and stem
Paeonia lactiflora	Radix Paeoniae lactiflorae	Bai Shao (Yao)	Baak Cheuk (Yeuk)	Byakushaku (yaku)	White peony root
Paeonia lactiflora, P. obovata, P. veitchii	Radix Paeoniae rubrae	Chi Shao (Yao)	Chek Cheuk (Yeuk)	Sekishaku-(yaku)	Red peony root
Paeonia sinjiangensis	Radix Paeoniae sinjiangensis	Xin Jiang Bai Shao (Yao)	San Geung Chek Cheuk		Xinjiang peony root
Paeonia suffruticosa	Cortex radicis Paeoniae suffruticosae	Mu Dan Pi, Dan Pi	Maau Daan Pei, Daan Pei	Botanpi	Tree peony root bark
Panax ginseng	Radix Panacis ginsengis praeparatae	Bai Shen	Baak Sam	Hakujin	Rock candy cured Asian ginseng root
Panax ginseng	Radix Panacis ginsengis praeparatae	Hong Ren Shen	Hung Yan Sam	Koninjin	Red cured Asian ginseng root
Panax ginseng	Radix Panacis ginsengis	Ren Shen	Yan Sam	Ninjin	Asian ginseng root
Panax ginseng	Rhizoma Panacis ginsengis	Ren Shen Lu	Yan Sam Lu	Ninjinro	Asian ginseng neck
Panax ginseng	Folium Panacis ginsengis	Ren Shen Ye	Yan Sam Yip	Ninjinyo	Asian ginseng leaf

SCIENTIFIC	PHARMACEUTICAL	CANTONESE	MANDARIN	JAPANESE	ENGLISH
Panax ginseng	Extremas radicis Panacis ginsengis praeparatae	(Ren) Shen Xu	(Yan) Sam Son		Rock candy cured Asian ginseng root tail
Panax ginseng	Radix Panacis ginsengis	Sheng Shai Shen	Sang Sai Sam		Dried Asian ginseng root
Panax ginseng	Radix Panacis ginsengis	Ye Shan Shen	Gam San Sam		Wild Asian ginseng
Panax ginseng	Flos Panacis ginsengis	Ren Shen Hua	Yan Sam Fa		Asian ginseng flower
Panax japonicus	Radix Panacis japonici	Zhu Jie (Ren) Shen	Juk Jit (Yan) Sam	Tikusetu-ninjin	Japanese ginseng root
Panax major, P. repens	Radix Panacis majoris	Zhu Er Shen	Ju Yi Sam		Pearl ginseng root
Panax notoginseng	Radix Panacis notoginsengis	San Qi Tian Qi	Saam Chat Tin Chat	Sanshishi	Pseudogin-seng root
Panax notoginseng	Flos Panacis notoginsengis	San Qi Hua	Saam Chat Fa	Sanshishika	Pseudogins-eng flower
Panax quinquefolius	Radix Panacis quinquefolii	Xi Yang Shen	Fa Kei Sam, Sei Yang Sam	Seiyojin	American ginseng root
Panthera	Os Leopardis	Bao Gu			Leopard bone
Panthera	Os tigris	Hu Gu	Fu Gwat	Kokotsu	Tiger bone
Papaver somniferum	Pericarpium Papaveris	Ying Su Ke	Ngang Suk Hok	Ozokukoku	Opium poppy husk
Paratenodera sinensis and *augustipennis, Hierodula patellifera, Mantis religiosa, Statilia maculata*	Paratenodera seu Hierodula seu Mantis seu Statilia	Sang Piao Xiao	Song Piu Seu		Praying mantis egg case
Paris chinensis	Rhizoma Paris chinensis	Zhong Lou, Qi Ye Yi Zhi Hua	Jung Lau, Chat Yip Yat Ji Pa		Chinese paris root
Paris polyphylla, P. chinensis, P. formosana and var.	Rhizoma Paris	Qi Ye Yi Zhi Hua, Zao Xiu	Chak Yip Jek Ji Fa, Sat Yau	Kenjin	Paris root
Paris yunnanensis	Rhizoma Paris yunnanensis	Zhong Lou, Yun Nan Zhong Lou	Jung Lau, Wan Laam Jung Lau		Yunnan paris root
Parmelia tinctorum, P. reticulata	Thallus Parmeliae	Shi Er			Parmelia thallus
Parthenocissus tricuspidata	Caulis Parthenocissi	Pa Shan Hu, Di Jin	Pa San Fu, Dei Gam		Japanese creeper stem
Passiflora coeruleae	Herba Passiflorae coeruleae	Xi Fan Lian	Sai Faan Lin		Cerulean passionflower herb
Patrinia scabiosaefolia, P. villosa	Herba et rhizoma Patriniae	Bai Jiang Cao	Baai Jeung Chou	Haishoso	Patrinia herb and root
Paulownia tomentosa	Flos Paulowniae	Pao Tong Hua	Pau Tung Fa		Paulownia flower
Pavetta hongkongiensis	Herba Pavettae	Man Tian Xing	Mun Tin Sing, Daai Sa Yip		Pavetta herb
Pelargonium graveolens	Herba Pelargonii	Xiang Ye	Heung Yip		Rose geranium herb
Perilla frutescens	Ramulus Perillae	Zi Su Geng	Sou Gan		Perilla stem
Perilla frutescens	Folium Perillae	Zi Su Ye	Sou Yip	Shisoyo	Perilla leaf
Perilla frutescens	Fructus Perillae	Zi Su Zi	Sou Ji	Soshi	Perilla seed
Periploca sepium	Cortex radicis Periplocae	Gang Liu Pi, Xiang Liu Pi	Gong Lau Pei, Heung Lau Pei		Silk vine root bark

SCIENTIFIC	PHARMACEUTICAL	CANTONESE	MANDARIN	JAPANESE	ENGLISH
Petasites japonicus	Flos Petasitis	Feng Dou Cai	Fung Dau Choi		Japanese butterbur flower
Peucedanum japonicum	Radix Peucedani japonici	Fang Gui	Fong Kwai		Japanese masterwort root
Peucedanum praeruptorum, P. decursivum	Radix Peucedani	Qian Hu	Chin Wu	Zenko	Asian masterwort root
Pharbitis nil, P. purpurea and spp	Semen Pharbitis	Qian Niu Zi	Hin Ngau Ji		Japanese morning glory seed
Phaseolus calcaratus, P. angularis	Semen Phaseoli calcarati	Chi Xiao Dou	Chek Siu Dau	Sekishozu	Aduki bean
Phaseolus mungo	Flos Phaseoli	Lu Dou Hua	Luk Dau Fa		Mung bean flower
Phaseolus radiatum	Semen Phaseoli radiati	Lu Dou	Luk Dau	Ryokuzu	Mung bean
Phaseolus radiatum	Testa Phaseoli radiatae	Lu Dou Yi	Luk Dau Yip		Mung bean husk
Phellodendron amurense, P. chinense	Cortex Phellodendris	Huang Bai Chuan Bai	Wong Paak Chyun Paak	Obaku	Siberian cork tree bark
Pheretima aspergillum, Allolobophora caliginosa	Pheretima seu Allolobophora	Di Long	Dei Lung	Jiryu	Earthworm
Phlogopitum	Phlogopitum	Jin Meng Shi	Gam Mung Sek		Phlogopite, Red mica
Pholidota chinensis	Radix Pholidotae	Shi Xian Tao Gen	Sek Sin Tou Gan		Rattlesnake orchid root
Photinia serrulata	Caulis et folium Photiniae	Shi Nan Teng, Shi Nan Ye	Sek Naam Tang, Sek Naam Yip		Photinia stem or leaf
Phragmites communis	Radix Phragmitis	Lu Gen	Lou Gan	Rokon	Water-reed root
Phragmites communis	Ramulus Phragmitis	Wei Jing	Lou Ging		Water-reed twig
Phyllostachys nigra var. *henonis* and spp	Concretio silicea bambusae	Tian Zhu Huang	Tin Juk Wong		Tabasheer
Phyllostachys nigra var. *henonis* and spp	Succus Phyllostachis	Zhu Li	Juk Lai	Chikureki	Black bamboo sap
Phyllostachys nigra var. *henonis* and spp	Caulis Phyllostachis in taeniis	Zhu Ru	Juk Yu	Chikujo	Black bamboo shaving
Phyllostachys nigra var. *henonis* and spp	Folium Phyllostachis	Zhu Ye	Juk Yip		Black bamboo leaf
Phyllostachys nigra var. *henonis* and spp	Radix Phyllostachis	Zi Zhu Gen	Ji Juk Gan		Black bamboo root
*Physalis alkakengi (*var. *franchetii)*	Rhizoma Physalis	Suan Jiang Gen	Syun Jeung Gan		Chinese lantern root
Physalis alkekengi (var. *franchetii)*	Calyx seu fructus Physalis	Suan Jiang, Jing Deng Long	Syun Jeung, Ching Dang Lung		Chinese lantern calyx or fruit
Physalis peruviana	Herba Physalis peruvianae	Deng Long Cao	Dang Lung Chou		Peru lantern herb

SCIENTIFIC	PHARMACEUTICAL	CANTONESE	MANDARIN	JAPANESE	ENGLISH
Phytolacca acinosa, P. esculenta	Radix Phytolaccae acinosae	Shang Lu	Seung Luk	Shoriku	Asian poke root
Picrasma quassioides	Cortex Picrassiae	Ku Shu Pi	Fu Syu Pei		Quassiawood bark
Picrasma quassioides	Ramulus et folium Picrasmae	Ku (Shu) Mu	Fu (Syu) Muk		Quassiawood twig and leaf
Picrorrhiza kurroa	Radix Picrorrhizae	Hu Huang Lian	Wu Wong Lin	Kooren	Picrorrhiza root
Pinellia pedatisecta	Rhizoma Pinelliae pedatisectae	Zhang Ye Ban Xia, Wu Zhang Nan Xing	Jeung Yip Bun Ha, Fu Jeung Lam Sing		Pedatisect pinellia corm
Pinellia ternata	Rhizoma Pinelliae fermentatae	Ban Xia Qu	Bun Ha Chau		Fermented Pinellia corm
Pinellia ternata	Rhizoma Pinelliae ternatae preparatae	Ban Xia Fa Ban Xia	Bun Ha, Faat Bun Ha	Hange, Kohange	Prepared pinellia corm
Pinellia ternata	Rhizoma pinelliae ternatae	Sheng Ban Xia	Sang Bun Ha, So Bun Ha	Shohange	Raw pinellia corm
Pinus massoniana, P. tabulaeformis and spp	Pollen Pini	Song Hua Fen	Chung Fa Fan		Pine pollen
Pinus massoniana, P. tabulaeformis and spp, *Larix* spp	Resina Pini prparatae, Colophonium	Song Xiang	Chung Heung		Pine resin
Pinus succinifera	Resina Pini succiniferae (Succinum)	Hu Po	Fu Po		Amber resin
Pinus tabulaeformis and spp	Semen Pini	Song Zi	Chung Ji		Pine kernel
Pinus tabulaeformis, P. massoniana, P. yunnannensis	Lignum Pini nodi	Song Jie, You Song Jie	Chung Jit, Yao Chung Jit	Shosetsu	Knotty pine wood shaving
Piper betle	Folium Piperis betlis	Ju Jiang Ye, Qing Lou Ye	Geui Jeung Yip		Betel pepper leaf
Piper hancei	Caulis Piperis hanceis	Hai Feng Teng	Hoi Fung Tang		Kadsura pepper stem
Piper hancei var. *squamiglandiferu m*	Caulis Piperis squamiglandiferi	Hai Feng Teng, Xian Lin Ju	Hoi Fung Tang		Fujian kadsura pepper stem
Piper longum	Fructus Piperis longis	Bi Ba	Bat Pa	Hihatsu	Long pepper fruit spike
Piper nigrum	Radix Piperis nigri	Hu Jiao Gen	Wu Jiu Gan		Black pepper root
Piper nigrum	Fructus Piperis nigri	Hu Jiao, Hei Hu Jiao	Wu Jiu, Mai Wu Jiu	Kosho	Black pepper corn
Piper wallichii	Ramulus Piperis wallichii	Shi Nan Teng	Sek Naam Tang		Wild pepper twig
Pistacia chinensis	Folium Pistaciae	Huang Lian Ya	Wong Lin Nga		Pistachio leaf
Pittosporum pentandrum	Radix Pittospori	Qi Li Xiang	Chat Lei Heung		Pittosporum root
Plantago asiatica, P. depressa and spp	Semen Plantaginis	Che Qian Zi	Che Chin Ji	Shazenshi	Asian plantain seed
Plantago asiatica, P. depressa and spp	Folium Plantaginis	Che Qian Cao	Che Chin Chou	Shazenso	Asian plantain leaf
Platycodon grandiflorum	Radix Platycodonis	Jie Geng, Ku Jie Geng	Gat Gan	Kikyo	Balloonflower root

SCIENTIFIC	PHARMACEUTICAL	CANTONESE	MANDARIN	JAPANESE	ENGLISH
Pleioblastus amarus	Folium Pleioblasti	Ku Zhu Ye	Fu Juk Yip		Bitter bamboo leaf
Pleione bulbocodioides	Rhizoma Pleionis	Shan Ci Gu	Saan Chi Gu		Pleione corm
Plumbago zeylanicum	Herba Plumbaginis	Hei Mian Ma, Bai Hua Dan	Baak Fa Daan		Ceylon leadwort
Plumeria rubra var. *acutifolia*	Flos Plumeriae	Ji Dan Hua	Gai Daan Fa		Frangipani flower
Podophyllum emodi	Rhizoma Podophylli emodii	Tao Er Qi	Tou Yi Chat		Emodi's podophullum root
Podophyllum pleianthum	Rhizoma Podophylli pleianthi	Ba Jiao Lian	Ba Gok Lin		Pleianth podophyllum root
Pogonatherum crinitum	Herba Pogonatheri	Bi Zi Cao	Bat Jai Chou		Golden Hair grass
Pogostemon cablin	Herba Pogostemis	Guang Huo Xiang	Gwong Fok Heung		Patchouli herb
Polistes mandarinus, Parapolybia varia	Nidus Polistis seu Parapolybiae	Lu Feng Fang	Lou Fun Fong		Hornet nest
Pollen	Granum floris pollinis	Feng Hua Fen	Fung Fa Fan		Flower (bee) pollen
Polygala japonica	Herba Polygalae japonicae	Gua Zi Jin	Gwa Ji Gam		Japanese milkwort herb
Polygala sibirica	Radix Polygalae sibiricae	Tian Yuan Zhi	Tin Yun Ji		Siberian milkwort root
Polygala tenuifolia	Radix Polygalae	Yuan Zhi	Yun Ji	Onji	Thin-leaf milkwort root
Polygonatum odoratum var. *pluriflorum, P. plurifolium*	Rhizoma Polygonati odorati	Yu Zhu	Yuk Juk	Gyokuchiku	Fragrant Solomon's seal root
Polygonatum sibiricum, P. cyrtonema, P. kingianum	Rhizoma Polygonati	Huang Jing	Wong Jing	Osei	Siberian Solomon's-seal root
Polygonum aviculare	Herba Polygoni avicularis	Bian Xu	Bin Chuk	Henchiku	Knotgrass herb
Polygonum bistorta	Radix Polygoni bistortae	Quan Shen	Kyun Sam		Bistort root
Polygonum chinense	Herba Polygoni chinensis	Huo Tan Mu (Cao), Qing Fan Teng	Fo Tan Mou (Chou)		Chinese knotweed herb
Polygonum cuspidatum	Radix et folium Polygoni cuspidati	Hu Zhang	Fu Jeung		Japanese Knotweed root and leaf
Polygonum cymosum	Radix et rhizoma Polygoni cymosi	Kai Jin Suo	Hoi Gam So		Cymose knotweed Root
Polygonum hydropiper	Fructus Polygoni hydropiperis	Liao Shi	Lou Sek		Water pepper fruit
Polygonum hydropiper	Herba et radix Polygoni hydropiperis	Shui Liao	Seui Liu		Water pepper herb and root
Polygonum lapathifolium	Herba Polygoni lapathifolii	La Liao Cao	La Lou Chou		Knotweed herb
Polygonum multiflorum	Radix Polygoni multiflori	He Shou Wu	Ho Sau Wu	Kashuu	Flowery knotweed root
Polygonum multiflorum	Caulis Polygoni multiflori	Ye Jiao Teng	Ye Gou Tang	Yakoto	Flowery knotweed stem

SCIENTIFIC	PHARMACEUTICAL	CANTONESE	MANDARIN	JAPANESE	ENGLISH
Polygonum orientale	Herba Polygoni orientalis	Shui Tong Hua Cao Hong Cao	Seui Tung Fa Chou Hung Chou		Prince's feather herb
Polygonum orientale	Fructus Polygoni orientalis	Shui Tong Hua Zi	Seui Tung Fa Ji		Prince's feather berry
Polygonum perfoliatum	Herba Polygoni perfoliati	Gang Ban Gui, Guan Ye Liao	Gong Bun Gwai, Gwan Yip Lou		Perfoliate knotweed herb
Polygonum tinctorium	Herba Polygoni tinctorii	Lan Shi	Laam Sat		Chinese indigo herb
Polypodium hastatum	Herba Polypodii	Qi Xing Cao	Chat Sing Chou		Polypody herb
Polyporus umbellatus	Sclerotium Polypori	Zhu Ling	Ju Ling	Chorei	Umbel polypore mushroom
Poncirus trifoliata	Fructus Ponciri	Gou Ju	Gau Gwat		Trifoliate orange fruit
Poncirus trifoliata	Fructus Ponciri immaturi	Lu Yi Zhi Qiao, Gou Yuan	Luk Ji Ji Hok, Gau Yun		Immature trifoliate orange fruit
Populus euphratica **and spp**	Resina Populi	Hu Tong Lei	Wu Tung Leui		Poplar resin
Poria cocos	Sclerotium Poriae rubrae	Chi Fu Ling	Chek Fuk Ling	Sekibikuryo	Red hoelen
Poria cocos	Sclerotium Poriae	Fu Ling	(Wong) Fuk Ling, Waan Ling	Bukuryo	Hoelen fungus
Poria cocos	Cortex Poriae	Fu Ling Pi	Wong Ling Pei, Fuk Ling Pei	Bukuryoshi	Hoelen skin
Poria cocos	Sclerotium Poriae paradicis	Fu Shen	Pou Fuk Sam	Bukushin	Hoelen spirit
Porites nigrescens	Os Poritis	Shi Hua	Sek Fa		Coral skeleton
Porphyra tenera	Herba Porphyrae	Zi Cai	Ji Choi		Porphyra herb
Portulacca oleracea	Herba Portulaccae	Ma Chi Xian	Ma Chi Yin	Bashiken	Purslane herb
Potentilla chinensis	Herba Potentillae chinensis	Wei Ling Cai	Wai Ling Choi		Chinese cinquefoil herb
Potentilla discolor	Herba Potentillae discoloris	Fan Bai Cao	Faan Baak Chou		Discolored cinquefoil herb
Potentilla fragarioides	Radix Potentillae fragarioidis	Mei Ye Wei Ling Cai	Mui Yip Wai Ling Choi		Strawberry-leaf cinquefoil
Prinsepia uniflora	Semen Prinsepiae	Rui Ren (Rou)	Seui Yan (Yuk)		Prinsepia seed
Protohermes grandis	Vermiculus Protohermis	Sun Tai Lang Chun	Syun Taai Long Chung	Magotaro-mushi	Protohermes larva
Prunella vulgaris	Spica Prunellae	Xia Ku Cao	Ha Fu Chou	Kagoso	Selfheal spike
Prunus armeniaca **and var.**	Semen Pruni armeniacae	Xing Ren, Ku Xing Ren	Baak Hang Yan	Kyonin	Bitter apricot kernel
Prunus armeniaca **and var.**	Semen Pruni armeniacae dulcis	Tian Xing Ren, Nan Xing Ren	Tim Hang Yan, Naam Hang Yan		Sweet apricot kernel
Prunus humilis	Semen Pruni humili	Yu Li Ren, Ou Li	Yuk Lei Yan, Ngao Lei		Dwarf cherry kernel
Prunus jamasakura, P. yedoensis	Cortex Pruni	Ying Pi	Ying Pei	Ouhi	Plum tree bark
Prunus japonica	Semen Pruni japonicae	Yu Li Ren	Yuk Lei Yan	Ikurinin	Bush cherry kernel

SCIENTIFIC	PHARMACEUTICAL	CANTONESE	MANDARIN	JAPANESE	ENGLISH
Prunus mume	Fructus Mumis immaturis preparatae	Bai Mei	Baak Mui		Unripe prepared black plum fruit
Prunus mume	Flos Pruni mumis	Lu Er Mei, Lu Mei Hua	Lat Mui Fa		Black plum flower
Prunus mume	Fructus Pruni mumis	Wu Mei (Rou)	Wu Mui (Yuk)	Ubai	Black plum fruit
Prunus persica and spp	Semen Pruni persicae	Tao Ren	Tou Yan	Tonin	Peach kernel
Prunus persica, P. davidiana	Fructus persicae immaturi	Bi Tao Gan			Unripe peach fruit
Prunus salicina	Cortex radicis Pruni salicinae	Li Gen Bai Pi	Lei Gan Baak Pei		Willow plum root bark
Pseudodrynaria fortunei, D. baronii	Rhizoma Pseudodrynariae	Gu Sui Bu	Gwat Seui Bou	Kotsusaiho	Boneknit root
Pseudolarix amabilis. P. kaempferi	Cortex radicis Pseudolaricis	Tu Jing Pi	Tou Ging Pei		Golden larch root bark
Pseudosciaena crocea, P. polyactis, Sciaena schlegeli	Otozithum Sciaenae	Yu Nao Shi	Yu Nou Sek		Fish otolith
Pseudostellaria heterophylla	Radix Pseudostellariae	Tai Zi Shen	Yi Sam, Taai Ji Sam	Taishijin	Prince ginseng root
Psidium guajava	Folium Psidii	Fan Shi Liu Gan Ye	Faan Sek Lau Gon Yip		Guava leaf
Psoralea corylifolia	Fructus Psoraleae	Bu Gu Zhi	Bou Gwat Ji	Hokotsushi	Scurf pea berry
Psychotria serpens	Herba Psychotriae serpentis	Chuan Gen Teng, Bo Gu Cao	Chyun Gen Tang		Twining psychotria herb
Pteria margaritifera and spp	Concha Pteriae	Zhen Zhu Mu	Chan Ju Mou		Mother of pearl shell
Pteria margaritiferae	Fructus conchae Pteriae	Zhen Zhu	Chan Ju	Shinju	Pearl
Pteris multifida and spp	Herba Pterii	Feng Wei Cao	Fung Mei Chou		Phoenix-tail fern
Pterocarpus indicus	Lignum Pterocarpi	Zi Tan	Ji Taan		Malay padauk wood, Burma rosewood
Pterospermum heterophyllum	Radix Pterospermi	Ban Feng He Gen	Bun Fung Ho Gan		Pterospermum root
Pueraria lobata, P. omeiensis and spp	Radix Puerariae	Ge Gen	Got Gan	Kakkon	Kudzu root
Pueraria lobata, P. omeiensis and spp	Flos Puerariae	Ge Hua	Got Fa		Kudzu flower
Pulsatilla chinensis, P. cernua, P. turczaninovii, P. ambigua and spp	Radix Pulsatillae	Bai Tou Weng	Baak Tau Yung	Hakutoo	Asian pasqueflower root
Pulsatilla dahurica	Radix Pulsatillae dahuricae	Bai Tou Weng, Xing An Bai Tou Weng	Baak Tau Yung, Ing On Baak Tau Yung		Dahurian pasqueflower root
Pumus	Lapis Pumicis	Fu Hai Shi	Fau Hoi Sek	Kaifuseki	Pumice
Punica granatum	Cortex Radicis Punicae	Shi Liu Gen Pi	Sek Lau Gan Pei	Sekiryu-kombi	Pomegranate root bark

SCIENTIFIC	PHARMACEUTICAL	CANTONESE	MANDARIN	JAPANESE	ENGLISH
Punica granatum	Pericarpium Punicae	Shi Liu Pi	Sek Lau Pei	Sekiryuhi	Pomegranate husk
Pycnostelma paniculatum	Herba Pycnostelmae	Shan Diao Zhu, Xu Chang Jing	Cheui Cheung Hing		Paniculate swallowwort herb
Pyrethrum cinerariifolium	Flos Pyrethri	Chu Chong Ju	Cheui Chung Guk		Dalmatia pellitory flower
Pyritum	Pyritum	Zi Ran Tong	Ji Yin Tung	Shizendo	Pyrite
Pyritum rotundum	Pyritum rotundum	She Han Shi			Iron pyrite
Pyrola rotundifolia subsp. chinensis, P. Japonica	Radix et herba Pyrolae	Lu Xian Cao, Lu Ti Cao	Luk Haam Chou, Luk Tai Chou	Rokuteiso	Asian wintergreen root and herb
Pyrolusitum	Pyrolusitum	Wu Ming Zi	Mou Ming Ji		Pyrolusite
Pyrrosia lingua, P. petiolosa **and spp**	Folium Pyrrosiae	Shi Wei	Sek Wai		Felt fern leaf
Pyrrosia sheareri	Folium Pyrrosiae sheareri	Shi Wei, Lu Shan Shi Wei	Sek Wai, Lou San Sek Wai	Sekii	Shearer's felt fern leaf
Pyrus betulaefolia	Pericarpium Pyri	Li Pi	Lei Pei		Chinese pear rind
Quercus acutissima	Fructus Querci acutissimae	Xiang Shi	Jeung Sat		Oak fruit
Quercus dentata, Q. acutissima	Ramulus et cortex Querci	Pu Suo	Pok Sau	Bokuso	Oak twig and bark
Quercus infectoria	Galla Querci	Mo Shi Zi	Mut Sik Ji		Oak gall
Quercus salicina, Q. myrsinaefolium	Folium Querci	Zhu Zi Ye	Jyu Ji	Urajirokashi	Oak leaf
Quisqualis indica	Fructus Quisqualis	Shi Jun Zi	Si Gwan Ji	Shikunshi	Rangoon creeper nut
Rabdosia rubescens **and spp**	Herba Rabdosiae	Dong Ling Cao	Dun Ling Chou		Rabdosia herb
Ranunculus japonicus	Radix et herba Ranunculi japonicae	Mao Gen	Maau Gan		Japanese buttercup root and herb
Ranunculus ternatus	Radix Ranunculi	Mao Zhao Cao, Mao Zhua Cao	Maau Jau Chou		Ternate buttercup root
Raphanus sativus	Radix Raphani	Di Gu Luo			Radish root
Raphanus sativus	Semen Raphani	Lai Fu Zi	Loi Fuk Ji		Radish seed
Raphanus sativus	Radix Raphani recentis	Luo Bo Gen	Lo Ba Gan		Fresh radish root
Raphanus sativus	Folium Raphani	Luo Bo Ye	Lo Ba Yip		Radish leaf
Rauvolfia verticillata, R. yunnanensis, R. latifrons, R. serpentina **& spp**	Radix Rauvolfiae	Luo Fu Mu	Lo Fu Mou		Rauvolfia root
Realgar	Realgar	Xiong Huang	Song Wong	Yuo	Realgar
Rehmannia glutinosa	Radix Rehmanniae	Sheng Di (Huang)	Sang Dei (Wong)	Shojio	Fresh Rehmannia root
Rehmannia glutinosa	Radix Rehmanniae preparatae	Shu Di (Huang)	Suk Dei (Wong)	Jukujio	Prepared Rehmannia root
Rhaponticum uniflorum	Radix Rhapontici	Lou Lu	Lau Lou	Roro	Swiss centaury root
Rheum palmatum, R. tanguticum, R. officinale	Rhizoma Rhei	Da Huang	Daai Wong	Daio	Rhubarb root

SCIENTIFIC	PHARMACEUTICAL	CANTONESE	MANDARIN	JAPANESE	ENGLISH
Rhinoceros unicornis, R. bicornis	Cornu Rhinoceri	Xi Jiao	Sai Gok		Rhinoceros horn
Rhodea japonica	Herba Rhodeae	Wan Nian Xing			Rhodea herb
Rhododendron dauricum, R. mariesii	Folium Rhododendri daurici	Man Shan Hong	Mun Saan Hung		Daurian rhododendron leaf
Rhododendron molle	Fructus Rhododendris mollis	Ba Li Ma	Baat Lei Ma		Yellow azalea fruit
Rhododendron molle	Flos Rhododendri mollis	Nao Yang Hua, Huang Du Juan	Naau Yeung Fa, Wong Dou Gun		Yellow azalea flower
Rhodomyrtus tomentosa	Radix Rhodomyrti	Shui Duo Nian, Shan Nian Gen	Seui Do Lin, San Nim Gan		Downy rosemyrtle root
Rhodomyrtus tomentosa	Semen Rhodomyrti	Shan Ren Zi	Saan Nam Ji		Rosemyrtle seed
Rhopilema esculenta	Tentaculum Rhopilema	Hai Zhe	Hoi Jit		Jellyfish tentacle
Rhus chinensis	Radix Rhudis chinensis	Pu Yan Pian	Pou Yim Pin		Chinese sumac root
Rhus chinensis	Cortex Rhudis chinensis	Yan Fu Mu	Yim Fo Muk	Gobaishi	Chinese sumac bark
Rhus sinensis **and spp, *Schlechtendaria chinensis***	Galla Rhudis sinensis	Wu Bei Zi	Ng Pan Ji		Chinese sumac gallnut
Rhus verniciflua	Succus exsiccatus Rhudis	Gan Qi	Gon Chat		Lacquer
Ricinus communis	Semen Ricini	Bi Ma Zi	Bei Ma Ji		Castor bean
Rorippa montana, R. indica	Herba Rorippae	Han Cai	Hon Choi		Nasturtium herb
Rosa chinensis	Radix Rosae chinensis	Yue Ji Gen	Yut Gwai Gan		Moonseason rose root
Rosa chinensis	Gemma Rosae chinensis	Yue Ji Hua	Yut Gwai Fa	Gekkika	Moonseason rose bud
Rosa cymosa	Cortex radicis Rosae cymosae	Hong Ci Teng, Hong Gen, Xiao Jin Ying	Hung Chi Teng, Siu Gam Ying		Cymose rose root bark
Rosa laevigata	Fructus Rosae laevigatae	Jin Ying Zi	Gam Ying Ji	Kinoshi	Cherokee rosehip
Rosa multiflora	Radix Rosae multiflorae	Ye Qiang Wei Gen	Ye Cheung Mei Gan		Wild rose root
Rosa polyantha **and spp**	Radix Rosae polyanthae	Qiang Wei Gen			Polyanth rose root
Rosa rugosa	Flos Rosae rugosae	Mei Gui Hua	Mui Gwai Fa	Maikaika	Japanese rose flower
Rosa rugosa	Fructus Rosae rugosae	Mei Gui Zi	Mui Gwai Ji		Japanese rosehip
Rosmarinus officinalis	Herba Rosmarini	Mi Die Xiang	Mai Dit Heung		Rosemary herb
Rostellulariae procumbens	Herba Rostellulariae	Jue Chuang	Jeuk Chong		Creeping rostellularia herb
Rubia cordifolia	Radix Rubiae cordifoliae	Qian Cao Gen	Sin Chou Gan	Seisokon	Heart-leaf madder root
Rubia cordifolia	Caulis Rubiae cordifoliae	Lu Gu Dan	Lu Gwat Daan		Heart-leaf madder stem
Rubus chingii	Fructus Rubi chingii	Fu Pen Zi	Fuk Pun Ji	Fukubonshi	Chinese raspberry fruit

SCIENTIFIC	PHARMACEUTICAL	CANTONESE	MANDARIN	JAPANESE	ENGLISH
Rubus coreanus	Fructus Rubi coreani	Dao Sheng Gen	Dou Sang Gan		Korean raspberry fruit
Rubus parvifolius	Folium Rubi parvifolii	Mao Mei, Hao Tian Biao	Mau Mui		Small-leaf raspberry leaf
Rumex crispus	Radix Rumicis crispi	Niu Er Da Huang	Ngau Yi Daai Wong		Yellow dock root
Rumex japonicus, R. nepalensis	Radix Rumicis japonici	Yang Ti	Yeung Tai		Japanese dock root
Rungia pectinata	Herba Rungiae	Hai Er Cao	Haai Yi Chou		Rungia herb
Ruta graveolens	Herba Rutae	Chou Cao	Chau Chou		Rue herb
Sabia japonica	Ramulus Sabiae	Qi Feng Teng	Ching Fung Tang		Sabia twig
Sagina japonica	Herba Saginae	Qi Gu Cao	Chat Gu Chou		Japanese pearlwort herb
Saiga tatarica	Cornu Saigae	Ling Yang Jiao	Ling Yeung Gok	Reiyokaku	Antelope horn
Salammonitum and *Halitum*	Salmiacum	Nao Sha	Lou Sa		Salmiac, Sal ammoniac
Salix babylonica, S. gracilistyla	Folium Salicis	Liu Ye	Lau Yip		Weeping willow twig
Salix babylonica, S. gracilistyla	Ramulus Salicis	Liu Zhi	Lau Ji		Weeping willow twig
Salix purpurea	Ramulus Salicis purpureae	Shui Yang Zhi	Seui Yeung Ji		Purple willow twig
Salsola collina, S. ruthenica, S. richteri	Radix et herba Salsolae	Zhu Mao Cai	Jyu Mou Choi		Salsola root and herb
Salvia bowleyana	Radix Salviae bowleyanae	Dan Shen, Nan Dan Shen	Daan Sam, Naam Dam Sam		Southern cinnabar sage root
Salvia chinensis	Radix et herba Salviae chinensis	Shi Jian Chuan, Chai Shen, Zi Shen	Sek Gin Chyun, Toi Sam, Ji Sam		Chinese sage root and herb
Salvia miltiorrhiza	Radix Salviae miltiorrhizae	Dan Shen	Daan Sam	Tanjin	Cinnabar sage root
Salvia plebeia	Herba et radix Salviae plebeiae	Li Zhi Cao	Lai Jik Chou		Plebeian sage herb and root
Salvia przelwalskii	Radix	Dan Shen, Gan Xi Shu Wei	Daan Sam, Gam Sai Syu Mei		Gan Xi cinnabar sage root
Sambucus formosana/taiwaniana	Caulis et folium Sambuci formosanae	Mao Gu Xiao	Mon Gwat Siu		Taiwan elder stem and leaf
Sambucus chinensis and spp	Caulis et folium Sambuci chinensis	Shuo Zhuo	Sok Dik		Chinese elder stem and leaf
Sambucus japonicus	Cortex Sambuci japonici	Lu Ying		Rakutokuda	Japanese elder bark
Sambucus javanica	Caulis et folium Sambuci javanici	Shuo Diao	Sok Duk		Java elder stem and leaf
Sanguisorba officinalis	Radix Sanguisorbae	Di Yu	Dei Yu	Jiyu	Great burnet root
Santalum album	Lignum Santalum	Tan Xiang	Taan Heung		Sandalwood
Sapindus mukorossi	Semen Sapindi	Wu Huan Zi, Mu Huan Zi	Mou Waan Ji		Soapnut seed, Bodhi seed
Sapindus mukorossi	Radix Sapindi	Wu Huan Gen, Mu Huan Gen	Mou Waan Gan		Soapnut tree root
Sapium sebiferum	Cortex radicis Sapii sebiferi	Wu Jiu (Mu) Gen Pi	Wu Kau Muk Gan Pei	Ukyukompi	Chinese tallow tree root bark
Sarcandra glabra	Herba Sarcandrae	Jiu Jie Feng	Gau Jit Fung		Smooth sarcandra herb
Sargassum fusiforme and spp	Herba Sargassi	Hai Zao	Hoi Chou	Kaiso	Sargassum seaweed
Sargentodoxa cuneata	Caulis Sargentodoxae	Da Xue Teng	Daai Hyut Tang		Sargentodoxa stem

SCIENTIFIC	PHARMACEUTICAL	CANTONESE	MANDARIN	JAPANESE	ENGLISH
Sauropus rostratus, S. changianus	Folium Sauropi	Long Li Ye	Lung Lei Yip		Lizardtail leaf
Saururus chinensis	Herba Saururi	San Bai Cao	Saam Baak Chou		Chinese lizardtail herb
Saussurea laniceps, S. involucrata and spp	Herba Saussureae lanicepsis	Xue Lian Hua	Hat Ling Fa		Snow lotus herb
Saussurea laniceps, S. involucrata & spp	Radix Saussureae lanicepsis	Xue Lian Gen	Hat Ling Gan		Snow lotus root
Saussurea lappa	Radix Saussureae lappae	Mu Xiang, Yun Mu Xiang	Muk Heung	Mokko	Wood aromatic root
Saxifraga stolonifera	Herba Saxifragae stoloniferae	Hu Er Cao	Fu Yi Chou		Saxifrage herb
Schefflera arboricola, S. kwangsiensis, S. venulosa	Folium et caulis Schefflerae	Qi Ye Lian	Chat Yip Lin		Taiwan schefflera leaf and stem
Schefflera octophylla	Cortex Schefflerae octophyllae	Ya Jiao Mu Pi	Ngaap Geuk Muk Pei		Umbrella tree bark
Schisandra chinensis	Fructus Schisandrae	Wu Wei Zi	Ng Mei Ji	Gomishi	Schisandra berry
Schizandra sphenantera	Fructus Schisandrae sphenanterae	Wu Wei Zi, Hua Zheng Wu Wei Zi	Ng Mei Ji, Wa Jung Ng Mei Ji	Gomishi	Central China schisandra berry
Schizonepeta tenuifolia	Herba Schizonepetae	Jing Jie	Ging Gaai	Keigai	Japanese catnip herb
Schizophragma integrifolium	Cortex radicis Schizophragmae	Zuan Di Feng	Jyun Dei Fung		Schizophrag-ma root bark
Scolopendra subspinipes mutilans	Scolopendra	Wu Gong	Ng Gung	Gosho	Centipede
Scoparia dulcis	Radix Scopariae	Ye Gan Cao, Zhu Cai Cao Gen	Ye Gam Chou, Chu Jai Chou Gan		Scoparia root
Scrophularia ningpoensis, S. buergeriana	Radix Scrophulariae ningpoensis	Xuan Shen, Yuan Shen	Yun Sam, Yun Sam	Genjin	Black figwort root
Scurrula ritozanensis	Ramulus Scurrulae	Tai Wan Ji Sheng	Toi Waan Ji Sang		Taiwan mistletoe twig
Scutellaria baicalensis, S. viscidula, S. amoena	Radix Scutellariae baicalensis	Huang Qin	Wong Kam	Ogon	Baikal skullcap root
Scutellaria barbata, B. rivularis	Radix et herba Scutellariae barbatae	Ban Zhi Lian	Bun Ji Lin		Barbed skullcap root and herb
Scutellaria indica	Herba Scutellariae indicae	Han Xin Cao	Hon Sam Chou		India skullcap herb
Securinega suffruticosa	Gemma et radix Securinegae	Yi Ye Qiu	Yat Yip Chau		Securinega shoot and root
Sedum aizoon	Herba Sedi aizoonis	Jing Tian San Qi	Ging Tin Saam Chat		Aizoon stonecrop herb
Sedum erythrostictum	Herba Sedi erythrosticti	Jing Tian (San Qi)	Ging Tin		Red stonecrop herb
Sedum erythrosticum	Flos Sedi erythrostici	Jing Tian Hua	Ging Ting Fa		Red stonecrop flower
Sedum sarmentosum	Radix et herba Sedi sarmentosi	Chui Pen Cao	Chai Pan Chou		Stringy stonecrop root and herb

SCIENTIFIC	PHARMACEUTICAL	CANTONESE	MANDARIN	JAPANESE	ENGLISH
Selaginella doederleinii, S. involvens	Herba Selaginellae	Shi Shang Bai	Sek Song Paap		Spikemoss herb
Selaginella moellendorfii	Herba Selaginella moellendorfii	Jiang Nan Juan Bai	Gong Naam Kyun Paap		Moellendorf's spikemoss herb
Selaginella tamariscina	Herba Selaginellae tamariscinae	Juan Bai	Kyun Paap		Resurrection plant herb
Selenitum	Selenitum	Xuan Jing Shi	San Ching Sek		Selenite
Semiaquilegia adoxoides	Radix Semiaquilegiae	Tian Kui	Tin Kwai		Semiaquilegia root
Semiaquilegia adoxoides	Herba Semiaquilegiae	Tian Kui	Tin Kwai		Semiaquilegia herb
Senecio kirilowii	Herba Senecionis kirilowii	Kou She Cao	Gau Sit Chou		Kirilow's ragwort herb
Senecio scandens	Herba Senecionis scandens	Qian Li Guang	Chin Lei Gwong		Climbing ragwort herb
Senna acutifolia, S. angustifolia	Folium Sennae	Fan Xie Ye	Faan Sie Yip		Senna leaf
Sepia esculenta, Sepiella maindroni	Os Sepiae seu Sapiellae	Hai Piao Xiao, Wu Zei Gu	Hoi Piu Seui		Cuttlefish bone
Serratula chinensis	Radix Serratulae	Guang Dong Sheng Ma	Gwong Dung Jing Ma		Serratula root
Sesamum indicum	Fructus Sesami	Hei Zhi Ma Hu Ma Ren	Hak Ji Ma		Black sesame seed
Setaria italica	Fructus germinatus Setariae	Su Ya	Suk Nga		Sprouted millet grain
Setaria italica	Fructus Setariae	Xiao Mi	Suk Mai		Millet grain
Siegesbeckia pubescens, S. orientalis, S. glabrescens	Herba Siegesbeckiae	Xi Xian Cao	Hei Lim Chou		Hairy siegesbeckia herb
Silybum marianum	Herba Silybi	Shui Fei Ji	Seui Fei Gai		Blessed thistle herb
Sinapis alba	Semen Sinapis albae	Bai Jie Zi	Baak Gaai Ji		White mustard seed
Sinomenium acutum	Radix Sinomenii	Qing Feng Teng	Ching Fung Tang		Sinomenium root
Skimmia reevesiana, S. japonica	Caulis et folium Skimmiae	Yin Yu	Yan Wu		Skimmia stem and leaf
Smilax china	Rhizoma Smilacis chinensis	Jin Gang Teng, Ba Qi	Gam Gong Tang, Bat Kai		Chinese green-brier root, China root
Smilax glabra	Rhizoma Smilacis glabrae	Tu Fu Ling	Tou Fuk Ling		Glabrous greenbrier root
Solanum dulcamara	Caulis Solani dulcamari	Ku Qie	Fu Ke		Bittersweet stem
Solanum lyratum	Herba Solani lyrati	Bai Ying, Shu Yang Quan, Bai Mao Teng	Baak Ying, Baak Mou Tang		Climbing nightshade herb
Solanum melongena	Radix et rhizoma Solani melongenae	Qie Gen	Ke Gan		Eggplant root
Solanum nigrum	Herba Solani nigri	Long Kui	Lung Kwai		Winter cherry herb
Solanum surratense	Herba Solani surattensis	Ye Dian Jie	Ye Din Ke		Soda-apple nightshade herb

SCIENTIFIC	PHARMACEUTICAL	CANTONESE	MANDARIN	JAPANESE	ENGLISH
Solanum verbascifolium	Radix Solani verbascifolii	Ye Yan Ye Gen, Tu Yen Tou	Ye Yin Yip Gan, Tou Yin Tau		Tobacco nightshade root
Solanum xanthocarpum	Herba Solani xanthocarpi	Huang Shui Qie	Wong Seui Ke		Prickly nightshade fruit
Solenognathus spp, *Syngna-thoid-es biaculeatus*	Solenognathus	Hai Long	Hoi Lung		Pipefish
Solidago virgaurea, S. derurrens	Herba Solidaginis	Yi Zhi Huang Hua, Liu Zhi Huang	Yat Ji Wong Fa, Lau Ji Wong		Goldenrod herb
Sonchus oleraceus	Herba Sonchi	Ku Cai	Fu Choi		Annual sowthistle herb
Sophora flavescens	Radix Sophorae flavescentis	Ku Shen	Fu Sam		Yellow pagoda tree root
Sophora flavescens	Radix Sophorae flavescentis	Ku Shen Zi	Fu Sam Ji		Yellow pagoda tree berry
Sophora japonica	Gemma Sophorae japonicae	Huai (Hua) Mi	Waai (Fa) Mai		Japanese pagoda tree bud
Sophora japonica	Flos Sophorae japonicae	Huai Hua	Waai Fa		Japanese pagoda tree flower
Sophora japonica	Fructus Sophorae japonicae	Huai Jiao (Zi)	Wai Jiu (Ji)		Japanese pagoda tree fruit
Sophora subprostata	Radix Sophorae subprostatae	Shan Dou Gen	Saan Dau Gan		Pigeon-pea root
Sparganium simplex, S. stoloniferum, S. stenophyllum	Rhizoma Sparganii	San Leng	Saam Ling		Bur-reed root
Spatholobus suberectus	Gelatinum Spatholobi	Ji Xue Teng Jiao	Gai Yut Tang Gaau		Spatholobus gel
Spatholobus suberectus	Caulis Spatholobi	Ji Xue Teng, Mi Hua Dou	Gai Yut Tang, Mat Fa Dau		Spatholobus stem
Speranskia tuberculata	Herba Speranskiae	Tou Gu Cao	Tau Gwat Chou		Speranskia herb
Spilanthes acmella var. *oleracea*	Flos Spilanthis	Liu Shen Hua	Lau Sam Fa		Six god flower
Spiranthes sinensis	Herba Spiranthis	Pan Long Shen	Pun Lung Sam		Chinese pearltwist herb
Spirodela polyrrhiza	Herba Spirodelae	Fu Ping	Fau Ping		Duckweed herb
Stalactitum, Balanophylla spp	Stalactitum	E Guan Shi, Shi Zhong Ru	Ngo Gun Sek		Stalactite tip
Statice sinensis	Radix Staticis	Hong Mao Cha	Hung Maau Cha		Statice root
Stegodon orientalis et al.	Dens Stegodontis	Long Chi	Lung Ji		Dragon tooth
Stegodon orientalis et al.	Os Stegodontis calcinatum	Duan Long Gu, Shu Long Gu	Taan Lung Gwat		Calcined dragon bone
Stegodon orientalis, S. rhinocerus sinensis, Hipparion	Os Stegodontis	Long Gu	Lung Gwat	Ryukotsu	Dragon bone

SCIENTIFIC	PHARMACEUTICAL	CANTONESE	MANDARIN	JAPANESE	ENGLISH
Stellaria aquatica	Herba Stellariae aquaticae	Cha Chi Huang	Cha Si Wong		Water chickweed herb
Stellaria dichotoma var. *lanceolata*	Radix Stellariae	Yin Chai Hu	Ngan Chaai Wu	Ginsaiko	Stellaria root
Stellera chamaejasme	Radix Stellerae	Hong Lang Du, Lang Du	Hung Long Duk, Long Duk		Stellara root
Stemona japonia	Radix Stemonae japonicae	Bai Bu, Man Sheng Bai Bu	Baak Bou, Maan Sang Baak Bou	Hyakubu	Japanese stemona root
Stemona sessilifolia	Radix Stemonae sessilifoliae	Bai Bu, Zhi Li Bai Bu	Baak Bou, Chek Lap Baak Bou		Sessile stemona root
Stemona tuberosa	Radix Stemonae tuberosae	Bai Bu, Dui Ye Bai Bu	Baak Bou, Deui Yip Baak Bou		Tuberous stemona root
Stephania japonica	Caulis Stephaniae japonicae	Qian Jin Teng	Chin Gam Tang		Japanese stephania stem
Stephania sinica	Caulis Stephaniae sinicae	Jin Bu Huan	Gam Bat Wun		Chinese stephania stem
Stephania tetrandra	Radix Stephaniae tetrandrae	Han Fang Ji, Fang Ji	Haan Fong Gei Fong Gei	Kamboi	Stephania root
Sterculia staphigera, S. lychnophera	Semen Sterculiae	Pang Da Hai	Bun Daai Hoi	Bantaikai	Sterculia seed
Stichopus japonicus	Stichopus	Hai Shen	Hoi Sam		Sea cucumber
Striga asiatica	Herba Strigae	Du Jiao Gan	Duk Geuk Gam		Witchweed herb
Strobilanthes flaccidifolius	Radix Strobilanthis	Ma Lan Gen	Ma Laam Gan		Strobilanthes root
Strophanthus divaricatus	Semen Strophanthi	Yang Jiao Yao	Yeung Gok Aau		Strophanthus seed
Strychnos pierrana, S. nux-vomica and spp	Semen Strychnotis preparatae	(Zhi) Ma Qian Zi	Ma Chin Ji	Basenshi	Prepared vomit nut
Styrax benzoin	Benzoinum	An Xi Xiang	Ngon Sik Heung	Ansokuko	Benzoin
Sulphurum	Sulphurum	Liu Huang, Shi Liu Huang	Lau Wong, Sek Lau Wong	Io	Sulphur
Sus scrofa domestica	Fel Suidis	Zhu Dan	Ju Daam		Pig gallbladder
Swertia pseudochinensis and spp	Radix Swertiae	Dang Yao	Dong Yeuk		Asian green gentian root
Swertia japonica, S. pseudochinensis	Herba Swertiae	Dang Yao Cao	Dong Yeuk Chou	Toyaku	Japanese green gentian herb
Syringa manchuriensis	Cortex Syringae	Bao Ma Zi			Manchurian lilac bark
Tabanus bivittatus	Tabanus	Meng Chong	Mung Chung		Gadfly
Tagetes erecta	Flos Tagetis	Wan Shou Ju	Maan Sau Guk		African marigold flower
Talcum	Talcum	Hua Shi	Wat Sek	Kasseki	Talc
Talinum paniculatum	Radix Talini	Tu Ren Shen	Tou Yan Sam		Fameflower root
Tamarix chinensis	Cacumen Tamaricis	Xi He Liu	Sei Ho Lau	Seikaryu	Chinese tamarisk tip

SCIENTIFIC	PHARMACEUTICAL	CANTONESE	MANDARIN	JAPANESE	ENGLISH
Taraxacum mongolicum	Radix et herba Taraxaci	Pu Gong Ying	Pou Gung Ying	Hokoei	Mongolian dandelion root and herb
Taxillus yadoriki, T. chinensis	Ramulus Taxilli	Shi Ji Sheng	Chi Gei Sang		Asian mistletoe twig
Terminalia chebula and var.	Fructus Terminaliae immaturi	Cang Qing Guo			Unripe myrobalan fruit
Terminalia chebula and var.	Fructus Terminaliae	He Zi (Rou)	Ho Ji (Yuk)	Kashi	Myrobalan fruit
Tetragonia tatragonoides	Herba Tetragoniae	Fan Xing	Faan Haang	Bankyo, Mantsai	Tetragonia herb
Tetrapanax papyrifera	Medulla Tetrapanacis	Tong Cao	Tong Chou, Bai Tong Chou	Toso	Rice paper pith
Thalictrum foliolosum	Herba Thalictri	Tang Song Cao			Meadow rue herb
Thevetia peruviana	Folium et semen Thevetiae	Huang Hua Jia Zhu Tao (Ye)	Wong Fa Gaap Juk Tou (Yip)		Peruvian thevetia leaf and seed
Thladiantha dubia	Fructus Thladianthae	Zhi Pao	Chek Pau		Thladiantha fruit
Thlaspi arvense	Herba Thlaspis	Xi Ming	Sik Ming		Boor's mustard herb
Thymus mongolicus	Herba Thymi mongolici	Di Jiao	Dei Jiu		Mongolian thyme herb
Tilia cordata	Flos Tiliae	Duan Shu Hua			Linden flower
Tinospora sagittata, T. capillipes	Radix Tinosporae	Jin Guo Lan	Gam Gwo Laam	Kinkaran	Tinospora root
Tinospora sinensis	Caulis Tinosporae sinensis	Kuan Jin Teng	Gwan Gam Tang	Kankinto	Chinese tinospora stem
Toddalia asiatica	Radix Toddaliae	Fei Long Zhang Xue	Fei Lung Jeung Hyut		Asian toddalia root
Torreya grandis, T. nucifera	Semen Torreyae	Fei Zi	Fei Ji		Japanese torreya nut
Trachelospermum jasminoides	Caulis Trachelospermi	Luo Shi Teng	Lok Sek Tang	Chikusekito	Star jasmine stem
Trachycarpus excelsa, T. fortunei	Fibra Stipulae Trachycarpi carbonisata	Zong Lu Pi Tan	Jung Leui Pei Daan		Charred windmill palm petiole
Trachycarpus excelsa, T. fortunei	Fructus Trachycarpi	Zong Lu Zi	Jung Leui Ji		Windmill palm seed
Trapa bispinosa, T. bicornis	Fructus Trapae	Ling Qiao	Ling Gok		Water caltrop fruit
Tremella fuciformis	Sclerotium Tremellae fucimormis	Bai Mu Er	Baak Muk Yi	Hakumokuji	Silver ear mushroom
Tremella mesenterica	Sclerotium Tremellae mesentericae	Huang Mu Er	Wong Muk Yi		Yellow ear mushroom
Tribulus terrestris	Fructus Tribuli	Bai Ji Li	Baak Jat Lai	Byakishitsuri	Caltrop fruit
Trichosanthes kirilowii, T. japonica, T. uniflora	Radix Trichosanthis	Tian Hua Fen	Tin Fa Fun	Tenkafun	Snakegourd root
Trichosanthes kirilowii, T. japonica, T. uniflora	Fructus Tricosanthis	Gua Lou (Shi)	Kwut Lau	Karo	Snakegourd fruit

SCIENTIFIC	PHARMACEUTICAL	CANTONESE	MANDARIN	JAPANESE	ENGLISH
Trichosanthes kirilowii, T. japonica, T. uniflora	Pericarpium Tricosanthis	Gua Lou Pi	Kwut Lau Pei	Karohi	Snakegourd rind
Trichosanthes kirilowii, T. japonica, T. uniflora	Semen Trichosanthis	Gua Lou Ren	Kwut Lau Yan	Karonin	Snakegourd seed
Trichosporum acuminatum	Herba Trichospori	Bai Mian Feng	Baak Ming Fung		Trichosporum herb
Trigonella foenum-graecum	Semen Trigonellae	Hu Lu Ba	Wu Lou Ba		Fenugreek seed
Tripterygium hypoglaucum	Radix Tripterygii hypoglauci decorticati	Kun Ming Shan Hai Tang, Diao Mao Cao	Kwan Ming Saan Hoi Tong		Peeled Tripterygium root
Tripterygium wilfordii	Medulla radicis Tripterygii	Lei Gong Teng	Leui Gung Tang		Yellow vine root pith
Triticum aestivum	Fructus Tritici	Fu Xiao Mai	Fau Siu Mak	Fushobaku	Wheat berry
Trogopterus xanthipes and spp, *Pteromys volans* and spp	Excrementum Trogopteri seu Pteromi	Wu Ling Zhi	Ng Ling Ji		Flying squirrel dropping
Tulipa edulis	Rhizoma et radix Tulipae	Shan Ci Gu, Guang Ci Gu	San Chi Gu, Gwong Chi Gu		Chinese tulip bulb
Tussilago farfara	Flos Tussilaginis	Kuan Dong Hua	Fun Dung Fa	Kantoka	Coltsfoot flower
Typha latifolia, T. angustifolia and spp	Pollen Typhae carbonisatus	Pu Huang Tan	Pou Wong Taan		Charred cattail pollen
Typha latifolia, T. angustifolia and spp	Pollen Typhae	Pu Huang, Xiang Pu	Pou Wong, Heung Pou	Hoo	Cattail pollen
Typhonium divaricatum	Rhizoma Typhonii divaricatii	Li Tou Jian	Lai Tau Jim		Divaricate typhonium root
Typhonium flagelliforme	Rhizoma Typhonii flagelliformis preparata	Shui Ban Xia	Seui Bun Ha		Prepared flagellate typhonium root
Typhonium giganteum	Rhizoma Typhonii gigantei preparata	Bai Fu Zi, Yu Bai Fu	Baak Fu Ji	Byakubushi	Prepared giant typhonium root
Typhonium giganteum	Radix Typhonii	Du Jiao Lan	Duk Gok Lin		Typhonium root
Ulmus macrocarpa	Praeparatio fructus Ulmi	Wu Yi	Mon Yi	Bui	Stinking elm fruit paste
Ulmus parvifolia	Cortex Ulmi parvifoliae	Lang Yu Pi	Long Yu Pei		Chinese elm bark
Ulmus pumila	Cortex Ulmi pumilae	Yu Qian	Yu Chin		White elm bark
Umbilicaria esculenta	Sclerotium Umbilicariae	Shi Er	Sek Yi		Stone ear mushroom
Uncaria gambir and spp	Pasta Uncaria seu Acaciae	Er Cha	Yi Cha		Catechu paste
Uncaria rhynchophylla, U. hirsuta, U. macrophylla and spp	Ramulus et uncus Uncariae	Gou Teng	Ngau Tang, Sheung Ngau (Tang)	Choto	Gambir vine twig
Uraria lagopodioides	Herba Urariae	Hu Li Wei, Tong Tian Cao	Tung Tin Chou		Uraria herb

SCIENTIFIC	PHARMACEUTICAL	CANTONESE	MANDARIN	JAPANESE	ENGLISH
Ursus arctos and spp	Fel Ursi	Xiong Dan	Hung Daam	Yutan	Bear gallbladder
Usnea diffracta and spp	Thallus Usneae	Song Luo	Chung Lo		Beard lichen thallus
Vaccaria segetalis	Semen Vaccariae	Wang Bu Liu Xing	Wong Bat Lau Hang	Ofurugyo	Cowcockle seed
Valeriana officinalis, V. hardwickii	Rhizoma Valerianae	Xie Cao	Kit Chou		Valerian root
Vanieria cochinchinensis	Caulis Vanieriae	Huang Jin Kui, Chuan Po Shi	Wong Jin Kwai		Vanieria stem
Ventilago leiocarpa	Radix et rhizoma Ventilaginis	Xue Feng Teng, Qing Pi Mao	Hyut Fung Tang		Ventilago root and stem
Veratrum nigrum and spp	Radix et rhizoma Veratri	Li Lu	Lai Lou	Riro	False hellebore root
Verbena officinalis	Herba Verbenae	Ma Bian Cao	Ma Bin Chou		Vervain herb
Vernonia cinerea	Herba Vernoniae	Yi Zhi Xiang	Yat Ji Heung		Vernonia herb
Veronica peregrina	Herba et radix Veronicae	Jie Gu Xian Tao	Jip Gwat Sin Tou		Peregrine speedwell herb and root
Vespertilium murinum	Excrementum Vespertilii	Ye Ming Sha	Ye Ming Sa	Yamyosha	Bat dropping
Viola collina	Radix et herba Violae collinae	Di He Tao	Dei Hat Tou		Collina violet root and herb
Viola diffusa	Radix et herba Violae diffusae	Di Bai Cao	Dei Baak Chou		Spreading violet root and herb
Viola japonica	Radix et herba Violae japonicae	Li Tou Cao	Lai Tau Chou		Japanese violet root and herb
Viola patrinii	Herba Violae patriniae	Hua Tou Cao	Wa Tau Chou		Patrinium violet herb
Viola yedoensis, V. japonica	Radix et herba Violae yedoensis	Zi Hua Di Ding	Ji Fa Dei Ding	Shikajicho	Asian violet root and herb
Viscum liquidambaricum	Ramulus Visci liquidambarici	Bian Ji Sheng	Bin Gei Sang		Asian mistletoe twig
Viscum coloratum, V. album	Herba Visci	Hu Ji Sheng	Wu Gei Sang		Western mistletoe herb
Vitex negundo	Fructus Viticis negundonis	Huang Jing Zi	Wong Ging Ji		Negundo chastetree berry
Vitex negundo var. *cannabifolia*	Fructus Viticis negundonis	Mu Jing Zi	Maau Ging Ji		Five-leaf chastetree berry
Vitex negundo var. *cannabifolia*	Folium Viticis negundonis	Mu Jing Ye	Maau Ging Yip		Five-leaf chastetree leaf
Vitex quinata	Radix Viticis quinatae	Pu Jiang Gen	Pou Geung Gan		Quinate chasteberry root
Vitex rotundifolia, V. trifolia	Fructus Viticis rotundifoliae	Man Jing Zi	Maan Ging Ji	Mankeishi	Seashore chastetree berry
Vitis amurensis	Radix Vitis amurensis	Shan Teng Teng Yang	Saan Tang Tang Yeung		Amur grape root
Vitis flexuosa	Radix Vitis flexuosis	Ge Lei Zhi Gen	Got Leui Jap Gan		Flexuose grape root
Vitis thunbergii and spp	Radix Vitis	Ye Pu Tao	Ye Pou Tou		Wild grape root
Wedelia chinensis	Herba Wedeliae	Ma Lan Jin, Peng Qi Ju	Paang Kei Guk		Wedelia herb

SCIENTIFIC	PHARMACEUTICAL	CANTONESE	MANDARIN	JAPANESE	ENGLISH
Wickstroemia indica	Radix Wickstroemiae	Liao Ge Wang (Gen)	Liu Go Wong	Ryokao	Wikstroemia root
Wikstroemia chamaedaphne	Flos Wikstroaemiae chamaedaphnis	Rao Hua	Iu Fa		Wikstroemia flower
Wisteria sinensis, W. floribunda	Galla Wisteriae	Zi Teng Zi, Teng Liu	Ji Tang Ji, Tang Lau	Figikobu	Asian wisteria gall
Woodwardia japonica, W. unigemmata	Rhizoma Woodwardiae	Guan Zhong, Gou Ji Guan Zhong	Gwun Jung, Gau Jek Gun Jung		Chain-fern root
Xanthium sibiricum, X. strumarium	Fructus Xanthii	Cang Er Zi	Chong Yi Ji	Sojishi	Siberian cocklebur
Zanthoxylum ailanthoides	Cortex Zanthoxyli ailanthoidis	Zhe Tong Pi	Jit Tung Pei		Zhejiang prickly ash bark
Zanthoxylum avicennae	Radix Zanthoxyli avicennae	Niao Bu Su, Bai Ma Niao	Niu Bat Suk		Prickly ash root
Zanthoxylum bungeanum	Fructus Zanthoxyli bungeani	Chuan Jiao, Hua Jiao	Chyun Jiu, Fa Jiu	Shokusho	Sichuan peppercorn
Zanthoxylum nitidum	Radix Zanthoxyi nitidi	Ru Di Jin Niu, Liang Mian Zhen	Yap Dei Gam Ngau		Shiny bramble root
Zanthoxylum planispinum	Fructus Zanthoxyli planispini	Zhu Ye Jiao	Juk Yip Jiu		Prickly ash berry
Zanthoxylum simulans	Fructus Zanthoxyli simulansis	Ye Hua Jiao	Ye Fa Jiu		Sichuan peppercorn
Zaocys dhumnades	Zaocys	Wu Shao She	U Sau Se	Ushoda	Black grass-snake
Zea mays	Stylus Zeae	Yu Mi Xu, Yu Mi Rui	Yuk Mai So, Yuk Mai Yeui	Gyokuma-ishu	Cornsilk style
Zea mays	Fructus Zeae	Yu Shu Shu	Yuk Suk Syu		Corn grain
Zea mays	Medulla Zeae	Yu Mi Xin	Yuk Mai Sam		Corn cob
Zingiber mioga	Rhizoma Zingiberis miogae	Rang He	Yeung Ho		Mioga ginger root
Zingiber officinalis	Rhizoma Zingiberis	(Sheng) Jiang Pi	Saang Geung Pei		Fresh ginger root skin
Zingiber officinalis	Rhizoma Zingiberis	Gan Jiang	Gaan Geung	Kankyo	Dried ginger root
Zingiber officinalis	Rhizoma Zingiberis	Pao Jiang	Bou Geung	Hokyo	Quick-fried ginger root
Zingiber officinalis	Rhizoma Zingiberis recentis	Sheng Jiang	Saang Geung	Shokyo	Fresh ginger root
Zizyphus jujuba var. ***inermis***	Fructus Zizyphi jujubae	Da Zao	Daai Jou	Taiso	Black jujube berry
Zizyphus jujuba var. ***inermis***	Fructus Zizyphi jujubae	Hong Zao	Hung Jou	Koso	Red jujube berry
Zizyphus jujuba var. ***inermis***	Fructus Zizyphi jujubae praeparatae	Mi Zao	Mat Jou		Honey-preserved jujube berry
Zizyphus mauritiana	Semen Zizyphi mauritianae	Mian Zao Ren	Mai Jou Yan		Mauritius jujube seed
Zizyphus spinosa	Semen Zizyphi spinosae	Suan Zao Ren, Jin Zao Ren	Syun Jou Yan	Sansonin	Sour jujube seed
Zizyphus spinosa	Semen Zizyphi spinosae preparatae	Chao Suan Zao Ren	Syu Jou Yan		Roasted sour jujube seed

Cross Index of Pharmaceutical Remedy Names

PHARMACEUTICAL	SCIENTIFIC	MANDARIN	CANTONESE	JAPANESE	ENGLISH
Actinolitum	***Actinolitum***	Yang Qi Shi	Yeung Hei Sek		Actinolite
Agate	***Agate***	Ma Nao			Agate
Agkistrodon	***Agkistrodon halys***	Fan Bi	Faan Bei		Viper
Agkistrodon seu Bungarus	***Agkistrodon acutus*** **and** ***Bungarus multicinctus***	Bai Hua She	Baak Fa Se	Hakkada	Multibanded krait
Alumen	***Alumen***	Ming Fan	Ming Faan	Myoban	Alum
Alumen praeparatum	***Alumen***	Ku Fan	Gu Faan		Prepared alum
Arillus Euphoriae	***Euphoria longan***	Long Yan Rou	Lung Ngaan Yuk	Ryuganniku	Longan fruit pulp
Armadillidium	***Armadillidium vulgare, Porcellio scaber***	Shu Fu	Syu Fu		Wood louse
Arsenolitum	***Arsenicum album***	Pi Shi, Xin Shi			White arsenic
Aspongopus	***Aspongopus***	Jiu Xiang Chong	Gau Heung Chung		Stinkbug
Benzoinum	***Styrax benzoin***	An Xi Xiang	Ngon Sik Heung	Ansokuko	Benzoin
Bombyx beauveriatus	***Bombyx mori artificially*** **infected with** ***Beauveria bassiana***	Jiang Yong	Geung Yung		Silkworm larva
Bombyx beauveriatus	***Bombyx mori*** **infected with** ***Beauveria bassiana***	Jiang Can	Geung Chaam		Silkworm larva
Borax	***Borax***	Peng Sha	Pang Sa	Hosha	Borax
Borax	***Borax***	Shu Peng Sha	Syu Pang Sa		Roasted borax
Borneolum	***Dryobalanops camphora***	Bing Pian	Bing Pin	Ryuno	Borneo camphor
Bulbus Allii fistulosi	***Allium fistulosum***	Cong Bai	Chung Baak		Fresh scallion bulb
Bulbus Allii macrostemonis	***Allium macrostemon***	Xie Bai	Se Baak	Gaihaku	Chinese chive bulb
Bulbus Allii sativi	***Allium sativum***	Da Suan	Daai Syun	Taisan	Garlic bulb
Bulbus Fritillariae cirrhosae	***Fritillaria cirrhosa***	Chuan Bei Mu	Chyun Bui Mou	Senbaimo	Sichuan fritillary bulb
Bulbus Fritillariae hupehensis	***Fritillaria hupehensis***	Hu Bei Bei Mu	Wu Bak Bui Mou		Hubei fritillary bulb
Bulbus Fritillariae pallidiflorae	***Fritillaria pallidiflora***	Yi Bei Mu	Yi Bui Mou		Pale-flower fritillary bulb
Bulbus Fritillariae puqiensis	***Fritillaria puqiensis***	Hu Bei Bei Mu, Pu Qi Bei Mu	Wu Bak Bui Mou, Pou Kei Bui Mou		Puqi fritillary bulb
Bulbus Fritillariae taipaiensis	***Fritillaria taipaiensis***	Chuan Bei Mu, Tai Bai Bei Mu	Chyun Bui Mou, Taai Baak Bui Mou		Taipei fritillary bulb
Bulbus Fritillariae thunbergii	***Fritillaria thunbergii***	Zhe Bei Mu	Chit Bui Mou	Setsubaimo	Zhejiang fritillary bulb
Bulbus Fritillariae tortifoliae	***Fritillaria tortifolia***	Yi Bei Mu, Tuo Li Bei Mu	Yi Bui Mou, Tok Lei Bui Mou		Twist-leaf fritillary bulb

PHARMACEUTICAL	SCIENTIFIC	MANDARIN	CANTONESE	JAPANESE	ENGLISH
Bulbus Fritillariae unibracteatae	***Fritillaria unibracteata***	Chuan Bei Mu, An Zi Bei Mu	Chyun Bui Mou, Am Ji Bui Mou		Single-bract fritillary bulb
Bulbus Fritillariae yuminensis	***Fritillaria yuminensis***	Yi Bei Mu, Yu Min Bei Mu	Yi Bui Mou, Yu Man Bui Mou		Yumin fritillary bulb
Bulbus Iphigeniae	***Iphigenia indica***	Shan Ci Gu	San Chi Gok		Iphigenia bulb
Bulbus Lilii	***Lilium brownii*** var. ***colchesteri***	Bai He	Baak Hap	Hyakugo	Brown's lily bulb
Bulbus Liliii concoloris	***Lilium concolor***	Shan Dan	Saan Daan		Japanese red star lily bulb
Bulbus Liliii lancifolii	***Lilium lancifolium***	Bai He, Juan Duan	Baak Hap, Gyun Daan		Lance-leaf lily bulb
Bulbus Narcissi	***Narcissus tazetta*** var. ***chinensis***	Shui Xian Gen	Seui Sin Gan		Chinese sacred lily bulb
Buthus	***Buthus Martensi***	Quan Xie	Chyun Kit	Zenkatsu	Scorpion
Cacumen Biotae orientalis	***Biota orientalis***	Ce Bai Ye	Jak Paak Yip	Sokuhakuyo	Oriental arborvitae tip
Cacumen Breyniae	***Breynia fruticosa***	Hei Mian Ye	Haak Min Yip		Breynia tip
Cacumen Glyptostrobi	***Glyptostrobus pensilis***	Shui Song Mao	Seui Chung Ma		Chinese water pine tip
Cacumen Tamaricis	***Tamarix chinensis***	Xi He Liu	Sei Ho Lau	Seikaryu	Chinese tamarisk tip
Calamina, Smithsonitum	***Calamina, Smithsonitum***	Lu Gan Shi	Lou Gam Sek	Rokanseki	Calamine
Calcaria	***Calcaria***	Chen Shi Hui	Chan Sek Wei		Calcium hydroxide
Calcitum	***Calcitum***	Han Shui Shi, Fang Jie Shi	Hon Seui Sek	Kansuiseki	Calcite
Calculus Bovis	***Bos taurus domesticus, Bubalis bubalis***	Niu Huang	Ngau Wong	Goo	Ox gallstone
Calculus Equi	***Equus caballos***	Ma Bao	Ma Bou		Horse bezoar
Calculus Macacae	***Macaca mulatta***	Hou Zao	Hau Jou	Koso	Macaque bezoar
Calomelas	***Calomelas***	Qing Fen	Ching Fan	Keifun	Calomel
Calyx Diospyri	***Diospyros kaki***	Shi Di	Chi Dai	Shitei	Persimmon calyx
Calyx seu fructus Physalis	***Physalis alkekengi (var. franchetii)***	Suan Jiang, Jing Deng Long	Syun Jeung, Ching Dang Lung		Chinese lantern calyx or fruit
Camphora	***Cinnamomum camphora***	Zhang Nao	Jeung Naau	Shono	Camphor flake
Cantharis	***Cantharis vesicatoria***	Ban Mao	Ban Mou	Hanmyo	Cantharides
Caput Angelicae sinensis	***Angelica sinensis, A. acutiloba***	Dang Gui Tou	Dong Gwai Tou	Tokito	Dong quai head
Carapax Amydae seu Trionis	***Amyda sinensis, Trionix sinensis***	Bie Jia	Bit Gaap	Bekko	Asian soft-shell turtle shell
Catharsius seu Xylotrupes	***Catharsius molossus, Xylotrupes dichotomus***	Jiang Lan Chong	Jeung Long Chung		Dung beetle
Cauda Cervi	***Cervus nippon*** and spp	Lu Wei Ba	Luk Mei Ba		Mature deer tail
Caudex Musae	***Musa basjoo***	Ba Jiao Gen	Ba Jiu Gan		Ryukyu banana root
Caulis Trachelospermi	***Trachelospermum jasminoides***	Luo Shi Teng	Lok Sek Tang	Chikusekito	Star jasmine stem
Caulis Akebiae	***Akebia quinata, A. trifoliata***	Mu Tong, Bai Mu Tong	Baak Muk Tong	Mokutsu	Akebia stem

PHARMACEUTICAL	SCIENTIFIC	MANDARIN	CANTONESE	JAPANESE	ENGLISH
Caulis Aristolochiae contortae	***Aristolochia contorta, A. debilis***	Tian Xian Teng	Tin Sin Tang	Tensendo	Green birthwort stem
Caulis Aristolochiae manshuriensis	***Aristolochia manshuriensis, A. moupinensis***	Guan Mu Tong	Gwaan Muk Tung		Manchurian birthwort stem
Caulis bauhiniae championi	***Bauhinia championi***	Jiu Long Teng, Wu Teng	Gaau Lung Tang, Lung Sou Tang		Bauhinia stem
Caulis Cissi	***Cissus pteroclada***	Kuan Jin Teng	Gwan Gam Tang		Cissus stem
Caulis Clematis montanae	***Clematis montana, C. armandii***	Chuan Mu Tong	Chyun Muk Tong		Mountain clematis stem
Caulis Cucumis	***Cucumis melo***	Tian Gua Di	Tim Gwa Dai	Katei	Young cantaloupe stalk
Caulis Dendrobii miniliformis	***Dendrobium moniliforme***	Xi Jing Shi Hu, Xiao Wan Chai	Sai Ging Sek Wu		Stonebushel stem
Caulis et folium Mussaendae	***Mussaenda pubescens, M. parviflora***	Shan Gan Cao	Saan Gam Chou		Mountain licorice stem and leaf
Caulis et folium Photiniae	***Photinia serrulata***	Shi Nan Teng, Shi Nan Ye	Sek Naam Tang, Sek Naam Yip		Photinia stem or leaf
Caulis et folium Sambuci chinensis	***Sambucus chinensis* and spp**	Shuo Zhuo	Sok Dik		Chinese elder stem and leaf
Caulis et folium Sambuci formosanae	***Sambucus formosana/taiwa niana***	Mao Gu Xiao	Mon Gwat Siu		Taiwan elder stem and leaf
Caulis et folium Sambuci javanici	***Sambucus javanica***	Shuo Diao	Sok Duk		Java elder stem and leaf
Caulis et folium Skimmiae	***Skimmia reevesiana, S. japonica***	Yin Yu	Yan Wu		Skimmia stem and leaf
Caulis et radix Gymnemae	***Gymnema sylvestre* and spp**	Wu Xue Teng	Mou Heu Tang		Gymnema stem and root
Caulis Kadsurae coccineae	***Kadsura coccinea***	Fan Tuan Teng	Faan Tyun Tang		Scarlet kadsura stem
Caulis Kadsurae heteroclitae	***Kadsura heteroclita***	Hai Feng Teng	Hoi Fung Tang		Heteroclite kadsura stem
Caulis Parthenocissi	***Parthenocissus tricuspidata***	Pa Shan Hu, Di Jin	Pa San Fu, Dei Gam		Japanese creeper stem
Caulis Phyllostachis in taeniis	***Phyllostachys nigra* var. *henonis* and spp**	Zhu Ru	Juk Yu	Chikujo	Black bamboo shaving
Caulis Piperis squamiglandiferi	***Piper hancei* var. *squamiglandiferu m***	Hai Feng Teng, Xian Lin Ju	Hoi Fung Tang		Fujian kadsura pepper stem
Caulis Piperis hanceis	***Piper hancei***	Hai Feng Teng	Hoi Fung Tang		Kadsura pepper stem
Caulis Polygoni multiflori	***Polygonum multiflorum***	Ye Jiao Teng	Ye Gou Tang	Yakoto	Flowery knotweed stem
Caulis Rubiae cordifoliae	***Rubia cordifolia***	Lu Gu Dan	Lu Gwat Daan		Heart-leaf madder stem
Caulis Sargentodoxae	***Sargentodoxa cuneata***	Da Xue Teng	Daai Hyut Tang		Sargentodoxa stem
Caulis Solani dulcamari	***Solanum dulcamara***	Ku Qie	Fu Ke		Bittersweet stem
Caulis Spatholobi	***Spatholobus suberectus***	Ji Xue Teng, Mi Hua Dou	Gai Yut Tang, Mat Fa Dau		Spatholobus stem

PHARMACEUTICAL	SCIENTIFIC	MANDARIN	CANTONESE	JAPANESE	ENGLISH
Caulis Stephaniae japonicae	***Stephania japonica***	Qian Jin Teng	Chin Gam Tang		Japanese stephania stem
Caulis Stephaniae sinicae	***Stephania sinica***	Jin Bu Huan	Gam Bat Wun		Chinese stephania stem
Caulis Tinosporae sinensis	***Tinospora sinensis***	Kuan Jin Teng	Gwan Gam Tang	Kankinto	Chinese tinospora stem
Caulis Vanieriae	***Vanieria cochinchinensis***	Huang Jin Kui, Chuan Po Shi	Wong Jin Kwai		Vanieria stem
Cera flava	***Apis cerana*** and spp	Feng La	Fung Laap		Beeswax
Cerussa	***Cerussa***	Qian Fen	Yun Fan		Cerusite
Chalcanthitum	***Chalcanthitum***	Dan Fan, Shi Dan	Daan Faan	Tanban	Crystallized blue vitriol
Chloris	***Chloris***	Jin Meng Shi	Gam Mein Sek		Mica schist
Chloris	***Chloris***	Qing Meng Shi	Ching Mein Sek		Chlorite schist
Cinnabarum	***Cinnabarum***	Zhu Sha	Ju Sa	Shusha	Cinnabar
Colla cornu Cervi	***Cervus nippon*** and spp	Lu Jiao Jiao	Luk Gok Gaau	Rokkakukyo	Mature deer antler glue
Colla piscis	***Acipenser sinensis, Miichthys*** spp	Yu Biao Jiao	Yu Biu Gaau		Fish airbladder
Compositum hydragyrum chloratum	***Hydragyrum chloratum***	Bai Jiang Dan	Baak Geung Dun		Mercury chloride
Compositum hydragyrum oxydatum crudum	***Hydragyrum chloratum***	San Xian Dan	Baak Gong Daan		Mercury oxide (crude)
Concha Arcae	***Arca inflata*** and spp	Wa Leng Zi	Nga Ling Ji	Garyoshi	Cockle shell
Concha Cyclinae	***Cyclina sinensis***	Hai Ge Ke, Ke Li	Hoi Gap Hok	Kaigokaku	Clam shell
Concha Cypraeae	***Cypraea moneta, C. macula*** and spp	Bei Zi	Chan Bu Chi		Cowrie shell
Concha Haliotis	***Haliotis diversicolor, H. gigantea*** and spp	Shi Jue Ming	Sek Kyut Ming	Sekketsumei	Abalone shell
Concha Mactrae	***Mactra sulcataria***	Ge	Hok	Jiseki	Mactra shell
Concha Metretris	***Meretrix meretrix***	Wen Ge	Man Gap		Asian venus clam shell
Concha Ostreae	***Ostrea gigas*** and spp	Mu Li	Mou Lai	Borei	Oyster shell
Concha Ostreae calcinati	***Ostrea gigas***	Duan Mu Li	Taan Mou Lai		Calcined oyster shell
Concha Pteriae	***Pteria margaritifera*** and spp	Zhen Zhu Mu	Chan Ju Mou		Mother of pearl shell
Concretio silicea bambusae	***Phyllostachys nigra*** var. ***henonis*** and spp	Tian Zhu Huang	Tin Juk Wong		Tabasheer
Corium Bovis	***Bos taurus domesticus, Bubalis bubalis***	Niu Pi	Ngau Pei		Ox hide
Corium Erinacei	***Erinaceaus europoeus, Hemichianum dauricus***	Ci Wei Pi	Chi Wai Pei		Hedgehog hide
Cornu Bubali	***Bubalus bubalis***	Shui Niu Jiao	Seui Ngau Gok		Water buffalo horn
Cornu Cervi	***Cervus nippon*** and spp	Lu Jiao	Luk Gok	Rokkaku	Mature deer antler
Cornu Cervi degelatinatum	***Cervus nippon*** and spp	Lu Jiao Shuang, Rong Mo	Luk Gok Shuen	Rokkakuso	Mature deer antler powder

PHARMACEUTICAL	SCIENTIFIC	MANDARIN	CANTONESE	JAPANESE	ENGLISH
Cornu cervi parvum	***Cervus nippon*** **and spp**	Lu Rong, Rong Tou, Nen Lu Rong	Luk Yan	Rokujo	Velvet deer antler
Cornu Naemorrhedis	***Naemorrhedis***	Shan Yang Jiao	San Yeung Gok	Sanyokaku	Goat horn
Cornu Rhinoceri	***Rhinoceros unicornis, R. bicornis***	Xi Jiao	Sai Gok		Rhinoceros horn
Cornu Saigae	***Saiga tatarica***	Ling Yang Jiao	Ling Yeung Gok	Reiyokaku	Antelope horn
Cortex Ailanthi	***Ailanthus altissima***	Chun (Bai) Pi	Chan (Baak) Pei		Tree of heaven bark
Cortex Albizziae	***Albizzia julibrissin, A. lebbak*** **and spp**	He Huan Pi	Hap Fun Pei	Gokanhi	Mimosa bark
Cortex Araliae elatate	***Aralia elata, A. elata*** **var.** ***suninermis***	Ci Lao Ya Pi	Chu Lou Nga	Taranoki	Aralia bark
Cortex Bauhiniae variegatae	***Bauhinia variegata***	Lao Bai Hua Pi	Lou Baak Fa Pei		Orchid tree bark
Cortex Betulae	***Betula platyphylla***	Hua Mu Pi	Wa Muk Pei		Asian birch bark
Cortex Catalpae	***Catalpa bungei***	Zi Bai Pi, Qiu Mu Pi	San Baak Pei, Chau Muk Pei		Catalpa bark
Cortex Cercis	***Cercis chinensis***	Zi Jing Pi	Ji Ging Pei		Chinese redbud bark
Cortex Cinchonae	***Cinchona succiruba*** **and spp**	Jin Ji Le, Jin Ji Na Pi	Gam Gai Laak		Cinchona bark
Cortex Cinnamomi cassiae	***Cinnamomum cassia***	Rou Gui (Pi)	Yuk Gwai (Pei)	Nikkei	Cassia Cinnamon bark
Cortex Cinnamomi japonici	***Cinnamomum japonicum, C. zeylanicum, C. obtusifolium***	Gui Pi	Gwai Pei		Cinnamon bark
Cortex Cinnamomi zeylanici	***Cinnamomum zeylanicum***	Rou Gui, Xi Lan Rou Gui	Yuk Gwai, Sek Laan Yuk Gwai		Ceylon cinnamon bark
Cortex Daphnis giraldii	***Daphne giraldii, D. tangutica, D. retusa***	Zu Shi Ma	Jou Si Ma		Giraldi's daphne bark
Cortex Erythrinae	***Erythrina variegata*** **var.** ***orientalis***	Hai Tong Pi	Hoi Tung Pei	Kaitohi	Asian coral tree bark
Cortex Eucommiae	***Eucommia ulmoides***	Du Zhong	Dou Jung	Tochu	Eucommia bark
Cortex Fraxini	***Fraxinus rhynchophyllae, F. bungeana, F. chinensis*** **and spp**	Qin Pi	Cheun Pei		Korean ash bark
Cortex Holarrheniae	***Holarrhenia antidysenterica***	Zhi Xie Mu Pi	Ji Se Muk Pei		Conessi bark
Cortex intimum Cinnamomi cassiae	***Cinnamomum cassia***	Rou Gui Xin	Yuk Gwai San		Cassia cinnamon inner bark
Cortex Kadsurae peltigerae	***Kadsura peltigera***	Zi Jing Pi	Ji Ging Pei		Chinese redbud bark
Cortex Loropetali	***Loropetalum chinense***	Ji Mu	Gai Muk		Strap flower bark
Cortex Magnoliae officinalis	***Magnolia officinalis, M. biloba, M. obovata***	Hou Po Chuan Po	Hau Pok, Chyun Pok	Koboku	Magnolia bark

PHARMACEUTICAL	SCIENTIFIC	MANDARIN	CANTONESE	JAPANESE	ENGLISH
Cortex Myricae rubrae	***Myrica rubra***	Yang Mei Pi	Yeung Miu Pei		Red bayberry bark
Cortex Phellodendris	***Phellodendron amurense, P. chinense***	Huang Bai Chuan Bai	Wong Paak Chyun Paak	Obaku	Siberian cork tree bark
Cortex Picrassiae	***Picrasma quassioides***	Ku Shu Pi	Fu Syu Pei		Quassiawood bark
Cortex Poriae	***Poria cocos***	Fu Ling Pi	Wong Ling Pei, Fuk Ling Pei	Bukuryoshi	Hoelen skin
Cortex Pruni	***Prunus jamasakura, P. yedoensis***	Ying Pi	Ying Pei	Ouhi	Plum tree bark
Cortex radicis Punicae	***Punica granatum***	Shi Liu Gen Pi	Sek Lau Gan Pei	Sekiryu-kombi	Pomegranate root bark
Cortex radicis Acanthopanacis gracilistylus	***Acanthopanax gracilistylus***	Wu Jia Pi, Xi Zhu Wu Jia	Ng Ga Pei, Sai Chu Ng Ga		Five additions root bark
Cortex radicis Acanthopanacis	***Acanthopanax gracilistylus, A. spinosus, A. sessiliflorus*** **and spp**	Wu Jia Pi	Ng Ga Pei	Gokahi	Five additions root bark
Cortex radicis Acanthopanacis trifoliati	***Acanthopanax trifoliatus***	Wu Jia Pi, Bai Le	Ng Ga Pei, Baak Lak		Three-leaf acanthopanax root bark
Cortex radicis Schizophragmae	***Schizophragma integrifolium***	Zuan Di Feng	Jyun Dei Fung		Schizophrag-ma root bark
Cortex radicis Ailanthi	***Ailanthus altissima***	Chun Gen Pi	Chan Gan Pei		Tree of heaven root bark
Cortex radicis Camptothecae	***Camptotheca acuminata***	Xi Shu	Hei Syu		Happy tree root bark
Cortex radicis Cedrelae	***Cedrela sinensis***	Chun Gen Bai Pi	Jung Gan Baak Pei		Cedrela root bark
Cortex radicis Dictamni	***Dictamnus dasycarpus***	Bai Xian Pi	Baak Sin Pei	Hakusempi	Asian dittany root bark
Cortex radicis Gossypii	***Gossypium hirsutum, G. herbaceum***	Mian Hua Gen	Min Fa Gan		Cotton root bark
Cortex radicis Hibisci syriacus	***Hibiscus syriacus***	Mu Jin Pi	Mut Gan Pei		Rose of Sharon root bark
Cortex radicis Lycii	***Lycium chinense***	Di Gu Pi	Dei Gwat Pei	Jikoppi	Wolfberry root bark
Cortex radicis Meliae	***Melia azedarach, M. toosendan***	Ku Lian (Gen) Pi	Fu Lin (Gan) Pei	Kurenkombi	Bead tree root bark
Cortex radicis Mori	***Morus alba***	Sang Bai Pi	Song Baak Pei	Sohakuhi	Mulberry root bark
Cortex radicis Paeoniae suffruticosae	***Paeonia suffruticosa***	Mu Dan Pi, Dan Pi	Maau Daan Pei, Daan Pei	Botanpi	Tree peony root bark
Cortex radicis Periplocae	***Periploca sepium***	Gang Liu Pi, Xiang Liu Pi	Gong Lau Pei , Heung Lau Pei		Silk vine root bark
Cortex radicis Pruni salicinae	***Prunus salicina***	Li Gen Bai Pi	Lei Gan Baak Pei		Willow plum root bark
Cortex radicis Pseudolaricis	***Pseudolarix amabilis. P. kaempferi***	Tu Jing Pi	Tou Ging Pei		Golden larch root bark
Cortex radicis Rosae cymosae	***Rosa cymosa***	Hong Ci Teng, Hong Gen, Xiao Jin Ying	Hung Chi Teng, Siu Gam Ying		Cymose rose root bark
Cortex radicis Sapii sebiferi	***Sapium sebiferum***	Wu Jiu (Mu) Gen Pi	Wu Kau Muk Gan Pei	Ukyukompi	Chinese tallow tree root bark

PHARMACEUTICAL	SCIENTIFIC	MANDARIN	CANTONESE	JAPANESE	ENGLISH
Cortex ramuli Osmanthi	***Osmanthus fragrans***	Gui Hua Pi	Gwai Fa Pei		Osmanthus twig bark
Cortex Rhudis chinensis	***Rhus chinensis***	Yan Fu Mu	Yim Fo Muk	Gobaishi	Chinese sumac bark
Cortex Sambuci japonici	***Sambucus japonicus***	Lu Ying		Rakutokuda	Japanese elder bark
Cortex Schefflerae octophyllae	***Schefflera octophylla***	Ya Jiao Mu Pi	Ngaap Geuk Muk Pei		Umbrella tree bark
Cortex Septemlobi	***Kalopanax septemlobus***	Chuan Tong Pi	Chyun Tung Pei		Kalopanax bark
Cortex Syringae	***Syringa manchuriensis***	Bao Ma Zi			Manchurian lilac bark
Cortex Ulmi parvifoliae	***Ulmus parvifolia***	Lang Yu Pi	Long Yu Pei		Chinese elm bark
Cortex Ulmi pumilae	***Ulmus pumila***	Yu Qian	Yu Chin		White elm bark
Cortex Zanthoxyli ailanthoidis	***Zanthoxylum ailanthoides***	Zhe Tong Pi	Jit Tung Pei		Zhejiang prickly ash bark
Crinis carbonisatus Hominis	***Homo sapiens***	Xue Yu Tan	Hyut Yu Taan		Charred human hair
Cyprinus	***Cyprinus carpio***	Li Yu	Lei Yu		Carp
Dens Stegodontis	***Stegodon orientalis et al.***	Long Chi	Lung Ji		Dragon tooth
Endothelium corneum gigeriae Galli	***Gallus gallus domesticus***	Ji Nei Jin	Gai Na Gam	Keinaikin	Chicken gizzard lining
Epicarpium Benincasae	***Benincasa hispida***	Dong Gua Pi	Dung Gwa Pei	Tokahi	Waxgourd fruit rind
Epicentrum seminis Nelumbinis	***Nelumbo nucifera***	Lian Zi Xin	Lin Ji Sam		Lotus seed heart
Ericerus	***Ericerus pela***	Chong Bai La	Chung Baak Laap		Ericerus worm
Eriocheir	***Eriocheir sinensis, E. japonicus***	Jin Xie	Jeun Haai	Zukani	Tianjin crab
Eulota	***Eulota peliomphala***	Gua Niu	Wo Ngau		Snail
Eupolyphaga	***Eupolyphaga sinensis***	Tu Bie Chong	Dei Bit Chung	Shachu	Cockroach
Excrementum Bombicis	***Bombyx mori***	Can Sha	Chaam Sa	Sansha	Silkworm dropping
Excrementum Lepi	***Lepus*** spp	Wang Yue Sha	Mong Yut Sa		Rabbit dropping
Excrementum Trogopteri seu Pteromi	***Trogopterus xanthipes*** and spp, ***Pteromys volans*** and spp	Wu Ling Zhi	Ng Ling Ji		Flying squirrel dropping
Excrementum Vespertilii	***Vespertilium murinum***	Ye Ming Sha	Ye Ming Sa	Yamyosha	Bat dropping
Exocarpium rubrum Citri	***Citrus grandis*** and spp	Ju Hong (Pi), Hua Ju Pi	Gwat Heung (Pei), Fa Gwat Pei		Red citrus outer rind
Extremas radicis Angelicae sinensis	***Angelica sinensis, A. acutiloba***	Dang Gui Wei	Dong Gwai Mai	Tokio	Dong quai tail
Extremas radicis Panacis ginsengis praeparatae	***Panax ginseng***	(Ren) Shen Xu	(Yan) Sam Son		Rock candy cured Asian ginseng root tail
Fasciculus vascularis Citri, Endocarpium Citri	***Citrus*** spp	Ju Luo, Ju Bai	Gwat Lok		Citrus fibre

PHARMACEUTICAL	SCIENTIFIC	MANDARIN	CANTONESE	JAPANESE	ENGLISH
Fasciculus vascularis Luffae	***Luffa cylindrica, L. acutangula***	Si Gua Luo	Si Gwa Lou	Shikaraku	Spongegourd
Fel Najae seu Bungari seu Elaphis	***Naja naja atra, Bungarus fasciatus, Elaphe radiata***	She Dan	Se Daam		Viper gallbladder
Fel Suidis	***Sus scrofa domestica***	Zhu Dan	Ju Daam		Pig gallbladder
Fel Ursi	***Ursus arctos*** **and spp**	Xiong Dan	Hung Daam	Yutan	Bear gallbladder
Fibra Stipulae Trachycarpi carbonisata	***Trachycarpus excelsa, T. fortunei***	Zong Lu Pi Tan	Jung Leui Pei Daan		Charred windmill palm petiole
Flos Adinae	***Adina rubella***	Shui Yang Mei	Seui Yeung Mui		Red modelwood flower
Flos Albizziae	***Albizzia julibrissin, A. lebbek*** **and spp**	He Huan Hua	Hap Fun Fa	Gokanka	Mimosa flower
Flos Amomi cardamomi	***Amomum cardamomum***	(Bai) Dou Kou Hua	(Baak) Dau Kau Fa	Byakuzu-kuka	Cluster cardamom flower
Flos Amomi villosi	***Amomum villosum***	Sha Ren Hua, (Yang) Chun Sha Hua	Sa Yan Fa, (Yeung) Chyun Sa Fa	Saninka	Wild cardamom flower
Flos Arecae catechu	***Areca catechu, A. dicksonii***	Bing Lang Hua	Ban Long Fa	Binroka	Betel nut flower
Flos Averrhoae	***Averrhoa carambola***	Yang Tao Hua	Yeung Tou Fa		Carambola flower
Flos Buddleiae	***Buddleia officinalis***	Mi Meng Hua	Mat Mung Fa	Mitsumoka	Buddleia flower and bud
Flos Camelliae japonicae	***Camellia japonica***	Shan Cha Hua	Saan Cha Fa		Common camellia flower
Flos Campsis grandiflorae	***Campsis grandiflora***	Ling Xiao Hua	Ling Siu Fa		Asian trumpetcree-per flower
Flos Campsis radicantis	***Campsis radicans***	Ling Xiao Hua, Mei Jou Ling Xiao	Ling Siu Fa, Mei Jau Ling Siu		Common trumpetcree-per flower
Flos Caraganae	***Caragana sinica*** **and spp**	Jin Que Hua	Gam Jeuk Fa		Caragana flower
Flos Carthami tinctorii	***Carthamus tinctorius***	Hong Hua	Hung Fa	Koka	Safflower
Flos Chimonanthi	***Chimonanthus praecox***	La Mei Hua	Laap Mui Fa	Sakubaika	Wintersweet flower
Flos Chrysanthemi	***Chrysanthemum x morifolium***	Ju Hua, Gan Ju Hua	Guk Fa		Chrysanthe-mum flower
Flos Chrysanthemi indici	***Chrysanthemum indicum***	Ye Ju Hua	Gam Guk Fa, Ye Guk Fa	Nogikuka	Wild chrysanthe-mum flower
Flos Citri grandi	***Citrus grandis*** **and spp**	Ju Hong Hua	Gwat Heung Fa		Citrus flower
Flos Citri sarctodactylis	***Citrus medica*** **var.** ***sarctodactylus***	Fo Shou (Gan) Hua	Fut Sao Fa	Bushukan	Finger lemon flower
Flos Daphnis genkwae	***Daphne genkwa***	Yuan Hua	Yun Fa	Genka	Lilac daphne flower
Flos Daphnis odorae	***Daphne odora***	Rui Xiang Hua	Seui Heung Fa		Mezerum flower
Flos Daturae	***Datura metel***	Yang Jin Hua	Yeung Gam Fa		Jimsonweed flower

PHARMACEUTICAL	SCIENTIFIC	MANDARIN	CANTONESE	JAPANESE	ENGLISH
Flos Desmodii umbellati	***Desmodium umbellatum***	Gu Su Hua	Gu Sou Fa		Umbel desmodium flower
Flos Edgeworthiae chrysanthae	***Edgeworthiae chrysantha***	Jie Xiang Hua, Meng Hua	Git Heung Fa, Mung Fa		Oriental paperbush flower
Flos Euphoriae	***Euphoria longan***	Long Yan Hua	Lung Ngaan Fa		Longan flower
Flos Fici	***Ficus carica***	Wu Hua Guo	Wu Fa Gwat		Fig flower
Flos Gomphrenae	***Gomphrena globosa***	Qian Ri Hong	Jin Yat Hung		Globe amaranth flower
Flos Gossampini	***Gossampinus malabarica***	Mu Mian Hua	Muk Min Fa		Silk cotton tree flower
Flos Hemerocallis	***Hemerocallis fulva***	Xuan Cao Hua	Syun Chou Fa		Tawny day lily flower
Flos Hibisci mutabili	***Hibiscus mutabilis***	Fu Rong Hua	Fu Yung Fa		Cotton rose flower
Flos Hibisci rosa-sinensis	***Hibiscus rosa-sinensis***	Fu Sang Hua	Fu Song Fa		Shoe flower
Flos Hibisci syriaci	***Hibiscus syriacus***	Mu Jin Hua	Mut Gan Fa		Rose of Sharon flower
Flos Humuli lupuli	***Humulus lupulus***	Pi Jiu Hua	Be Jau Fa		Hops flower
Flos Hydrangeae	***Hydrangea macrophylla***	Ba Xian Hua	Baat Sin Fa		French hydrangea flower
Flos Hylocerei	***Hylocereus undatus***	Jian Hua, Ba Wang Hua	Gim Fa		Cereus flower
Flos Impatiensis	***Impatiens balsamina***	Ji Xing Hua	Jek Chin Fa		Garden balsam flower
Flos Imperatae	***Imperata cylindrica*** var. ***major***	Bai Mao Hua	Baak Maau Fa		Woolly grass flower
Flos Inulae	***Inula japonica, I. brittanica, I. linariaefolia***	Xuan Fu Hua	Syun Fuk Fa	Sembukuka	Elecampane flower
Flos Jasmini officinalis	***Jasminum officinale*** var. ***grandiflorum***	Su Xin Hua	Sou Hing Fa		Jasmine flower
Flos Jasmini sambacis	***Jasminum sambac***	Mo Li Hua	Mut Lei Fa		Jasmine sambac flower
Flos Junci	***Juncus effusus***	Deng Xin Hua	Ding Sam Fa		Bulrush flower
Flos Lilii	***Lilium brownii*** var. ***colchesteri***	Bai He Hua	Baak Hap Fa		Brown's lily flower
Flos Lithospermi	***Lithospermum erythrorhizon***	Zi Cao Rong	Ji Chou Yan		Purple groomwell flower
Flos Lonicerae confusae	***Lonicera confusa***	Tu Yin Hua, Shan Yin Hua	Tou Ngan Fa		Wild honeysuckle flower
Flos Lonicerae japonicae	***Lonicera japonica***	Jin Yin Hua, Ren Dong Hua	Gam Ngan Fa Yan Dung Fa	Kinginka	Japanese honeysuckle flower
Flos Loropetali	***Loropetalum chinense***	Ji Hua	Gai Fa		Strap flower
Flos Magnoliae officinalis	***Magnolia officinalis, M. biloba, M. obovata***	Hou Po Hua	Hau Pok Fa	Koboka, Kobokuka	Magnolia flower
Flos Micheliae	***Michelia alba***	Bai Lan Hua	Baak Laan Fa		White champac flower
Flos Nelumbinis	***Nelumbo nucifera***	Bai Lian Hua	Baak Lin Fa		Lotus flower

PHARMACEUTICAL	SCIENTIFIC	MANDARIN	CANTONESE	JAPANESE	ENGLISH
Flos Panacis ginsengis	*Panax ginseng*	Ren Shen Hua	Yan Sam Fa		Asian ginseng flower
Flos Panacis notoginsengis	*Panax notoginseng*	San Qi Hua	Saam Chat Fa	Sanshishika	Pseudoginseng flower
Flos Paulowniae	*Paulownia tomentosa*	Pao Tong Hua	Pau Tung Fa		Paulownia flower
Flos Petasitis	*Petasites japonicus*	Feng Dou Cai	Fung Dau Choi		Japanese butterbur flower
Flos Phaseoli	*Phaseolus mungo*	Lu Dou Hua	Luk Dau Fa		Mung bean flower
Flos Plumeriae	*Plumeria rubra* var. *acutifolia*	Ji Dan Hua	Gai Daan Fa		Frangipani flower
Flos Pruni mumis	*Prunus mume*	Lu Er Mei, Lu Mei Hua	Lat Mui Fa		Black plum flower
Flos Puerariae	*Pueraria lobata, P. omeiensis* and spp	Ge Hua	Got Fa		Kudzu flower
Flos Pyrethri	*Pyrethrum cinerariifolium*	Chu Chong Ju	Cheui Chung Guk		Dalmatia pellitory flower
Flos Rhododendri mollis	*Rhododendron molle*	Nao Yang Hua, Huang Du Juan	Naau Yeung Fa, Wong Dou Gun		Yellow azalea flower
Flos Rosae rugosae	*Rosa rugosa*	Mei Gui Hua	Mui Gwai Fa	Maikaika	Japanese rose flower
Flos Sedi erythrostici	*Sedum erythrosticum*	Jing Tian Hua	Ging Ting Fa		Red stonecrop flower
Flos Sophorae japonicae	*Sophora japonica*	Huai Hua	Waai Fa		Japanese pagoda tree flower
Flos Spilanthis	*Spilanthes acmella* var. *oleracea*	Liu Shen Hua	Lau Sam Fa		Six god flower
Flos Tagetis	*Tagetes erecta*	Wan Shou Ju	Maan Sau Guk		African marigold flower
Flos Tiliae	*Tilia cordata*	Duan Shu Hua			Linden flower
Flos Tussilaginis	*Tussilago farfara*	Kuan Dong Hua	Fun Dung Fa	Kantoka	Coltsfoot flower
Flos Wikstroaemiae chamaedaphnis	*Wikstroemia chamaedaphne*	Rao Hua	Iu Fa		Wikstroemia flower
Fluoritum	*Fluoritum*	Zi Shi Ying	Ji Sek Ying		Purple fluorite
Folium Clerodendronis bungeis	*Clerodendron bungei*	Chou Mu Dan	Chau Maau Daan		Bung's Clerodendron leaf
Folium Agavis americanae	*Agave americana*	Jin Bian Long She Lan	Gam Bin Lung Sit Laan		Agave leaf
Folium Andrographis	*Andrographis paniculata*	Chuan Xin Lian	Chyun Sam Lin	Senshinren	Heart-thread lotus leaf
Folium Artemisiae argyi	*Artemisia argyi*	Ai Ye	Ngaai Yang, Ngaai Yip	Gaiyo	Asian mugwort leaf
Folium at semen Actinostemmae	*Actinostemma lobata*	He Zi Cao	Hap Ji Chou		Actinostemma leaf and seed
Folium Aurantium	*Citrus* spp.	Ju Ye	Gwat Yip		Citrus leaf
Folium Auri	*Aurum*	Jin Bo	Gam Bok		Gold foil
Folium Baphicacanthi	*Baphicacanthus cusia*	Ma Lan Ye	Ma Laam Yip	Banranyo	Assam indigo leaf
Folium Callicarpae macrophyllae	*Callicarpa macrophylla*	Zi Zhu Ye, Ta Ye Zi Zhu	Ji Jyu Yip, Daai Yip Ji Jyu		Large-leaf Callicarpa leaf
Folium Callicarpae pedunculatae	*Callicarpa pedunculata*	Zi Zhu Ye	Ji Jyu Yip	Jijuso	Callicarpa leaf

PHARMACEUTICAL	SCIENTIFIC	MANDARIN	CANTONESE	JAPANESE	ENGLISH
Folium Camelliae sinensis	***Camellia sinensis***	Cha Ye	Cha Yip	Fujucha, Chayo	Tea leaf
Folium Cassiae alatae	***Cassia alata***	Dui Ye Dou Ye	Deui Yip Dau Yip		Ringworm bush leaf
Folium Centellae	***Centella asiatica***	Ji Xue Cao, Peng Da Wan	Jik Syut Chou, Pang Daai Yan		Gotu kola leaf
Folium Citri grandi immaturi	***Citrus grandis***	You Ye	Yau Yip		Pomelo leaf
Folium Clauseniae	***Clausenia lansium***	Huang Pi Ye	Wong Pei Yip		Wampi leaf
Folium Clerodendronis cyrtophylli	***Clerodendron cyrtophyllum***	Da Qing Ye	Daai Cheng Yip		Green-white clerodendron leaf
Folium Clerodendronis inermis	***Clerodendron inerme***	Shui Hu Man	Seui Wu Mun		Glorybower leaf
Folium Clerodendronis trichotomi	***Clerodendron trichotomum***	Chou Wu Tong (Ye)	Chau Ng Tung (Yip)		Forked glorybower leaf
Folium Coriariae	***Coriaria sinica***	Ma Sang Ye	Ma Song Yip		Coriaria leaf
Folium Cratoxyli	***Cratoxylon ligustrinum***	Huang Niu Cha	Wong Ngau Cha		Cratoxylon leaf
Folium Cycadis	***Cycas revoluta***	Tie Shu	Tit Syu		Sago palm leaf
Folium Cymbidii	***Cymbidium ensifolium***	Jian Lan Ye	Gin Laan Yip		Cymbidium orchid leaf
Folium Dalbergiae hupeanae	***Dalbergia hupeana***	Tan Gen	Taan Gan		Hupei rosewood
Folium Dichroae	***Dichroa febrifuga***	Shu Qi	Suk Chat	Shokushitsu	Feverflower leaf
Folium Diospyri	***Diospyros kaki***	Shi Ye	Chi Yip		Persimmon leaf
Folium Eleagni pungensis	***Eleagnus pungens***	Hu Tui (Zi) Ye	Wu Teui (Ji) Yip		Thorny eleagnus leaf
Folium Epimedii	***Epimedium saggitatum, E. macranthum*** and spp	Yin Yang Huo, Xian Ling Pi	Yam Yeung Fok, Sin Ling Pei	Inyokaku	Horny goat weed leaf
Folium Eriobotryae	***Eriobotrya japonica***	Pi Pa Ye	Pei Pa Yip	Biwayo	Loquat leaf
Folium et caulis Schefflerae	***Schefflera arboricola, S. kwangsiensis, S. venulosa***	Qi Ye Lian	Chat Yip Lin		Taiwan schefflera leaf and stem
Folium et radix Ilicis asprellae	***Ilex asprella***	Gang Mei (Gen), Wang Dian Jing	Gong Mui Gan, Maan Dim Gam		Rough holly leaf and root
Folium et semen Thevetiae	***Thevetia peruviana***	Huang Hua Jia Zhu Tao (Ye)	Wong Fa Gaap Juk Tou (Yip)		Peruvian thevetia leaf and seed
Folium Eucalypti globuli	***Eucalyptus globulus***	An Ye	Ngon Yip		Eucalyptus leaf
Folium Eucommiae	***Eucommia ulmoides***	Du Zhong Ye	Dou Jung Yip		Eucommia leaf
Folium Ginkgoidis	***Ginkgo biloba***	Yin Xing Ye, Bai Guo Ye	Ngan Hang Yip, Baak Gwo Yip	Ginkyoyo	Ginkgo leaf
Folium Gynurae	***Gynura segetum***	San Qi Cao, Ju San Qi	Sam Chat Chou		Canton sanchi leaf
Folium Hibisci mutabilis	***Hibiscus mutabilis***	Fu Rong Ye	Fu Yung Yip		Cotton rose leaf
Folium Hydrangeae	***Hydrangea serrata*** var. ***thunbergii***	Gan Cha	Gam Cha	Amatya, Dochouzan	Sweet tea leaf

PHARMACEUTICAL	SCIENTIFIC	MANDARIN	CANTONESE	JAPANESE	ENGLISH
Folium Ilicis chinensis	***Ilex chinensis***	Si Ji Qing, Dong Qing Ye	Sei Gwai Ching, Dung Ching Yip		Wintergreen holly leaf
Folium Ilicis cornutae	***Ilex cornuta***	Gou Gu Ye	Gau Gwat Yip		Cat thorn holly leaf
Folium Ilicis latifoliae	***Ilex latifolia***	Ku Ding Cha	Fu Ding Cha		Broadleaf holly leaf
Folium Ilicis rotundis	***Ilex rotunda***	Jiu Bi Ying	Gau Bit Ying		Round-leaf holly leaf
Folium Indigoferae	***Indigofera tinctoria***	Mu Lan Ye	Muuk Laam Yip		Indigo leaf
Folium Isatis indigoticae	***Isatis indigotica***	Song Lan Ye	Song Laan Yip		Woad leaf
Folium Isatis tinctoriae	***Isatis tinctoria***	Da Qing Ye	Daai Ching Yip		Woad leaf
Folium Juglandis	***Juglans regia***	Hu Tao Ye	Wu Tou Yip		Walnut leaf
Folium Lopatheri	***Lopatherum gracile***	Dan Zhu Ye	Daam Juk Yip	Tanchikuyo	Bamboo grass leaf
Folium Lycii chinensis	***Lycium chinense, L. barbarum***	Gou Qi Ye	Gau Ji Yip		Wolfberry leaf
Folium Mahoniae bealei	***Mahonia bealei***	Shi Da Gong Lao Ye, Kuo Ye Shi Da Gong Lao Ye	Sap Daai Gung Lou Yip, Fut Yip Sap Daai Gung Lou Yip	Judaikoro	Leather-leaf mahonia leaf
Folium Mahoniae fortunei	***Mahonia fortunei***	Shi Da Gong Lao Ye, Xi Ye Shi Da Gong Lao Ye	Gung Lou Yip, Sai Yip Sap Daai Gung Lou Yip	Judaikoro	Mahonia leaf
Folium Marsileae	***Marsilea quaddrifolia***	Ping	Ping		European water clover leaf
Folium Melaleucae leucadendronis	***Melaleuca leucadendron***	Bai Qian Ceng	Baak Chin Chang		Cajeput leaf
Folium Menyanthis	***Menyanthes trifoliata***	Shui Cai Ye	Seui Choi Yip	Suisayo, Meisai	Bogbean leaf
Folium Microcotis	***Microcos paniculata***	Bu Zha Ye	Bou Jai Yip		Microcos leaf
Folium Momordicae grosvenorii	***Momordica grosvenori***	Luo Han Ye	Lou Haan Yip	Rakankayo	Arhat leaf
Folium Mori	***Morus alba***	Sang Ye	Song Yip	Soyo	Mulberry leaf
Folium Nandinae	***Nandina domestica***	(Nan) Tian Zhu Ye	(Naam) Tin Juk Yip		Sacred bamboo leaf
Folium Nelumbinis	***Nelumbo nucifera***	He Ye, Lian Lie	Ho Yip	Kayo	Lotus leaf
Folium Nerii	***Nerium indicum***	Jiao Zhu Tao Ye	Gap Juk Tou Yip		Indian oleander leaf
Folium Panacis ginsengis	***Panax ginseng***	Ren Shen Ye	Yan Sam Yip	Ninjinyo	Asian ginseng leaf
Folium Perillae	***Perilla frutescens***	Zi Su Ye	Sou Yip	Shisoyo	Perilla leaf
Folium Phyllostachis	***Phyllostachys nigra* var. *henonis* and spp**	Zhu Ye	Juk Yip		Black bamboo leaf
Folium Piperis betlis	***Piper betle***	Ju Jiang Ye, Qing Lou Ye	Geui Jeung Yip		Betel pepper leaf
Folium Pistaciae	***Pistacia chinensis***	Huang Lian Ya	Wong Lin Nga		Pistachio leaf
Folium Plantaginis	***Plantago asiatica, P. depressa* and spp**	Che Qian Cao	Che Chin Chou	Shazenso	Asian plantain leaf
Folium Pleioblasti	***Pleioblastus amarus***	Ku Zhu Ye	Fu Juk Yip		Bitter bamboo leaf
Folium Psidii	***Psidium guajava***	Fan Shi Liu Gan Ye	Faan Sek Lau Gon Yip		Guava leaf

PHARMACEUTICAL	SCIENTIFIC	MANDARIN	CANTONESE	JAPANESE	ENGLISH
Folium Pyrrosiae	***Pyrrosia lingua, P. petiolosa*** **and spp**	Shi Wei	Sek Wai		Felt fern leaf
Folium Pyrrosiae sheareri	***Pyrrosia sheareri***	Shi Wei, Lu Shan Shi Wei	Sek Wai, Lou San Sek Wai	Sekii	Shearer's felt fern leaf
Folium Querci	***Quercus salicina, Q. myrsinaefolium***	Zhu Zi Ye	Jyu Ji	Urajirokashi	Oak leaf
Folium Raphani	***Raphanus sativus***	Luo Bo Ye	Lo Ba Yip		Radish leaf
Folium Rhododendri daurici	***Rhododendron dauricum, R. mariesii***	Man Shan Hong	Mun Saan Hung		Daurian rhododendron leaf
Folium Rubi parvifolii	***Rubus parvifolius***	Mao Mei, Hao Tian Biao	Mau Mui		Small-leaf raspberry leaf
Folium Salicis	***Salix babylonica, S. gracilistyla***	Liu Ye	Lau Yip		Weeping willow twig
Folium Sauropi	***Sauropus rostratus, S. changianus***	Long Li Ye	Lung Lei Yip		Lizardtail leaf
Folium Sennae	***Senna acutifolia, S. angustifolia***	Fan Xie Ye	Faan Sie Yip		Senna leaf
Folium Viticis negundonis	***Vitex negundo*** **var. *cannabifolia***	Mu Jing Ye	Maau Ging Yip		Five-leaf chastetree leaf
Fructrus Aesculi	***Aesculus wilsonii, A. chinensis***	Suo Luo Zi	So Lo Ji		Chinese horse chestnut
Fructus Actinidiae chinensis	***Actinidia chinensis***	Mi Hou Tao, Teng Li	Nei Hau Tou		Kiwi fruit
Fructus Actinidiae chinensis	***Actinidia chinensis***	Teng Li Gen	Tang Li Gan		Kiwi root
Fructus Ailanthi	***Ailanthus altissima***	Feng Yen Cao	Fung Ngaan Chou		Tree of heaven fruit
Fructus Akebiae	***Akebia quinata***	Ba Yue Zha, Yu Zhi Zi	Baat Yut Jaat, Yu Ji Ji		Akebia fruit
Fructus Alpiniae Galangae	***Alpinia galanga***	Hong Dou Kou	Hung Dau Kau		Greater galangal berry
Fructus Alpiniae oxyphyllae	***Alpinia oxyphylla***	Yi Zhi Ren	Yik Ji Yan	Yakuchinin	Sharp-leaf galangal berry
Fructus Alpiniae zerumbetsis	***Alpinia zerumbet***	Da Cao Kou	Daai Chou Kau		Beautiful galangal berry
Fructus Amomi cardamomi	***Amomum cardamomum***	Bai Dou Kou	Baak Dau Kau	Byakuzuku	Cluster cardamom pod
Fructus Amomi longiligularis	***Amomum longiligulare***	Sha Ren, Hai Nan Sha Ren	Sai Yan, Hoi Naam Sa Yan		Hainan cardamom pod
Fructus Amomi tsao-konis	***Amomum tsao-ko***	Cao Guo (Ren)	Chou Gwat (Yan)	Soka	Cochin cardamom fruit
Fructus Amomi villosi	***Amomum villosum***	Sha Ren, (Yang) Chun Sha Ren	Sa Yan, (Yeung) Chyun Sa Yan	Sanin	Wild cardamom pod (fruit)
Fructus Amomi xanthioidis	***Amomum xanthioides***	Sha Ren, Suo Sha Mi	Sa Yan, Suk Sa Mat		Cocklebur cardamom pod
Fructus Arctii	***Arctium lappa***	Niu Bang Zi	Ngau Pong Ji	Goboshi	Burdock seed
Fructus Aristolochiae	***Aristolochia contorta, A. debilis***	Ma Dou Ling	Ma Dau Ling	Batorei	Green birthwort capsule
Fructus Artemisiae keiskeanae	***Artemisia keiskeana***	An Lu Zi	Am Leui Ji		Keiskeana mugwort seed
Fructus Averrhoae	***Averrhoa carambola***	Yang Tao	Yeung Tou		Carambola fruit

PHARMACEUTICAL	SCIENTIFIC	MANDARIN	CANTONESE	JAPANESE	ENGLISH
Fructus Broussonetiae	***Broussonetia papyrifera***	Chu Shi Zi	Chyu Sat Ji		Paper mulberry fruit
Fructus Bruceae	***Brucea javanica***	Ya Dan Zi	Nga Daan Ji	Atanshi	Brucea berry
Fructus Camptothecae	***Camptotheca acuminata***	Xi Shu Guo	Hei Syu Gwo		Happy tree seed
Fructus Canarii	***Canarium album***	Gan Lan, Jing Guo	Gaam Laam		Asian olive fruit
Fructus Castaneae	***Castanea mollissima***	Li Zi, Feng Li Gu	Leut Ji	Furitsukaku	Chinese chestnut
Fructus Catalpae	***Catalpa ovata***	Zhi Shi	San Sat	Kisasage	Catalpa fruit
Fructus Chaenomelis lagenariae	***Chaenomeles lagenaria***	Mu Gua, Chuan Mu Gua	Muk Gwa, Chyun Muk Gwa	Mokka	Chinese quince fruit
Fructus Chaenomelis sinensis	***Chaenomeles sinensis***	Mu Gua, Ming Za	Muk Gwa		Chinese quince fruit
Fructus Chaenomelis speciosae	***Chaenomeles speciosa***	Mu Gua, Tie Geng Hai Tang	Muk Gwa, Tip Gang Hoi Teng		Flowering quince fruit
Fructus Citri aurantii amarae	***Citrus aurantium*** var. ***amara***	Zhi Ke, Zhi Qiao, Dai Dai Hua Zhi Qiao	Ji Hok, Doi Doi Fa Ji Hok	Kikoku	Ripe bitter orange fruit
Fructus Citri aurantii immaturi	***Citrus aurantium, C. wilsonii***	Zhi Shi	Ji Sat	Kijitsu	Unripe bitter orange fruit
Fructus Citri grandi immaturi	***Citrus grandis*** and spp.	Ju Hong Zhu	Gwat Heung		Unripe citrus fruit
Fructus Citri medicae	***Citrus medica*** var. ***sarcodactylis***	Fo Shou (Gan)	Fut Sau (Gam)		Finger lemon fruit
Fructus Citri medicae	***Citrus medica, C. wilsonii***	Xiang Yuan, Gou Yuan	Heung Yun		Citron fruit
Fructus Citri sinensis	***Citrus sinensis***	Tian Chen	Tim Chaang		Sweet orange fruit
Fructus Citrulli	***Citrullus vulgaris***	Xi Gua	Sai Gwa	Seika	Watermelon fruit
Fructus Cnidii	***Cnidium monnieri***	She Chuang Zi	Se Chong Ji	Jashoshi	Cnidium seed
Fructus conchae Pteriae	***Pteria margaritiferae***	Zhen Zhu	Chan Ju	Shinju	Pearl
Fructus Coriandri	***Coriandrum sativum***	Yan Sui Zi	Yun Sai Ji		Coriander seed
Fructus Corni	***Cornus officinalis***	Shan Zhu Yu, Shan Yu Rou	San Jyu Yu, San Yu Yuk	Sanshuyu	Japanese dogwood berry
Fructus Crataegi	***Crataegus pinnatifida, C. cuneata*** and spp	Shan Zha (Rou)	Saan Ja (Yuk)	Sanzashi	Asian hawthorn berry
Fructus Crataegi carbonisatus	***Crataegus pinnatifida, C. cuneata*** and spp	Shan Zha Tan	Saan Ja Tan		Charred Asian hawthorn berry
Fructus Crataegus cuneatae	***Crataegus cuneata***	Ye Shan Zha	Ye Saan Ja		Wild hawthorn berry
Fructus Dauci	***Daucus carota***	Nan He Zao	Naam Hok Sat		Wild carrot seed
Fructus Diospyri	***Diospyros kaki***	Shi Shuang Bing	Chi Shuen Bing		Persimmon frosted fruit
Fructus Dipsaci	***Dipsacus chinensis*** and spp	Ju Sheng Zi	Geui Sing Ji		Chinese teasel fruit
Fructus Eriobotryae	***Eriobotrya japonica***	Pi Pa	Pei Pa		Loquat fruit
Fructus Eriocaulonis	***Eriocaulon buergerianum, E. sieboldianum***	Gu Jing Zi	Guk Jing Ji		Pipewort seed

PHARMACEUTICAL	SCIENTIFIC	MANDARIN	CANTONESE	JAPANESE	ENGLISH
Fructus Evodiae rutecarpae	***Evodia rutaecarpa***	Wu Zhu Yu	Ng Jyu Yu	Goshuyu	Evodia berry
Fructus Fici pumilae	***Ficus pumila***	Bi Li, Mu Man Tou	Bai La		Creeping fig fruit
Fructus Foeniculi	***Foeniculum vulgare***	Xiao Hui Xiang	Siu Wui Heung	Shouikyo	Fennel seed
Fructus Forsythiae	***Forsythia suspensa***	Lian Qiao	Lin Kiu	Rengyo	Forsythia valve
Fructus Gardeniae	***Gardenia jasminoides***	Zhi Zi Shan Zhi Zi	Ji Ji, Saan Ji Ji	Sanshishi	Gardenia pod
Fructus germinatus Hordei	***Hordeum vulgare***	Mai Ya	San Man Nga	Bakuga	Sprouted barley grain
Fructus germinatus Setariae	***Setaria italica***	Su Ya	Suk Nga		Sprouted millet grain
Fructus Ginkgoidis	***Ginkgo biloba***	Bai Guo, Yin Xing He	Baak Gwo, Ngan Hang Wat	Ginkyo	Ginkgo nut
Fructus Gleditsiae	***Gleditsia sinensis* and spp**	Zao Jiao, Zao Jia	Jou Gok, Jou Gaap	Sokaku	Honeylocust pod
Fructus Gymnocladi	***Gymnocladus chinensis***	Fei Zao Jia	Fei Jou Choi		Chinese gymnocladus berry
Fructus Hippophae	***Hippophae rhamnoides***	Sha Ji	Sa Jik		Sea buckthorn berry
Fructus Illicii	***Illicium verum***	Ba Jiao Hui Xiang	Baat Gok Wui Heung		Star anise fruit
Fructus Lagenariae	***Lagenaria siceraria***	Hu Lu Ke	Wu Lok Hok		Bottle gourd fruit
Fructus Ligustri	***Ligustrum japonicum, L. lucidum***	Nu Zhen Zi	Neui Jing Ji	Joteishi	Glossy privet berry
Fructus Liquidambaris	***Liquidambar taiwaniana***	Lu Lu Tong	Lou Lou Tung	Rorotsu	Taiwan maple fruit
Fructus Litseae	***Litsea cubeba***	Bi Cheng Qie	Bat Ching Ke		Cubeb peppercorn
Fructus Lycii	***Lycium chinense, L. barbarum***	Gou Qi Zi	Gau Gei Ji, Gei Ji	Kukoshi	Wolfberry
Fructus Meliae toosendanis	***Melia toosendan***	Chuan Lian Zi	Chyun Lin Ji		Sichuan bead tree berry
Fructus Melodini	***Melodinus suaveolens***	Shan Chen, Qu Tou Ji	Saan Chaang		Melodinus fruit
Fructus Metaplexis	***Metaplexis japonica***	Tian Qiang Ke	Tin Cheung Hok		Metaplexis fruit
Fructus Momordicae charantiae	***Momordica charantia***	Ku Gua (Gan)	Fu Gwa (Gam)		Bitter melon fruit
Fructus Momordicae grosvenorii	***Momordica grosvenori***	Luo Han Guo	Lou Haan Kwo	Rakanka	Arhat fruit
Fructus Mori	***Morus alba***	Sang Shen (Zi)	Song Sam (Ji)	Sojin	Mulberry fruit
Fructus Mumis immaturis preparatae	***Prunus mume***	Bai Mei	Baak Mui		Unripe prepared black plum fruit
Fructus Nandinae	***Nandina domestica***	(Nan) Tian Zhu Zi	(Naam) Tin Juk Ji		Sacred bamboo fruit
Fructus Narcissi	***Narcissus tazetta* var. *chinensis***	Shui Xian Zi	Seui Sin Ji		Chinese sacred lily seed
Fructus Nephelii	***Nephelium lappaceum***	Shao Zi	Siu Ji		Rambutan fruit

PHARMACEUTICAL	SCIENTIFIC	MANDARIN	CANTONESE	JAPANESE	ENGLISH
Fructus Ocimi	***Ocimum Basilicum***	Guang Ming Zi	Gwong Ming Ji		Basil seed
Fructus Oryzae	***Oryza sativa***	Nuo Mi	Lo Mai		Sweet rice
Fructus Oryzae	***Oryza sativa***	Jing Mi	Gang Mai		Rice grain
Fructus Oryzae fermentatus cum Monasco	***Oryza sativa*** and ***Monascus purpureus***	Hong Qu Mi	Hung Ju Mai		Fermented rice with red yeast
Fructus Oryzae germinatus	***Oryza sativa***	Gu Ya	Gu Nga	Kokuga	Sprouted rice grain
Fructus Perillae	***Perilla frutescens***	Zi Su Zi	Sou Ji	Soshi	Perilla seed
Fructus persicae immaturi	***Prunus persica, P. davidiana***	Bi Tao Gan			Unripe peach fruit
Fructus Piperis longis	***Piper longum***	Bi Ba	Bat Pa	Hihatsu	Long pepper fruit spike
Fructus Piperis nigri	***Piper nigrum***	Hu Jiao, Hei Hu Jiao	Wu Jiu, Mai Wu Jiu	Kosho	Black pepper corn
Fructus Polygoni hydropiperis	***Polygonum hydropiper***	Liao Shi	Lou Sek		Water pepper fruit
Fructus Polygoni orientalis	***Polygonum orientale***	Shui Tong Hua Zi	Seui Tung Fa Ji		Prince's feather berry
Fructus Ponciri	***Poncirus trifoliata***	Gou Ju	Gau Gwat		Trifoliate orange fruit
Fructus Ponciri immaturi	***Poncirus trifoliata***	Lu Yi Zhi Qiao, Gou Yuan	Luk Ji Ji Hok, Gau Yun		Immature trifoliate orange fruit
Fructus Pruni mumis	***Prunus mume***	Wu Mei (Rou)	Wu Mui (Yuk)	Ubai	Black plum fruit
Fructus Psoraleae	***Psoralea corylifolia***	Bu Gu Zhi	Bou Gwat Ji	Hokotsushi	Scurf pea berry
Fructus Querci acutissimae	***Quercus acutissima***	Xiang Shi	Jeung Sat		Oak fruit
Fructus Quisqualis	***Quisqualis indica***	Shi Jun Zi	Si Gwan Ji	Shikunshi	Rangoon creeper nut
Fructus Rhododendris mollis	***Rhododendron molle***	Ba Li Ma	Baat Lei Ma		Yellow azalea fruit
Fructus Rosae laevigatae	***Rosa laevigata***	Jin Ying Zi	Gam Ying Ji	Kinoshi	Cherokee rosehip
Fructus Rosae rugosae	***Rosa rugosa***	Mei Gui Zi	Mui Gwai Ji		Japanese rosehip
Fructus Rubi chingii	***Rubus chingii***	Fu Pen Zi	Fuk Pun Ji	Fukubonshi	Chinese raspberry fruit
Fructus Rubi coreani	***Rubus coreanus***	Dao Sheng Gen	Dou Sang Gan		Korean raspberry fruit
Fructus Schisandrae	***Schisandra chinensis***	Wu Wei Zi	Ng Mei Ji	Gomishi	Schisandra berry
Fructus Schisandrae sphenanterae	***Schizandra sphenantera***	Wu Wei Zi, Hua Zheng Wu Wei Zi	Ng Mei Ji, Wa Jung Ng Mei Ji	Gomishi	Central China schisandra berry
Fructus Sesami	***Sesamum indicum***	Hei Zhi Ma Hu Ma Ren	Hak Ji Ma		Black sesame seed
Fructus Setariae	***Setaria italica***	Xiao Mi	Suk Mai		Millet grain
Fructus seu semen Carpesii	***Carpesium abrotanoides***	He Shi	Hok Sat	Kakushitsu	Starwort fuit or seed
Fructus Sophorae flavescentis	***Sophora flavescens***	Ku Shen Zi	Fu Sam Ji		Yellow pagoda tree berry
Fructus Sophorae japonicae	***Sophora japonica***	Huai Jiao (Zi)	Wai Jiu (Ji)		Japanese pagoda tree fruit
Fructus Terminaliae	***Terminalia chebula*** and var.	He Zi (Rou)	Ho Ji (Yuk)	Kashi	Myrobalan fruit

PHARMACEUTICAL	SCIENTIFIC	MANDARIN	CANTONESE	JAPANESE	ENGLISH
Fructus Terminaliae immaturi	***Terminalia chebula*** and var.	Cang Qing Guo			Unripe myrobalan fruit
Fructus Thladianthae	***Thladiantha dubia***	Zhi Pao	Chek Pau		Thladiantha fruit
Fructus Trachycarpi	***Trachycarpus excelsa, T. fortunei***	Zong Lu Zi	Jung Leui Ji		Windmill palm seed
Fructus Trapae	***Trapa bispinosa, T. bicornis***	Ling Qiao	Ling Gok		Water caltrop fruit
Fructus Tribuli	***Tribulus terrestris***	Bai Ji Li	Baak Jat Lai	Byakishitsuri	Caltrop fruit
Fructus Tricosanthis	***Trichosanthes kirilowii, T. japonica, T. uniflora***	Gua Lou (Shi)	Kwut Lau	Karo	Snakegourd fruit
Fructus Tritici	***Triticum aestivum***	Fu Xiao Mai	Fau Siu Mak	Fushobaku	Wheat berry
Fructus Viticis negundonis	***Vitex negundo***	Huang Jing Zi	Wong Ging Ji		Negundo chastetree berry
Fructus Viticis negundonis	***Vitex negundo*** var. ***cannabifolia***	Mu Jing Zi	Maau Ging Ji		Five-leaf chastetree berry
Fructus Viticis rotundifoliae	***Vitex rotundifolia, V. trifolia***	Man Jing Zi	Maan Ging Ji	Mankeishi	Seashore chastetree berry
Fructus Xanthii	***Xanthium sibiricum, X. strumarium***	Cang Er Zi	Chong Yi Ji	Sojishi	Siberian cocklebur
Fructus Zanthoxyli bungeani	***Zanthoxylum bungeanum***	Chuan Jiao, Hua Jiao	Chyun Jiu, Fa Jiu	Shokusho	Sichuan peppercorn
Fructus Zanthoxyli planispini	***Zanthoxylum planispinum***	Zhu Ye Jiao	Juk Yip Jiu		Prickly ash berry
Fructus Zanthoxyli simulansis	***Zanthoxylum simulans***	Ye Hua Jiao	Ye Fa Jiu		Sichuan peppercorn
Fructus Zeae	***Zea mays***	Yu Shu Shu	Yuk Suk Syu		Corn grain
Fructus Zizyphi jujubae	***Zizyphus jujuba*** var. ***inermis***	Da Zao	Daai Jou	Taiso	Black jujube berry
Fructus Zizyphi jujubae	***Zizyphus jujuba*** var. ***inermis***	Hong Zao	Hung Jou	Koso	Red jujube berry
Fructus Zizyphi jujubae praeparatae	***Zizyphus jujuba*** var. ***inermis***	Mi Zao	Mat Jou		Honey-preserved jujube berry
Frusta Ferrum	***Ferrum***	Sheng Tie Luo	Sang Tit Lo		Iron filing/cinder
Funis umbilici Hominis	***Homo sapiens***	Qi Dai	Chi Daai		Umbilical cord
Galla fructi Actinidiae	***Actinidia polygama***	Mu Tian Lian	Muk Tin Lin	Mokutenryo	Actinidia gall
Galla Querci	***Quercus infectoria***	Mo Shi Zi	Mut Sik Ji		Oak gall
Galla Rhudis sinensis	***Rhus sinensis*** and spp, ***Schlechtendaria chinensis***	Wu Bei Zi	Ng Pan Ji		Chinese sumac gallnut
Galla Wisteriae	***Wisteria sinensis, W. floribunda***	Zi Teng Zi, Teng Liu	Ji Tang Ji, Tang Lau	Figikobu	Asian wisteria gall
Gecko	***Gecko gecko, G. verticilatus***	Ge Jie	Gap Gaai	Gokai	Toad-headed lizard
Gecko chinensis	***Gecko chinensis, G. japonicus*** and spp	Shou Gong, Bi Hu	Sau Gung, Bik Fu		House lizard

PHARMACEUTICAL	SCIENTIFIC	MANDARIN	CANTONESE	JAPANESE	ENGLISH
Gelatinum carapaxis Chinemis	***Chinemys reevesii***	Gui Ban Jiao	Gwai Baan Gaau		Tortoise shell gel
Gelatinum corii Equi asini	***Equus asinus*** **and spp**	E Jiao	O Gaau	Akyo	Ass hide glue
Gelatinum Macacae	***Macaca mulatta***	Hou Jiao	Hao Gaau		Macaque gel
Gelatinum Spatholobi	***Spatholobus suberectus***	Ji Xue Teng Jiao	Gai Yut Tang Gaau		Spatholobus gel
Gemma Agrimoniae pilosae	***Agrimonia pilosa*** **var. *japonica***	He Cao Ya	Hok Chou Nga		Furry agrimony winter bud
Gemma Cleistocalycis	***Cleistocalyx operculatus***	Shui Weng Hua	Seui Yung Fa		Cleistolcalyx bud
Gemma Dolichis	***Dolichos lablab***	Bian Dou Hua	Bin Dau Fa	Henzuka	Hyacinth bean bud
Gemma et radix Securinegae	***Securinega suffruticosa***	Yi Ye Qiu	Yat Yip Chau		Securinega shoot and root
Gemma Eugeniae	***Eugenia caryophyllata***	Ding Xiang	Ding Heung	Choko	Clove bud
Gemma Magnoliae	***Magnolia liliflora, M. denudata, M. yulan*** **and spp**	Xin Yi Hua	San Yi Fa	Shinika	Yulan magnolia bud
Gemma Rosae chinensis	***Rosa chinensis***	Yue Ji Hua	Yut Gwai Fa	Gekkika	Moonseason rose bud
Gemma Sophorae japonicae	***Sophora japonica***	Huai (Hua) Mi	Waai (Fa) Mai		Japanese pagoda tree bud
Granum floris pollinis	***Pollen***	Feng Hua Fen	Fung Fa Fan		Flower (bee) pollen
Gryllulus	***Gryllulus chinensis, G. mitratus, Gampsocleis buergeri***	Xi Shuai	Sik Seut		Cricket
Gypsum	***Gypsum fibrosum***	Shi Gao	Sek Gou	Sekko	Gypsum
Gypsum dehydratum	***Gypsum fibrosum***	Shu Shi Gao	Chek Sek Gou		Dehydrated gypsum
Gypsum rubrum	***Gypsum rubrum***	Han Shui Shi, Hong Shi Gao	Hon Seui Sek, Hung Sek Gau		Red gypsum
Haematitum	***Haematitum***	Dai Zhe Shi	Doi Jyu Sek	Taishaseki	Hematite
Halitum	***Halitum***	Da Qing Yan	Daai Ching Yim		Rock salt
Halloysitum	***Halloysitum rubrum***	Chi Shi Zhi	Chek Sek Chi	Shakuse-kishi	Red kaolin
Halloysitum	***Halloysitum rubrum***	Shu Chi Shi	Chek Sek Ji		Roasted red kaolin
Halloysitum album	***Halloysitum album***	Bai Shi Zhi	Baak Sek Ji		White kaolin
Herba Adenostemmae	***Adenostemma lavenia***	Ma Zhi Hu, Feng Qi Cao	Ma Ji Wu, Fung Hei Chou		Adenostemma herb
Herba Clerodendranthi	***Clerodendranthus spicatus***	Mao Xu Cao	Maau Sao Chou		Orthosiphon herb
Herba Cymbopogonis	***Cymbopogon citratus***	Xiang Mao	Heung Maau		Lemongrass herb
Herba Cymbopogonis distansis	***Cymbopogon distans***	Yun Xiang Cao	Yun Heung Chou		Distant lemongrass herb
Herba Ephemeranthae	***Ephemerantha fimbriata***	Shi Hu	Sek Hap	Sekkoku	Ephemerantha stem
Herba Euphorbiaehelioscopiae	***Euphorbia helioscopia***	Ze Qi	Jaak Chat	Takushitsu	Sunspurge herb

PHARMACEUTICAL	SCIENTIFIC	MANDARIN	CANTONESE	JAPANESE	ENGLISH
Herba Abri	***Abrus precatorius, A. cantoniensis***	Ji Gu Cao	Gai Gwat Chou		Licorice bean herb
Herba Abutilonis indici	***Abutilon indicum***	Mo Pan Cao, Mi Lan Cao	Mo Bun Chou		Country mallow herb
Herba Acalyphae	***Acalypha australis***	Tie Xian (Cai)	Tit Yin		Annual copperleaf herb
Herba Adenosmae glutinosi	***Adenosma glutinosum***	Mao She Xiang	Mou Se Heung		Adenosma herb
Herba Adonis	***Adonis amurensis***	Fu Shou Cao	Fuk Sau Chou		Amur adonis herb
Herba Aeginetiae	***Aeginetia indica***	Guan Zhen Huang, Ye Gu	Gwon Jam Wong, Ye Gu		Aeginetia herb
Herba Agastachis	***Agastache rugosa***	Huo Xiang	Fok Heung	Kakko	Rugose giant hyssop herb
Herba Agrimoniae pilosae	***Agrimonia pilosa*** var. ***japonica***	Xian He Cao	Sin Hok Chou	Senkakuso	Furry agrimony herb
Herba Ajugae	***Ajuga decumbens***	Bai Mao Xia Ku Cao, Jing Gu Cao	Baak Mou Ha Fu Chou, Gan Gwat Chou		Bugleweed herb
Herba Alternantherae	***Alternanthera philoxeroides***	Kong Xiu Lian Zi Cao	Hung Sam Lin Ji Chou		Alligator Alternanthera herb
Herba Anagallis	***Anagallis arvensis***	Jian Feng Hong	Gin Fung Hung		Scarlet pimpernel herb
Herba Androsacae	***Androsaca umbellata***	Dian Di Mei			Androsaca herb
Herba Anemonis hupehensis	***Anemone hupehensis***	Da Po Wan Hua Hua	Da Po Wun Fa Fa		Hubei anemone herb
Herba Ardisiae crispae	***Ardisia crispa***	Bai Liang Jin	Baak Leung Gam		Crisp ardisia herb
Herba Aristolochiae mollissimae	***Aristolochia mollissima***	Xun Gu Feng, Mian Mao Ma Dou Ling	Cham Gwat Fung, Min Mou Ma Dou Ling		Soft birthwort herb
Herba Artemisiae annuae	***Artemisia annua***	Huang Hua Hao Qing Hao	Wong Fa Hou, Ching Hou		Annual wormwood herb
Herba Artemisiae anomalae	***Artemisia anomala***	Liu Ji Niu	Lau Gei Nou	Ryukido	Anomalous wormwood herb
Herba Artemisiae apiaceae	***Artemisia apiacea***	Qing Hao	Ching Hou	Seiko	Celery wormwood herb
Herba Artemisiae capillaris	***Artemisia capillaris, A. scoparia***	Yin Chen (Hao), Mian Yin Chen	Yan Chan (Hou), Min Yan Chan	Inchinko	Downy wormwood herb
Herba Artemisiae scopariae	***Artemisia scoparia***	Bei Yin Chen	Bak Yan Chan		Northern wormwood herb
Herba Asari heterotropoidis	***Asarum heterotropoides***	Xi Xin, Bei Xi Xin	Bak Sai San		Northern wild ginger root
Herba Asari maximi	***Asarum maximum***	Ta Hua Xi Xin	Daai Fa Sai San		Large flower wild ginger herb
Herba Asari sieboldii	***Asarum sieboldii***	Xi Xin, Hua Xi Xin	Wa Sai San		Siebold's wild ginger herb
Herba Asteris indici	***Aster indicus*** and spp	Ma Lan	Ma Laan		Indian aster herb
Herba Bauhiniae paraglaucae	***Bauhinia paraglauca***	Hu Die Cao			Green bauhinia herb

PHARMACEUTICAL	SCIENTIFIC	MANDARIN	CANTONESE	JAPANESE	ENGLISH
Herba Begoniae crassirostris	***Begonia crassirostris***	Hong Ban Bian Lian	Hung Bun Bin Lin		Begonia herb
Herba Begoniae fimbristipulae	***Begonia fimbristipula***	Zi Bei Tian Kuei Hong Tian Kui	Ji Mai Tin Kwai, Hung Tin Kwai		Begonia herb
Herba Belamcandae	***Belamcanda chinensis***	She Gan Miao	Se Gon Miu		Leopard flower herb
Herba Bidentis bipinnatae	***Bidens bipinnata***	Gui Zhen Cao	Gwai Jam Chou		Beggartick herb
Herba Bidentis pilosae	***Bidens pilosa* var. *minor* and spp**	Xian Feng Cao	Heun Fung Chou		Hairy beggartick herb
Herba Bidentis pilosae	***Bodens pilosa***	San Ye Gui Zhen Cao	Sam Yip Gwai Jam Chou		
Herba Blumeae balsamiferae	***Blumea balsamifera***	Ai Na Xiang, Da Feng Cao	Ngaai Naap Heung	Daifuso	Camphor plant
Herba Buchnerae	***Buchnera cruciata***	Gui Yu Jian	Gwai Yu Jin		Cruciate bluehart herb
Herba Capsellae	***Capsella bursa-pastoris***	Ji Cai	Chai Choi	Seisai	Shepherd's purse herb
Herba Carpesii	***Carpesium abrotanoides***	Tian Ming Jing	Tin Ming Jing		Starwort herb
Herba Cayratiae	***Cayratia japonica***	Wu Lian Mei	Wu Lin Mui		Cayratia herb
Herba Celosiae cristatae	***Celosia cristata***	Ji Guan Hua	Gai Gun Fa		Cock'scomb herb
Herba Centipedae	***Centipeda minima***	E Bu Shi Cao	Ngo Bat Sik Chou	Sekikozui, Gabusho-kuso	Centipeda herb
Herba Chelidonii	***Chelidonium majus* var. *asiaticum***	Bai Qu Cai	Baak Wat Choi	Hakkutusai	Asian celandine herb
Herba Chenopodii ambrosioidis	***Chenopodium ambrosioides***	Tu Jing Jie	Tou Ging Gai		Wormseed herb
Herba Cirsii japonici	***Cirsium japonicum***	Da Ji	Daai Gai	Taikei	Japanese thistle herb
Herba Cistanchis	***Cistanche salsa* and spp**	Rou Cong Rong	Yuk Chung Yung	Nikujuyo	Fleshy broomrape herb
Herba Clematis floridae	***Clematis florida***	Tie Xian Lian	Ti Chik Lin		Flowering clematis herb
Herba Clinopodii	***Clinopodium confine***	Jian Dao Cao	Jin Dou Chou		Clinopodium herb
Herba Commelinae	***Commelina benghalensis***	Tang Shi Song	Tong Sek Chung		Bengal dayflower hb
Herba Commelinae	***Commelina communis***	Ya Zhi Cao	Ngaap Jek Chou		Common dayflower herb
Herba Coniogrammis	***Coniogramme japonica***	Huo Xue Lian	Fo Hyut Lin		Bamboo fern herb
Herba Coriandri	***Coriandrum sativum***	Hu Sui	Wu Sai		Coriander herb
Herba Corydalis decumbensis	***Corydalis decumbens***	Xia Tian Wu	Ha Tin Mou		Decumbent corydalis herb
Herba Crossostephii	***Crossostephium chinense***	Fu Rong	Fu Yung		Crossosteph-ium herb
Herba Crotalariae	***Crotalaria sessiliflora***	Ye Bai He	Ye Baak Hap		Thin-leaf rattlebox herb
Herba Cynomorii	***Cynomorium songaricum***	Suo Yang	Soi Yeung	Sayo	Lock yang stem
Herba Cypripedii	***Cypripedium formosanum***	Yi Dian Hong	Yut Dim Hung		Formosa lady' slipper herb

PHARMACEUTICAL	SCIENTIFIC	MANDARIN	CANTONESE	JAPANESE	ENGLISH
Herba Dendrobii	***Dendrobium nobile, D. linawianum, D. officinale*** **and spp**	Shi Hu	Sek Wu	Sekkoku	Stonebushel stem
Herba Dendrobii chrysanthi	***Dendrobium chrysanthum***	Shi Hu, Shu Hua Shi Hu	Sek Wu, Chuk Fa Shi Hu		Stonebushel stem
Herba Dendrobii fimbriati	***Dendrobium fimbriatum***	Shi Hu, Ma Bian Shi Hu	Sek Wu, Ma Bin Sek Wu		Stonebushel stem
Herba Dendrobii loddigesii	***Dendrobium loddigesii***	Shi Hu, Wan Cao Shi Hu	Sek Wu, Waan Chou Sek Wu		Stonebushel stem
Herba Dendrobii nobilis	***Dendrobium nobile***	Shi Hu, Jin Sha Shi Hu	Sek Wu, Gam Ja Sek Wu		Stonebushel stem
Herba Dendrobii officinalis	***Dendrobium officinalis***	Shi Hu, Tie Pi Shi Hu	Sek Wu, Tit Pei Sek Wu		Stonebushel stem
Herba Desmodii pseudotriquetrii	***Desmodium pseudotriquetrum, D. triquetrum***	Long Shi Huang	Lung Sek Wong		Bottlegourd herb
Herba Desmodii	***Desmodium styracifolium***	Guang Dong (Jin) Qian Cao	Gwong Dung (Gam) Chin Chou	Kinsenso	Coin-leaf desmodium herb
Herba Desmodii sinnati	***Desmodium sinnatum***	Guo Lu Huang, Nian Ren Hua	Lim Yan Fa		Sinnate desmodium herb
Herba Dianthi	***Dianthus superbus, D. chinensis***	Qu Mai	Geui Mak	Kubaku	Proud pink herb
Herba Dianthi chinensis	***Dianthus chinensis***	Qu Mai, Shi Zhu	Geui Mak, Sek Juk		Chinese pink herb
Herba Dichondrae	***Dichondra repens***	Ma Di Jin	Ma Dei Jing	Kinsenso	Dichondra herb
Herba Droserae	***Drosera burmanni***	Jin Di Luo	Gam Dei Lo		Sundew herb
Herba Duchesneae	***Duchesnea indica***	She Mei	Se Mui		Mock strawberry herb
Herba Ecliptae	***Eclipta prostata, E. alba***	Han Lian Cao, Mo Han Lian	Hon Lin Chou	Kanrenso	Field lotus herb
Herba Elephantopi	***Elephantopus scaber***	Di Dan Tou, Ku Di Dan, Tu Gong Ying	Fu Dei Daam		Rough elephant's foot herb
Herba Elsholtziae	***Elsholtzia splendens, E. stauntonii***	Xiang Ru (Cao)	Heung Yu (Chou)	Koju	Aromatic madder herb
Herba Emiliae	***Emilia sonchifolia***	Yang Ti Cao	Yeung Tai Chou		Red tassel-flower herb
Herba Ephedrae	***Ephedra sinica***	Ma Huang	Ma Wong	Mao	Ephedra stem
Herba Equiseti hiemalis	***Equisetum hiemale***	Mu Zei	Muuk Chaak	Mokuzoku	Horsetail herb
Herba Equiseti ramosissimi	***Equisetum ramosissimum***	Bi Tong Cao	Bat Tung Chou		Ramose horsetail herb
Herba Eriocaulonis	***Eriocaulon buergerianum, E. sieboldianum***	Gu Jing Cao	Guk Jing Chou	Kokuseiso	Pipewort herb
Herba Erodii seu Geranii	***Erodium stephaniarum, Geranium*** **spp**	Lao Guan Cao	Lou Gwun Chou		Storksbill or cranesbill herb
Herba Ervatamiae	***Ervatamia divaricata, E. hainaensis***	Gou Ya Hua	Gaau Nga Fa		Crepe jasmine herb
Herba et radix Cymbidii	***Cymbidium ensifolium***	Jian Lan Hua	Gin Laan Fa		Cymbidium orchid herb and root

PHARMACEUTICAL	SCIENTIFIC	MANDARIN	CANTONESE	JAPANESE	ENGLISH
Herba et radix Lobeliae chinensis	***Lobelia chinensis***	Ban Bian Lian	Bau Bin Ling	Hanbanren	Rooting lobelia herb and root
Herba et radix Polygoni hydropiperis	***Polygonum hydropiper***	Shui Liao	Seui Liu		Water pepper herb and root
Herba et radix Salviae plebeiae	***Salvia plebeia***	Li Zhi Cao	Lai Jik Chou		Plebeian sage herb and root
Herba et radix Veronicae	***Veronica peregrina***	Jie Gu Xian Tao	Jip Gwat Sin Tou		Peregrine speedwell herb and root
Herba et rhizoma Patriniae	***Patrinia scabiosaefolia, P. villosa***	Bai Jiang Cao	Baai Jeung Chou	Haishoso	Patrinia herb and root
Herba Eupatorii	***Eupatorium lindleyanum*** **var.** ***tripartum***	Ye Ma Zhui, Jian Pei Lan	Ye Ma Jeui, Jim Pui Laan		Lindley's eupatorium herb
Herba Eupatorii fortunei	***Eupatorium fortunei***	Pei Lan	Pui Laan	Haikan	Orchid-grass herb
Herba Eupatorii lindleyani	***Eupatorium lindleyanum***	Cheng Gan Sheng Ma	Ping Gon Sing Ma		Lindley's eupatorium herb
Herba Euphorbiae humifusae	***Euphorbia humifusa***	Di Jin Cao	Dei Gam Chou		Wolf'smilk herb
Herba Euphorbiae milii	***Euphorbia milii***	Ci Peng Hua	Chi Fung Fa		Prickly spurge herb
Herba Fissistigmae	***Fissistigma glaucescens***	Wu Gu Teng	Wu Gwat Tang		Fissistigma herb
Herba Galii aparinis	***Galium aparine***	Ba Xian Cao, Zhu Yang Yang	Baat Sin Chou		Cleavers herb
Herba Gendarussae	***Gendarussa vulgaris***	Bo Gu Dan	Bok Gwat Daam		Gendarussa herb
Herba Geranii	***Geranium wilfordii, G. thunbergii***	Lao He Cao	Lou Hap Chou	Gennoshio-uko	Geranium herb
Herba Glechomae	***Glechoma hederacea, G. longituba***	Lian Qian Cao	Ling Chin Chou		Ground ivy herb
Herba Glossogyne	***Glossogyne tenuifolia***	Shan Shen Zi	Saan Sam Jai		Thin-leaf glossgyne herb
Herba Gnaphalii	***Gnaphalium affine***	Shu Qu Cao	Syu Guk Chou		Cudweed herb
Herba Gynostemmae	***Gynostemma pentaphyllum***	Jiao Gu Lan	Gaan Gu Laam		Gynostemma herb
Herba Hederae nepalensis	***Hedera nepalensis*** **var.** ***sinensis***	Chang Chun Teng	Seung Cheun Tang		Nepalese ivy leaf
Herba Heleocharis	***Heleocharis plantaginea***	Bi Qi	But Chai	Bossai	Water chestnut herb
Herba Helicteres	***Helicteres angustifolia***	Shan Zhi Ma	Saan Ji Ma		Helicteres herb
Herba Heliotropi	***Heliotropium indicum***	Da Wei Yao, Er Gou Cao	Daai Mei Yiu		Heliotrope herb
Herba Heliotropi	***Heliotropium indicum***	Er Gou Cao	Yi Ngau Chou		Indian heliotrope herb
Herba Houttuyniae	***Houttuynia cordata***	Yu Xing Cao	Yu Seng Chou	Juyakuso	Fishwort herb
Herba Humuli scandentis	***Humulus scandens***	Lu Cao	Leut Chou		Climbing hops flower

PHARMACEUTICAL	SCIENTIFIC	MANDARIN	CANTONESE	JAPANESE	ENGLISH
Herba Hydrocotylis	***Hydrocotyle sibthorpioides***	Tian Hu Sui	Tin Wu Seui		Lawn (water) pennywort herb
Herba Hyperici ascyronis	***Hypericum ascyron***	Hong Han Lian	Hung Hon Lin		St. John's wort
Herba Hyperici chinensis	***Hypericum chinense***	Jin Si Tao			Chinese St. John's wort herb
Herba Hyperici japonici	***Hypericum japonicum***	Tian Ji Huang, Di Er Cao	Tin Jik Wong, Dei Yi Chou		Japanese St. John's wort herb
Herba Hyperici sampsonii	***Hypericum sampsonii***	Yuan Bao Cao	Yun Bou Chou		South China St. John's wort herb
Herba Impatientis	***Impatiens balsamina***	Tou Gu Cao	Tau Gwat Chou		Garden balsam herb
Herba Inulae	***Inula japonica, I. brittanica, I. linariaefolia***	Jin Fei Cao	Gam Fai Chou	Kinfutsuso	Elecampane herb
Herba Inulae cappae	***Inula cappa***	Bai Niu Dan, Bai Mian Feng	Baak Ngau Daam		Goatear herb
Herba Ipomoeae cairicae	***Ipomoea cairica***	Wu Zhao Long	Ng Jaau Lung		Cairo morning-glory herb
Herba Isodonis	***Isodon japonicus***	Ye Ming Cao	Yin Ming Chou	Enmeiso	Isodon herb
Herba Ixeris	***Ixeris denticulata***	Mu Dou Hui	Mou Tau Wui		Ixeris herb
Herba Jussiaeae	***Jussiaea repens***	Kuo Tang She	Gwo Tong Se		Clove strip herb
Herba Justiciae	***Justicia procumbens***	Jue Chuang Cao, Shu Wei Huang	Jeuk Chong, Syu Mei Wong		Justicia herb
Herba Kyllingae	***Kyllinga brevifolia***	Shui Wu Gong	Seui Ng Gung		Kyllinga herb
Herba Laminariae	***Laminaria*** spp	Hai Dai	Hoi Daai		Algae
Herba Lantanae	***Lantana camara***	Wu Se Mei	Ng Sik Mui		Wild sage herb
Herba Lemnae	***Lemna minor***	Fu Ping	Fau Ping		Duckweed herb
Herba Leonori	***Leonorus heterophyllus, L. japonicus, L. sibiricus*** and spp	Yi Mu Cao, Chong Wei	Yik Mou Chou, Chong Wai	Yakumoso	Asian motherwort herb
Herba Lespedezae	***Lespedeza cuneata***	Ye Guan Men	Ye Gwaan Mun		Perennial lespedeza herb
Herba Leuci	***Leucas mollissima***	Bai Hua Zi Cao, Hu Yao Huang	Baak Fa Ji Chou, Fu Ngao Wong		Leucas herb
Herba Limnophilae	***Limnophila sessiliflora***	Shuang Liu Huang	Seung Lan Wong		Limnophila herb
Herba Linderniae	***Lindernia anagallis***	Ding Jing Cao	Ding Ging Chou		Lindernia herb
Herba Lippiae	***Lippia nodiflora***	Peng Lai Cao, Ya She Huang	Fung Loi Chou, Ngaap Sit Wong		Frogfruit herb
Herba Ludwigiae	***Ludwigia prostata***	Shui Ding Xiang	Seui Ding Heung		Water clove herb
Herba Lycopi	***Lycopus lucidus***	Ze Lan	Jaak Laan	Takuran	Bright bugleweed herb
Herba Lycopodi	***Lycopodium clavatum***	Shen Jin Cao	Sam Gam Chou		Clubmoss herb

PHARMACEUTICAL	SCIENTIFIC	MANDARIN	CANTONESE	JAPANESE	ENGLISH
Herba Lycopodii serrati	***Lycopodium serratum*** **and** ***varieties***	Jin Bu Huan	Gam Bat Wun		Serrated clubmoss
Herba Lygodii	***Lygodium japonicum***	Hai Jin Sha Teng	Hoi Gam Sa Tang	Kaikinshato	Japanese climbing fern herb
Herba Lyoniae	***Lyonia ovafolia, L. neziki***	Nan Zhu	Naam Juk		Lyonia herb
Herba Lysimachiae	***Lysimachia christinae, L. hemsleyana***	Jin Qian Cao, Guo Lu Huang	Gam Chin Chou, Gwo Lou Wong	Kinsenso	Asian moneywort herb
Herba Lysimachiae candidae	***Lysimachia candida***	Dan Tian Cao	Daan Tiu Chou		White lysimachia herb
Herba Lysimachiae congestiflorae	***Lysimachia congestiflora***	Xiao Guo Lu Huang	Siu Gwo Lou Wong		Full-flowered lysimachia
Herba Lysimachiae sikokianae	***Lysimachia sikokiana***	Ling Ling Xiang	Ling Ling Heung		Lysimachia herb
Herba Lysinoti	***Lysionotus pauciflora***	Shi Diao Lan	Sek Diu Laan		Lysionotus herb
Herba Lythri salicariae	***Lythrum salicaria***	Qian Cu Cai	Jin Wat Choi		Loosestrife herb
Herba Macleayae	***Macleaya cordata***	Bo Luo Hui	Bok Lok Wui		Plum poppy herb
Herba Marsdeniae	***Marsdenia tenacissima***	Wu Gu Teng	Wu Gwat Tang		Marsdenia herb
Herba Melastomae candidae	***Melastoma candidum***	Ye Mu Dan	Ye Maau Daan		Melastoma herb
Herba Menthae arvensis	***Mentha arvensis***	Bo He	Bok Ho	Hakka	Asian fieldmint herb
Herba Menthae spicatae	***Mentha spicata***	Xiang Hua Cai, Liu Lan Xiang	Heung Fa Choi, Lou Laan Heung		Spearmint herb
Herba Mesonae	***Mesona chinensis***	Xian Cao, Liang Fen Cao	Heun Chou, Leung Fan Chou		Jellywort herb
Herba Metaplexis	***Metaplexis japonica***	Guo Lu Huang, Luo Mo	Lo Mo		Metaplexis herb
Herba Microsorii	***Microsorium hancockii, M. dilatatum***	Lu Ji Wei	Luk Gai Mei		Microsorium herb
Herba mimosae pudicae	***Mimosa pudica***	Han Xiu Cao	Ham Sau Chou		Mimosa herb
Herba Miscanthi	***Miscanthus sinensis***	Mang Jing	Mong Hong		Miscanthus herb
Herba Nepenthis	***Nepenthes mirabilis***	Zhu Long Cao	Jyu Lung Chou		Pitcher plant herb
Herba Nerviliae	***Nervilia fordii***	Qing Tian Kui	Ching Tin Kwai		Nervilia herb
Herba Ocimi	***Ocimum basilicum***	Jiu Ceng Ta, Luo Le	Lo Lak		Basil herb
Herba Oenanthis	***Oenanthe javanica***	Shui Qin	Seui Kan		Water dropwort
Herba Oldenlandiae	***Oldenlandia diffusa***	Bai Hua She She Cao	Baak Fa Se Sit Chou	Byakka-jazesso	Snaketongue grass herb
Herba Ophioglossi	***Ophioglossum vulgatum***	Ping Er Xiao Cao	Ping Yi Siu Chou		Adder's tongue herb
Herba Origani vulgaris	***Origanum vulgare***	Tu Yin Chen, Tu Xiang Ru	Tou Gam Chan, Tou Heung Yu		Oregano herb

PHARMACEUTICAL	SCIENTIFIC	MANDARIN	CANTONESE	JAPANESE	ENGLISH
Herba Orobanchis	***Orobanche caerulescens*** and spp	Lie Dang	Lit Dong		Orobanche herb
Herba Orostachis	***Orostachys fimbriatus***	Wa Song	Nga Chung		Fimbriate orostachys herb
Herba Orostachis	***Orostachys japonica, O. fimbriatus***	Wa Song	Nga Chung		Hens-and-chickens herb
Herba Orthosiphonis	***Orthosiphon aristatus, O. grandiflorus***	Mao Xu Kao, Hua Shi Cao	Maau Sou Chou, Fa Sek Chou		Orthosiphon herb
Herba Osbeckiae	***Osbeckia chinensis***	Tian Xiang Lu, Jin Shi Lu	Tin Heung Lou		Chinese osbeckia herb
Herba Oxalis	***Oxalis corniculata***	Cu Jiang Cao	Chou Jeung Chou		Indian sorrel herb
Herba Passiflorae coeruleae	***Passiflora coeruleae***	Xi Fan Lian	Sai Faan Lin		Cerulean passionflower herb
Herba Pavettae	***Pavetta hongkongiensis***	Man Tian Xing	Mun Tin Sing, Daai Sa Yip		Pavetta herb
Herba Pelargonii	***Pelargonium graveolens***	Xiang Ye	Heung Yip		Rose geranium herb
Herba Physalis peruvianae	***Physalis peruviana***	Deng Long Cao	Dang Lung Chou		Peru lantern herb
Herba Plumbaginis	***Plumbago zeylanicum***	Hei Mian Ma, Bai Hua Dan	Baak Fa Daan		Ceylon leadwort
Herba Pogonatheri	***Pogonatherum crinitum***	Bi Zi Cao	Bat Jai Chou		Golden Hair grass
Herba Pogostemis	***Pogostemon cablin***	Guang Huo Xiang	Gwong Fok Heung		Patchouli herb
Herba Polygalae japonicae	***Polygala japonica***	Gua Zi Jin	Gwa Ji Gam		Japanese milkwort herb
Herba Polygoni avicularis	***Polygonum aviculare***	Bian Xu	Bin Chuk	Henchiku	Knotgrass herb
Herba Polygoni chinensis	***Polygonum chinense***	Huo Tan Mu (Cao), Qing Fan Teng	Fo Tan Mou (Chou)		Chinese knotweed herb
Herba Polygoni lapathifolii	***Polygonum lapathifolium***	La Liao Cao	La Lou Chou		Knotweed herb
Herba Polygoni orientalis	***Polygonum orientale***	Shui Tong Hua Cao Hong Cao	Seui Tung Fa Chou Hung Chou		Prince's feather herb
Herba Polygoni perfoliati	***Polygonum perfoliatum***	Gang Ban Gui, Guan Ye Liao	Gong Bun Gwai, Gwan Yip Lou		Perfoliate knotweed herb
Herba Polygoni tinctorii	***Polygonum tinctorium***	Lan Shi	Laam Sat		Chinese indigo herb
Herba Polypodii	***Polypodium hastatum***	Qi Xing Cao	Chat Sing Chou		Polypody herb
Herba Porphyrae	***Porphyra tenera***	Zi Cai	Ji Choi		Porphyra herb
Herba Portulaccae	***Portulacca oleracea***	Ma Chi Xian	Ma Chi Yin	Bashiken	Purslane herb
Herba Potentillae chinensis	***Potentilla chinensis***	Wei Ling Cai	Wai Ling Choi		Chinese cinquefoil herb
Herba Potentillae discoloris	***Potentilla discolor***	Fan Bai Cao	Faan Baak Chou		Discolored cinquefoil herb
Herba Psychotriae serpentis	***Psychotria serpens***	Chuan Gen Teng, Bo Gu Cao	Chyun Gen Tang		Twining psychotria herb

PHARMACEUTICAL	SCIENTIFIC	MANDARIN	CANTONESE	JAPANESE	ENGLISH
Herba Pterii	***Pteris multifida*** and spp	Feng Wei Cao	Fung Mei Chou		Phoenix-tail fern
Herba Pycnostelmae	***Pycnostelma paniculatum***	Shan Diao Zhu, Xu Chang Jing	Cheui Cheung Hing		Paniculate swallowwort herb
Herba Rabdosiae	***Rabdosia rubescens*** and spp	Dong Ling Cao	Dun Ling Chou		Rabdosia herb
Herba Rhodeae	***Rhodea japonica***	Wan Nian Xing			Rhodea herb
Herba Rorippae	***Rorippa montana, R. indica***	Han Cai	Hon Choi		Nasturtium herb
Herba Rosmarini	***Rosmarinus officinalis***	Mi Die Xiang	Mai Dit Heung		Rosemary herb
Herba Rostellulariae	***Rostellulariae procumbens***	Jue Chuang	Jeuk Chong		Creeping rostellularia herb
Herba Rungiae	***Rungia pectinata***	Hai Er Cao	Haai Yi Chou		Rungia herb
Herba Rutae	***Ruta graveolens***	Chou Cao	Chau Chou		Rue herb
Herba Saginae	***Sagina japonica***	Qi Gu Cao	Chat Gu Chou		Japanese pearlwort herb
Herba Sarcandrae	***Sarcandra glabra***	Jiu Jie Feng	Gau Jit Fung		Smooth sarcandra herb
Herba Sargassi	***Sargassum fusiforme*** and spp	Hai Zao	Hoi Chou	Kaiso	Sargassum seaweed
Herba Saururi	***Saururus chinensis***	San Bai Cao	Saam Baak Chou		Chinese lizardtail herb
Herba Saussureae lanicepsis	***Saussurea laniceps, S. involucrata*** and spp	Xue Lian Hua	Hat Ling Fa		Snow lotus herb
Herba Saxifragae stoloniferae	***Saxifraga stolonifera***	Hu Er Cao	Fu Yi Chou		Saxifrage herb
Herba Schizonepetae	***Schizonepeta tenuifolia***	Jing Jie	Ging Gaai	Keigai	Japanese catnip herb
Herba Scutellariae indicae	***Scutellaria indica***	Han Xin Cao	Hon Sam Chou		India skullcap herb
Herba Sedi aizoonis	***Sedum aizoon***	Jing Tian San Qi	Ging Tin Saam Chat		Aizoon stonecrop herb
Herba Sedi erythrosticti	***Sedum erythrostictum***	Jing Tian (San Qi)	Ging Tin		Red stonecrop herb
Herba Selaginella moellendorfii	***Selaginella moellendorfii***	Jiang Nan Juan Bai	Gong Naam Kyun Paap		Moellendorf's spikemoss herb
Herba Selaginellae	***Selaginella doederleinii, S. involvens***	Shi Shang Bai	Sek Song Paap		Spikemoss herb
Herba Selaginellae tamariscinae	***Selaginella tamariscina***	Juan Bai	Kyun Paap		Resurrection plant herb
Herba Semiaquilegiae	***Semiaquilegia adoxoides***	Tian Kui	Tin Kwai		Semiaquilegia herb
Herba Senecionis kirilowii	***Senecio kirilowii***	Kou She Cao	Gau Sit Chou		Kirilow's ragwort herb
Herba Senecionis scandens	***Senecio scandens***	Qian Li Guang	Chin Lei Gwong		Climbing ragwort herb
Herba Siegesbeckiae	***Siegesbeckia pubescens, S. orientalis, S. glabrescens***	Xi Xian Cao	Hei Lim Chou		Hairy siegesbeckia herb
Herba Silybi	***Silybum marianum***	Shui Fei Ji	Seui Fei Gai		Blessed thistle herb
Herba Solani lyrati	***Solanum lyratum***	Bai Ying, Shu Yang Quan, Bai Mao Teng	Baak Ying, Baak Mou Tang		Climbing nightshade herb

PHARMACEUTICAL	SCIENTIFIC	MANDARIN	CANTONESE	JAPANESE	ENGLISH
Herba Solani nigri	*Solanum nigrum*	Long Kui	Lung Kwai		Winter cherry herb
Herba Solani surattensis	*Solanum surratense*	Ye Dian Jie	Ye Din Ke		Soda-apple nightshade herb
Herba Solani xanthocarpi	*Solanum xanthocarpum*	Huang Shui Qie	Wong Seui Ke		Prickly nightshade fruit
Herba Solidaginis	*Solidago virgaurea, S. derurrens*	Yi Zhi Huang Hua, Liu Zhi Huang	Yat Ji Wong Fa, Lau Ji Wong		Goldenrod herb
Herba Sonchi	*Sonchus oleraceus*	Ku Cai	Fu Choi		Annual sowthistle herb
Herba Speranskiae	*Speranskia tuberculata*	Tou Gu Cao	Tau Gwat Chou		Speranskia herb
Herba Spiranthis	*Spiranthes sinensis*	Pan Long Shen	Pun Lung Sam		Chinese pearltwist herb
Herba Spirodelae	*Spirodela polyrrhiza*	Fu Ping	Fau Ping		Duckweed herb
Herba Stellariae aquaticae	*Stellaria aquatica*	Cha Chi Huang	Cha Si Wong		Water chickweed herb
Herba Strigae	*Striga asiatica*	Du Jiao Gan	Duk Geuk Gam		Witchweed herb
Herba Swertiae	*Swertia japonica, S. pseudochinensis*	Dang Yao Cao	Dong Yeuk Chou	Toyaku	Japanese green gentian herb
Herba Tetragoniae	*Tetragonia tatragonoides*	Fan Xing	Faan Haang	Bankyo, Mantsai	Tetragonia herb
Herba Thalictri	*Thalictrum foliolosum*	Tang Song Cao			Meadow rue herb
Herba Thlaspis	*Thlaspi arvense*	Xi Ming	Sik Ming		Boor's mustard herb
Herba Thymi mongolici	*Thymus mongolicus*	Di Jiao	Dei Jiu		Mongolian thyme herb
Herba Trichospori	*Trichosporum acuminatum*	Bai Mian Feng	Baak Ming Fung		Trichosporum herb
Herba Urariae	*Uraria lagopodioides*	Hu Li Wei, Tong Tian Cao	Tung Tin Chou		Uraria herb
Herba Verbenae	*Verbena officinalis*	Ma Bian Cao	Ma Bin Chou		Vervain herb
Herba Vernoniae	*Vernonia cinerea*	Yi Zhi Xiang	Yat Ji Heung		Vernonia herb
Herba Violae patriniae	*Viola patrinii*	Hua Tou Cao	Wa Tau Chou		Patrinium violet herb
Herba Visci	*Viscum coloratum, V. album*	Hu Ji Sheng	Wu Gei Sang		Western mistletoe herb
Herba Wedeliae	*Wedelia chinensis*	Ma Lan Jin, Peng Qi Ju	Paang Kei Guk		Wedelia herb
Hippocampus	*Hippocampus kelloggiand* spp	Hai Ma	Hoi Ma	Kaiba	Sea horse
Hirudo seu Whitmania	*Hirudo nipponia, Whitmania pigra* and spp	Shui Zhi	Seui Jik		Leech
Holotrichia	*Holotrichia diomphalia*	Qi Cao	Chai Chou		June beetle grub (larva)
Huechys	*Huechys sanguinea, H, philaemata*	Hong Niang Zi	Hung Leung Ji		Red cicada
Hydragyrum	*Hydragyrum*	Shui Yin	Seui Yin		Mercury

PHARMACEUTICAL	SCIENTIFIC	MANDARIN	CANTONESE	JAPANESE	ENGLISH
Indigo pulverata levis	***Isatis tinctoria*** **and spp,** ***Baphicacanthus cusia, Indigofera suffruticosa, Polygonum tinctorium***	Qing Dai	Ching Doi		Woad pigment
Jecur Lutrae	***Lutra lutra***	Ta Gan	Taap Gon		Otter liver
Lapis Pumicis	***Pumus***	Fu Hai Shi	Fau Hoi Sek	Kaifuseki	Pumice
Larva Chrysomyiae	***Chrysomyia megacephala*** **and spp**	Wu Gu Chong	Ng Guk Chung		Maggot
Lignum Acronychiae	***Acronychia laurifolia***	Sha Tang Mu, Jiang Xiang	Sa Tong Muk		Acronychia heartwood
Lignum Aquilariae	***Aquilaria agallocha, A. sinensis***	Chen Xiang	Cham Heung	Jinko	Aloeswood
Lignum Berberis thunbergii	***Berberis thunbergii***	Xiao Nie	Siu Maak	Megi	Barberry wood
Lignum Caesalpiniae	***Caesalpinia sappan***	Su Mu	Sou Muk	Soboku	Sappanwood
Lignum Cinnamomi camphorae	***Cinnamomum camphora***	Zhang Mu	Jeung Muk		Camphor wood
Lignum Cudraniae tricuspidatae	***Cudrania tricuspidata***	Da Ding Huang, Zhe Mu	Je Muk		Cudrania heartwood
Lignum Dalbergiae odoriferae	***Dalbergia odorifera***	Jiang Xiang	Geung Heung		Asian rosewood
Lignum Pini nodi	***Pinus tabulaeformis, P. massoniana, P. yunnannensis***	Song Jie, You Song Jie	Chung Jit, Yao Chung Jit	Shosetsu	Knotty pine wood shaving
Lignum Pterocarpi	***Pterocarpus indicus***	Zi Tan	Ji Taan		Malay padauk wood, Burma rosewood
Lignum Santalum	***Santalum album***	Tan Xiang	Taan Heung		Sandalwood
Limax	***Limax agrestic***	Guo Yu	Gwat Kut		Slug
Limonitum	***Limonitum***	Yu Liang Shi	Yu Leung Sek	Uyoryo	Clay ironstone
Lithagyrum	***Lithargyrum***	Mi Tuo Seng	Muk Toi Sang	Mitsudaso	Litharge
Magnetitum	***Magnetitum***	Ci Shi	Chi Sek		Magnetite
Malachitum	***Malachitum***	Tong Lu	Tung Luk		Copper rust
Manganitum	***Manganitum***	Wu Ming Yi	Mon Ming Yi		Manganite
Massa fermentata		Shen Qu	Sam Chau	Shinkiku	Medicated leaven
Massa fermentata		Shen Qu Cha	Sam Chau Cha		Medicated leaven tea
Medulla Junci	***Juncus effusus***	Deng Xin Cao	Dang Sam Chou	Toshinso	Bulrush pith
Medulla radicis Tripterygii	***Tripterygium wilfordii***	Lei Gong Teng	Leui Gung Tang		Yellow vine root pith
Medulla Tetrapanacis	***Tetrapanax papyrifera***	Tong Cao	Tong Chou, Bai Tong Chou	Toso	Rice paper pith
Medulla Zeae	***Zea mays***	Yu Mi Xin	Yuk Mai Sam		Corn cob
Mel	***Apis cerana*** **and spp**	Feng Mi	Fung Mat		Honey
Melanteritum	***Melanteritum***	Zao Fan, Lu Fan	Jou Faan		Green vitriol
Membrana follicularis ovi	***Gallus gallus domesticus***	Feng Huang Yi			Chicken egg membrane
Mica, Chloritum	***Mica, Chloritum***	Meng Shi, Jin Meng Shi	Mung Sek, Ching Mung Sek		Mica, Chlorite schist

PHARMACEUTICAL	SCIENTIFIC	MANDARIN	CANTONESE	JAPANESE	ENGLISH
Minium	***Minium***	Qian Dan, Huang Dan	Chin Daan, Wong Daan	Entan	Red lead oxide
Mirabilitum	***Mirabilitum***	Mang Xiao	Mong Seu	Bosho	Mirabilite
Mirabilitum purum	***Mirabilitum***	Xuan Ming Fan	San Ming Fun	Bosho	Glauber's salt, Pure mirabilite
Mogera carbonisatus	***Mogera robusta*** **and spp.,** ***Scaptochirus moschatus***	Yan Shu Shuang	Yim Syu Seung	Ensosu	Carbonized mogera
Muscovitum	***Muscovitum***	Yun Mu Shi	Wan Mou Sek		Muscovite
Mylabris	***Mylabris***	Ban Mao	Ban Mou	Hanmyo	Asian cantharides
Mytilus	***Mytilus crassitesta*** **and spp**	Dan Cai	Daam Choi		Mussel
Nidus Polistis seu Parapolybiae	***Polistes mandarinus, Parapolybia varia***	Lu Feng Fang	Lou Fun Fong		Hornet nest
Niter	***Niter***	Xiao Shi	Siu Sek	Shoseki	Potassium nitrate
Ophicalcitum	***Ophicalcitum***	Hua Rui Shi	Fa Yeui Sek	Kazuiseki	Dolomite
Orpimentum	***Orpimentum***	Ci Huang, Xiong Huang	Chi Wong		Orpiment
Os Leopardis	***Panthera***	Bao Gu			Leopard bone
Os Poritis	***Porites nigrescens***	Shi Hua	Sek Fa		Coral skeleton
Os Sepiae seu Sapiellae	***Sepia esculenta, Sepiella maindroni***	Hai Piao Xiao, Wu Zei Gu	Hoi Piu Seui		Cuttlefish bone
Os Stegodontis	***Stegodon orientalis, S. rhinocerus sinensis, Hipparion***	Long Gu	Lung Gwat	Ryukotsu	Dragon bone
Os Stegodontis calcinatum	***Stegodon orientalis et al.***	Duan Long Gu, Shu Long Gu	Taan Lung Gwat		Calcined dragon bone
Os tigris	***Panthera***	Hu Gu	Fu Gwat	Kokotsu	Tiger bone
Otozithum Sciaenae	***Pseudosciaena crocea, P. polyactis, Sciaena schlegeli***	Yu Nao Shi	Yu Nou Sek		Fish otolith
Paratenodera seu Hierodula seu Mantis seu Statilia	***Paratenodera sinensis*** **and** ***augustipennis, Hierodula patellifera, Mantis religiosa, Statilia maculata***	Sang Piao Xiao	Song Piu Seu		Praying mantis egg case
Pasta Acaciae seu Uncariae	***Acacia catechu***	Er Cha	Yi Cha	Asenyaku	Catechu paste
Pasta Uncaria seu Acaciae	***Uncaria gambir*** **and spp**	Er Cha	Yi Cha		Catechu paste
Pericarpium Amomi villosi	***Amomum villosum***	Sha Ren Ke	Sa Yan Hok		Wild cardamom shell
Pericarpium Arachis	***Arachis hypogaea***	Hua Sheng Pi	Fa Sang Pei	Kashohi	Peanut skin
Pericarpium Arecae	***Areca catechu, A. dicksonii***	Da Fu Pi	Daai Fuk Pei	Daifukuhi	Betel husk
Pericarpium Citri grandi immaturi	***Citrus grandis***	You Pi (Ju Hong), Hua Ju Hong	Yau Pei (Gwat Hung), Fa Gwat Hung		Pomelo rind

PHARMACEUTICAL	SCIENTIFIC	MANDARIN	CANTONESE	JAPANESE	ENGLISH
Pericarpium Citri medicae	***Citrus medica, C. wilsonii***	Xiang Yuan Pi, Gou Yuan Pi	Heung Yun Pei, Gau Yun Pei		Citron rind
Pericarpium Citri reticulatae	***Citrus reticulata, C. tangerina, C. erythrosa***	Chen Pi, Ju Pi	Chan Pei, Gwat Pei	Chimpi	Ripe tangerine rind
Pericarpium Citri reticulatae viride	***Citrus reticulata, C. tangerina, C. erythrosa***	Qing Pi	Ching Pei	Johi	Unripe tangerine rind
Pericarpium Citrulli	***Citrullus vulgaris***	Xi Gua Pi	Sai Pa Pei		Watermelon rind
Pericarpium Clauseniae	***Clausenia lansium***	Huang Pi Guo	Wong Pei Gwo		Wampi fruit
Pericarpium Glycinis	***Glycine max***	Hei Dou Yi	Haak Dau Yi		Soybean husk
Pericarpium Litchis	***Litchi chinensis***	Li Zhi Ke	Lai Ji Hok		Lychee rind
Pericarpium Luffae	***Luffa cylindrica, L. acutangula***	Si Gua Pi	Si Gwa Pei		Luffa skin
Pericarpium Papaveris	***Papaver somniferum***	Ying Su Ke	Ngang Suk Hok	Ozokukoku	Opium poppy husk
Pericarpium Punicae	***Punica granatum***	Shi Liu Pi	Sek Lau Pei	Sekiryuhi	Pomegranate husk
Pericarpium Pyri	***Pyrus betulaefolia***	Li Pi	Lei Pei		Chinese pear rind
Pericarpium Tricosanthis	***Trichosanthes kirilowii, T. japonica, T. uniflora***	Gua Lou Pi	Kwut Lau Pei	Karohi	Snakegourd rind
Periostracum Cryptotympanae	***Cryptotympana atrata*** **and spp**	Chan Tui	Sim Teui, Sim Tyut	Sentai	Cicada slough
Periostracum Bombycis	***Bombyx mori***	Ma Ming Dui	Ma Ming Teui		Silkworm slough
Periostracum/Exuviae Elephis	***Elephe taeniurus*** **and spp,** ***Dinodon rufozonatum***	She Tui (Pi)	Se Teui (Pei)	Dataihi	Snakeskin slough
Pheretima seu Allolobophora	***Pheretima aspergillum, Allolobophora caliginosa***	Di Long	Dei Lung	Jiryu	Earthworm
Phlogopitum	***Phlogopitum***	Jin Meng Shi	Gam Mung Sek		Phlogopite, Red mica
Placenta Hominis	***Homo sapiens***	Zi He Che	Ji Ho Je	Shikasha	Human placenta
Plastrum Chinemis	***Chinemys reevesii***	Gui Ban	Gwai Baan	Kiban	Tortoise shell
Plastrum Eretmochelis	***Eretmochelys imbricata***	Dai Mao	Doi Mou	Taimai	Hawksbill turtle shell
Plumula Nelumbinis	***Nelumbo nucifera***	Lian Xin	Lin Sam		Lotus plumule
Pollen Lycopodii	***Lycopodium serratum*** **and spp**	Qian Cang Ta, Pu Di Wu Gong, Guo Jiang Long, Yu Bai	Jin Jang Tap		Lycopodium pollen
Pollen Pini	***Pinus massoniana, P. tabulaeformis*** **and spp**	Song Hua Fen	Chung Fa Fan		Pine pollen
Pollen Typhae	***Typha latifolia, T. angustifolia*** **and spp**	Pu Huang, Xiang Pu	Pou Wong, Heung Pou	Hoo	Cattail pollen
Pollen Typhae carbonisatus	***Typha latifolia, T. angustifolia*** **and spp**	Pu Huang Tan	Pou Wong Taan		Charred cattail pollen

PHARMACEUTICAL	SCIENTIFIC	MANDARIN	CANTONESE	JAPANESE	ENGLISH
Praeparatio fructus Ulmi	***Ulmus macrocarpa***	Wu Yi	Mon Yi	Bui	Stinking elm fruit paste
Pulvis Arisaemae cum felle Bovis	***Arisaema consanguineum, A. amurense*** and spp	Dan Nan Xing	Daam Naam Sing	Tannansho	Powdered dragon arum corm with ox bile
Pulvis ferri	***Ferrum***	Chen Sha	Chan Sa		Black iron oxide
Pulvis ferri	***Ferrum***	Chen Sha	San Sa		Black ferric oxide
Pulvus fumi carbonisati		Bai Cao Shuang	Baak Chou Sheung		Boiler or chimney soot
Pyritum	***Pyritum***	Zi Ran Tong	Ji Yin Tung	Shizendo	Pyrite
Pyritum rotundum	***Pyritum rotundum***	She Han Shi			Iron pyrite
Pyrolusitum	***Pyrolusitum***	Wu Ming Zi	Mou Ming Ji		Pyrolusite
Radix Campanumoeae	***Campanumoea javanica***	Tu Dang Shen	Tou Dong Sam		Java bellflower root
Radix Daemonoropsis	***Daemonorops margaritae***	Huang Teng Gen	Wong Tang Gan		Daemonorops root
Radix Pseudostellariae	***Pseudostellaria heterophylla***	Tai Zi Shen	Yi Sam, Taai Ji Sam	Taishijin	Prince ginseng root
Radix	***Salvia przelwalskii***	Dan Shen, Gan Xi Shu Wei	Daan Sam, Gam Sai Syu Mei		Gan Xi cinnabar sage root
Radix Abri	***Abrus precatorius, A. cantoniensis***	Xiang Si Zi Gen	Seung Si Ji Gan		Licorice bean root
Radix Acanthi ilicifolii	***Acanthus ilicifolius***	Lao Shu Le	Lou Syu Laak		Holly-leaf acanthus root
Radix Achyranthis	***Achyranthes bidentata***	Niu Xi, Huai Niu Xi	Ngau Sat, Wai Ngau Sat	Goshitsu	White oxknee Root
Radix Achyranthis asperae	***Achyranthes aspera***	Wei Niu Xi, Ju Niu Xi, Dou Kou Cao	Wai Ngau Sat, Dou Kau Chou		Rough oxknee root
Radix Achyranthis longae	***Achyranthes longifolia***	Tu Niu Xi	Tou Ngau Sat		Long-leaf oxknee root
Radix Aconiti brachypodi	***Aconitum brachypodum*** and spp	Xue Shang Yi Zhi Yao	Syu Seung Yat Ji Hou		Brachypode aconite root
Radix Aconiti carmichaeli	***Aconitum carmichaeli***	Chuan Wu Wu Tou	Chyun Wu, Wu Tau	Uzu	Prepared Sichuan aconite root tuber
Radix Aconiti chinensis	***Aconitum chinense, A. kusnezoffii*** and spp	Cao Wu, Bei Wu Tou	Chou Wu, Mai Wu Tau	So-u	Prepared wild aconite root tuber
Radix Adenophorae strictae	***Adenophora stricta, A. capillaris, A. tetraphylla*** and spp	Nan Sha Shen	Naam Sa Sam	Nanshajin	Upright ladybell root
Radix Adenophorae trachelioidis	***Adenophora trachelioides***	Gan Jie Geng	Gam Gaat Gan, Ai Ji Sam		Sweet ladybell root
Radix Adenophorae trachelioidis	***Adenophora trachelioides, A. remotifolia***	Ji Ni	Chai Ni		Common harebell root
Radix Alangii	***Alangium chinense***	Ba Jiao Feng	Baat Gok Fung		Alangium root
Radix Alpiniae galangae	***Alpinia galanga***	Da Liang Jiang	Daai Leung Geung		Greater galangal root

PHARMACEUTICAL	SCIENTIFIC	MANDARIN	CANTONESE	JAPANESE	ENGLISH
Radix Ampelopsis	***Ampelopsis japonica***	Bai Lian	Baak Lim	Byakuran	Japanese peppervine root
Radix Anemarrhenae	***Anemarrhena asphodeloides***	Zhi Mu	Ji Mou	Chimo	Know mother root
Radix Angelicae acutilobae	***Angelica acutiloba***	Dang Gui	Dong Gwai		Dong quai root
Radix Angelicae dahuricae	***Angelica dahurica, A. anomala, A. taiwaniana***	Bai Zhi	Baak Ji	Byakushi	White angelica Root
Radix Angelicae pubescentis	***Angelica pubescens, A. laxiflora*** and spp	Du Huo	Duk Wut	Dokkatsu	Hairy angelica Root
Radix Angelicae sinensis	***Angelica sinensis***	Dang Gui	Dong Gwai	Toki	Dong quai root
Radix Araliae chinensis	***Aralia chinensis***	Song Mu Bai Pi	Sung Muk Baak Pei		Chinese aralia root
Radix Araliae cordatae	***Aralia cordata***	Tu Dang Gui	Tou Dong Gwai		Heart-leaf aralia root
Radix Ardisiae crenatae	***Ardisia crenata, A. bicolor***	Da Lo San, Zhu Sha Gen	Jyu Sa Gan	Shushakon	Coralberry root
Radix Aristolochiae	***Aristolochia contorta, A. debilis***	Qing Mu Xiang, Ma Dou Ling Gen	Ching Muk Heung	Seimokko	Green birthwort root
Radix Aristolochiae fangchis	***Aristolochia fangchi, A. westlandii***	Fang Ji, Guang Fang Ji	Fong Gei, Gwong Fong Gei		Fangchi birthwort root
Radix Arnebiae	***Arnebia euchroma, A. guttata***	Zi Cao, Xin Jiang Zi Cao	Ji Chou, San Geung Ji Chou	Shikon	Arnebia root
Radix Asteris tatarici	***Aster tataricus***	Zi Wan	Ji Yun	Shion	Tartary aster root
Radix Astragali	***Astragalus membranaceus, A. mongholicus*** and spp	Huang Qi	Wong Kei, Paak Kei	Ogi	Astragalus root
Radix Atalantiae	***Atalantia buxifolia***	Dong Feng Ju Gen	Dung Fung Gwat Gan	Tofukitsu	Atalantia root
Radix Baphicacanthi	***Baphicacanthus cusia***	Ma Lan Gen	Ma Laam Gan	Banrankon	Assam indigo root
Radix Berberis sargentianae	***Berberis sargentiana, B. wilsonae, B. vernae*** and spp	San Ke Zhen	Saam Gwo Jam		Three-needle barberry root
Radix Berchemiae	***Berchemia lineata***	Tie Bao Jin	Tit Bau Gam		Supplejack root
Radix Boehmeriae	***Boehmeria nivea***	Zhu Ma Gen	Chyu Ma Gan		Ramie root
Radix Buddleiae asiaticae	***Buddleia asiatica***	Bai Pu Jiang	Baak Pou Geung		Asian Buddleia root
Radix Buddleiae lindleyanae	***Buddleia lindleyana***	Qi Li Xiang	Chat Lei Heung		Buddleia root
Radix Bupleuri	***Bupleurum chinense, B. falcatum, B. longiradiatum*** and spp	Chai Hu	Chaai Wu	Saiko	Asian buplever root
Radix Bupleuri scorzonerifolii	***Bupleurum scorzonerifolium***	Chai Hu, Xia Ye Chai Hu	Chaai Wu, Hap Yip Chaai Wu		Thin-leaf buplever root
Radix Campsis grandiflorae	***Campsis grandiflora***	Ling Xiao Gen	Ling Siu Gan	Ryoshoka	Asian trumpetcreeper root

PHARMACEUTICAL	SCIENTIFIC	MANDARIN	CANTONESE	JAPANESE	ENGLISH
Radix Caraganae	***Caragana sinica, C., microphylla*** **and spp**	Jin Ji Er	Gam Jik Yi		Caragana root
Radix Changii	***Changium smyrnioides***	Ming Dang Shen	Ming Dong Sam	Mintojin	Bright changium root
Radix Chloranthi	***Chloranthus serratus***	Ji Ji	Kap Gei		Serrate-leaf chloranthus
Radix Cimicifugae dahuricae	***Cimicifuga dahurica***	Sheng Ma, Xing An Sheng Ma	Sing Ma, Hing On Sing Ma	Shoma	Dahurian rising hemp root
Radix Cimicifugae foetidae	***Cimicifuga foetida***	Sheng Ma	Sing Ma	Shoma	Rising hemp root
Radix Cimicifugae heracleifoliae	***Cimicifuga heracleifolia***	Sheng Ma, Ta San Ye Sheng Ma	Sing Ma, Da Sam Yip Sing Ma	Shoma	Heraclean rising hemp root
Radix Cissampeli	***Cissampelos pareira***	Xi Sheng Teng	Sak Sang Tang		Ice vine root
Radix Clematis chinensis	***Clematis chinensis, C. hexapetala*** **and spp**	Wei Ling Xian	Wai Ling Sin	Ireisen	Chinese clematis root
Radix Clematis hexapetalae	***Clematis hexapetala***	Wei Ling Xian, Mian Tuan Tie Xian Lian	Wai Ling Sin, Min Tyun Ti Chik Lin		Six-petal clematis root
Radix Clerodendronis paniculati	***Clerodendron paniculatum***	Bai Long Chuan Gen	Baak Lung Chyun Gan		Panicled clerodendron root
Radix Cocculi	***Cocculus trilobus***	Mu Fang Ji	Muk Fong Gei		Three-leaf cocculus root
Radix Codonopsis	***Codonopsis pilosula, C. tangshen, C. nervosa***	Dang Shen	Fong Dong Sam	Tojin	Downy bellflower root
Radix Codonopsis lanceolatae	***Codonopsis lanceolata***	Yang Ju, Shi Ye Shen	Yang Guk, Sei Yip Sam	Yonyu, Shiyojin	Goat's-tit bellflower root
Radix Codonopsis subglobosae	***Codonopsis subglobosa***	Dang Shen, Qiu Hua Dang Shen	Dong Sam, Kau Fa Dong Sam		Subglobular bellflower root
Radix Codonopsis tangshenis	***Codonopsis tangshen***	Dang Shen, Chuan Dang Shen	Chyun Dong Sam		Sichuan bellflower root
Radix Coicis	***Coix lachryma-jobi*** **var.** ***Ma-yuen***	Yi Yi Gen	Yi Yi Gan		Job's-tears root
Radix Colocasiae	***Colocasia esculenta***	Yu Tou Gen	Wu Tau Gan		Taro root
Radix Crotonis crassifolii	***Croton crassifolius***	Ji Gu Xiang	Gai Gwat Heung		Thick-leaf croton root
Radix Cuccubalae bacciferis	***Cuccubala baccifer***	Bai Niu Xi	Baak Ngao Sat		White oxknee root
Radix Cudraniae cochinchinensis	***Cudrania cochinchinensis***	Chuan Po Shi	Chyun Po Sek		Cochin cudrania root
Radix Cyathulae	***Cyathula officinalis,. C. officinalis***	Chuan Niu Xi	Chyun Ngau Sat		Hookweed root
Radix Cymbidii	***Cymbidium ensifolium***	Jian Lan Gen	Gin Laan Gan		Cymbidium orchid root
Radix Cynanchi atrati	***Cynanchum atratum, C. versicolor***	Bai Wei	Baak Mei	Byakubi	Swallow-wort root
Radix Cynanchi auriculati	***Cynanchum auriculatum***	Bai Shou Wu, Niu Pi Xiao	Baak Sau Wu, Ngau Pei Siu		Auricle dogbane root

PHARMACEUTICAL	SCIENTIFIC	MANDARIN	CANTONESE	JAPANESE	ENGLISH
Radix Dichroae	***Dichroa febrifuga***	Chang Shan	Seung Saan	Joszan	Feverflower root
Radix Dipsaci asperoides	***Dipsacus asperoides***	Xu Duan, Chuan Duan	Juk Dyun, Chyun Dyun		Sichuan teasel root
Radix Dipsaci japonicae	***Dipsacus japonica***	Xu Duan	Juk Dyun	Zokudan	Japanese teasel root
Radix Dolichoris	***Dolichos lablab***	Rou Dou Gen	Yuk Dau Gan		Hyacinth bean root
Radix Dolomiaea berardioidea	***Dolomiaea berardioidea***	Hou Ye Chuan Mu Xiang	Hau Yip Chyun Muk Heung		Thick-leaf Dolomiaea root
Radix Dolomiaeae souliei	***Dolomiaea souliei***	Chuan Mu Xiang	Chyun Muk Heung		Sichuan Dolomiaea root
Radix Echinopsis	***Echinops latifolius, E. gmelinii***	Lou Lu	Lau Lou		Globe thistle root
Radix Eleagni oldhamii	***Eleagnus oldhamii***	Yi Wu Gen	Yi Ng Gan		Oldham's eleagnus root
Radix Ephedrae	***Ephedra sinica***	Ma Huang Gen	Ma Wong Gan	Maokon	Ephedra root
Radix et caulis Erycibis	***Erycibes obtusifolia***	Ding Gong Teng	Ding Gung Tang		Erycibe root and stem
Radix et caulis Litseae	***Litsea cubeba***	Dou Chi Jiang	Dau Chek Geung	Toshikyo	Cubeb root and stem
Radix et caulis Millettiae dielsianae	***Millettia dielsiana, M. reticulata, M. nitida***	Ji Xue Teng	Gai Yut Tang	Keiketto	Millettia root and stem
Radix et caulis Millettiae reticulatae	***Millettia reticulata***	Ji Xue Teng, Kun Ming Ji Xue Teng	Kwan Ming Gai Yut Tang		Millettia root and stem
Radix et caulis Mucunae	***Mucuna birdwoodiana, M. sempervirens***	Ji Xue Teng, Chang Chun You Ma Teng	Gei Hat Tang, Seung Cheun Yao Ma Tang		Mucuna root and stem
Radix et caulis Nandinae	***Nandina domestica***	(Nan) Tian Zhu Gen	(Naam) Tin Juk Gan		Sacred bamboo root and stem
Radix et caulis Paederiae	***Paederia scandens***	Ji Shi Teng	Gai Niu Tang	Hakumokeis hito	Chicken dung vine root and stem
Radix et folium Ampelopsis brevipedunculatae	***Ampelopsis brevipedunculata***	She Pu Tao, Shan Pu Tao	Se Pou Tou, Saan Pou Tou		Snake grape root and leaf
Radix et folium Polygoni cuspidati	***Polygonum cuspidatum***	Hu Zhang	Fu Jeung		Japanese Knotweed root and leaf
Radix et herba Apocyni	***Apocynum lancifolium, A. venetum, A. hendersonii***	Luo Bu Ma	Lo Bou Ma		Dogbane root and herb
Radix et herba Ardisiae japonicae	***Ardisia japonica***	Zi Jin Niu, Jin Niu Cao	Ji Gam Ngau		Marlberry root and herb
Radix et herba Asari	***Asarum sieboldii, A. heterotropoides* and spp**	Xi Xin	Sai San	Saishin	Asian wild ginger root and herb
Radix et herba Catharanthi	***Catharanthus roseus***	Chang Chun Hua	Cheung Cheun Fa		Madagascar periwinkle root and herb
Radix et herba Cephalanoplis	***Cephalanoplos segetum***	Xiao Ji	Siu Gai		Field thistle herb and root
Radix et herba Cynanchi paniculati	***Cynanchum paniculatum***	Xu Chang Qing, Liao Diao Zhu	Cheui Cheung Hing		Panicled dogbane root and herb

PHARMACEUTICAL	SCIENTIFIC	MANDARIN	CANTONESE	JAPANESE	ENGLISH
Radix et herba Pyrolae	***Pyrola rotundifolia subsp. chinensis, P. Japonica***	Lu Xian Cao, Lu Ti Cao	Luk Haam Chou, Luk Tai Chou	Rokuteiso	Asian wintergreen root and herb
Radix et herba Ranunculi japonicae	***Ranunculus japonicus***	Mao Gen	Maau Gan		Japanese buttercup root and herb
Radix et herba Salsolae	***Salsola collina, S. ruthenica, S. richteri***	Zhu Mao Cai	Jyu Mou Choi		Salsola root and herb
Radix et herba Salviae chinensis	***Salvia chinensis***	Shi Jian Chuan, Chai Shen, Zi Shen	Sek Gin Chyun, Toi Sam, Ji Sam		Chinese sage root and herb
Radix et herba Scutellariae barbatae	***Scutellaria barbata, B. rivularis***	Ban Zhi Lian	Bun Ji Lin		Barbed skullcap root and herb
Radix et herba Sedi sarmentosi	***Sedum sarmentosum***	Chui Pen Cao	Chai Pan Chou		Stringy stonecrop root and herb
Radix et herba Taraxaci	***Taraxacum mongolicum***	Pu Gong Ying	Pou Gung Ying	Hokoei	Mongolian dandelion root and herb
Radix et herba Violae collinae	***Viola collina***	Di He Tao	Dei Hat Tou		Collina violet root and herb
Radix et herba Violae diffusae	***Viola diffusa***	Di Bai Cao	Dei Baak Chou		Spreading violet root and herb
Radix et herba Violae japonicae	***Viola japonica***	Li Tou Cao	Lai Tau Chou		Japanese violet root and herb
Radix et herba Violae yedoensis	***Viola yedoensis, V. japonica***	Zi Hua Di Ding	Ji Fa Dei Ding	Shikajicho	Asian violet root and herb
Radix et rhizoma Cynanchi stauntoni	***Cynanchum stauntoni, C. glaucescens***	Bai Qian	Baak Chin	Byakuzen	Prime white root
Radix et rhizoma Polygoni cymosi	***Polygonum cymosum***	Kai Jin Suo	Hoi Gam So		Cymose knotweed Root
Radix et rhizoma Solani melongenae	***Solanum melongena***	Qie Gen	Ke Gan		Eggplant root
Radix et rhizoma Ventilaginis	***Ventilago leiocarpa***	Xue Feng Teng, Qing Pi Mao	Hyut Fung Tang		Ventilago root and stem
Radix et rhizoma Veratri	***Veratrum nigrum* and spp**	Li Lu	Lai Lou	Riro	False hellebore root
Radix Euphorbiae ebracteolatae	***Euphorbia ebracteolata***	Lang Du, Yue Xian Da Ji	Long Duk, Yu Sin Daai Gik		Bractless spurge root
Radix Euphorbiae fischerianae	***Euphorbia fischeriana***	Lang Du, Lang Du Da Ji	Long Duk, Long Duk Daai Gik		Fischer's spurge root
Radix Euphorbiae kansui	***Euphorbia kansui***	Gan Sui	Gam Seui	Kansui	Sweet spurge root
Radix Euphorbiae nematocyphae	***Euphorbia nematocypha***	Lang Du, Da Lang Du	Long Duk, Daai Long Duk		Gigantic spurge root
Radix Euphorbiae pallasii seu ebracteolatae	***Euphorbia pallasii, E. abracteolatae, E. fischerianae***	(Bai) Lang Du	(Baak) Long Duk		White spurge root
Radix Euphorbiae pekinensis	***Euphorbia pekinensis***	Jing Da Ji	Ging Daai Gik	Taigeki	Peking spurge root

PHARMACEUTICAL	SCIENTIFIC	MANDARIN	CANTONESE	JAPANESE	ENGLISH
Radix Euphorbiae proliferae	***Euphorbia prolifera***	Lang Du, Ji Chang Lang Du	Long Duk, Gai Cheung Long Duk		Prolific spurge root
Radix Evodiae leptae	***Evodia lepta***	San Ya Ku (Gen)	Sam Nga Fu (Gan)		Bitter evodia root
Radix Fici microcarpae seu retusae	***Ficus microcarpa, F. retusa***	Lao Gong Xu, Rong Shu Xu	Lou Gung Chuk		Aerial fig root
Radix Gelsemii	***Gelsemium elegans***	Gou Wen	Au Man		Chinese gelsemium
Radix Gentianae macrophyllae	***Gentiana macrophylla, G. tibetica, G. dahurica*** **and spp**	Qin Jiao	Cheun Gau	Jingyo	Large-leaf gentian root
Radix Gentianae scabrae	***Gentiana scabra, G. triflora, G. manshurica***	Long Dan Cao	Lung Daam Chou	Ryutan	Scabrous gentian root
Radix Glehniae	***Glehnia littoralis***	Bei Sha Shen	Mai Sa Sam	Shajin	Northern sandroot
Radix Glycirrhizae	***Glycirrhiza uralensis, G. glabra*** **and spp**	Gan Cao	Gam Chou	Kanzo	Ural licorice root
Radix Glycirrhizae preparatae	***Glycirrhiza uralensis, G. glabra*** **and spp**	Zhi Gan Cao	Jek Gam Chou	Shakanzo	Honey-fried licorice root
Radix Glycirrhizae preparatae cum urino	***Glycirrhiza uralensis, G. glabra*** **and spp**	Ren Zhong Huang	Yan Chung Wong		Urine-prepared licorice root
Radix Gypsophylae	***Gypsophyla oldhamiana***	Yin Chai Hu	Ngan Chaai Wu		Gypsophyla root
Radix Hedysari polybotris	***Hedysarum polybotrys*** **and spp**	Huang Qi, Hong Qi	Wong Kei		Hedysarum root
Radix Hemerocallis	***Hemerocallis fulva***	Xuan Cao (Gen)	Syun Chou Gan		Tawny day lily root
Radix Hemsleyae	***Hemsleya amabilis, H. macrosperma*** **and spp.**	Xue Dan	Hat Daam		Hemsleya tuber
Radix Heraclei candicantis	***Heracleum candicans***	Du Huo	Duk Wut		White cow parsnip root
Radix Ilicis pubescentis	***Ilex pubescens***	Mao Dong Qing	Mou Dung Ching	Motosei	Furry holly root
Radix Inula helenii	***Inula helenium***	Tu Mu Xiang	Tou Muk Heung		Elecampane root
Radix Inulae racemosae	***Inula racemosa***	Tu Mu Xiang, Zong Zhuang Tu Mu Xiang	Tou Muk Heung, Chung Ching Tou Muk Heung		Racemose elecampane root
Radix Isatis tinctoriae	***Isatis tinctoria, I. indigotica***	Ban Lan Gen	Baan Laam Gan		Woad root
Radix Jasmini sambacis	***Jasminum sambac***	Mo Li Gen	Mut Lei Gan		Jasmine sambac root
Radix Kadsurae longipedunculatae	***Kadsura longipedunculata***	Hong Mu Xiang	Hung Muk Heung		Long-stalk kadsura root
Radix Knoxiae	***Knoxia valerianoides***	Hong Da Ji	Hung Daai Gik	Kogataigeki	Knoxia root
Radix lateralis Aconiti carmichaeli praeparatae	***Aconitum carmichaeli***	Fu Zi	Fu Ji	Bushi	Prepared Sichuan aconite root

PHARMACEUTICAL	SCIENTIFIC	MANDARIN	CANTONESE	JAPANESE	ENGLISH
Radix Ledebouriellae	***Ledebouriella divaricata, L. seseloides***	Fang Feng	Fong Fung	Bofu	Wind-protector root
Radix Leonticis	***Leontice robustum***	Hong Mao Qi	Hung Mou Chat		Leontice root
Radix Ligustici levistici	***Ligusticum levisticum***	Ou Dang Gui	Au Dong Gwai		Garden lovage root
Radix Ligustici sinensis	***Ligusticum sinense, L. jeholense***	Gao Ben	Gou Bun	Kohon	Chinese lovage root
Radix Ligustici walichii	***Ligusticum walichii***	Chuan Xiong, Xiong Qiong	Chyun Gung	Senkyu	Sichuan lovage root
Radix Lilii	***Lilium brownii*** var. ***colchesteri***	Bai He Gen	Baak Hap Gan		Brown's lily root
Radix Linderae	***Lindera strychnifolia***	Wu Yao, Tai Wu	Wu Yeuk, Toi Wu	Uyaku	Lindera root
Radix Liriopis platyphyllae	***Liriope platyphylla***	Mai Men Dong	Mak (Mun) Dung		Broad-leaf liriope root
Radix Liriopis spicatae	***Liriope spicata***	Mai (Men) Dong, Hu Bei Mai Men Dong	Mak (Mun) Dung, Wu Ba Mak Dung		Lance-leaf liriope root
Radix Lithospermi	***Lithospermum erythrorhizon***	Zi Cao	Ji Chou	Shikon	Purple groomwell root
Radix Lopatheri	***Lopatherum gracile***	Dan Zhu Gen	Daam Juk Gan		Bamboo grass root
Radix Macrotomiae	***Macrotomia euchroma***	Zi Cao	Ji Chou	Shikon	Macrotomia root
Radix Mahoniae japonicae	***Mahonia japonica***	Shi Da Gong Lao Gen	Sap Daai Gung Lou Gan		Japanese mahonia root
Radix Melothriae mederospatanae	***Melothria mederospatana***	Diao Jin Zhong	Diu Gam Jung		Melothria root
Radix Melothriae heterolphyllae	***Melothria heterophylla***	Tu Bai Lian	Taou Baak Lin		Native peppervine root
Radix Menispermi	***Menispermum dauricum***	Bei Dou Gen	Pan Dau Gan		Siberian moonseed root
Radix Millettiae philipinensis	***Millettia philipinensis***	Niu Da Li	Ngao Daai Lik		Millettia root
Radix Moghaniae	***Moghania macrophylla, M. philippinensis***	Yi Tiao Gen	Yat Tiu Gan		Moghania root
Radix Morindae	***Morinda officinalis***	Ba Ji Tian	Ba Gik Tin	Hagekiten	Morinda root
Radix Nardostachis	***Nardostachys jatamansi, N. chinensis***	Gan Song	Gam Chung		Indian spikenard root
Radix Onosmae	***Onosma paniculatum***	Zi Cao	Ji Chou		Onosma root
Radix Ophiopogonis	***Ophiopogon japonicus***	Mai (Men) Dong	Mak (Mun) Dung	Bakumondo	Dwarf lilyturf root
Radix Oryzae	***Oryza sativa***	Nuo Dao Gen (Xu)	No Du Gan	Jubeikon	Sweet rice root
Radix Paeoniae lactiflorae	***Paeonia lactiflora***	Bai Shao (Yao)	Baak Cheuk (Yeuk)	Byakushaku -(yaku)	White peony root
Radix Paeoniae rubrae	***Paeonia lactiflora, P. obovata, P. veitchii***	Chi Shao (Yao)	Chek Cheuk (Yeuk)	Sekishaku-(yaku)	Red peony root
Radix Paeoniae sinjiangensis	***Paeonia sinjiangensis***	Xin Jiang Bai Shao (Yao)	San Geung Chek Cheuk		Xinjiang peony root

PHARMACEUTICAL	SCIENTIFIC	MANDARIN	CANTONESE	JAPANESE	ENGLISH
Radix Panacis ginsengis	***Panax ginseng***	Ren Shen	Yan Sam	Ninjin	Asian ginseng root
Radix Panacis ginsengis	***Panax ginseng***	Sheng Shai Shen	Sang Sai Sam		Dried Asian ginseng root
Radix Panacis ginsengis	***Panax ginseng***	Ye Shan Shen	Gam San Sam		Wild Asian ginseng
Radix Panacis ginsengis praeparatae	***Panax ginseng***	Bai Shen	Baak Sam	Hakujin	Rock candy cured Asian ginseng root
Radix Panacis ginsengis praeparatae	***Panax ginseng***	Hong Ren Shen	Hung Yan Sam	Koninjin	Red cured Asian ginseng root
Radix Panacis japonici	***Panax japonicus***	Zhu Jie (Ren) Shen	Juk Jit (Yan) Sam	Tikusetu-ninjin	Japanese ginseng root
Radix Panacis majoris	***Panax major, P. repens***	Zhu Er Shen	Ju Yi Sam		Pearl ginseng root
Radix Panacis notoginsengis	***Panax notoginseng***	San Qi Tian Qi	Saam Chat Tin Chat	Sanshishi	Pseudogin-seng root
Radix Panacis quinquefolii	***Panax quinquefolius***	Xi Yang Shen	Fa Kei Sam, Sei Yang Sam	Seiyojin	American ginseng root
Radix Peucedani	***Peucedanum praeruptorum, P. decursivum***	Qian Hu	Chin Wu	Zenko	Asian masterwort root
Radix Peucedani japonici	***Peucedanum japonicum***	Fang Gui	Fong Kwai		Japanese masterwort root
Radix Pholidotae	***Pholidota chinensis***	Shi Xian Tao Gen	Sek Sin Tou Gan		Rattlesnake orchid root
Radix Phragmitis	***Phragmites communis***	Lu Gen	Lou Gan	Rokon	Water-reed root
Radix Phyllostachis	***Phyllostachys nigra*** var. ***henonis*** and spp	Zi Zhu Gen	Ji Juk Gan		Black bamboo root
Radix Phytolaccae acinosae	***Phytolacca acinosa, P. esculenta***	Shang Lu	Seung Luk	Shoriku	Asian poke root
Radix Picrorrhizae	***Picrorrhiza kurroa***	Hu Huang Lian	Wu Wong Lin	Kooren	Picrorrhiza root
Radix Piperis nigri	***Piper nigrum***	Hu Jiao Gen	Wu Jiu Gan		Black pepper root
Radix Pittospori	***Pittosporum pentandrum***	Qi Li Xiang	Chat Lei Heung		Pittosporum root
Radix Platycodonis	***Platycodon grandiflorum***	Jie Geng, Ku Jie Geng	Gat Gan	Kikyo	Balloonflower root
Radix Polygalae	***Polygala tenuifolia***	Yuan Zhi	Yun Ji	Onji	Thin-leaf milkwort root
Radix Polygalae sibiricae	***Polygala sibirica***	Tian Yuan Zhi	Tin Yun Ji		Siberian milkwort root
Radix Polygoni bistortae	***Polygonum bistorta***	Quan Shen	Kyun Sam		Bistort root
Radix Polygoni multiflori	***Polygonum multiflorum***	He Shou Wu	Ho Sau Wu	Kashuu	Flowery knotweed root
Radix Potentillae fragarioidis	***Potentilla fragarioides***	Mei Ye Wei Ling Cai	Mui Yip Wai Ling Choi		Strawberry-leaf cinquefoil root
Radix Pterospermi	***Pterospermum heterophyllum***	Ban Feng He Gen	Bun Fung Ho Gan		Pterospermum root
Radix Puerariae	***Pueraria lobata, P. omeiensis*** and spp	Ge Gen	Got Gan	Kakkon	Kudzu root

PHARMACEUTICAL	SCIENTIFIC	MANDARIN	CANTONESE	JAPANESE	ENGLISH
Radix Pulsatillae	***Pulsatilla chinensis, P. cernua, P. turczaninovii, P. ambigua*** and spp	Bai Tou Weng	Baak Tau Yung	Hakutoo	Asian pasqueflower root
Radix Pulsatillae dahuricae	***Pulsatilla dahurica***	Bai Tou Weng, Xing An Bai Tou Weng	Baak Tau Yung, Ing On Baak Tau Yung		Dahurian pasqueflower root
Radix Ranunculi	***Ranunculus ternatus***	Mao Zhao Cao, Mao Zhua Cao	Maau Jau Chou		Ternate buttercup root
Radix Raphani	***Raphanus sativus***	Di Gu Luo			Radish root
Radix Raphani recentis	***Raphanus sativus***	Luo Bo Gen	Lo Ba Gan		Fresh radish root
Radix Rauvolfiae	***Rauvolfia verticillata, R. yunnanensis, R. latifrons, R. serpentina*** and spp	Luo Fu Mu	Lo Fu Mou		Rauvolfia root
Radix Rehmanniae	***Rehmannia glutinosa***	Sheng Di (Huang)	Sang Dei (Wong)	Shojio	Fresh Rehmannia root
Radix Rehmanniae preparatae	***Rehmannia glutinosa***	Shu Di (Huang)	Suk Dei (Wong)	Jukujio	Prepared Rehmannia root
Radix Rhapontici	***Rhaponticum uniflorum***	Lou Lu	Lau Lou	Roro	Swiss centaury root
Radix Rhodomyrti	***Rhodomyrtus tomentosa***	Shui Duo Nian, Shan Nian Gen	Seui Do Lin, San Nim Gan		Downy rosemyrtle root
Radix Rhudis chinensis	***Rhus chinensis***	Pu Yan Pian	Pou Yim Pin		Chinese sumac root
Radix Rosae chinensis	***Rosa chinensis***	Yue Ji Gen	Yut Gwai Gan		Moonseason rose root
Radix Rosae multiflorae	***Rosa multiflora***	Ye Qiang Wei Gen	Ye Cheung Mei Gan		Wild rose root
Radix Rosae polyanthae	***Rosa polyantha*** and spp.	Qiang Wei Gen			Polyanth rose root
Radix Rubiae cordifoliae	***Rubia cordifolia***	Qian Cao Gen	Sin Chou Gan	Seisokon	Heart-leaf madder root
Radix Rumicis crispi	***Rumex crispus***	Niu Er Da Huang	Ngau Yi Daai Wong		Yellow dock root
Radix Rumicis japonici	***Rumex japonicus, R. nepalensis***	Yang Ti	Yeung Tai		Japanese dock root
Radix Salviae bowleyanae	***Salvia bowleyana***	Dan Shen, Nan Dan Shen	Daan Sam, Naam Dam Sam		Southern cinnabar sage root
Radix Salviae miltiorrhizae	***Salvia miltiorrhiza***	Dan Shen	Daan Sam	Tanjin	Cinnabar sage root
Radix Sanguisorbae	***Sanguisorba officinalis***	Di Yu	Dei Yu	Jiyu	Great burnet root
Radix Sapindi	***Sapindus mukorossi***	Wu Huan Gen, Mu Huan Gen	Mou Waan Gan		Soapnut tree root
Radix Saussureae lanicepsis	***Saussurea laniceps, S. involucrata*** and spp	Xue Lian Gen	Hat Ling Gan		Snow lotus root
Radix Saussureae lappae	***Saussurea lappa***	Mu Xiang, Yun Mu Xiang	Muk Heung	Mokko	Wood aromatic root
Radix Scopariae	***Scoparia dulcis***	Ye Gan Cao, Zhu Cai Cao Gen	Ye Gam Chou, Chu Jai Chou Gan		Scoparia root

PHARMACEUTICAL	SCIENTIFIC	MANDARIN	CANTONESE	JAPANESE	ENGLISH
Radix Scrophulariae	***Scrophularia ningpoensis, S. buergeriana***	Xuan Shen, Yuan Shen	Yun Sam, Yun Sam	Genjin	Black figwort root
Radix Scutellariae baicalensis	***Scutellaria baicalensis, S. viscidula, S. amoena***	Huang Qin	Wong Sam	Ogon	Baikal skullcap root
Radix Semiaquilegiae	***Semiaquilegia adoxoides***	Tian Kui	Tin Kwai		Semiaquilegia root
Radix Serratulae	***Serratula chinensis***	Guang Dong Sheng Ma	Gwong Dung Jing Ma		Serratula root
Radix seu caulis Aristolochiae moupiensis	***Aristolochia moupiensis***	Huai Tong	Waai Tung		Birthwort root or stem
Radix seu cortex radicis Eleutherococci senticosi	***Eleutherococcus senticosus***	Ci Wu Jia (Gen Pi)	Chi Ng Ga (Gan Pei)		Eleuthero ginseng root
Radix Sinomenii	***Sinomenium acutum***	Qing Feng Teng	Ching Fung Tang		Sinomenium root
Radix Solani verbascifolii	***Solanum verbascifolium***	Ye Yan Ye Gen, Tu Yen Tou	Ye Yin Yip Gan, Tou Yin Tau		Tobacco nightshade root
Radix Sophorae flavescentis	***Sophora flavescens***	Ku Shen	Fu Sam		Yellow pagoda tree root
Radix Sophorae subprostatae	***Sophora subprostata***	Shan Dou Gen	Saan Dau Gan		Pigeon-pea root
Radix Staticis	***Statice sinensis***	Hong Mao Cha	Hung Maau Cha		Statice root
Radix Stellariae	***Stellaria dichotoma*** var. ***lanceolata***	Yin Chai Hu	Ngan Chaai Wu	Ginsaiko	Stellaria root
Radix Stellerae	***Stellera chamaejasme***	Hong Lang Du, Lang Du	Hung Long Duk, Long Duk		Stellara root
Radix Stemonae japonicae	***Stemona japonia***	Bai Bu, Man Sheng Bai Bu	Baak Bou, Maan Sang Baak Bou	Hyakubu	Japanese stemona root
Radix Stemonae sessilifoliae	***Stemona sessilifolia***	Bai Bu, Zhi Li Bai Bu	Baak Bou, Chek Lap Baak Bou		Sessile stemona root
Radix Stemonae tuberosae	***Stemona tuberosa***	Bai Bu, Dui Ye Bai Bu	Baak Bou, Deui Yip Baak Bou		Tuberous stemona root
Radix Stephaniae tetrandrae	***Stephania tetrandra***	Han Fang Ji, Fang Ji	Haan Fong Gei Fong Gei	Kamboi	Stephania root
Radix Strobilanthis	***Strobilanthes flaccidifolius***	Ma Lan Gen	Ma Laam Gan		Strobilanthes root
Radix Swertiae	***Swertia pseudochinensis*** and spp	Dang Yao	Dong Yeuk		Asian green gentian root
Radix Talini	***Talinum paniculatum***	Tu Ren Shen	Tou Yan Sam		Fameflower root
Radix Tinosporae	***Tinospora sagittata, T. capillipes***	Jin Guo Lan	Gam Gwo Laam	Kinkaran	Tinospora root
Radix Toddaliae	***Toddalia asiatica***	Fei Long Zhang Xue	Fei Lung Jeung Hyut		Asian toddalia root
Radix Trichosanthis	***Trichosanthes kirilowii, T. japonica, T. uniflora***	Tian Hua Fen	Tin Fa Fun	Tenkafun	Snakegourd root

PHARMACEUTICAL	SCIENTIFIC	MANDARIN	CANTONESE	JAPANESE	ENGLISH
Radix Tripterygii hypoglauci decorticati	***Tripterygium hypoglaucum***	Kun Ming Shan Hai Tang, Diao Mao Cao	Kwan Ming Saan Hoi Tong		Peeled Tripterygium root
Radix Typhonii	***Typhonium giganteum***	Du Jiao Lan	Duk Gok Lin		Typhonium root
Radix Viticis quinatae	***Vitex quinata***	Pu Jiang Gen	Pou Geung Gan		Quinate chasteberry root
Radix Vitis	***Vitis thunbergii*** and spp	Ye Pu Tao	Ye Pou Tou		Wild grape root
Radix Vitis amurensis	***Vitis amurensis***	Shan Teng Teng Yang	Saan Tang Tang Yeung		Amur grape root
Radix Vitis flexuosis	***Vitis flexuosa***	Ge Lei Zhi Gen	Got Leui Jap Gan		Flexuose grape root
Radix Wickstroemiae	***Wickstroemia indica***	Liao Ge Wang (Gen)	Liu Go Wong	Ryokao	Wikstroemia root
Radix Zanthoxyli avicennae	***Zanthoxylum avicennae***	Niao Bu Su, Bai Ma Niao	Niu Bat Suk		Prickly ash root
Radix Zanthoxyli nitidi	***Zanthoxylum nitidum***	Ru Di Jin Niu, Liang Mian Zhen	Yap Dei Gam Ngau		Shiny bramble root
Radox Ixorae	***Ixora chinensis***	Long Chuan Hua Gen	Lung Syun Fa Gan		Ixora root
Ramulus Cinnamomi cassiae	***Cinnamomum cassia***	Gui Zhi , Rou Gui Zhi	Gwai Ji	Keishi	Cassia cinnamon twig
Ramulus et cortex Querci	***Quercus dentata, Q. acutissima***	Pu Suo	Pok Sau	Bokuso	Oak twig and bark
Ramulus et folium Cephalotaxi	***Cephalotaxus fortunei***	San Jian Shan	Saam Jim Chaam		Yew twig and leaf
Ramulus et folium Cephalotaxi sinensis	***Cephalotaxus sinensis***	Tu Xiang Fei	Tou Heung Fei		Plum yew twig and leaf
Ramulus et folium Murrayae	***Murraya paniculata***	Jiu Li Xiang	Gau Lei Heung		Burma boxwood twig and leaf
Ramulus et folium Picrasmae	***Picrasma quassioides***	Ku (Shu) Mu	Fu (Syu) Muk		Quassiawood twig and leaf
Ramulus et uncus Uncariae	***Uncaria rhynchophylla, U. hirsuta, U. macrophylla*** and spp	Gou Teng	Ngau Tang, Sheung Ngau (Tang)	Choto	Gambir vine twig
Ramulus Eunymi alati	***Euonymus alata***	Gui Jian Yu	Gwai Jin Yu		Winged spindletree twig
Ramulus Juglandis	***Juglans regia***	Hu Tao Zhi	Wu Tou Ji		Walnut twig
Ramulus Loranthi	***Loranthus parasiticus, L. yadorici*** and spp	Sang Ji Sheng	Song Gei Sang	Sokisei	Asian mistletoe twig
Ramulus Mori	***Morus alba***	Sang Zhi	Song Ji	Soshi	Mulberry twig
Ramulus Nelumbinis	***Nelumbo nucifera***	Lian Geng	Lin Gang		Lotus stem
Ramulus Perillae	***Perilla frutescens***	Zi Su Geng	Sou Gan		Perilla stem
Ramulus Phragmitis	***Phragmites communis***	Wei Jing	Lou Ging		Water-reed twig
Ramulus Piperis wallichii	***Piper wallichii***	Shi Nan Teng	Sek Naam Tang		Wild pepper twig
Ramulus Sabiae	***Sabia japonica***	Qi Feng Teng	Ching Fung Tang		Sabia twig
Ramulus Salicis	***Salix babylonica, S. gracilistyla***	Liu Zhi	Lau Ji		Weeping willow twig

PHARMACEUTICAL	SCIENTIFIC	MANDARIN	CANTONESE	JAPANESE	ENGLISH
Ramulus Salicis purpureae	*Salix purpurea*	Shui Yang Zhi	Seui Yeung Ji		Purple willow twig
Ramulus Scurrulae	*Scurrula ritozanensis*	Tai Wan Ji Sheng	Toi Waan Ji Sang		Taiwan mistletoe twig
Ramulus Taxilli	*Taxillus yadoriki, T. chinensis*	Shi Ji Sheng	Chi Gei Sang		Asian mistletoe twig
Ramulus Visci liquidambarici	*Viscum liquidambaricum*	Bian Ji Sheng	Bin Gei Sang		Asian mistletoe twig
Ramus et folium Lonicerae japonicae	*Lonicera japonica*	Jin Yin Teng, Ren Dong Teng	Gam Ngan Tang, Yan Dung Tang		Japanese honeysuckle stem and leaf
Realgar	*Realgar*	Xiong Huang	Song Wong	Yuo	Realgar
Receptaculum Helianthi	*Helianthus annuus*	Xian Ji Gui Hua Pan	Heung Yat Kwai Fa Bun		Sunflower receptacle
Receptaculum Nelumbinis	*Nelumbo nucifera*	Lian Fang	Lin Fong	Renshin	Lotus receptacle
Redix seu semen Anisodi	*Anisodus tanguticus*	Zang Qie	Jong Ke		Anisodus root or seed
Resina Daemonoropsis (Sanguis draconis)	*Daemonorops draco*	Xue Jie	Hyut Kit	Kekketsu	Dragon's-blood resin
Resina Aloidis	*Aloe vera* var. *chinensis*	Lu Hui	Lou Wui		Aloe resin
Resina Boswelliae	*Boswellia carterii* and spp.	Ru Xiang	Yu Heung	Nyuko	Frankincense resin
Resina Calophylli	*Calophyllum inophyllum*	Hu Tong Lei	Ng Tung Leui		Foraha resin
Resina Commiphorae	*Commiphora myrrha*	Mo Yao	Mut Yeuk	Motsuyaku	Myrrh resin
Resina Ferulae (Asafoetidae)	*Ferula foetida*	A Wei	A Ngai	Agi	Asafoetida resin
Resina Garciniae	*Garcinia morella*	Teng Huang	Tang Wong		Gamboge resin
Resina Liquidambaris (Styrax liquidis)	*Liquidambar orientalis*	Su He Xiang	Sou Hap Heung	Sogoko	Storax resin
Resina Liquidambaris taiwaninanae	*Liquidambar taiwaniana*	Bai Jiao Xiang	Baak Gaau Heung		Taiwan maple fruit resin
Resina Pini preparatae, Colophonium	*Pinus massoniana, P. tabulaeformis* and spp, *Larix* spp	Song Xiang	Chung Heung		Pine resin
Resina Pini succiniferae (Succinum)	*Pinus succinifera*	Hu Po	Fu Po		Amber resin
Resina Populi	*Populus euphratica* and spp	Hu Tong Lei	Wu Tung Leui		Poplar resin
Rhizoma Helminthostachys	*Helminthostachys zeylanica*	Di Wu Song	Dei Ng Gung		Helmintho-stachys root
Rhizoma Pseudodrynariae	*Pseudodrynaria fortunei, D. baronii*	Gu Sui Bu	Gwat Seui Bou	Kotsusaiho	Boneknit root
Rhizoma Aconiti coreani	*Aconitum coreanum*	Bai Fu Zi, Guan Bai Fu	Baak Fu Ji, Gwan Baak Fu Ji		Prepared Korean aconite root
Rhizoma Acori calami	*Acorus calamus*	Shui Chang Pu, Bai Chang Pu	Seui Cheung Pou, Baak Cheung Pou	Shobu	Sweetflag root
Rhizoma Acori graminei	*Acorus gramineus*	Shi Chang Pu	Sek Cheung Pou		Rock sweetflag root

PHARMACEUTICAL	SCIENTIFIC	MANDARIN	CANTONESE	JAPANESE	ENGLISH
Rhizoma Acori tatarinowii	***Acorus tatarinowii***	Jie Chang Pu	Jik Cheung Pou		Tatarinow's sweetflag root
Rhizoma Alismae	***Alisma orientalis***	Ze Xie	Jaak Se	Takusha	Water plantain root
Rhizoma Alocasiae	***Alocasia odora***	Guang Lang Du, Hai Yu	Hoi Wu		Alocasia root
Rhizoma Alpiniae officinari	***Alpinia officinarum***	Gao Liang Jiang	Gou Leung Geung	Koryokyo	Galangal root
Rhizoma Amorphophalli	***Amorphophallus rivieri, A. sinensis, A. knojac***	Ju Ruo	Geui Yeuk		Amorpho-phallus root
Rhizoma Anemoni altaicae	***Anemone altaica***	Jiu Jie Chang Pu	Gau Jit Cheung Pou	Arutai ginrenkon	Altai anemone root
Rhizoma Anemonis raddeanae	***Anemone raddeana***	Liang Tou Jian	Leung Tau Jim		Anemone root
Rhizoma Ardisiae gigantifoliae	***Ardisia gigantifolia***	Zou Ma Tai	Jau Ma Toi		Ardisia root
Rhizoma Arisaemae preparatae	***Arisaema consanguineum, A. amurense*** **and spp**	Tian Nan Xing, Zhi Nan Xing	Tin Naam Sing, Jek Naam Sing		Prepared dragon arum corm
Rhizoma Asari forbesii	***Asarum forbesii***	Du Heng	Dou Hang		Forbes' wild ginger root
Rhizoma Asparagi cochinensis	***Asparagus cochinchinensis***	Tian (Men) Dong	Tin (Mun) Dung	Tenmondo	Shiny asparagus root
Rhizoma Asparagi officinalis	***Asparagus officinalis***	Shi Diao Bai	Sek Diu Baak		Asparagus root
Rhizoma Astilbis	***Astilbe chinensis***	Luo Xin Fu	Lok San Fu		Astilbe root
Rhizoma Atractylodis japonicae	***Atractylodes japonica***	Cang Zhu, Guan Cang Zhu	Chong Seut, Gwan Chong Seut		Japanese black Atractylodes root
Rhizoma Atractylodis lanceae	***Atractylodes lancea, A. sinensis*** **and spp**	Cang Zhu, Mao Cang Zhu	Chong Seut, Mau Chong Seut	Sojutsu	Black atractylodes root
Rhizoma Atractylodis macrocephalae	***Atractylodes macrocephala***	Bai Zhu	Baak Seut	Byakujutsu	White atractylodes root
Rhizoma Belamcandae	***Belamcanda chinensis***	She Gan	Se Gon	Yakan	Leopard flower root
Rhizoma Blechni	***Blechnum orientale***	Guan Zhong, Wu Mao Jue Guan Zhong, Dong Fang Wu Mao Jue Ye	Gwun Jung, Dung Fong Wu Mou Kyut Yip	Kanju	Oriental hammock fern root
Rhizoma Bletillae	***Bletilla striata***	Bai Ji	Baak Gap	Byakukyu	Amethyst orchid root
Rhizoma Cannae	***Canna indica***	Mei Ren Jiao (Gen)	Mei Yan Jiu (Gan)	Dandoku	Canna lily root
Rhizoma Cibotii	***Cibotium barometz***	Gou Ji	Gau Jek	Kuseki	Dogspine root
Rhizoma Coptis	***Coptis chinensis, C. omeiensis*** **and spp**	Huang Lian, Chuan Lian	Wong Lin, Chyun Wong Lin	Oren	Goldthread root
Rhizoma Corydalis	***Corydalis turtschaninovii***	Yan Hu Suo, Chi Ban Yan Hu Suo	Yin Wu Sok, Chi Faan Yin Wu Sok	Engosaku	Dentate-leaf corydalis corm
Rhizoma Corydalis ambiguae	***Corydalis ambigua*** **var.** ***amurensis***	Yan Hu Suo, Dong Bei Yan Hu Suo	Yin Wu Sok, Dung Bak Yin Wu Sok		Amur corydalis corm

PHARMACEUTICAL	SCIENTIFIC	MANDARIN	CANTONESE	JAPANESE	ENGLISH
Rhizoma Curculigonis	***Curculigo orchioides***	Xian Mao	Sin Maau	Sembo	Golden eye-grass root
Rhizoma Curcumae	***Curcuma longa. C. aromatica***	Jiang Huang	Geung Wong	Kyoo	Turmeric root
Rhizoma Curcumae kwangsiensis	***Curcuma kwangsiensis***	E Zhu, Guang Xi Er Zhu	Ngo Seut, Gwong Sai Ngo Seut		Guangxi turmeric root
Rhizoma Curcumae zedoariae	***Curcuma zedoaria, C. aeruginosa*** and spp	E Zhu, Peng Er Zhu	Ngo Seut, Fung Ngo Seut	Gajutsu	Zedoary root
Rhizoma Cyatheae	***Cyathea spinulosa***	Guan Zhong	Gwun Jung		Cyathea root
Rhizoma Cyperi	***Cyperus rotundus***	Xiang Fu	Heung Fu	Kobushi	Purple nutsedge root
Rhizoma Cyrtomi	***Cyrtomium fortunei***	Guan Zhong, Hun Ji Tou,	Gwun Jung, Fan Gai Tau		Boss fern root
Rhizoma Davalliae	***Davallia divaricata***	Gu Sui Bu	Gwat Seui Bou	Kotsusaiho	Boneknit root
Rhizoma Dioscoreae bulbiferae	***Dioscorea bulbifera***	Huang Yao Zi	Wong Yeuk Ji	Oyakushi	Potato yam root
Rhizoma Dioscoreae cirrhosae	***Dioscorea cirrhosa***	Shu Liang	Syu Leung		Dyer's yam root
Rhizoma Dioscoreae hypoglaucae	***Dioscorea hypoglauca***	Bi Xie, Fen Bi Xie, Bei Xie	Bei Gaai, Fan Bei Gaai	Hikai	Long yam root
Rhizoma Dioscoreae japonicae	***Dioscorea japonica***	Feng Che Er	Fung Che Yi		Japanese yam root
Rhizoma Dioscoreae nipponicae	***Dioscorea nipponica***	Chuan Shan Long	Chyun Saan Lung		Nippon yam root
Rhizoma Dioscoreae oppositae	***Dioscorea opposita, D. batatas***	Shan Yao Shu Yu	Wai Saan, Saan Yeuk	Sanyaku	Mountain yam root
Rhizoma Dioscoreae septemlobae	***Dioscorea septemloba***	Bi Xie, Mian Bi Xie	Bei Gaai, Min Bei Gaai		Seven-lobe yam root
Rhizoma Dioscoreae zingiberis	***Dioscorea zingiberensis***	Dun Ye Shu Yu	Teun Yip Syu Yu		Shield-leaf yam root
Rhizoma Drynariae	***Drynaria fortunei*** and spp	Gu Sui Bu	Gwat Seui Bou	Kotsusaiho	Boneknit root
Rhizoma Dryopteris	***Dryopteris crassirhizoma***	Guan Zhong, Mian Ma Guan Zhong	Gwun Jung, Min Ma Gwun Jung	Tohoku-kanju	Shield fern root
Rhizoma Dysosmae pleianthae	***Dysosma pleiantha***	Ba Jiao Lian	Baat Gok Lin		Pleianth dysosma root
Rhizoma Dysosmae versipellis	***Dysosma versipellis***	Gui Jiu	Gwai Kau		Common dysosma root
Rhizoma et radix Cremastrae	***Cremastra variabilis***	Shan Ci Gu	Saan Chi Gu		Cremastra corm
Rhizoma et radix Hemerocallis thunbergii	***Hemerocallis thunbergii***	Li Lu	Lai Lou		Day lily root
Rhizoma et radix Notopterigii	***Notopterygium incisum, N. forbesii, N. francherii***	Qiang Huo	Geung Wut	Kyokatsu	Notopterygium root

PHARMACEUTICAL	SCIENTIFIC	MANDARIN	CANTONESE	JAPANESE	ENGLISH
Rhizoma et radix Tulipae	***Tulipa edulis***	Shan Ci Gu, Guang Ci Gu	San Chi Gu, Gwong Chi Gu		Chinese tulip bulb
Rhizoma Fagopyri	***Fagopyrum cymosum***	Jin Qiao Mai Gen	Gam Kiu Mak Gan		Buckwheat root
Rhizoma Gastrodiae	***Gastrodia elata***	Tian Ma	Tin Ma	Temma	Celestial hemp corm
Rhizoma Homalomenae	***Homalomena occulta***	Qian Nian Jian	Chin Nin Gin	Sennenken	Homalomena root
Rhizoma Imperatae	***Imperata cylindrica*** var. ***major***	Bai Mao Gen	Baak Maau Gan	Bokon	Woolly grass root
Rhizoma Iris tectoris	***Iris tectorum***	Yuan Wei	Yun Mei		Kite-tail iris root
Rhizoma Kaempferiae	***Kaempferia galanga***	Shan Nai, Sha Jiang	Saan Noi		Galanga root
Rhizoma Lunathyri	***Lunathyrum vegetius, L. giraldii***	Guan Zhong	Gwun Jung		Lunathyrum fern root
Rhizoma Lycopi lucidi	***Lycopus lucidus***	Di Sun	Dei Seun		Bright bugleweed root
Rhizoma Lycoris	***Lycoris radiata***	Shi Suan	Sek Syun		Red spiderlily corm
Rhizoma Matteuciae	***Matteucia struthiopteris***	Guan Zhong, Jia Guo Jue Guan Zhong	Gwun Jung, Ying Gwo Kyut Gwun Jung		Ostrich-feather fern root
Rhizoma nodi Nelumbinis	***Nelumbo nucifera***	Ou Jie	Ngau Jit		Lotus root node
Rhizoma Nupharis	***Nuphar japonicum, N. pumilum***	Ping Peng Cao Gan	Ping Fung Chou Gan	Senkotu	Yellow pond lily root
Rhizoma Opuntiae	***Opuntia dillenii*** and spp	Xian Ren Zhang	Sin Yan Jeung		Prickly pear root
Rhizoma Osmundae	***Osmunda japonica***	Guan Zhong, Zi Qi Guan Zhong	Gwun Jung, Ji Kei Gwun Jung	Tohoku-kanju	Japanese flowering fern root
Rhizoma Panacis ginsengis	***Panax ginseng***	Ren Shen Lu	Yan Sam Lu	Ninjinro	Asian ginseng neck
Rhizoma Paris	***Paris polyphylla, P. chinensis, P. formosana*** and var.	Qi Ye Yi Zhi Hua, Zao Xiu	Chak Yip Jek Ji Fa, Sat Yau	Kenjin	Paris root
Rhizoma Paris chinensis	***Paris chinensis***	Zhong Lou, Qi Ye Yi Zhi Hua	Jung Lau, Chat Yip Yat Ji Pa		Chinese paris root
Rhizoma Paris yunnanensis	***Paris yunnanensis***	Zhong Lou, Yun Nan Zhong Lou	Jung Lau, Wan Laam Jung Lau		Yunnan paris root
Rhizoma Physalis	***Physalis alkakengi*** (var. ***franchetii)***	Suan Jiang Gen	Syun Jeung Gan		Chinese lantern root
Rhizoma Pinelliae fermentatae	***Pinellia ternata***	Ban Xia Qu	Bun Ha Chau		Fermented Pinellia corm
Rhizoma Pinelliae pedatisectae	***Pinellia pedatisecta***	Zhang Ye Ban Xia, Wu Zhang Nan Xing	Jeung Yip Bun Ha, Fu Jeung Lam Sing		Pedatisect pinellia corm
Rhizoma Pinelliae ternatae preparatae	***Pinellia ternata***	Ban Xia Fa Ban Xia	Bun Ha, Faat Bun Ha	Hange, Kohange	Prepared pinellia corm
Rhizoma pinelliae ternatae	***Pinellia ternata***	Sheng Ban Xia	Sang Bun Ha, So Bun Ha	Shohange	Raw pinellia corm
Rhizoma Pleionis	***Pleione bulbocodioides***	Shan Ci Gu	Saan Chi Gu		Pleione corm

PHARMACEUTICAL	SCIENTIFIC	MANDARIN	CANTONESE	JAPANESE	ENGLISH
Rhizoma Podophylli emodii	***Podophyllum emodi***	Tao Er Qi	Tou Yi Chat		Emodi's podophullum root
Rhizoma Podophylli pleianthi	***Podophyllum pleianthum***	Ba Jiao Lian	Ba Gok Lin		Pleianth podophyllum root
Rhizoma Polygonati	***Polygonatum sibiricum, P. cyrtonema, P. kingianum***	Huang Jing	Wong Jing	Osei	Siberian Solomon's-seal root
Rhizoma Polygonati odorati	***Polygonatum odoratum*** var. ***pluriflorum, P. plurifolium***	Yu Zhu	Yuk Juk	Gyokuchiku	Fragrant Solomon's seal root
Rhizoma Rhei	***Rheum palmatum, R. tanguticum, R. officinale***	Da Huang	Daai Wong	Daio	Rhubarb root
Rhizoma seu herba Lysimachiae capillipis	***Lysimachia capillipes***	Man Shan Xiang	Mun Sam Heung		Lysimachia root or herb
Rhizoma Smilacis chinensis	***Smilax china***	Jin Gang Teng, Ba Qi	Gam Gong Tang, Bat Kai		Chinese greenbrier root, China root
Rhizoma Smilacis glabrae	***Smilax glabra***	Tu Fu Ling	Tou Fuk Ling		Glabrous greenbrier root
Rhizoma Sparganii	***Sparganium simplex, S. stoloniferum, S. stenophyllum***	San Leng	Saam Ling		Bur-reed root
Rhizoma Typhonii divaricatii	***Typhonium divaricatum***	Li Tou Jian	Lai Tau Jim		Divaricate typhonium root
Rhizoma Typhonii flagelliformis preparata	***Typhonium flagelliforme***	Shui Ban Xia	Seui Bun Ha		Prepared flagellate typhonium root
Rhizoma Typhonii gigantei preparata	***Typhonium giganteum***	Bai Fu Zi, Yu Bai Fu	Baak Fu Ji	Byakubushi	Prepared giant typhonium root
Rhizoma Valerianae	***Valeriana officinalis, V. hardwickii***	Xie Cao	Kit Chou		Valerian root
Rhizoma Woodwardiae	***Woodwardia japonica, W. unigemmata***	Guan Zhong, Gou Ji Guan Zhong	Gwun Jung, Gau Jek Gun Jung		Chain-fern root
Rhizoma Zingiberis	***Zingiber officinalis***	(Sheng) Jiang Pi	Saang Geung Pei		Fresh ginger root skin
Rhizoma Zingiberis	***Zingiber officinalis***	Gan Jiang	Gaan Geung	Kankyo	Dried ginger root
Rhizoma Zingiberis	***Zingiber officinalis***	Pao Jiang	Bou Geung	Hokyo	Quick-fried ginger root
Rhizoma Zingiberis miogae	***Zingiber mioga***	Rang He	Yeung Ho		Mioga ginger root
Rhizoma Zingiberis recentis	***Zingiber officinalis***	Sheng Jiang	Saang Geung	Shokyo	Fresh ginger root
Rizoma Corydalis yanhusuoidis	***Corydalis yanhusuo***	Yan Hu Suo, Yuan Hu	Yin Wu Sok, Yun Wu	Engosaku	Asian corydalis corm
Saccharum Diospyris	***Diospyros kaki***	Shi Bing Shuang	Chi Beng Sheung		Persimmon frost
Saccharum Hordei	***Hordeum vulgare***	Yi Tang, Jiao Yi	Yi Tong		Barley malt sugar

PHARMACEUTICAL	SCIENTIFIC	MANDARIN	CANTONESE	JAPANESE	ENGLISH
Saccharum Oryzae	***Oryza sativa***			Koi	Rice malt (syrup)
Salmiacum	***Salammonitum*** **and *Halitum***	Nao Sha	Lou Sa		Salmiac, Sal ammoniac
Sclerotium Armillariae	***Armillaria mellea***	Mi Huan Jun			Honey mushroom
Sclerotium Auriculariae	***Auricularia auricula***	Mu Er	Muk Yi	Kikurage	Wood ear mushroom
Sclerotium Cordycepsis scotianus	***Cordyceps scotianus*** **and *host Cryptotympana atrata*** **and spp**	Chan Hua, Jin Chan Hua	Sim Fa, Gam Sim Fa		Cicada fungus
Sclerotium Cordycepsis sinensis	***Cordyceps sinensis*** **and host larvae *Hepialus armoricanus or Holotrichia koraiensis***	Dong Chong Xia Cao	Dung Chung Ha Chou	Tochukaso	Chinese caterpillar mushroom
Sclerotium Corioli versicolori	***Coriolus versicolor (syn. Trametes versicolor)***	Yun Zhi	Wan Ji		Turkey tail mushroom
Sclerotium Fomis	***Fomes applanatus*** **and *host fruit Euphoria longana***	Long Yan Gu	Lung Ngan Gu		Longan fungus
Sclerotium Ganodermae	***Ganoderma lucidum, G. sinense, G applanatum*** **and spp**	Ling Zhi (Cao)	Ling Ji (Chou)	Reishi	Reishi mushroom
Sclerotium Grifolae frondosae	***Grifola frondosa***			Maitake	Maitake, Hen of the woods mushroom
Sclerotium Hericii	***Hericium erinaceus***	Hou Gu			Hedgehog fungus
Sclerotium Lasiosphaerae seu Calvatiae	***Lasiosphaera fenslii*** **and spp, *Calvatia lilacina, C. fenzlii, C. gigantea***	Ma Bo	Ma But	Babotsu	Puffball mushroom
Sclerotium Lentinulae	***Lentinula edodes***	Xiang Gu	Heung Gu	Shiitake	Shiitake mushroom
Sclerotium Mylittae	***Mylitta lapidescens***	Lei Wan	Leui Yun		Thunder ball fungus
Sclerotium Polypori	***Polyporus umbellatus***	Zhu Ling	Ju Ling	Chorei	Umbel polypore mushroom
Sclerotium Poriae	***Poria cocos***	Fu Ling	(Wong) Fuk Ling, Waan Ling	Bukuryo	Hoelen fungus
Sclerotium Poriae paradicis	***Poria cocos***	Fu Shen	Pou Fuk Sam	Bukushin	Hoelen spirit
Sclerotium Poriae rubrae	***Poria cocos***	Chi Fu Ling	Chek Fuk Ling	Sekibikuryo	Red hoelen
Sclerotium Tremellae fucimormis	***Tremella fuciformis***	Bai Mu Er	Baak Muk Yi	Hakumokuji	Silver ear mushroom
Sclerotium Tremellae mesentericae	***Tremella mesenterica***	Huang Mu Er	Wong Muk Yi		Yellow ear mushroom
Sclerotium Umbilicariae	***Umbilicaria esculenta***	Shi Er	Sek Yi		Stone ear mushroom

PHARMACEUTICAL	SCIENTIFIC	MANDARIN	CANTONESE	JAPANESE	ENGLISH
Scolopendra	*Scolopendra subspinipes mutilans*	Wu Gong	Ng Gung	Gosho	Centipede
Secretio Bufonis	*Bufo gargarizans, B. melanostictus*	Chan Su	Sim Sou	Senjo	Toad venom
Secretio Moschi	*Moschus berezovskii* and spp	She Xiang	Se Heung	Jako	Musk
Sedimen urinae Hominis	*Homo sapiens*	Ren Zhong Bai, Qiu Shi Dan	Yan Jung Baak		Human urine sediment
Selenitum	*Selenitum*	Xuan Jing Shi	San Ching Sek		Selenite
Semen Abutili theophrasti	*Abutilon theophrastii*	Qing Ma (Zi)	King Ma (Ji)		China jute seed
Semen Aleuritis	*Aleurites fordii*	You Tong Zi	Yau Tung Ji		Tung seed
Semen Alii tuberosi	*Allium tuberosum*	Jiu Cai Zi	Gau Choi Ji	Kyushi	Asian leek seed
Semen Allii fistulosi	*Allium fistulosum*	Cong Zi	Chung Ji	Sohaku	Scallion seed
Semen Alpiniae katsumadis	*Alpinia katsumadai*	Cao Dou Kou	Chou Dau Kau	Sozuku	Katsumada's galangal seed
Semen Amomi villosi	*Amomum villosum*	Guang Sha Ren	Gwong Sa Yan		Wild cardamom seed
Semen Arecae catechu	*Areca catechu, A. dicksonii*	Bing Lang	Ban Long	Binroji	Betel nut
Semen Astragali complanati	*Astragalus complanatus* and spp	Sha Yuan Zi, Sha Yuan Ji Li	Sa Yun Ji, Sa Yun Jek Lai	Saenshi, Toshitsuri	Flat milkvetch seed
Semen Benincasae	*Benincasa hispida*	Dong Gua Ren	Dong Gwa Yan	Tokanin	Waxgourd seed
Semen Biotae orientalis	*Biota orientalis*	Bai Zi Ren	(Baak) Ji Yan	Hakushinin	Oriental arborvitae berry
Semen Caesalpiniae minacis	*Caesalpinia minax*	Ku Shi Lian (Zi)	Fu Sek Lin (Ji)		Caesalpinia seed
Semen Cajani	*Cajanus cajan*	Mu Dou Zi	Muk Dau Ji		Pigeon pea seed
Semen Canavaliae	*Canavalia gladiata, C. ensiformis*	Dao Dou	Dou Dau		Swordbean seed
Semen Cannabis	*Cannabis sativa*	Huo Ma Ren	Fo Ma Yan	Mashinin	Cannabis seed
Semen Capparis	*Capparis masaikai*	Ma Bin Lang	Ma Ban Long	Kuttokei	Capparis berry
Semen Cassiae occidentalis	*Cassia occidentalis*	Wang Jiang Nan Zi	Mong Gong Naam	Banshashi	Coffee senna seed
Semen Cassiae torae	*Cassia tora, C. obtusifolia* and spp	Jue Ming Zi, Cao Jue Ming	Kyut Ming Ji, Chou Kyut Ming	Ketsumeishi	Sickle senna seed
Semen Celosiae argenteae	*Celosia argentea*	Qing Xiang Zi	Ching Seung Ji	Seisoshi	Silver quail-grass seed
Semen Citri grandi immaturi	*Citrus grandis*	You He	Yau Hat		Pomelo seed
Semen Citri reticulatae	*Citrus reticulata, C. tangerina, C. erythrosa*	Ju He	Gwat Hat		Tangerine seed
Semen Clauseniae	*Clausenia lansium*	Huang Pi He	Wong Pei Ho		Wampi seed
Semen Coicis	*Coix lachryma-jobi* var. *Ma-yuen*	Yi Yi Ren	San Yi Mai, Yi Yi Yan	Yokuinin	Job's-tears seed

PHARMACEUTICAL	SCIENTIFIC	MANDARIN	CANTONESE	JAPANESE	ENGLISH
Semen Coicis preparatae	*Coix lachryma-jobi* var. *Ma-yuen*	Shu Yi Ren	Suk Yi Mai		Dry-fried Job's-tears seed
Semen Crotonis	*Croton tiglium*	Ba Dou	Ba Dau		Croton seed
Semen Cucumis	*Cucumis melo*	Tian Gua Zi	Tim Gwa Ji		Cantaloupe seed
Semen Cucurbitae	*Cucurbita moschata*	Nan Gua Zi	Naam Gwa Ji	Nankashi	Red squash seed
Semen Cuscutae	*Cuscuta chinensis , C. japonica*	Tu Si Zi	Tou Si Ji	Toshishi	Asian dodder seed
Semen Cycadis	*Cycas revoluta*	Su Tie Zi	Sou Tit Ji		Sago palm seed
Semen Descurainiae	*Descurainia sophia*	Ting Li Zi	Ting Lai Ji	Teirekishi	Tansy mustard seed
Semen Dolichis	*Dolichos lablab*	Bai Bian Dou	Baak Bin Dau	Hakuhenzu	Hyacinth bean
Semen et fructus Hoveniae	*Hovenia dulcis*	Zhi Ju Zi	Ji Gwat Ji		Hovenia seed and fruit
Semen Euphorbiae lathyris	*Euphorbia lathyris*	Qian Jin Zi	Chin Gam Ji	Zokuzuishi	Caper spurge seed
Semen Euphoriae	*Euphoria longan*	Long Yan He	Lung Ngaan Ho		Longan seed
Semen Euryalis	*Euryale ferox*	Qian Shi	Him Sat	Kenjitsu	Foxnut
Semen Firmianae	*Firmiana simplex*	Wu Tong Zi	Ng Tung Ji		Chinese parasol tree seed
Semen Gleditsiae	*Gleditsia sinensis* and spp.	Zao Jiao Zi	Jou Gok Ji		Honeylocust fruit
Semen Glycinis germinati	*Glycene max*	Dou (Huang) Juan	Dau (Wong) Geun		Sprouting soybean
Semen Glycinis preparatum	*Glycine max*	Dan Dou Chi	Taam Dau Si	Tantoshi	Fermented soybean
Semen Gossypii	*Gossypium hirsutum, G. herbaceum*	Mian Hua Zi	Min Fa Ji		Cotton seed
Semen Hydnocarpi	*Hydnocarpus anthelmintica, H. hainanensis*	Da Feng Zi	Daai Fung Ji	Daifushi	Chaulmoogra seed
Semen Hyoscyami	*Hyoscyamus niger*	Tian Xian Zi	Tin Sin Ji		Black henbane seed
Semen Impatiensis	*Impatiens balsamina*	Ji Xing Zi	Jek Chin Ji	Kyuseishi	Garden balsam seed
Semen Iris pallasii	*Iris pallasii* var. *chinensis*	Ma Lin Zi	Ma Leun Ji		North China iris seed
Semen Juglandis	*Juglans regia*	Hu Tao Ren	Wu Tou Yan	Kotoniku	Walnut meat
Semen Kochiae	*Kochia scoparia*	Di Fu Zi	Dei Fu Ji	Jibushi	Kochia seed
Semen Leonori	*Leonorus heterophyllus* and spp	Chong Wei Zi	Chong Wai Ji		Asian motherwort seed
Semen Lepidii	*Lepidium apetalum, L. virginicum*	Ting Li Zi	Ting Lai Ji	Teirekishi	Wood whitlow grass seed
Semen Lini	*Linum usitatissimum*	Ya Ma Zi	A Ma Ji		Flax seed
Semen Litchis	*Litchi chinensis*	Li Zhi He	Lai Ji Ho		Lychee seed
Semen Livistonae	*Livistona chinensis*	Kui Shu Zi	Kwai Sat Ji		Fan palm seed
Semen Malvae	*Malva verticillata*	Dong Kui Zi	Dung Kwai Ji		Musk mallow seed
Semen Mangiferae	*Mangifera indica*	Mang Guo Zi	Man Gou Wat		Mango seed
Semen Momordicae cochinchinensis	*Momordica cochinchinensis*	Mu Bie Zi	Muk Bit Ji	Mokubesshi	Cochin bitter melon seed
Semen Myristicae	*Myristica fragrans*	Rou Dou Kou	Yuk Dau Kau	Nikuzuku	Nutmeg seed

PHARMACEUTICAL	SCIENTIFIC	MANDARIN	CANTONESE	JAPANESE	ENGLISH
Semen Nelumbinis	***Nelumbo nucifera***	Lian Zi	Lin Ji	Renshi	Lotus seed
Semen Oroxyli	***Oroxylum indicum***	Mu Hu Die	Muk Wu Dip	Mokukocho	Oroxylum seed
Semen Pharbitis	***Pharbitis nil, P. purpurea*** **and spp**	Qian Niu Zi	Hin Ngau Ji		Japanese morning glory seed
Semen Phaseoli calcarati	***Phaseolus calcaratus, P. angularis***	Chi Xiao Dou	Chek Siu Dau	Sekishozu	Aduki bean
Semen Phaseoli radiati	***Phaseolus radiatum***	Lu Dou	Luk Dau	Ryokuzu	Mung bean
Semen Pini	***Pinus tabulaeformis*** **and spp**	Song Zi	Chung Ji		Pine kernel
Semen Plantaginis	***Plantago asiatica, P. depressa*** **and spp**	Che Qian Zi	Che Chin Ji	Shazenshi	Asian plantain seed
Semen Prinsepiae	***Prinsepia uniflora***	Rui Ren (Rou)	Seui Yan (Yuk)		Prinsepia seed
Semen Pruni armeniacae	***Prunus armeniaca*** **and var.**	Xing Ren, Ku Xing Ren	Baak Hang Yan	Kyonin	Bitter apricot kernel
Semen Pruni armeniacae dulcis	***Prunus armeniaca*** **and var.**	Tian Xing Ren, Nan Xing Ren	Tim Hang Yan, Naam Hang Yan		Sweet apricot kernel
Semen Pruni humili	***Prunus humilis***	Yu Li Ren, Ou Li	Yuk Lei Yan, Ngao Lei		Dwarf cherry kernel
Semen Pruni japonicae	***Prunus japonica***	Yu Li Ren	Yuk Lei Yan	Ikurinin	Bush cherry kernel
Semen Pruni persicae	***Prunus persica*** **and spp**	Tao Ren	Tou Yan	Tonin	Peach kernel
Semen Raphani	***Raphanus sativus***	Lai Fu Zi	Loi Fuk Ji		Radish seed
Semen Rhodomyrti	***Rhodomyrtus tomentosa***	Shan Ren Zi	Saan Nam Ji		Rosemyrtle seed
Semen Ricini	***Ricinus communis***	Bi Ma Zi	Bei Ma Ji		Castor bean
Semen Sapindi	***Sapindus mukorossi***	Wu Huan Zi, Mu Huan Zi	Mou Waan Ji		Soapnut seed, Bodhi seed
Semen seu herba Crotalariae assamicae	***Crotalaria assamica***	Da Zhu Shi Dou, Zi Xiao Rong	Daai Ju Si Dau		Assam crotalaria seed or herb
Semen Sinapis albae	***Sinapis alba***	Bai Jie Zi	Baak Gaai Ji		White mustard seed
Semen Sterculiae	***Sterculia staphigera, S. lychnophera***	Pang Da Hai	Bun Daai Hoi	Bantaikai	Sterculia seed
Semen Strophanthi	***Strophanthus divaricatus***	Yang Jiao Yao	Yeung Gok Aau		Strophanthus seed
Semen Strychnotis preparatae	***Strychnos pierrana, S. nux-vomica*** **and spp**	(Zhi) Ma Qian Zi	Ma Chin Ji	Basenshi	Prepared vomit nut
Semen Torreyae	***Torreya grandis, T. nucifera***	Fei Zi	Fei Ji		Japanese torreya nut
Semen Trichosanthis	***Trichosanthes kirilowii, T. japonica, T. uniflora***	Gua Lou Ren	Kwut Lau Yan	Karonin	Snakegourd seed
Semen Trigonellae	***Trigonella foenum-graecum***	Hu Lu Ba	Wu Lou Ba		Fenugreek seed
Semen Vaccariae	***Vaccaria segetalis***	Wang Bu Liu Xing	Wong Bat Lau Hang	Ofurugyo	Cowcockle seed
Semen Zizyphi mauritianae	***Zizyphus mauritiana***	Mian Zao Ren	Mai Jou Yan		Mauritius jujube seed

PHARMACEUTICAL	SCIENTIFIC	MANDARIN	CANTONESE	JAPANESE	ENGLISH
Semen Zizyphi spinosae	***Zizyphus spinosa***	Suan Zao Ren, Jin Zao Ren	Syun Jou Yan	Sansonin	Sour jujube seed
Semen Zizyphi spinosae preparatae	***Zizyphus spinosa***	Chao Suan Zao Ren	Syu Jou Yan		Roasted sour jujube seed
Solenognathus	***Solenognathus* spp, *Syngnathoides biaculeatus***	Hai Long	Hoi Lung		Pipefish
Spica Prunellae	***Prunella vulgaris***	Xia Ku Cao	Ha Fu Chou	Kagoso	Selfheal spike
Spina Gleditsiae	***Gleditsia sinensis* and spp**	Zao Jiao Ci	Jou Gok Chi	Sokakushi	Honeylocust spine
Spora Lygodii	***Lygodium japonicum***	Hai Jin Sha	Hoi Gam Sa	Kaikinsha	Japanese climbing fern spore
Squama manis	***Manis pentadactyla***	Chuan Shan Jia	Chyun San Gaap	Senzanko	Pangolin scale
Stalactitum	***Stalactitum, Balanophylla* spp.**	E Guan Shi, Shi Zhong Ru	Ngo Gun Sek		Stalactite tip
Stamen Nelumbinis	***Nelumbo nucifera***	Lian Xu	Lin Sou	Renshu	Lotus stamen
Stichopus	***Stichopus japonicus***	Hai Shen	Hoi Sam		Sea cucumber
Stigma Croci	***Crocus sativus***	Xi Hong Hua, Fan Hong Hua	Fun Hung Fa	Bankoka	Saffron stigma
Stylus Zeae	***Zea mays***	Yu Mi Xu, Yu Mi Rui	Yuk Mai So, Yuk Mai Yeui	Gyoku-maishu	Cornsilk style
Succus exsiccatus Rhudis	***Rhus verniciflua***	Gan Qi	Gon Chat		Lacquer
Succus Phyllostachis	***Phyllostachys nigra* var. *henonis* and spp**	Zhu Li	Juk Lai	Chikureki	Black bamboo sap
Sulphurum	***Sulphurum***	Liu Huang, Shi Liu Huang	Lau Wong, Sek Lau Wong	Io	Sulphur
Tabanus	***Tabanus bivittatus***	Meng Chong	Mung Chung		Gadfly
Talcum	***Talcum***	Hua Shi	Wat Sek	Kasseki	Talc
Tentaculum Rhopilema	***Rhopilema esculenta***	Hai Zhe	Hoi Jit		Jellyfish tentacle
Terra flava usta, Bolus usta		Fu Long Gan	Fuk Lung Gon	Bukuryukan	Wood stove clay
Testa Dolichoris	***Dolichos lablab***	Bian Dou Yi	Bin Dau Yi		Hyacinth bean capsule
Testa Phaseoli radiatae	***Phaseolus radiatum***	Lu Dou Yi	Luk Dau Yip		Mung bean husk
Testes et penis Callorhini seu Phocae	***Callorhinus ursinus, Phoca vitulina***	Hai Gou Shen	Hoi Gau Sam	Kaikujin	Seal genitals
Testes et penis canis	***Canis***	Guang Gou Shen	Gwong Gau Sam	Kujin	Male dog genitals
Testes et penis Cervi	***Cervus nippon* and spp**	Hua Lu Shen	Fa Luk Sam		Male deer genitals
Thallus Laminariae	***Laminaria japonica* and spp**	Kun Bu	Gwan Bou	Kombu	Kelp seaweed
Thallus Parmeliae	***Parmelia tinctorum, P. reticulata***	Shi Er			Parmelia thallus
Thallus Usneae	***Usnea diffracta* and spp**	Song Luo	Chung Lo		Beard lichen thallus
Tuber Curcumae	***Curcuma longa, C. aromatica***	Yu Jin	Yuk Gam	Ukon	Turmeric tuber
Urina Hominis	***Homo sapiens***	Ren Niao	Yan Niu		Human urine
Vermiculus Protohermis	***Protohermes grandis***	Sun Tai Lang Chun	Syun Taai Long Chung	Magotaro-mushi	Protohermes larva

PHARMACEUTICAL	SCIENTIFIC	MANDARIN	CANTONESE	JAPANESE	ENGLISH
Vesica fellae Bovis	***Bos taurus domesticus, Bubalis bubalis***	Niu Dan	Ngau Daam	Gyutan	Ox gallbladder
Vitellus Galli	***Gallus gallus domesticus***	Ji Zi Huang	Gai Ji Wong		Egg yolk
Zaocys	***Zaocys dhumnades***	Wu Shao She	U Sau Se	Ushoda	Black grass-snake

Cross Index of Mandarin Remedy Names

MANDARIN	SCIENTIFIC	PHARMACEUTICAL	CANTONESE	JAPANESE	ENGLISH
	Grifola frondosa	Sclerotium Grifolae frondosae		Maitake	Maitake, Hen of the woods mushroom
	Oryza sativa	Saccharum Oryzae		Koi	Rice malt (syrup)
A Wei	*Ferula foetida*	Resina Ferulae (Asafoetidae)	A Ngai	Agi	Asafoetida resin
Ai Na Xiang, Da Feng Cao	*Blumea balsamifera*	Herba Blumeae balsamiferae	Ngaai Naap Heung	Daifuso	Camphor plant
Ai Ye	*Artemisia argyi*	Folium Artemisiae argyi	Ngaai Yang, Ngaai Yip	Gaiyo	Asian mugwort leaf
An Lu Zi	*Artemisia keiskeana*	Fructus Artemisiae keiskeanae	Am Leui Ji		Keiskeana mugwort seed
An Xi Xiang	*Styrax benzoin*	Benzoinum	Ngon Sik Heung	Ansokuko	Benzoin
An Ye	*Eucalyptus globulus*	Folium Eucalypti	Ngon Yip		Eucalyptus leaf
Ba Dou	*Croton tiglium*	Semen Crotonis	Ba Dau		Croton seed
Ba Ji Tian	*Morinda officinalis*	Radix Morindae	Ba Gik Tin	Hagekiten	Morinda root
Ba Jiao Feng	*Alangium chinense*	Radix Alangii	Baat Gok Fung		Alangium root
Ba Jiao Gen	*Musa basjoo*	Caudex Musae	Ba Jiu Gan		Ryukyu banana root
Ba Jiao Hui Xiang	*Illicium verum*	Fructus Illicii	Baat Gok Wui Heung		Star anise fruit
Ba Jiao Lian	*Dysosma pleiantha*	Rhizoma Dysosmae pleianthae	Baat Gok Lin		Pleianth dysosma root
Ba Jiao Lian	*Podophyllum pleianthum*	Rhizoma Podophylli pleianthi	Ba Gok Lin		Pleianth podophyllum root
Ba Li Ma	*Rhododendron molle*	Fructus Rhododendris mollis	Baat Lei Ma		Yellow azalea fruit
Ba Xian Cao, Zhu Yang Yang	*Galium aparine*	Herba Galii aparinis	Baat Sin Chou		Cleavers herb
Ba Xian Hua	*Hydrangea macrophylla*	Flos Hydrangeae	Baat Sin Fa		French hydrangea flower
Ba Yue Zha, Yu Zhi Zi	*Akebia quinata*	Fructus Akebiae	Baat Yut Jaat, Yu Ji Ji		Akebia fruit
Bai Bian Dou	*Dolichos lablab*	Semen Dolichis	Baak Bin Dau	Hakuhenzu	Hyacinth bean
Bai Bu, Dui Ye Bai Bu	*Stemona tuberosa*	Radix Stemonae tuberosae	Baak Bou, Deui Yip Baak Bou		Tuberous stemona root
Bai Bu, Man Sheng Bai Bu	*Stemona japonia*	Radix Stemonae japonicae	Baak Bou, Maan Sang Baak Bou	Hyakubu	Japanese stemona root
Bai Bu, Zhi Li Bai Bu	*Stemona sessilifolia*	Radix Stemonae sessilifoliae	Baak Bou, Chek Lap Baak Bou		Sessile stemona root
Bai Cao Shuang		Pulvus fumi carbonisati	Baak Chou Sheung		Boiler or chimney soot

MANDARIN	SCIENTIFIC	PHARMACEUTICAL	CANTONESE	JAPANESE	ENGLISH
Bai Dou Kou	***Amomum cardamomum***	Fructus Amomi cardamomi	Baak Dau Kau	Byakuzuku	Cluster cardamom pod
(Bai) Dou Kou Hua	***Amomum cardamomum***	Flos Amomi cardamomi	(Baak) Dau Kau Fa	Byakuzu-kuka	Cluster cardamom flower
Bai Fu Zi, Guan Bai Fu	***Aconitum coreanum***	Rhizoma Aconiti coreani	Baak Fu Ji, Gwan Baak Fu Ji		Prepared Korean aconite root
Bai Fu Zi, Yu Bai Fu	***Typhonium giganteum***	Rhizoma Typhonii gigantei preparata	Baak Fu Ji	Byakubushi	Prepared giant typhonium root
Bai Guo Ye	***Ginkgo biloba***	Folium Ginkgoidis	Baak Gwo Yip	Ginkyoyo	Ginkgo leaf
Bai Guo, Yin Xing He	***Ginkgo biloba***	Fructus Ginkgoidis	Baak Gwo, Ngan Hang Wat	Ginkyo	Ginkgo nut
Bai He	***Lilium brownii* var. *colchesteri***	Bulbus Lilii	Baak Hap	Hyakugo	Brown's lily bulb
Bai He Gen	***Lilium brownii* var. *colchesteri***	Radix Lilii	Baak Hap Gan		Brown's lily root
Bai He Hua	***Lilium brownii* var. *colchesteri***	Flos Lilii	Baak Hap Fa		Brown's lily flower
Bai He, Juan Duan	***Lilium lancifolium***	Bulbus Liliii lancifolii	Baak Hap, Gyun Daan		Lance-leaf lily bulb
Bai Hua She	***Agkistrodon acutus* and *Bungarus multicinctus***	Agkistrodon seu Bungarus	Baak Fa Se	Hakkada	Multibanded krait
Bai Hua She She Cao	***Oldenlandia diffusa***	Herba Oldenlandiae	Baak Fa Se Sit Chou	Byakkaja-zesso	Snaketongue grass herb
Bai Hua Zi Cao, Hu Yao Huang	***Leucas mollissima***	Herba Leuci	Baak Fa Ji Chou, Fu Ngao Wong		Leucas herb
Bai Ji	***Bletilla striata***	Rhizoma Bletillae	Baak Gap	Byakukyu	Amethyst orchid root
Bai Ji Li	***Tribulus terrestris***	Fructus Tribuli	Baak Jat Lai	Byakishitsuri	Caltrop fruit
Bai Jiang Cao	***Patrinia scabiosaefolia, P. villosa***	Herba et rhizoma Patriniae	Baai Jeung Chou	Haishoso	Patrinia herb and root
Bai Jiang Dan	***Hydragyrum chloratum***	Compositum Hydragyri chlorati	Baak Geung Daan		Mercury chloride
Bai Jiao Xiang	***Liquidambar taiwaniana***	Resina Liquidambaris taiwaninanae	Baak Gaau Heung		Taiwan maple fruit resin
Bai Jie Zi	***Sinapis alba***	Semen Sinapis albae	Baak Gaai Ji		White mustard seed
Bai Lan Hua	***Michelia alba***	Flos Micheliae	Baak Laan Fa		White champac flower
(Bai) Lang Du	***Euphorbia pallasii, E. abracteolatae, E. fischerianae***	Radix Euphorbiae pallasii seu ebracteolatae	(Baak) Long Duk		White spurge root
Bai Lian	***Ampelopsis japonica***	Radix Ampelopsis	Baak Lim	Byakuran	Japanese peppervine root
Bai Lian Hua	***Nelumbo nucifera***	Flos Nelumbinis	Baak Lin Fa		Lotus flower
Bai Liang Jin	***Ardisia crispa***	Herba Ardisiae crispae	Baak Leung Gam		Crisp ardisia herb
Bai Long Chuan Gen	***Clerodendron paniculatum***	Radix Clerodendronis paniculati	Baak Lung Chyun Gan		Panicled clerodendron root

MANDARIN	SCIENTIFIC	PHARMACEUTICAL	CANTONESE	JAPANESE	ENGLISH
Bai Mao Gen	***Imperata cylindrica*** var. ***major***	Rhizoma Imperatae	Baak Maau Gan	Bokon	Woolly grass root
Bai Mao Hua	***Imperata cylindrica*** var. ***major***	Flos Imperatae	Baak Maau Fa		Woolly grass flower
Bai Mao Xia Ku Cao, Jing Gu Cao	***Ajuga decumbens***	Herba Ajugae	Baak Mou Ha Fu Chou, Gan Gwat Chou		Bugleweed herb
Bai Mei	***Prunus mume***	Fructus Mumis immaturis preparatae	Baak Mui		Unripe prepared black plum fruit
Bai Mian Feng	***Trichosporum acuminatum***	Herba Trichospori	Baak Ming Fung		Trichosporum herb
Bai Mu Er	***Tremella fuciformis***	Sclerotium Tremellae fucimormis	Baak Muk Yi	Hakumokuji	Silver ear mushroom
Bai Niu Dan, Bai Mian Feng	***Inula cappa***	Herba Inulae cappae	Baak Ngau Daam		Goatear herb
Bai Niu Xi	***Cuccubala baccifer***	Radix Cuccubalae bacciferis	Baak Ngao Sat		White oxknee root
Bai Pu Jiang	***Buddleia asiatica***	Radix Buddleiae asiaticae	Baak Pou Geung		Asian Buddleia root
Bai Qian	***Cynanchum stauntoni, C. glaucescens***	Radix et rhizoma Cynanchi stauntoni	Baak Chin	Byakuzen	Prime white root
Bai Qian Ceng	***Melaleuca leucadendron***	Folium Melaleucae leucadendronis	Baak Chin Chang		Cajeput leaf
Bai Qu Cai	***Chelidonium majus*** var. ***asiaticum***	Herba Chelidonii	Baak Wat Choi	Hakkutusai	Asian celandine herb
Bai Shao (Yao)	***Paeonia lactiflora***	Radix Paeoniae lactiflorae	Baak Cheuk (Yeuk)	Byakushaku (yaku)	White peony root
Bai Shen	***Panax ginseng***	Radix Panacis ginsengis praeparatae	Baak Sam	Hakujin	Rock candy cured Asian ginseng root
Bai Shi Zhi	***Halloysitum album***	Halloysitum album	Baak Sek Ji		White kaolin
Bai Shou Wu, Niu Pi Xiao	***Cynanchum auriculatum***	Radix Cynanchi auriculati	Baak Sau Wu, Ngau Pei Siu		Auricle dogbane root
Bai Tou Weng	***Pulsatilla chinensis, P. cernua, P. turczaninovii, P. ambigua*** and spp	Radix Pulsatillae	Baak Tau Yung	Hakutoo	Asian pasqueflower root
Bai Tou Weng, Xing An Bai Tou Weng	***Pulsatilla dahurica***	Radix Pulsatillae dahuricae	Baak Tau Yung, Ing On Baak Tau Yung		Dahurian pasqueflower root
Bai Wei	***Cynanchum atratum, C. versicolor***	Radix Cynanchi atrati	Baak Mei	Byakubi	Swallow-wort root
Bai Xian Pi	***Dictamnus dasycarpus***	Cortex radicis Dictamni	Baak Sin Pei	Hakusempi	Asian dittany root bark
Bai Ying, Shu Yang Quan, Bai Mao Teng	***Solanum lyratum***	Herba Solani lyrati	Baak Ying, Baak Mou Tang		Climbing nightshade herb
Bai Zhi	***Angelica dahurica, A. anomala, A. taiwaniana***	Radix Angelicae dahuricae	Baak Ji	Byakushi	White angelica Root

MANDARIN	SCIENTIFIC	PHARMACEUTICAL	CANTONESE	JAPANESE	ENGLISH
Bai Zhu	***Atractylodes macrocephala***	Rhizoma Atractylodis macrocephalae	Baak Seut	Byakujutsu	White atractylodes root
Bai Zi Ren	***Biota orientalis***	Semen Biotae orientalis	(Baak) Ji Yan	Hakushinin	Oriental arborvitae berry
Ban Bian Lian	***Lobelia chinensis***	Herba et radix Lobeliae chinensis	Bau Bin Ling	Hanbanren	Rooting lobelia herb and root
Ban Feng He Gen	***Pterospermum heterophyllum***	Radix Pterospermi	Bun Fung Ho Gan		Pterospermum root
Ban Lan Gen	***Isatis tinctoria, I. indigotica***	Radix Isatis tinctoriae	Baan Laam Gan		Woad root
Ban Mao	***Cantharis vesicatoria***	Cantharis	Ban Mou	Hanmyo	Cantharides
Ban Mao	***Mylabris***	Mylabris	Ban Mou	Hanmyo	Asian cantharides
Ban Xia Qu	***Pinellia ternata***	Rhizoma Pinelliae fermentatae	Bun Ha Chau		Fermented Pinellia corm
Ban Xia, Fa Ban Xia	***Pinellia ternata***	Rhizoma Pinelliae ternatae preparatae	Bun Ha, Faat Bun Ha	Hange, Kohange	Prepared pinellia corm
Ban Zhi Lian	***Scutellaria barbata, B. rivularis***	Radix et herba Scutellariae barbatae	Bun Ji Lin		Barbed skullcap root and herb
Bao Gu	***Panthera***	Os Leopardis			Leopard bone
Bao Ma Zi	***Syringa manchuriensis***	Cortex Syringae			Manchurian lilac bark
Bei Dou Gen	***Menispermum dauricum***	Radix Menispermi	Pan Dau Gan		Siberian moonseed root
Bei Sha Shen	***Glehnia littoralis***	Radix Glehniae	Mai Sa Sam	Shajin	Northern sandroot
Bei Wu Tou	***Aconitum chinense, A. kusnezoffii*** **and spp**	Radix Aconiti chinensis	Chou Wu, Mai Wu Tau	So-u	Prepared wild aconite root tuber
Bei Xie, Bi Xie	***Dioscorea hypoglauca***	Rhizoma Dioscoreae hypoglaucae	Bei Gaai, Fan Bei Gaai	Hikai	Long yam root
Bei Yin Chen	***Artemisia scoparia***	Herba Artemisiae scopariae	Bak Yan Chan		Northern wormwood herb
Bei Zi	***Cypraea moneta, C. macula*** **and spp**	Concha Cypraeae	Chan Bu Chi		Cowrie shell
Bi Ba	***Piper longum***	Fructus Piperis longis	Bat Pa	Hihatsu	Long pepper fruit spike
Bi Cheng Qie	***Litsea cubeba***	Fructus Litseae	Bat Ching Ke		Cubeb peppercorn
Bi Li, Mu Man Tou	***Ficus pumila***	Fructus Fici pumilae	Bai La		Creeping fig fruit
Bi Ma Zi	***Ricinus communis***	Semen Ricini	Bei Ma Ji		Castor bean
Bi Qi	***Heleocharis plantaginea***	Herba Heleocharis	But Chai	Bossai	Water chestnut herb
Bi Tao Gan	***Prunus persica, P. davidiana***	Fructus persicae immaturi			Unripe peach fruit
Bi Tong Cao	***Equisetum ramosissimum***	Herba Equiseti ramosissimi	Bat Tung Chou		Ramose horsetail herb
Bi Xie, Fen Bi Xie, Bei Xie	***Dioscorea hypoglauca***	Rhizoma Dioscoreae hypoglaucae	Bei Gaai, Fan Bei Gaai	Hikai	Long yam root

MANDARIN	SCIENTIFIC	PHARMACEUTICAL	CANTONESE	JAPANESE	ENGLISH
Bi Xie, Mian Bi Xie	***Dioscorea septemloba***	Rhizoma Dioscoreae septemlobae	Bei Gaai, Min Bei Gaai		Seven-lobe yam root
Bi Zi Cao	***Pogonatherum crinitum***	Herba Pogonatheri	Bat Jai Chou		Golden Hair grass
Bian Dou Hua	***Dolichos lablab***	Gemma Dolichis	Bin Dau Fa	Henzuka	Hyacinth bean bud
Bian Dou Yi	***Dolichos lablab***	Testa Dolichoris	Bin Dau Yi		Hyacinth bean capsule
Bian Ji Sheng	***Viscum liquidambaricum***	Ramulus Visci liquidambarici	Bin Gei Sang		Asian mistletoe twig
Bian Xu	***Polygonum aviculare***	Herba Polygoni avicularis	Bin Chuk	Henchiku	Knotgrass herb
Bie Jia	***Amyda sinensis, Trionix sinensis***	Carapax Amydae seu Trionis	Bit Gaap	Bekko	Asian soft-shell turtle shell
Bing Lang	***Areca catechu, A. dicksonii***	Semen Arecae catechu	Ban Long	Binroji	Betel nut
Bing Lang Hua	***Areca catechu, A. dicksonii***	Flos Arecae catechu	Ban Long Fa	Binroka	Betel nut flower
Bing Pian	***Dryobalanops camphora***	Borneolum	Bing Pin	Ryuno	Borneo camphor
Bo Gu Dan	***Gendarussa vulgaris***	Herba Gendarussae	Bok Gwat Daam		Gendarussa herb
Bo He	***Mentha arvensis***	Herba Menthae arvensis	Bok Ho	Hakka	Asian fieldmint herb
Bo Luo Hui	***Macleaya cordata***	Herba Macleayae	Bok Lok Wui		Plum poppy herb
Bu Gu Zhi	***Psoralea corylifolia***	Fructus Psoraleae	Bou Gwat Ji	Hokotsushi	Scurf pea berry
Bu Zha Ye	***Microcos paniculata***	Folium Microcotis	Bou Jai Yip		Microcos leaf
Can Sha	***Bombyx mori***	Excrementum Bombicis	Chaam Sa	Sansha	Silkworm dropping
Cang Er Zi	***Xanthium sibiricum, X. strumarium***	Fructus Xanthii	Chong Yi Ji	Sojishi	Siberian cocklebur
Cang Qing Guo	***Terminalia chebula*** **and var.**	Fructus Terminaliae immaturi			Unripe myrobalan fruit
Cang Zhu, Guan Cang Zhu	***Atractylodes japonica***	Rhizoma Atractylodis japonicae	Chong Seut, Gwan Chong Seut		Japanese black Atractylodes root
Cang Zhu, Mao Cang Zhu	***Atractylodes lancea, A. sinensis*** **and spp**	Rhizoma Atractylodis lanceae	Chong Seut, Mau Chong Seut	Sojutsu	Black atractylodes root
Cao Dou Kou	***Alpinia katsumadai***	Semen Alpiniae katsumadis	Chou Dau Kau	Sozuku	Katsumada's galangal seed
Cao Guo (Ren)	***Amomum tsao-ko***	Fructus Amomi tsao-konis	Chou Gwat (Yan)	Soka	Cochin cardamom fruit
Cao Wu, Bei Wu Tou	***Aconitum chinense, A. kusnezoffii*** **and spp**	Radix Aconiti chinensis	Chou Wu, Mai Wu Tau	So-u	Prepared wild aconite root tuber
Ce Bai Ye	***Biota orientalis***	Cacumen Biotae orientalis	Jak Paak Yip	Sokuhakuyo	Oriental arborvitae tip
Cha Chi Huang	***Stellaria aquatica***	Herba Stellariae aquaticae	Cha Si Wong		Water chickweed herb
Cha Ye	***Camellia sinensis***	Folium Camelliae sinensis	Cha Yip	Fujucha, Chayo	Tea leaf

MANDARIN	SCIENTIFIC	PHARMACEUTICAL	CANTONESE	JAPANESE	ENGLISH
Chai Hu	***Bupleurum chinense, B. falcatum, B. longiradiatum* and spp**	Radix Bupleuri	Chaai Wu	Saiko	Asian buplever root
Chai Hu, Xia Ye Chai Hu	***Bupleurum scorzonerifolium***	Radix Bupleuri scorzonerifolii	Chaai Wu, Hap Yip Chaai Wu		Thin-leaf buplever root
Chan Hua, Jin Chan Hua	***Cordyceps scotianus* and host *Cryptotympana atrata* and spp**	Sclerotium Cordycepsis scotianus	Sim Fa, Gam Sim Fa		Cicada fungus
Chan Su	***Bufo gargarizans, B. melanostictus***	Secretio Bufonis	Sim Sou	Senjo	Toad venom
Chan Tui	***Cryptotympana atrata* and spp**	Periostracum Cryptotympanae	Sim Teui, Sim Tyut	Sentai	Cicada slough
Chang Chun Hua	***Catharanthus roseus***	Radix et herba Catharanthi	Cheung Cheun Fa		Madagascar periwinkle root and herb
Chang Chun Teng	***Hedera nepalensis* var. *sinensis***	Herba Hederae nepalensis	Seung Cheun Tang		Nepalese ivy leaf
Chang Shan	***Dichroa febrifuga***	Radix Dichroae	Seung Saan	Joszan	Feverflower root
Chao Suan Zao Ren	***Zizyphus spinosa***	Semen Zizyphi spinosae preparatae	Syu Jou Yan		Roasted sour jujube seed
Che Qian Cao	***Plantago asiatica, P. depressa* and spp**	Folium Plantaginis	Che Chin Chou	Shazenso	Asian plantain leaf
Che Qian Zi	***Plantago asiatica, P. depressa* and spp**	Semen Plantaginis	Che Chin Ji	Shazenshi	Asian plantain seed
Chen Pi, Ju Pi	***Citrus reticulata, C. tangerina, C. erythrosa***	Pericarpium Citri reticulatae	Chan Pei, Gwat Pei	Chimpi	Ripe tangerine rind
Chen Sha	***Ferrum***	Pulvis ferri	Chan Sa		Black iron oxide
Chen Sha	***Ferrum***	Pulvis ferri	San Sa		Black ferric oxide
Chen Shi Hui	***Calcaria***	Calcaria	Chan Sek Wei		Calcium hydroxide
Chen Xiang	***Aquilaria agallocha, A. sinensis***	Lignum Aquilariae	Cham Heung	Jinko	Aloeswood
Cheng Gan Sheng Ma	***Eupatorium lindleyanum***	Herba Eupatorii lindleyani	Ping Gon Sing Ma		Lindley's eupatorium herb
Chi Fu Ling	***Poria cocos***	Sclerotium Poriae rubrae	Chek Fuk Ling	Sekibikuryo	Red hoelen
Chi Shao (Yao)	***Paeonia lactiflora, P. obovata, P. veitchii***	Radix Paeoniae rubrae	Chek Cheuk (Yeuk)	Sekishaku-(yaku)	Red peony root
Chi Shi Zhi	***Halloysitum rubrum***	Halloysitum	Chek Sek Chi	Shakusek-ishi	Red kaolin
Chi Xiao Dou	***Phaseolus calcaratus, P. angularis***	Semen Phaseoli calcarati	Chek Siu Dau	Sekishozu	Aduki bean
Chong Bai La	***Ericerus pela***	Ericerus	Chung Baak Laap		Ericerus worm
Chong Wei Zi	***Leonorus heterophyllus* and spp**	Semen Leonori	Chong Wai Ji		Asian motherwort seed
Chou Cao	***Ruta graveolens***	Herba Rutae	Chau Chou		Rue herb

MANDARIN	SCIENTIFIC	PHARMACEUTICAL	CANTONESE	JAPANESE	ENGLISH
Chou Mu Dan	***Clerodendron bungei***	Folium Clerodendronis bungeis	Chau Maau Daan		Bung's Clerodendron leaf
Chou Wu Tong (Ye)	***Clerodendron trichotomum***	Folium Clerodendronis trichotomi	Chau Ng Tung (Yip)		Forked glorybower leaf
Chu Chong Ju	***Pyrethrum cinerariifolium***	Flos Pyrethri	Cheui Chung Guk		Dalmatia pellitory flower
Chu Shi Zi	***Broussonetia papyrifera***	Fructus Broussonetiae	Chyu Sat Ji		Paper mulberry fruit
Chuan Bai, Huang Bai	***Phellodendron amurense, P. chinense***	Cortex Phellodendris	Chyun Paak, Wong Paak	Obaku	Siberian cork tree bark
Chuan Bei Mu	***Fritillaria cirrhosa***	Bulbus Fritillariae cirrhosae	Chyun Bui Mou	Senbaimo	Sichuan fritillary bulb
Chuan Bei Mu, An Zi Bei Mu	***Fritillaria unibracteata***	Bulbus Fritillariae unibracteatae	Chyun Bui Mou, Am Ji Bui Mou		Single-bract fritillary bulb
Chuan Bei Mu, Tai Bai Bei Mu	***Fritillaria taipaiensis***	Bulbus Fritillariae taipaiensis	Chyun Bui Mou, Taai Baak Bui Mou		Taipei fritillary bulb
Chuan Gen Teng, Bo Gu Cao	***Psychotria serpens***	Herba Psychotriae serpentis	Chyun Gen Tang		Twining psychotria herb
Chuan Jiao, Hua Jiao	***Zanthoxylum bungeanum***	Fructus Zanthoxyli bungeani	Chyun Jiu, Fa Jiu	Shokusho	Sichuan peppercorn
Chuan Lian Zi	***Melia toosendan***	Fructus Meliae toosendanis	Chyun Lin Ji		Sichuan bead tree berry
Chuan Mu Tong	***Clematis montana, C. armandii***	Caulis Clematis montanae	Chyun Muk Tong		Mountain clematis stem
Chuan Mu Xiang	***Dolomiaea souliei***	Radix Dolomiaeae souliei	Chyun Muk Heung		Sichuan Dolomiaea root
Chuan Niu Xi	***Cyathula officinalis,. C. officinalis***	Radix Cyathulae	Chyun Ngau Sat		Hookweed root
Chuan Po Shi	***Cudrania cochinchinensis***	Radix Cudraniae cochinchinensis	Chyun Po Sek		Cochin cudrania root
Chuan Po, Hou Po	***Magnolia officinalis, M. biloba, M. obovata***	Cortex Magnoliae officinalis	Chyun Pok, Hau Pok	Koboku	Magnolia bark
Chuan Shan Jia	***Manis pentadactyla***	Squama manis	Chyun San Gaap	Senzanko	Pangolin scale
Chuan Shan Long	***Dioscorea nipponica***	Rhizoma Dioscoreae nipponicae	Chyun Saan Lung		Nippon yam root
Chuan Tong Pi	***Kalopanax septemlobus***	Cortex Septemlobi	Chyun Tung Pei		Kalopanax bark
Chuan Wu Wu Tou	***Aconitum carmichaeli***	Radix Aconiti carmichaeli	Chyun Wu, Wu Tau	Uzu	Prepared Sichuan aconite root tuber
Chuan Xin Lian	***Andrographis paniculata***	Folium Andrographis	Chyun Sam Lin	Senshinren	Heart-thread lotus leaf
Chuan Xiong, Xiong Qiong	***Ligusticum walichii***	Radix Ligustici walichii	Chyun Gung	Senkyu	Sichuan lovage root
Chui Pen Cao	***Sedum sarmentosum***	Radix et herba Sedi sarmentosi	Chai Pan Chou		Stringy stonecrop root and herb
Chun (Bai) Pi	***Ailanthus altissima***	Cortex Ailanthi	Chan (Baak) Pei		Tree of heaven bark

MANDARIN	SCIENTIFIC	PHARMACEUTICAL	CANTONESE	JAPANESE	ENGLISH
Chun Gen Bai Pi	***Cedrela sinensis***	Cortex radicis Cedrelae	Jung Gan Baak Pei		Cedrela root bark
Chun Gen Pi	***Ailanthus altissima***	Cortex radicis Ailanthi	Chan Gan Pei		Tree of heaven root bark
Ci Huang, Xiong Huang	***Orpimentum***	Orpimentum	Chi Wong		Orpiment
Ci Lao Ya Pi	***Aralia elata, A. elata*** **var.** ***suninermis***	Cortex Araliae elatate	Chu Lou Nga	Taranoki	Aralia bark
Ci Peng Hua	***Euphorbia milii***	Herba Euphorbiae milii	Chi Fung Fa		Prickly spurge herb
Ci Shi	***Magnetitum***	Magnetitum	Chi Sek		Magnetite
Ci Wei Pi	***Erinaceaus europoeus, Hemichianum dauricus***	Corium Erinacei	Chi Wai Pei		Hedgehog hide
Ci Wu Jia (Gen Pi)	***Eleutherococcus senticosus***	Radix seu cortex radicis Eleutherococci senticosi	Chi Ng Ga (Gan Pei)		Eleuthero ginseng root
Cong Bai	***Allium fistulosum***	Bulbus Allii fistulosi	Chung Baak		Fresh scallion bulb
Cong Zi	***Allium fistulosum***	Semen Allii fistulosi	Chung Ji	Sohaku	Scallion seed
Cu Jiang Cao	***Oxalis corniculata***	Herba Oxalis	Chou Jeung Chou		Indian sorrel herb
Da Cao Kou	***Alpinia zerumbet***	Fructus Alpiniae zerumbetsis	Daai Chou Kau		Beautiful galangal berry
Da Ding Huang, Zhe Mu	***Cudrania tricuspidata***	Lignum Cudraniae tricuspidatae	Je Muk		Cudrania heartwood
Da Feng Zi	***Hydnocarpus anthelmintica, H. hainanensis***	Semen Hydnocarpi	Daai Fung Ji	Daifushi	Chaulmoogra seed
Da Fu Pi	***Areca catechu, A. dicksonii***	Pericarpium Arecae	Daai Fuk Pei	Daifukuhi	Betel husk
Da Huang	***Rheum palmatum, R. tanguticum, R. officinale***	Rhizoma Rhei	Daai Wong	Daio	Rhubarb root
Da Ji	***Cirsium japonicum***	Herba Cirsii japonici	Daai Gai	Taikei	Japanese thistle herb
Da Liang Jiang	***Alpinia galanga***	Radix Alpiniae galangae	Daai Leung Geung		Greater galangal root
Da Lo San, Zhu Sha Gen	***Ardisia crenata, A. bicolor***	Radix Ardisiae crenatae	Jyu Sa Gan	Shushakon	Coralberry root
Da Po Wan Hua Hua	***Anemone hupehensis***	Herba Anemonis hupehensis	Da Po Wun Fa Fa		Hubei anemone herb
Da Qing Yan	***Halitum***	Halitum	Daai Ching Yim		Rock salt
Da Qing Ye	***Clerodendron cyrtophyllum***	Folium Clerodendronis cyrtophylli	Daai Cheng Yip		Green-white clerodendron leaf
Da Qing Ye	***Isatis tinctoria***	Folium Isatis tinctoriae	Daai Ching Yip		Woad leaf
Da Suan	***Allium sativum***	Bulbus Allii sativi	Daai Syun	Taisan	Garlic bulb
Da Wei Yao, Er Gou Cao	***Heliotropium indicum***	Herba Heliotropi	Daai Mei Yiu		Heliotrope herb
Da Xue Teng	***Sargentodoxa cuneata***	Caulis Sargentodoxae	Daai Hyut Tang		Sargentodoxa stem
Da Zao	***Zizyphus jujuba*** **var.** ***inermis***	Fructus Zizyphi jujubae	Daai Jou	Taiso	Black jujube berry

MANDARIN	SCIENTIFIC	PHARMACEUTICAL	CANTONESE	JAPANESE	ENGLISH
Da Zhu Shi Dou, Zi Xiao Rong	***Crotalaria assamica***	Semen seu herba Crotalariae assamicae	Daai Ju Si Dau		Assam crotalaria seed or herb
Dai Mao	***Eretmochelys imbricata***	Plastrum Eretmochelis	Doi Mou	Taimai	Hawksbill turtle shell
Dai Zhe Shi	***Haematitum***	Haematitum	Doi Jyu Sek	Taishaseki	Hematite
Dan Cai	***Mytilus crassitesta*** **and spp**	Mytilus	Daam Choi		Mussel
Dan Dou Chi	***Glycine max***	Semen Glycinis preparatum	Taam Dau Si	Tantoshi	Fermented soybean
Dan Fan, Shi Dan	***Chalcanthitum***	Chalcanthitum	Daan Faan	Tanban	Crystallized blue vitriol
Dan Nan Xing	***Arisaema consanguineum, A. amurense*** **and spp**	Pulvis Arisaemae cum felle Bovis	Daam Naam Sing	Tannansho	Powdered dragon arum corm with ox bile
Dan Shen	***Salvia miltiorrhiza***	Radix Salviae miltiorrhizae	Daan Sam	Tanjin	Cinnabar sage root
Dan Shen, Gan Xi Shu Wei	***Salvia przelwalskii***	Radix	Daan Sam, Gam Sai Syu Mei		Gan Xi cinnabar sage root
Dan Shen, Nan Dan Shen	***Salvia bowleyana***	Radix Salviae bowleyanae	Daan Sam, Naam Dam Sam		Southern cinnabar sage root
Dan Tian Cao	***Lysimachia candida***	Herba Lysimachiae candidae	Daan Tiu Chou		White lysimachia herb
Dan Zhu Gen	***Lopatherum gracile***	Radix Lopatheri	Daam Juk Gan		Bamboo grass root
Dan Zhu Ye	***Lopatherum gracile***	Folium Lopatheri	Daam Juk Yip	Tanchikuyo	Bamboo grass leaf
Dang Gui	***Angelica acutiloba***	Radix Angelicae acutilobae	Dong Gwai		Dong quai root
Dang Gui	***Angelica sinensis***	Radix Angelicae sinensis	Dong Gwai	Toki	Dong quai root
Dang Gui Tou	***Angelica sinensis, A. acutiloba***	Caput Angelicae sinensis	Dong Gwai Tou	Tokito	Dong quai head
Dang Gui Wei	***Angelica sinensis, A. acutiloba***	Extremas radicis Angelicae sinensis	Dong Gwai Mai	Tokio	Dong quai tail
Dang Shen	***Codonopsis pilosula, C. tangshen, C. nervosa***	Radix Codonopsis	Fong Dong Sam	Tojin	Downy bellflower root
Dang Shen, Chuan Dang Shen	***Codonopsis tangshen***	Radix Codonopsis tangshenis	Chyun Dong Sam		Sichuan bellflower root
Dang Shen, Qiu Hua Dang Shen	***Codonopsis subglobosa***	Radix Codonopsis subglobosae	Dong Sam, Kau Fa Dong Sam		Subglobular bellflower root
Dang Yao	***Swertia pseudochinensis*** **and spp**	Radix Swertiae	Dong Yeuk		Asian green gentian root
Dang Yao Cao	***Swertia japonica, S. pseudochinensis***	Herba Swertiae	Dong Yeuk Chou	Toyaku	Japanese green gentian herb
Dao Dou	***Canavalia gladiata, C. ensiformis***	Semen Canavaliae	Dou Dau		Swordbean seed
Dao Sheng Gen	***Rubus coreanus***	Fructus Rubi coreani	Dou Sang Gan		Korean raspberry fruit
Deng Long Cao	***Physalis peruviana***	Herba Physalis peruvianae	Dang Lung Chou		Peru lantern herb

MANDARIN	SCIENTIFIC	PHARMACEUTICAL	CANTONESE	JAPANESE	ENGLISH
Deng Xin Cao	***Juncus effusus***	Medulla Junci	Dang Sam Chou	Toshinso	Bulrush pith
Deng Xin Hua	***Juncus effusus***	Flos Junci	Ding Sam Fa		Bulrush flower
Di Bai Cao	***Viola diffusa***	Radix et herba Violae diffusae	Dei Baak Chou		Spreading violet root and herb
Di Dan Tou, Ku Di Dan, Tu Gong Ying	***Elephantopus scaber***	Herba Elephantopi	Fu Dei Daam		Rough elephant's foot herb
Di Fu Zi	***Kochia scoparia***	Semen Kochiae	Dei Fu Ji	Jibushi	Kochia seed
Di Gu Luo	***Raphanus sativus***	Radix Raphani			Radish root
Di Gu Pi	***Lycium chinense***	Cortex radicis Lycii	Dei Gwat Pei	Jikoppi	Wolfberry root bark
Di He Tao	***Viola collina***	Radix et herba Violae collinae	Dei Hat Tou		Collina violet root and herb
Di Jiao	***Thymus mongolicus***	Herba Thymi mongolici	Dei Jiu		Mongolian thyme herb
Di Jin Cao	***Euphorbia humifusa***	Herba Euphorbiae humifusae	Dei Gam Chou		Wolf'smilk herb
Di Long	***Pheretima aspergillum, Allolobophora caliginosa***	Pheretima seu Allolobophora	Dei Lung	Jiryu	Earthworm
Di Sun	***Lycopus lucidus***	Rhizoma Lycopi lucidi	Dei Seun		Bright bugleweed root
Di Wu Song	***Helminthostachys zeylanica***	Rhizoma Helminthostachys	Dei Ng Gung		Helmintho-stachys root
Di Yu	***Sanguisorba officinalis***	Radix Sanguisorbae	Dei Yu	Jiyu	Great burnet root
Dian Di Mei	***Androsaca umbellata***	Herba Androsacae			Androsaca herb
Diao Jin Zhong	***Melothria mederospatana***	Radix Melothriae mederospatanae	Diu Gam Jung		Melothria root
Ding Gong Teng	***Erycibes obtusifolia***	Radix et caulis Erycibis	Ding Gung Tang		Erycibe root and stem
Ding Jing Cao	***Lindernia anagallis***	Herba Linderniae	Ding Ging Chou		Lindernia herb
Ding Xiang	***Eugenia caryophyllata***	Gemma Eugeniae	Ding Heung	Choko	Clove bud
Dong Chong Xia Cao	***Cordyceps sinensis* and host larvae *Hepialus armoricanus*** or ***Holotrichia koraiensis***	Sclerotium Cordycepsis	Dung Chung Ha Chou	Tochukaso	Chinese caterpillar mushroom
Dong Feng Ju Gen	***Atalantia buxifolia***	Radix Atalantiae	Dung Fung Gwat Gan	Tofukitsu	Atalantia root
Dong Gua Pi	***Benincasa hispida***	Epicarpium Benincasae	Dung Gwa Pei	Tokahi	Waxgourd fruit rind
Dong Gua Ren	***Benincasa hispida***	Semen Benincasae	Dong Gwa Yan	Tokanin	Waxgourd seed
Dong Kui Zi	***Malva verticillata***	Semen Malvae	Dung Kwai Ji		Musk mallow seed
Dong Ling Cao	***Rabdosia rubescens* and spp**	Herba Rabdosiae	Dun Ling Chou		Rabdosia herb
Dou (Huang) Juan	***Glycene max***	Semen Glycinis germinati	Dau (Wong) Geun		Sprouting soybean
Dou Chi Jiang	***Litsea cubeba***	Radix et caulis Litseae	Dau Chek Geung	Toshikyo	Cubeb root and stem
Du Heng	***Asarum forbesii***	Rhizoma Asari forbesii	Dou Hang		Forbes' wild ginger root

MANDARIN	SCIENTIFIC	PHARMACEUTICAL	CANTONESE	JAPANESE	ENGLISH
Du Huo	***Angelica pubescens, A. laxiflora*** **and spp**	Radix Angelicae pubescentis	Duk Wut	Dokkatsu	Hairy angelica Root
Du Huo	***Heracleum candicans***	Radix Heraclei candicantis	Duk Wut		White cow parsnip root
Du Jiao Gan	***Striga asiatica***	Herba Strigae	Duk Geuk Gam		Witchweed herb
Du Jiao Lan	***Typhonium giganteum***	Radix Typhonii	Duk Gok Lin		Typhonium root
Du Zhong	***Eucommia ulmoides***	Cortex Eucommiae	Dou Jung	Tochu	Eucommia bark
Du Zhong Ye	***Eucommia ulmoides***	Folium Eucommiae	Dou Jung Yip		Eucommia leaf
Duan Long Gu, Shu Long Gu	***Stegodon orientalis et al.***	Os Stegodontis calcinatum	Taan Lung Gwat		Calcined dragon bone
Duan Mu Li	***Ostrea gigas***	Concha Ostreae calcinati	Taan Mou Lai		Calcined oyster shell
Duan Shu Hua	***Tilia cordata***	Flos Tiliae			Linden flower
Dui Ye Dou Ye	***Cassia alata***	Folium Cassiae alatae	Deui Yip Dau Yip		Ringworm bush leaf
Dun Ye Shu Yu	***Dioscorea zingiberensis***	Rhizoma Dioscoreae zingiberis	Teun Yip Syu Yu		Shield-leaf yam root
E Bu Shi Cao	***Centipeda minima***	Herba Centipedae	Ngo Bat Sik Chou	Sekikozui, Gabusho-kuso	Centipeda herb
E Guan Shi, Shi Zhong Ru	***Stalactitum, Balanophylla*** **spp.**	Stalactitum	Ngo Gun Sek		Stalactite tip
E Jiao	***Equus asinus*** **and spp**	Gelatinum corii Equi asini	O Gaau	Akyo	Ass hide glue
E Zhu, Guang Xi Er Zhu	***Curcuma kwangsiensis***	Rhizoma Curcumae kwangsiensis	Ngo Seut, Gwong Sai Ngo Seut		Guangxi turmeric root
E Zhu, Peng Er Zhu	***Curcuma zedoaria, C. aeruginosa*** **and spp**	Rhizoma Curcumae zedoariae	Ngo Seut, Fung Ngo Seut	Gajutsu	Zedoary root
Er Cha	***Acacia catechu***	Pasta Acaciae seu Uncariae	Yi Cha	Asenyaku	Catechu paste
Er Cha	***Uncaria gambir*** **and spp**	Pasta Uncaria seu Acaciae	Yi Cha		Catechu paste
Er Gou Cao	***Heliotropium indicum***	Herba Heliotropi	Yi Ngau Chou		Indian heliotrope herb
Fa Ban Xia	***Pinellia ternata***	Rhizoma Pinelliae ternatae preparatae	Faat Bun Ha	Hange, Kohange	Prepared pinellia corm
Fan Bai Cao	***Potentilla discolor***	Herba Potentillae discoloris	Faan Baak Chou		Discolored cinquefoil herb
Fan Bi	***Agkistrodon halys***	Agkistrodon	Faan Bei		Viper
Fan Shi Liu Gan Ye	***Psidium guajava***	Folium Psidii	Faan Sek Lau Gon Yip		Guava leaf
Fan Tuan Teng	***Kadsura coccinea***	Caulis Kadsurae coccineae	Faan Tyun Tang		Scarlet kadsura stem
Fan Xie Ye	***Senna acutifolia, S. angustifolia***	Folium Sennae	Faan Sie Yip		Senna leaf
Fan Xing	***Tetragonia tatragonoides***	Herba Tetragoniae	Faan Haang	Bankyo, Mantsai	Tetragonia herb
Fang Feng	***Ledebouriella divaricata, L. seseloides***	Radix Ledebouriellae	Fong Fung	Bofu	Wind-protector root

MANDARIN	SCIENTIFIC	PHARMACEUTICAL	CANTONESE	JAPANESE	ENGLISH
Fang Gui	***Peucedanum japonicum***	Radix Peucedani japonici	Fong Kwai		Japanese masterwort root
Fang Ji, Guang Fang Ji	***Aristolochia fangchi, A. westlandii***	Radix Aristolochiae fangchis	Fong Gei, Gwong Fong Gei		Fangchi birthwort root
Fei Long Zhang Xue	***Toddalia asiatica***	Radix Toddaliae	Fei Lung Jeung Hyut		Asian toddalia root
Fei Zao Jia	***Gymnocladus chinensis***	Fructus Gymnocladi	Fei Jou Choi		Chinese gymnocladus berry
Fei Zi	***Torreya grandis, T. nucifera***	Semen Torreyae	Fei Ji		Japanese torreya nut
Feng Che Er	***Dioscorea japonica***	Rhizoma Dioscoreae japonicae	Fung Che Yi		Japanese yam root
Feng Dou Cai	***Petasites japonicus***	Flos Petasitis	Fung Dau Choi		Japanese butterbur flower
Feng Hua Fen	***Pollen***	Granum floris pollinis	Fung Fa Fan		Flower (bee) pollen
Feng Huang Yi	***Gallus gallus domesticus***	Membrana follicularis ovi			Chicken egg membrane
Feng La	***Apis cerana*** and spp	Cera flava	Fung Laap		Beeswax
Feng Mi	***Apis cerana*** and spp	Mel	Fung Mat		Honey
Feng Wei Cao	***Pteris multifida*** and spp	Herba Pterii	Fung Mei Chou		Phoenix-tail fern
Feng Yen Cao	***Ailanthus altissima***	Fructus Ailanthi	Fung Ngaan Chou		Tree of heaven fruit
Fo Shou (Gan)	***Citrus medica*** var. ***sarcodactylis***	Fructus Citri medicae	Fut Sau (Gam)		Finger lemon fruit
Fo Shou (Gan) Hua	***Citrus medica*** var. ***sarctodactylus***	Flos Citri sarctodactylis	Fut Sao Fa	Bushukan	Finger lemon flower
Fu Hai Shi	***Pumus***	Lapis Pumicis	Fau Hoi Sek	Kaifuseki	Pumice
Fu Ling	***Poria cocos***	Sclerotium Poriae	(Wong) Fuk Ling, Waan Ling	Bukuryo	Hoelen fungus
Fu Ling Pi	***Poria cocos***	Cortex Poriae	Wong Ling Pei, Fuk Ling Pei	Bukuryoshi	Hoelen skin
Fu Long Gan		Terra flava usta, Bolus usta	Fuk Lung Gon	Bukuryukan	Wood stove clay
Fu Pen Zi	***Rubus chingii***	Fructus Rubi chingii	Fuk Pun Ji	Fukubonshi	Chinese raspberry fruit
Fu Ping	***Lemna minor***	Herba Lemnae	Fau Ping		Duckweed herb
Fu Ping	***Spirodela polyrrhiza***	Herba Spirodelae	Fau Ping		Duckweed herb
Fu Rong	***Crossostephium chinense***	Herba Crossostephii	Fu Yung		Crossosteph-ium herb
Fu Rong Hua	***Hibiscus mutabilis***	Flos Hibisci mutabili	Fu Yung Fa		Cotton rose flower
Fu Rong Ye	***Hibiscus mutabilis***	Folium Hibisci mutabilis	Fu Yung Yip		Cotton rose leaf
Fu Sang Hua	***Hibiscus rosa-sinensis***	Flos Hibisci rosa-sinensis	Fu Song Fa		Shoe flower
Fu Shen	***Poria cocos***	Sclerotium Poriae paradicis	Pou Fuk Sam	Bukushin	Hoelen spirit
Fu Shou Cao	***Adonis amurensis***	Herba Adonis	Fuk Sau Chou		Amur adonis herb
Fu Xiao Mai	***Triticum aestivum***	Fructus Tritici	Fau Siu Mak	Fushobaku	Wheat berry

MANDARIN	SCIENTIFIC	PHARMACEUTICAL	CANTONESE	JAPANESE	ENGLISH
Fu Zi	***Aconitum carmichaeli***	Radix lateralis Aconiti carmichaeli praeparatae	Fu Ji	Bushi	Prepared Sichuan aconite root
Gan Cao	***Glycirrhiza uralensis, G. glabra*** **and spp**	Radix Glycirrhizae	Gam Chou	Kanzo	Ural licorice root
Gan Cha	***Hydrangea serrata*** **var.** ***thunbergii***	Folium Hydrangeae	Gam Cha	Amatya, Dochouzan	Sweet tea leaf
Gan Jiang	***Zingiber officinalis***	Rhizoma Zingiberis	Gaan Geung	Kankyo	Dried ginger root
Gan Jie Geng	***Adenophora trachelioides***	Radix Adenophorae trachelioidis	Gam Gaat Gan, Ai Ji Sam		Sweet ladybell root
Gan Lan, Jing Guo	***Canarium album***	Fructus Canarii	Gaam Laam		Asian olive fruit
Gan Qi	***Rhus verniciflua***	Succus exsiccatus Rhudis	Gon Chat		Lacquer
Gan Song	***Nardostachys jatamansi, N. chinensis***	Radix Nardostachis	Gam Chung		Indian spikenard root
Gan Sui	***Euphorbia kansui***	Radix Euphorbiae kansui	Gam Seui	Kansui	Sweet spurge root
Gang Ban Gui, Guan Ye Liao	***Polygonum perfoliatum***	Herba Polygoni perfoliati	Gong Bun Gwai, Gwan Yip Lou		Perfoliate knotweed herb
Gang Liu Pi, Xiang Liu Pi	***Periploca sepium***	Cortex radicis Periplocae	Gong Lau Pei, Heung Lau Pei		Silk vine root bark
Gang Mei (Gen), Wang Dian Jing	***Ilex asprella***	Folium et radix Ilicis asprellae	Gong Mui Gan, Maan Dim Gam		Rough holly leaf and root
Gao Ben	***Ligusticum sinense, L. jeholense***	Radix Ligustici sinensis	Gou Bun	Kohon	Chinese lovage root
Gao Liang Jiang	***Alpinia officinarum***	Rhizoma Alpiniae officinari	Gou Leung Geung	Koryokyo	Galangal root
Ge	***Mactra sulcataria***	Concha Mactrae	Hok	Jiseki	Mactra shell
Ge Gen	***Pueraria lobata, P. omeiensis*** **and spp**	Radix Puerariae	Got Gan	Kakkon	Kudzu root
Ge Hua	***Pueraria lobata, P. omeiensis*** **and spp**	Flos Puerariae	Got Fa		Kudzu flower
Ge Jie	***Gecko gecko, G. verticilatus***	Gecko	Gap Gaai	Gokai	Toad-headed lizard
Ge Lei Zhi Gen	***Vitis flexuosa***	Radix Vitis flexuosis	Got Leui Jap Gan		Flexuose grape root
Gou Gu Ye	***Ilex cornuta***	Folium Ilicis cornutae	Gau Gwat Yip		Cat thorn holly leaf
Gou Ji	***Cibotium barometz***	Rhizoma Cibotii	Gau Jek	Kuseki	Dogspine root
Gou Ju	***Poncirus trifoliata***	Fructus Ponciri	Gau Gwat		Trifoliate orange fruit
Gou Qi Ye	***Lycium chinense, L. barbarum***	Folium Lycii chinensis	Gau Ji Yip		Wolfberry leaf
Gou Qi Zi	***Lycium chinense, L. barbarum***	Fructus Lycii	Gau Gei Ji, Gei Ji	Kukoshi	Wolfberry
Gou Teng	***Uncaria rhynchophylla, U. hirsuta, U. macrophylla*** **and spp**	Ramulus et uncus Uncariae	Ngau Tang, Sheung Ngau (Tang)	Choto	Gambir vine twig

MANDARIN	SCIENTIFIC	PHARMACEUTICAL	CANTONESE	JAPANESE	ENGLISH
Gou Wen	***Gelsemium elegans***	Radix Gelsemii	Au Man		Chinese gelsemium
Gou Ya Hua	***Ervatamia divaricata, E. hainaensis***	Herba Ervatamiae	Gaau Nga Fa		Crepe jasmine herb
Gu Jing Cao	***Eriocaulon buergerianum, E. sieboldianum***	Herba Eriocaulonis	Guk Jing Chou	Kokuseiso	Pipewort herb
Gu Jing Zi	***Eriocaulon buergerianum, E. sieboldianum***	Fructus Eriocaulonis	Guk Jing Ji		Pipewort seed
Gu Su Hua	***Desmodium umbellatum***	Flos Desmodii umbellati	Gu Sou Fa		Umbel desmodium flower
Gu Sui Bu	***Davallia divaricata***	Rhizoma Davalliae	Gwat Seui Bou	Kotsusaiho	Boneknit root
Gu Sui Bu	***Drynaria fortunei* and spp**	Rhizoma Drynariae	Gwat Seui Bou	Kotsusaiho	Boneknit root
Gu Sui Bu	***Pseudodrynaria fortunei, D. baronii***	Rhizoma Pseudodrynariae	Gwat Seui Bou	Kotsusaiho	Boneknit root
Gu Ya	***Oryza sativa***	Fructus Oryzae germinatus	Gu Nga	Kokuga	Sprouted rice grain
Gua Lou (Shi)	***Trichosanthes kirilowii, T. japonica, T. uniflora***	Fructus Tricosanthis	Kwut Lau	Karo	Snakegourd fruit
Gua Lou Pi	***Trichosanthes kirilowii, T. japonica, T. uniflora***	Pericarpium Tricosanthis	Kwut Lau Pei	Karohi	Snakegourd rind
Gua Lou Ren	***Trichosanthes kirilowii, T. japonica, T. uniflora***	Semen Trichosanthis	Kwut Lau Yan	Karonin	Snakegourd seed
Gua Niu	***Eulota peliomphala***	Eulota	Wo Ngau		Snail
Gua Zi Jin	***Polygala japonica***	Herba Polygalae japonicae	Gwa Ji Gam		Japanese milkwort herb
Guan Mu Tong	***Aristolochia manshuriensis, A. moupinensis***	Caulis Aristolochiae manshuriensis	Gwaan Muk Tung		Manchurian birthwort stem
Guan Zhen Huang, Ye Gu	***Aeginetia indica***	Herba Aeginetiae	Gwon Jam Wong, Ye Gu		Aeginetia herb
Guan Zhong	***Cyathea spinulosa***	Rhizoma Cyatheae	Gwun Jung		Cyathea root
Guan Zhong	***Lunathyrum vegetius, L. giraldii***	Rhizoma Lunathyri	Gwun Jung		Lunathyrum fern root
Guan Zhong, Gou Ji Guan Zhong	***Woodwardia japonica, W. unigemmata***	Rhizoma Woodwardiae	Gwun Jung, Gau Jek Gun Jung		Chain-fern root
Guan Zhong, Hun Ji Tou,	***Cyrtomium fortunei***	Rhizoma Cyrtomi	Gwun Jung, Fan Gai Tau		Boss fern root
Guan Zhong, Jia Guo Jue Guan Zhong	***Matteucia struthiopteris***	Rhizoma Matteuciae	Gwun Jung, Ying Gwo Kyut Gwun Jung		Ostrich-feather fern root
Guan Zhong, Mian Ma Guan Zhong	***Dryopteris crassirhizoma***	Rhizoma Dryopteris	Gwun Jung, Min Ma Gwun Jung	Tohoku-kanju	Shield fern root

MANDARIN	SCIENTIFIC	PHARMACEUTICAL	CANTONESE	JAPANESE	ENGLISH
Guan Zhong, Wu Mao Jue Guan Zhong, Dong Fang Wu Mao Jue Ye	***Blechnum orientale***	Rhizoma Blechni	Gwun Jung, Dung Fong Wu Mou Kyut Yip	Kanju	Oriental hammock fern root
Guan Zhong, Zi Qi Guan Zhong	***Osmunda japonica***	Rhizoma Osmundae	Gwun Jung, Ji Kei Gwun Jung	Tohoku-kanju	Japanese flowering fern root
Guang Dong (Jin) Qian Cao	***Desmodium styracifolium***	Herba Desmodii	Gwong Dung (Gam) Chin Chou	Kinsenso	Coin-leaf desmodium herb
Guang Dong Sheng Ma	***Serratula chinensis***	Radix Serratulae	Gwong Dung Jing Ma		Serratula root
Guang Gou Shen	***Canis***	Testes et penis canis	Gwong Gau Sam	Kujin	Male dog genitals
Guang Huo Xiang	***Pogostemon cablin***	Herba Pogostemis	Gwong Fok Heung		Patchouli herb
Guang Lang Du, Hai Yu	***Alocasia odora***	Rhizoma Alocasiae	Hoi Wu		Alocasia root
Guang Ming Zi	***Ocimum Basilicum***	Fructus Ocimi	Gwong Ming Ji		Basil seed
Guang Sha Ren	***Amomum villosum***	Semen Amomi villosi	Gwong Sa Yan		Wild cardamom seed
Gui Ban	***Chinemys reevesii***	Plastrum Chinemis	Gwai Baan	Kiban	Tortoise shell
Gui Ban Jiao	***Chinemys reevesii***	Gelatinum carapaxis Chinemis	Gwai Baan Gaau		Tortoise shell gel
Gui Hua Pi	***Osmanthus fragrans***	Cortex ramuli Osmanthi	Gwai Fa Pei		Osmanthus twig bark
Gui Jian Yu	***Euonymus alata***	Ramulus Eunymi alati	Gwai Jin Yu		Winged spindletree twig
Gui Jiu	***Dysosma versipellis***	Rhizoma Dysosmae versipellis	Gwai Kau		Common dysosma root
Gui Pi	***Cinnamomum japonicum, C. zeylanicum, C. obtusifolium***	Cortex Cinnamomi japonici	Gwai Pei		Cinnamon bark
Gui Yu Jian	***Buchnera cruciata***	Herba Buchnerae	Gwai Yu Jin		Cruciate bluehart herb
Gui Zhen Cao	***Bidens bipinnata***	Herba Bidentis bipinnatae	Gwai Jam Chou		Beggartick herb
Gui Zhi , Rou Gui Zhi	***Cinnamomum cassia***	Ramulus Cinnamomi cassiae	Gwai Ji	Keishi	Cassia cinnamon twig
Guo Lu Huang, Luo Mo	***Metaplexis japonica***	Herba Metaplexis	Lo Mo		Metaplexis herb
Guo Lu Huang, Nian Ren Hua	***Desmodium sinnatum***	Herba Desmodii sinnati	Lim Yan Fa		Sinnate desmodium herb
Guo Yu	***Limax agrestic***	Limax	Gwat Kut		Slug
Hai Dai	***Laminaria*** **spp**	Herba Laminariae	Hoi Daai		Algae
Hai Er Cao	***Rungia pectinata***	Herba Rungiae	Haai Yi Chou		Rungia herb
Hai Feng Teng	***Kadsura heteroclita***	Caulis Kadsurae heteroclitae	Hoi Fung Tang		Heteroclite kadsura stem
Hai Feng Teng	***Piper hancei***	Caulis Piperis hanceis	Hoi Fung Tang		Kadsura pepper stem

MANDARIN	SCIENTIFIC	PHARMACEUTICAL	CANTONESE	JAPANESE	ENGLISH
Hai Feng Teng, Xian Lin Ju	***Piper hancei*** var. ***squamiglandiferum***	Caulis Piperis squamiglandiferi	Hoi Fung Tang		Fujian kadsura pepper stem
Hai Ge Ke, Ke Li	***Cyclina sinensis***	Concha Cyclinae	Hoi Gap Hok	Kaigokaku	Clam shell
Hai Gou Shen	***Callorhinus ursinus, Phoca vitulina***	Testes et penis Callorhini seu Phocae	Hoi Gau Sam	Kaikujin	Seal genitals
Hai Jin Sha	***Lygodium japonicum***	Spora Lygodii	Hoi Gam Sa	Kaikinsha	Japanese climbing fern spore
Hai Jin Sha Teng	***Lygodium japonicum***	Herba Lygodii	Hoi Gam Sa Tang	Kaikinshato	Japanese climbing fern herb
Hai Long	***Solenognathus*** spp, ***Syngnathoides biaculeatus***	Solenognathus	Hoi Lung		Pipefish
Hai Ma	***Hippocampus kelloggiand*** spp	Hippocampus	Hoi Ma	Kaiba	Sea horse
Hai Piao Xiao, Wu Zei Gu	***Sepia esculenta, Sepiella maindroni***	Os Sepiae seu Sapiellae	Hoi Piu Seui		Cuttlefish bone
Hai Shen	***Stichopus japonicus***	Stichopus	Hoi Sam		Sea cucumber
Hai Tong Pi	***Erythrina variegata*** var. ***orientalis***	Cortex Erythrinae	Hoi Tung Pei	Kaitohi	Asian coral tree bark
Hai Zao	***Sargassum fusiforme*** and spp	Herba Sargassi	Hoi Chou	Kaiso	Sargassum seaweed
Hai Zhe	***Rhopilema esculenta***	Tentaculum Rhopilema	Hoi Jit		Jellyfish tentacle
Han Cai	***Rorippa montana, R. indica***	Herba Rorippae	Hon Choi		Nasturtium herb
Han Fang Ji, Fang Ji	***Stephania tetrandra***	Radix Stephaniae tetrandrae	Haan Fong Gei Fong Gei	Kamboi	Stephania root
Han Lian Cao, Mo Han Lian	***Eclipta prostata, E. alba***	Herba Ecliptae	Hon Lin Chou	Kanrenso	Field lotus herb
Han Shui Shi, Fang Jie Shi	***Calcitum***	Calcitum	Hon Seui Sek	Kansuiseki	Calcite
Han Shui Shi, Hong Shi Gao	***Gypsum rubrum***	Gypsum rubrum	Hon Seui Sek, Hung Sek Gau		Red gypsum
Han Xin Cao	***Scutellaria indica***	Herba Scutellariae indicae	Hon Sam Chou		India skullcap herb
Han Xiu Cao	***Mimosa pudica***	Herba mimosae pudicae	Ham Sau Chou		Mimosa herb
He Cao Ya	***Agrimonia pilosa*** var. ***japonica***	Gemma Agrimoniae pilosae	Hok Chou Nga		Furry agrimony winter bud
He Huan Hua	***Albizzia julibrissin, A. lebbek*** and spp	Flos Albizziae	Hap Fun Fa	Gokanka	Mimosa flower
He Huan Pi	***Albizzia julibrissin, A. lebbak*** and spp	Cortex Albizziae	Hap Fun Pei	Gokanhi	Mimosa bark
He Shi	***Carpesium abrotanoides***	Fructus seu semen Carpesii	Hok Sat	Kakushitsu	Starwort fuit or seed
He Shou Wu	***Polygonum multiflorum***	Radix Polygoni multiflori	Ho Sau Wu	Kashuu	Flowery knotweed root
He Ye, Lian Lie	***Nelumbo nucifera***	Folium Nelumbinis	Ho Yip	Kayo	Lotus leaf
He Zi (Rou)	***Terminalia chebula*** and var.	Fructus Terminaliae	Ho Ji (Yuk)	Kashi	Myrobalan fruit

MANDARIN	SCIENTIFIC	PHARMACEUTICAL	CANTONESE	JAPANESE	ENGLISH
He Zi Cao	***Actinostemma lobata***	Folium at semen Actinostemmae	Hap Ji Chou		Actinostemma leaf and seed
Hei Dou Yi	***Glycine max***	Pericarpium Glycinis	Haak Dau Yi		Soybean husk
Hei Mian Ma, Bai Hua Dan	***Plumbago zeylanicum***	Herba Plumbaginis	Baak Fa Daan		Ceylon leadwort
Hei Mian Ye	***Breynia fruticosa***	Cacumen Breyniae	Haak Min Yip		Breynia tip
Hei Zhi Ma, Hu Ma Ren	***Sesamum indicum***	Fructus Sesami	Hak Ji Ma		Black sesame seed
Hong Ban Bian Lian	***Begonia crassirostris***	Herba Begoniae crassirostris	Hung Bun Bin Lin		Begonia herb
Hong Ci Teng, Hong Gen, Xiao Jin Ying	***Rosa cymosa***	Cortex radicis Rosae cymosae	Hung Chi Teng, Siu Gam Ying		Cymose rose root bark
Hong Da Ji	***Knoxia valerianoides***	Radix Knoxiae	Hung Daai Gik	Kogataigeki	Knoxia root
Hong Dou Kou	***Alpinia galanga***	Fructus Alpiniae Galangae	Hung Dau Kau		Greater galangal berry
Hong Han Lian	***Hypericum ascyron***	Herba Hyperici ascyronis	Hung Hon Lin		St. John's wort
Hong Hua	***Carthamus tinctorius***	Flos Carthami tinctorii	Hung Fa	Koka	Safflower
Hong Lang Du, Lang Du	***Stellera chamaejasme***	Radix Stellerae	Hung Long Duk, Long Duk		Stellara root
Hong Mao Cha	***Statice sinensis***	Radix Staticis	Hung Maau Cha		Statice root
Hong Mao Qi	***Leontice robustum***	Radix Leonticis	Hung Mou Chat		Leontice root
Hong Mu Xiang	***Kadsura longipedunculata***	Radix Kadsurae longipedunculatae	Hung Muk Heung		Long-stalk kadsura root
Hong Niang Zi	***Huechys sanguinea, H, philaemata***	Huechys	Hung Leung Ji		Red cicada
Hong Qi, Huang Qi	***Hedysarum polybotrys*** and spp	Radix Hedysari polybotris	Hung Kei, Wong Kei		Hedysarum root
Hong Qu Mi	***Oryza sativa*** and ***Monascus purpureus***	Fructus Oryzae fermentatus cum Monasco	Hung Ju Mai		Fermented rice with red yeast
Hong Ren Shen	***Panax ginseng***	Radix Panacis ginsengis praeparatae	Hung Yan Sam	Koninjin	Red cured Asian ginseng root
Hong Zao	***Zizyphus jujuba*** var. ***inermis***	Fructus Zizyphi jujubae	Hung Jou	Koso	Red jujube berry
Hou Gu	***Hericium erinaceus***	Sclerotium Hericii			Hedgehog fungus
Hou Jiao	***Macaca mulatta***	Gelatinum Macacae	Hao Gaau		Macaque gel
Hou Po Hua	***Magnolia officinalis, M. biloba, M. obovata***	Flos Magnoliae officinalis	Hau Pok Fa	Koboka, Kobokuka	Magnolia flower
Hou Po, Chuan Po	***Magnolia officinalis, M. biloba, M. obovata***	Cortex Magnoliae officinalis	Hau Pok, Chyun Pok	Koboku	Magnolia bark
Hou Ye Chuan Mu Xiang	***Dolomiaea berardioidea***	Radix Dolomiaea berardioidea	Hau Yip Chyun Muk Heung		Thick-leaf Dolomiaea root
Hou Zao	***Macaca mulatta***	Calculus Macacae	Hau Jou	Koso	Macaque bezoar
Hu Bei Bei Mu	***Fritillaria hupehensis***	Bulbus Fritillariae hupehensis	Wu Bak Bui Mou		Hubei fritillary bulb

MANDARIN	SCIENTIFIC	PHARMACEUTICAL	CANTONESE	JAPANESE	ENGLISH
Hu Bei Bei Mu, Pu Qi Bei Mu	*Fritillaria puqiensis*	Bulbus Fritillariae puqiensis	Wu Bak Bui Mou, Pou Kei Bui Mou		Puqi fritillary bulb
Hu Die Cao	*Bauhinia paraglauca*	Herba Bauhiniae paraglaucae			Green bauhinia herb
Hu Er Cao	*Saxifraga stolonifera*	Herba Saxifragae stoloniferae	Fu Yi Chou		Saxifrage herb
Hu Gu	*Panthera*	Os tigris	Fu Gwat	Kokotsu	Tiger bone
Hu Huang Lian	*Picrorrhiza kurroa*	Radix Picrorrhizae	Wu Wong Lin	Kooren	Picrorrhiza root
Hu Ji Sheng	*Viscum coloratum, V. album*	Herba Visci	Wu Gei Sang		Western mistletoe herb
Hu Jiao Gen	*Piper nigrum*	Radix Piperis nigri	Wu Jiu Gan		Black pepper root
Hu Jiao, Hei Hu Jiao	*Piper nigrum*	Fructus Piperis nigri	Wu Jiu, Mai Wu Jiu	Kosho	Black pepper corn
Hu Li Wei, Tong Tian Cao	*Uraria lagopodioides*	Herba Urariae	Tung Tin Chou		Uraria herb
Hu Lu Ba	*Trigonella foenum-graecum*	Semen Trigonellae	Wu Lou Ba		Fenugreek seed
Hu Lu Ke	*Lagenaria siceraria*	Fructus Lagenariae	Wu Lok Hok		Bottle gourd fruit
Hu Po	*Pinus succinifera*	Resina Pini succiniferae (Succinum)	Fu Po		Amber resin
Hu Sui	*Coriandrum sativum*	Herba Coriandri	Wu Sai		Coriander herb
Hu Tao Ren	*Juglans regia*	Semen Juglandis	Wu Tou Yan	Kotoniku	Walnut meat
Hu Tao Ye	*Juglans regia*	Folium Juglandis	Wu Tou Yip		Walnut leaf
Hu Tao Zhi	*Juglans regia*	Ramulus Juglandis	Wu Tou Ji		Walnut twig
Hu Tong Lei	*Calophyllum inophyllum*	Resina Calophylli	Ng Tung Leui		Foraha resin
Hu Tong Lei	*Populus euphratica* and spp	Resina Populi	Wu Tung Leui		Poplar resin
Hu Tui (Zi) Ye	*Eleagnus pungens*	Folium Eleagni pungensis	Wu Teui (Ji) Yip		Thorny eleagnus leaf
Hu Zhang	*Polygonum cuspidatum*	Radix et folium Polygoni cuspidati	Fu Jeung		Japanese Knotweed root and leaf
Hua Jiao, Chuan Jiao	*Zanthoxylum bungeanum*	Fructus Zanthoxyli bungeani	Chyun Jiu, Fa Jiu	Shokusho	Sichuan peppercorn
Hua Lu Shen	*Cervus nippon* and spp	Testes et penis Cervi	Fa Luk Sam		Male deer genitals
Hua Mu Pi	*Betula platyphylla*	Cortex Betulae	Wa Muk Pei		Asian birch bark
Hua Rui Shi	*Ophicalcitum*	Ophicalcitum	Fa Yeui Sek	Kazuiseki	Dolomite
Hua Sheng Pi	*Arachis hypogaea*	Pericarpium Arachis	Fa Sang Pei	Kashohi	Peanut skin
Hua Shi	*Talcum*	Talcum	Wat Sek	Kasseki	Talc
Hua Tou Cao	*Viola patrinii*	Herba Violae patriniae	Wa Tau Chou		Patrinium violet herb
Huai (Hua) Mi	*Sophora japonica*	Gemma Sophorae japonicae	Waai (Fa) Mai		Japanese pagoda tree bud
Huai Hua	*Sophora japonica*	Flos Sophorae japonicae	Waai Fa		Japanese pagoda tree flower
Huai Jiao (Zi)	*Sophora japonica*	Fructus Sophorae japonicae	Wai Jiu (Ji)		Japanese pagoda tree fruit

MANDARIN	SCIENTIFIC	PHARMACEUTICAL	CANTONESE	JAPANESE	ENGLISH
Huai Niu Xi	***Achyranthes bidentata***	Radix Achyranthis	Ngau Sat, Wai Ngau Sat	Goshitsu	White oxknee Root
Huai Tong	***Aristolochia moupiensis***	Radix seu caulis Aristolochiae moupiensis	Waai Tung		Birthwort root or stem
Huang Bai, Chuan Bai	***Phellodendron amurense, P. chinense***	Cortex Phellodendris	Wong Paak, Chyun Paak	Obaku	Siberian cork tree bark
Huang Hua Hao, Qing Hao	***Artemisia annua***	Herba Artemisiae annuae	Wong Fa Hou, Ching Hou		Annual wormwood herb
Huang Hua Jia Zhu Tao (Ye)	***Thevetia peruviana***	Folium et semen Thevetiae	Wong Fa Gaap Juk Tou (Yip)		Peruvian thevetia leaf and seed
Huang Jin Kui, Chuan Po Shi	***Vanieria cochinchinensis***	Caulis Vanieriae	Wong Jin Kwai		Vanieria stem
Huang Jing	***Polygonatum sibiricum, P. cyrtonema, P. kingianum***	Rhizoma Polygonati	Wong Jing	Osei	Siberian Solomon's-seal root
Huang Jing Zi	***Vitex negundo***	Fructus Viticis negundonis	Wong Ging Ji		Negundo chastetree berry
Huang Lian Ya	***Pistacia chinensis***	Folium Pistaciae	Wong Lin Nga		Pistachio leaf
Huang Lian, Chuan Lian	***Coptis chinensis, C. omeiensis*** and spp	Rhizoma Coptis	Wong Lin, Chyun Wong Lin	Oren	Goldthread root
Huang Mu Er	***Tremella mesenterica***	Sclerotium Tremellae mesentericae	Wong Muk Yi		Yellow ear mushroom
Huang Niu Cha	***Cratoxylon ligustrinum***	Folium Cratoxyli	Wong Ngau Cha		Cratoxylon leaf
Huang Pi Guo	***Clausenia lansium***	Pericarpium Clauseniae	Wong Pei Gwo		Wampi fruit
Huang Pi He	***Clausenia lansium***	Semen Clauseniae	Wong Pei Ho		Wampi seed
Huang Pi Ye	***Clausenia lansium***	Folium Clauseniae	Wong Pei Yip		Wampi leaf
Huang Qi	***Astragalus membranaceus, A. mongholicus*** and spp	Radix Astragali	Wong Kei, Paak Kei	Ogi	Astragalus root
Huang Qi, Hong Qi	***Hedysarum polybotrys*** and spp	Radix Hedysari polybotris	Wong Kei, Hung Kei		Hedysarum root
Huang Qin	***Scutellaria baicalensis, S. viscidula, S. amoena***	Radix Scutellariae baicalensis	Wong Sam	Ogon	Baikal skullcap root
Huang Shui Qie	***Solanum xanthocarpum***	Herba Solani xanthocarpi	Wong Seui Ke		Prickly nightshade fruit
Huang Teng Gen	***Daemonorops margaritae***	Radix Daemonoropsis	Wong Tang Gan		Daemonorops root
Huang Yao Zi	***Dioscorea bulbifera***	Rhizoma Dioscoreae bulbiferae	Wong Yeuk Ji	Oyakushi	Potato yam tuber
Huo Ma Ren	***Cannabis sativa***	Semen Cannabis	Fo Ma Yan	Mashinin	Cannabis seed
Huo Tan Mu (Cao), Qing Fan Teng	***Polygonum chinense***	Herba Polygoni chinensis	Fo Tan Mou (Chou)		Chinese knotweed herb
Huo Xiang	***Agastache rugosa***	Herba Agastachis	Fok Heung	Kakko	Rugose giant hyssop herb

MANDARIN	SCIENTIFIC	PHARMACEUTICAL	CANTONESE	JAPANESE	ENGLISH
Huo Xue Lian	***Coniogramme japonica***	Herba Coniogrammis	Fo Hyut Lin		Bamboo fern herb
Ji Cai	***Capsella bursa-pastoris***	Herba Capsellae	Chai Choi	Seisai	Shepherd's purse herb
Ji Dan Hua	***Plumeria rubra*** **var.** ***acutifolia***	Flos Plumeriae	Gai Daan Fa		Frangipani flower
Ji Gu Cao	***Abrus precatorius, A. cantoniensis***	Herba Abri	Gai Gwat Chou		Licorice bean herb
Ji Gu Xiang	***Croton crassifolius***	Radix Crotonis crassifolii	Gai Gwat Heung		Thick-leaf croton root
Ji Guan Hua	***Celosia cristata***	Herba Celosiae cristatae	Gai Gun Fa		Cock'scomb herb
Ji Hua	***Loropetalum chinense***	Flos Loropetali	Gai Fa		Strap flower
Ji Ji	***Chloranthus serratus***	Radix Chloranthi	Kap Gei		Serrate-leaf chloranthus
Ji Mu	***Loropetalum chinense***	Cortex Loropetali	Gai Muk		Strap flower bark
Ji Nei Jin	***Gallus gallus domesticus***	Endothelium corneum gigeriae Galli	Gai Na Gam	Keinaikin	Chicken gizzard lining
Ji Ni	***Adenophora trachelioides, A. remotifolia***	Radix Adenophorae trachelioidis	Chai Ni		Common harebell root
Ji Shi Teng	***Paederia scandens***	Radix et caulis Paederiae	Gai Niu Tang	Hakumokeishito	Chicken dung vine root and stem
Ji Xing Hua	***Impatiens balsamina***	Flos Impatiensis	Jek Chin Fa		Garden balsam flower
Ji Xing Zi	***Impatiens balsamina***	Semen Impatiensis	Jek Chin Ji	Kyuseishi	Garden balsam seed
Ji Xue Cao, Peng Da Wan	***Centella asiatica***	Folium Centellae	Jik Syut Chou, Pang Daai Yan		Gotu kola leaf
Ji Xue Teng	***Millettia dielsiana, M. reticulata, M. nitida***	Radix et caulis Millettiae dielsianae	Gai Yut Tang	Keiketto	Millettia root and stem
Ji Xue Teng Jiao	***Spatholobus suberectus***	Gelatinum Spatholobi	Gai Yut Tang Gaau		Spatholobus gel
Ji Xue Teng, Chang Chun You Ma Teng	***Mucuna birdwoodiana, M. sempervirens***	Radix et caulis Mucunae	Gei Hat Tang, Seung Cheun Yao Ma Tang		Mucuna root and stem
Ji Xue Teng, Kun Ming Ji Xue Teng	***Millettia reticulata***	Radix et caulis Millettiae reticulatae	Kwan Ming Gai Yut Tang		Millettia root and stem
Ji Xue Teng, Mi Hua Dou	***Spatholobus suberectus***	Caulis Spatholobi	Gai Yut Tang, Mat Fa Dau		Spatholobus stem
Ji Zi Huang	***Gallus gallus domesticus***	Vitellus Galli	Gai Ji Wong		Egg yolk
Jian Dao Cao	***Clinopodium confine***	Herba Clinopodii	Jin Dou Chou		Clinopodium herb
Jian Feng Hong	***Anagallis arvensis***	Herba Anagallis	Gin Fung Hung		Scarlet pimpernel herb
Jian Hua, Ba Wang Hua	***Hylocereus undatus***	Flos Hylocerei	Gim Fa		Cereus flower
Jian Lan Gen	***Cymbidium ensifolium***	Radix Cymbidii	Gin Laan Gan		Cymbidium orchid root
Jian Lan Hua	***Cymbidium ensifolium***	Herba et radix Cymbidii	Gin Laan Fa		Cymbidium orchid herb and root
Jian Lan Ye	***Cymbidium ensifolium***	Folium Cymbidii	Gin Laan Yip		Cymbidium orchid leaf

MANDARIN	SCIENTIFIC	PHARMACEUTICAL	CANTONESE	JAPANESE	ENGLISH
Jiang Can	***Bombyx mori*** **infected with** ***Beauveria bassiana***	Bombyx beauveriatus	Geung Chaam		Silkworm larva
Jiang Huang	***Curcuma longa. C. aromatica***	Rhizoma Curcumae	Geung Wong	Kyoo	Turmeric root
Jiang Lan Chong	***Catharsius molossus, Xylotrupes dichotomus***	Catharsius seu Xylotrupes	Jeung Long Chung		Dung beetle
Jiang Nan Juan Bai	***Selaginella moellendorfii***	Herba Selaginella moellendorfii	Gong Naam Kyun Paap		Moellendorf's spikemoss herb
Jiang Xiang	***Dalbergia odorifera***	Lignum Dalbergiae odoriferae	Geung Heung		Asian rosewood
Jiang Yong	***Bombyx mori artificially*** **infected with** ***Beauveria bassiana***	Bombyx beauveriatus	Geung Yung		Silkworm larva
Jiao Gu Lan	***Gynostemma pentaphyllum***	Herba Gynostemmae	Gaan Gu Laam		Gynostemma herb
Jiao Zhu Tao Ye	***Nerium indicum***	Folium Nerii	Gap Juk Tou Yip		Indian oleander leaf
Jie Chang Pu	***Acorus tatarinowii***	Rhizoma Acori tatarinowii	Jik Cheung Pou		Tatarinow's sweetflag root
Jie Geng, Ku Jie Geng	***Platycodon grandiflorum***	Radix Platycodonis	Gat Gan	Kikyo	Balloonflower root
Jie Gu Xian Tao	***Veronica peregrina***	Herba et radix Veronicae	Jip Gwat Sin Tou		Peregrine speedwell herb and root
Jie Xiang Hua, Meng Hua	***Edgeworthiae chrysantha***	Flos Edgeworthiae chrysanthae	Git Heung Fa, Mung Fa		Oriental paperbush flower
Jin Bian Long She Lan	***Agave americana***	Folium Agavis americanae	Gam Bin Lung Sit Laan		Agave leaf
Jin Bo	***Aurum***	Folium Auri	Gam Bok		Gold foil
Jin Bu Huan	***Lycopodium serratum*** **and** ***varieties***	Herba Lycopodii serrati	Gam Bat Wun		Serrated clubmoss
Jin Bu Huan	***Stephania sinica***	Caulis Stephaniae sinicae	Gam Bat Wun		Chinese stephania stem
Jin Di Luo	***Drosera burmanni***	Herba Droserae	Gam Dei Lo		Sundew herb
Jin Fei Cao	***Inula japonica, I. brittanica, I. linariaefolia***	Herba Inulae	Gam Fai Chou	Kinfutsuso	Elecampane herb
Jin Gang Teng, Ba Qi	***Smilax china***	Rhizoma Smilacis chinensis	Gam Gong Tang, Bat Kai		Chinese greenbrier root, China root
Jin Guo Lan	***Tinospora sagittata, T. capillipes***	Radix Tinosporae	Gam Gwo Laam	Kinkaran	Tinospora root
Jin Ji Er	***Caragana sinica, C., microphylla*** **and spp**	Radix Caraganae	Gam Jik Yi		Caragana root
Jin Ji Le, Jin Ji Na Pi	***Cinchona succiruba*** **and spp**	Cortex Cinchonae	Gam Gai Laak		Cinchona bark
Jin Meng Shi	***Chloris***	Chloris	Gam Mein Sek		Mica schist
Jin Meng Shi	***Phlogopitum***	Phlogopitum	Gam Mung Sek		Phlogopite, Red mica

MANDARIN	SCIENTIFIC	PHARMACEUTICAL	CANTONESE	JAPANESE	ENGLISH
Jin Qian Cao, Guo Lu Huang	***Lysimachia christinae, L. hemsleyana***	Herba Lysimachiae	Gam Chin Chou, Gwo Lou Wong	Kinsenso	Asian moneywort herb
Jin Qiao Mai Gen	***Fagopyrum cymosum***	Rhizoma Fagopyri	Gam Kiu Mak Gan		Buckwheat root
Jin Que Hua	***Caragana sinica*** **and spp**	Flos Caraganae	Gam Jeuk Fa		Caragana flower
Jin Si Tao	***Hypericum chinense***	Herba Hyperici Chinensis			Chinese St. John's wort herb
Jin Xie	***Eriocheir sinensis, E. japonicus***	Eriocheir	Jeun Haai	Zukani	Tianjin crab
Jin Yin Hua, Ren Dong Hua	***Lonicera japonica***	Flos Lonicerae japonicae	Gam Ngan Fa Yan Dung Fa	Kinginka	Japanese honeysuckle flower
Jin Yin Teng, Ren Dong Teng	***Lonicera japonica***	Ramus et folium Lonicerae japonicae	Gam Ngan Tang, Yan Dung Tang		Japanese honeysuckle stem and leaf
Jin Ying Zi	***Rosa laevigata***	Fructus Rosae laevigatae	Gam Ying Ji	Kinoshi	Cherokee rosehip
Jing Da Ji	***Euphorbia pekinensis***	Radix Euphorbiae pekinensis	Ging Daai Gik	Taigeki	Peking spurge root
Jing Jie	***Schizonepeta tenuifolia***	Herba Schizonepetae	Ging Gaai	Keigai	Japanese catnip herb
Jing Mi	***Oryza sativa***	Fructus Oryzae	Gang Mai		Rice grain
Jing Tian (San Qi)	***Sedum erythrostictum***	Herba Sedi erythrosticti	Ging Tin		Red stonecrop herb
Jing Tian Hua	***Sedum erythrosticum***	Flos Sedi erythrostici	Ging Ting Fa		Red stonecrop flower
Jing Tian San Qi	***Sedum aizoon***	Herba Sedi aizoonis	Ging Tin Saam Chat		Aizoon stonecrop herb
Jiu Bi Ying	***Ilex rotunda***	Folium Ilicis rotundis	Gau Bit Ying		Round-leaf holly leaf
Jiu Cai Zi	***Allium tuberosum***	Semen Alii tuberosi	Gau Choi Ji	Kyushi	Asian leek seed
Jiu Ceng Ta, Luo Le	***Ocimum basilicum***	Herba Ocimi	Lo Lak		Basil herb
Jiu Jie Chang Pu	***Anemone altaica***	Rhizoma Anemoni altaicae	Gau Jit Cheung Pou	Arutai ginrenkon	Altai anemone root
Jiu Jie Feng	***Sarcandra glabra***	Herba Sarcandrae	Gau Jit Fung		Smooth sarcandra herb
Jiu Li Xiang	***Murraya paniculata***	Ramulus et folium Murrayae	Gau Lei Heung		Burma boxwood twig and leaf
Jiu Long Teng, Wu Teng	***Bauhinia championi***	Caulis bauhiniae championi	Gaau Lung Tang, Lung Sou Tang		Bauhinia stem
Jiu Xiang Chong	***Aspongopus***	Aspongopus	Gau Heung Chung		Stinkbug
Ju He	***Citrus reticulata, C. tangerina, C. erythrosa***	Semen Citri reticulatae	Gwat Hat		Tangerine seed
Ju Hong (Pi), Hua Ju Pi	***Citrus grandis*** **and spp**	Exocarpium rubrum Citri	Gwat Heung (Pei), Fa Gwat Pei		Red citrus outer rind
Ju Hong Hua	***Citrus grandis*** **and spp**	Flos Citri grandi	Gwat Heung Fa		Citrus flower
Ju Hong Zhu	***Citrus grandis*** **and spp.**	Fructus Citri grandi immaturi	Gwat Heung		Unripe citrus fruit

MANDARIN	SCIENTIFIC	PHARMACEUTICAL	CANTONESE	JAPANESE	ENGLISH
Ju Hua, Gan Ju Hua	***Chrysanthemum* x *morifolium***	Flos Chrysanthemi	Guk Fa		Chrysanthe-mum flower
Ju Jiang Ye, Qing Lou Ye	***Piper betle***	Folium Piperis betlis	Geui Jeung Yip		Betel pepper leaf
Ju Luo, Ju Bai	***Citrus* spp**	Fasciculus vascularis Citri, Endocarpium Citri	Gwat Lok		Citrus fibre
Ju Pi, Chen Pi	***Citrus reticulata, C. tangerina, C. erythrosa***	Pericarpium Citri reticulatae	Chan Pei, Gwat Pei	Chimpi	Ripe tangerine rind
Ju Ruo	***Amorphophallus rivieri, A. sinensis, A. knojac***	Rhizoma Amorphophalli	Geui Yeuk		Amorpho-phallus root
Ju Sheng Zi	***Dipsacus chinensis* and spp**	Fructus Dipsaci	Geui Sing Ji		Chinese teasel fruit
Ju Ye	***Citrus* spp.**	Folium Aurantium	Gwat Yip		Citrus leaf
Juan Bai	***Selaginella tamariscina***	Herba Selaginellae tamariscinae	Kyun Paap		Resurrection plant herb
Jue Chuang	***Rostellulariae procumbens***	Herba Rostellulariae	Jeuk Chong		Creeping rostellularia herb
Jue Chuang Cao, Shu Wei Huang	***Justicia procumbens***	Herba Justiciae	Jeuk Chong, Syu Mei Wong		Justicia herb
Jue Ming Zi, Cao Jue Ming	***Cassia tora, C. obtusifolia* and spp**	Semen Cassiae torae	Kyut Ming Ji, Chou Kyut Ming	Ketsumeishi	Sickle senna seed
Kai Jin Suo	***Polygonum cymosum***	Radix et rhizoma Polygoni cymosi	Hoi Gam So		Cymose knotweed Root
Kong Xiu Lian Zi Cao	***Alternanthera philoxeroides***	Herba Alternantherae	Hung Sam Lin Ji Chou		Alligator Alternanthera herb
Kou She Cao	***Senecio kirilowii***	Herba Senecionis kirilowii	Gau Sit Chou		Kirilow's ragwort herb
Ku (Shu) Mu	***Picrasma quassioides***	Ramulus et folium Picrasmae	Fu (Syu) Muk		Quassiawood twig and leaf
Ku Cai	***Sonchus oleraceus***	Herba Sonchi	Fu Choi		Annual sowthistle herb
Ku Ding Cha	***Ilex latifolia***	Folium Ilicis latifoliae	Fu Ding Cha		Broadleaf holly leaf
Ku Fan	***Alumen***	Alumen praeparatum	Gu Faan		Prepared alum
Ku Gua (Gan)	***Momordica charantia***	Fructus Momordicae charantiae	Fu Gwa (Gam)		Bitter melon fruit
Ku Lian (Gen) Pi	***Melia azedarach, M. toosendan***	Cortex radicis Meliae	Fu Lin (Gan) Pei	Kurenkombi	Bead tree root bark
Ku Qie	***Solanum dulcamara***	Caulis Solani dulcamari	Fu Ke		Bittersweet stem
Ku Shen	***Sophora flavescens***	Radix Sophorae flavescentis	Fu Sam		Yellow pagoda tree root
Ku Shen Zi	***Sophora flavescens***	Fructus Sophorae flavescentis	Fu Sam Ji		Yellow pagoda tree berry
Ku Shi Lian (Zi)	***Caesalpinia minax***	Semen Caesalpiniae minacis	Fu Sek Lin (Ji)		Caesalpinia seed
Ku Shu Pi	***Picrasma quassioides***	Cortex Picrassiae	Fu Syu Pei		Quassiawood bark

MANDARIN	SCIENTIFIC	PHARMACEUTICAL	CANTONESE	JAPANESE	ENGLISH
Ku Zhu Ye	***Pleioblastus amarus***	Folium Pleioblasti	Fu Juk Yip		Bitter bamboo leaf
Kuan Dong Hua	***Tussilago farfara***	Flos Tussilaginis	Fun Dung Fa	Kantoka	Coltsfoot flower
Kuan Jin Teng	***Cissus pteroclada***	Caulis Cissi	Gwan Gam Tang		Cissus stem
Kuan Jin Teng	***Tinospora sinensis***	Caulis Tinosporae sinensis	Gwan Gam Tang	Kankinto	Chinese tinospora stem
Kui Shu Zi	***Livistona chinensis***	Semen Livistonae	Kwai Sat Ji		Fan palm seed
Kun Bu	***Laminaria japonica*** and spp	Thallus Laminariae	Gwan Bou	Kombu	Kelp seaweed
Kun Ming Shan Hai Tang, Diao Mao Cao	***Tripterygium hypoglaucum***	Radix Tripterygii hypoglauci decorticati	Kwan Ming Saan Hoi Tong		Peeled Tripterygium root
Kuo Tang She	***Jussiaea repens***	Herba Jussiaeae	Gwo Tong Se		Clove strip herb
La Liao Cao	***Polygonum lapathifolium***	Herba Polygoni lapathifolii	La Lou Chou		Knotweed herb
La Mei Hua	***Chimonanthus praecox***	Flos Chimonanthi	Laap Mui Fa	Sakubaika	Wintersweet flower
Lai Fu Zi	***Raphanus sativus***	Semen Raphani	Loi Fuk Ji		Radish seed
Lan Shi	***Polygonum tinctorium***	Herba Polygoni tinctorii	Laam Sat		Chinese indigo herb
Lang Du, Da Lang Du	***Euphorbia nematocypha***	Radix Euphorbiae nematocyphae	Long Duk, Daai Long Duk		Gigantic spurge root
Lang Du, Ji Chang Lang Du	***Euphorbia prolifera***	Radix Euphorbiae proliferae	Long Duk, Gai Cheung Long Duk		Prolific spurge root
Lang Du, Lang Du Da Ji	***Euphorbia fischeriana***	Radix Euphorbiae fischerianae	Long Duk, Long Duk Daai Gik		Fischer's spurge root
Lang Du, Yue Xian Da Ji	***Euphorbia ebracteolata***	Radix Euphorbiae ebracteolatae	Long Duk, Yu Sin Daai Gik		Bractless spurge root
Lang Yu Pi	***Ulmus parvifolia***	Cortex Ulmi parvifoliae	Long Yu Pei		Chinese elm bark
Lao Bai Hua Pi	***Bauhinia variegata***	Cortex Bauhiniae variegatae	Lou Baak Fa Pei		Orchid tree bark
Lao Gong Xu, Rong Shu Xu	***Ficus microcarpa, F. retusa***	Radix Fici microcarpae seu retusae	Lou Gung Chuk		Aerial fig root
Lao Guan Cao	***Erodium stephaniarum, Geranium*** spp	Herba Erodii seu Geranii	Lou Gwun Chou		Storksbill or cranesbill herb
Lao He Cao	***Geranium wilfordii, G. thunbergii***	Herba Geranii	Lou Hap Chou	Gennoshio-uko	Geranium herb
Lao Shu Le	***Acanthus ilicifolius***	Radix Acanthi ilicifolii	Lou Syu Laak		Holly-leaf acanthus root
Lei Gong Teng	***Tripterygium wilfordii***	Medulla radicis Tripterygii	Leui Gung Tang		Yellow vine root pith
Lei Wan	***Mylitta lapidescens***	Sclerotium Mylittae	Leui Yun		Thunder ball fungus
Li Gen Bai Pi	***Prunus salicina***	Cortex radicis Pruni salicinae	Lei Gan Baak Pei		Willow plum root bark
Li Lu	***Hemerocallis thunbergii***	Rhizoma et radix Hemerocallis thunbergii	Lai Lou		Day lily root
Li Lu	***Veratrum nigrum*** and spp	Radix et rhizoma Veratri	Lai Lou	Riro	False hellebore root
Li Pi	***Pyrus betulaefolia***	Pericarpium Pyri	Lei Pei		Chinese pear rind

MANDARIN	SCIENTIFIC	PHARMACEUTICAL	CANTONESE	JAPANESE	ENGLISH
Li Tou Cao	***Viola japonica***	Radix et herba Violae japonicae	Lai Tau Chou		Japanese violet root and herb
Li Tou Jian	***Typhonium divaricatum***	Rhizoma Typhonii divaricatii	Lai Tau Jim		Divaricate typhonium root
Li Yu	***Cyprinus carpio***	Cyprinus	Lei Yu		Carp
Li Zhi Cao	***Salvia plebeia***	Herba et radix Salviae plebeiae	Lai Jik Chou		Plebeian sage herb and root
Li Zhi He	***Litchi chinensis***	Semen Litchis	Lai Ji Ho		Lychee seed
Li Zhi Ke	***Litchi chinensis***	Pericarpium Litchis	Lai Ji Hok		Lychee rind
Li Zi, Feng Li Gu	***Castanea mollissima***	Fructus Castaneae	Leut Ji	Furitsukaku	Chinese chestnut
Lian Fang	***Nelumbo nucifera***	Receptaculum Nelumbinis	Lin Fong	Renshin	Lotus receptacle
Lian Geng	***Nelumbo nucifera***	Ramulus Nelumbinis	Lin Gang		Lotus stem
Lian Qian Cao	***Glechoma hederacea, G. longituba***	Herba Glechomae	Ling Chin Chou		Ground ivy herb
Lian Qiao	***Forsythia suspensa***	Fructus Forsythiae	Lin Kiu	Rengyo	Forsythia valve
Lian Xin	***Nelumbo nucifera***	Plumula Nelumbinis	Lin Sam		Lotus plumule
Lian Xu	***Nelumbo nucifera***	Stamen Nelumbinis	Lin Sou	Renshu	Lotus stamen
Lian Zi	***Nelumbo nucifera***	Semen Nelumbinis	Lin Ji	Renshi	Lotus seed
Lian Zi Xin	***Nelumbo nucifera***	Epicentrum seminis Nelumbinis	Lin Ji Sam		Lotus seed heart
Liang Tou Jian	***Anemone raddeana***	Rhizoma Anemonis raddeanae	Leung Tau Jim		Anemone root
Liao Ge Wang (Gen)	***Wickstroemia indica***	Radix Wickstroemiae	Liu Go Wong	Ryokao	Wikstroemia root
Liao Shi	***Polygonum hydropiper***	Fructus Polygoni hydropiperis	Lou Sek		Water pepper fruit
Lie Dang	***Orobanche caerulescens*** **and spp**	Herba Orobanchis	Lit Dong		Orobanche herb
Ling Ling Xiang	***Lysimachia sikokiana***	Herba Lysimachiae sikokianae	Ling Ling Heung		Lysimachia herb
Ling Qiao	***Trapa bispinosa, T. bicornis***	Fructus Trapae	Ling Gok		Water caltrop fruit
Ling Xiao Gen	***Campsis grandiflora***	Radix Campsis grandiflorae	Ling Siu Gan	Ryoshoka	Asian trumpetcree-per root
Ling Xiao Hua	***Campsis grandiflora***	Flos Campsis grandiflorae	Ling Siu Fa		Asian trumpetcreep-er flower
Ling Xiao Hua, Mei Jou Ling Xiao	***Campsis radicans***	Flos Campsis radicantis	Ling Siu Fa, Mei Jau Ling Siu		Common trumpetcreep-er flower
Ling Yang Jiao	***Saiga tatarica***	Cornu Saigae	Ling Yeung Gok	Reiyokaku	Antelope horn
Ling Zhi (Cao)	***Ganoderma lucidum, G. sinen-se, G applanatum*** **and spp**	Sclerotium Ganodermae	Ling Ji (Chou)	Reishi	Reishi mushroom
Liu Huang, Shi Liu Huang	***Sulphurum***	Sulphurum	Lau Wong, Sek Lau Wong	Io	Sulphur
Liu Ji Niu	***Artemisia anomala***	Herba Artemisiae anomalae	Lau Gei Nou	Ryukido	Anomalous wormwood herb

MANDARIN	SCIENTIFIC	PHARMACEUTICAL	CANTONESE	JAPANESE	ENGLISH
Liu Shen Hua	***Spilanthes acmella*** var. ***oleracea***	Flos Spilanthis	Lau Sam Fa		Six god flower
Liu Ye	***Salix babylonica, S. gracilistyla***	Folium Salicis	Lau Yip		Weeping willow twig
Liu Zhi	***Salix babylonica, S. gracilistyla***	Ramulus Salicis	Lau Ji		Weeping willow twig
Long Chi	***Stegodon orientalis et al.***	Dens Stegodontis	Lung Ji		Dragon tooth
Long Chuan Hua Gen	***Ixora chinensis***	Radox Ixorae	Lung Syun Fa Gan		Ixora root
Long Dan Cao	***Gentiana scabra, G. triflora, G. manshurica***	Radix Gentianae scabrae	Lung Daam Chou	Ryutan	Scabrous gentian root
Long Gu	***Stegodon orientalis, S. rhinocerus sinensis, Hipparion***	Os Stegodontis	Lung Gwat	Ryukotsu	Dragon bone
Long Kui	***Solanum nigrum***	Herba Solani nigri	Lung Kwai		Winter cherry herb
Long Li Ye	***Sauropus rostratus, S. changianus***	Folium Sauropi	Lung Lei Yip		Lizardtail leaf
Long Shi Huang	***Desmodium pseudotriquetrum D. triquetrum***	Herba Desmodii pseudotriquetrii	Lung Sek Wong		Bottlegourd herb
Long Yan Gu	***Fomes applanatus*** **and *host fruit Euphoria longana***	Sclerotium Fomis	Lung Ngan Gu		Longan fungus
Long Yan He	***Euphoria longan***	Semen Euphoriae	Lung Ngaan Ho		Longan seed
Long Yan Hua	***Euphoria longan***	Flos Euphoriae	Lung Ngaan Fa		Longan flower
Long Yan Rou	***Euphoria longan***	Arillus Euphoriae	Lung Ngaan Yuk	Ryuganniku	Longan fruit pulp
Lou Lu	***Echinops latifolius, E. gmelinii***	Radix Echinopsis	Lau Lou		Globe thistle root
Lou Lu	***Rhaponticum uniflorum***	Radix Rhapontici	Lau Lou	Roro	Swiss centaury root
Lu Cao	***Humulus scandens***	Herba Humuli scandentis	Leut Chou		Climbing hops flower
Lu Dou	***Phaseolus radiatum***	Semen Phaseoli radiati	Luk Dau	Ryokuzu	Mung bean
Lu Dou Hua	***Phaseolus mungo***	Flos Phaseoli	Luk Dau Fa		Mung bean flower
Lu Dou Yi	***Phaseolus radiatum***	Testa Phaseoli radiatae	Luk Dau Yip		Mung bean husk
Lu Er Mei, Lu Mei Hua	***Prunus mume***	Flos Pruni mumis	Lat Mui Fa		Black plum flower
Lu Feng Fang	***Polistes mandarinus, Parapolybia varia***	Nidus Polistis seu Parapolybiae	Lou Fun Fong		Hornet nest
Lu Gan Shi	***Calamina, Smithsonitum***	Calamina, Smithsonitum	Lou Gam Sek	Rokanseki	Calamine
Lu Gen	***Phragmites communis***	Radix Phragmitis	Lou Gan	Rokon	Water-reed root
Lu Gu Dan	***Rubia cordifolia***	Caulis Rubiae cordifoliae	Lu Gwat Daan		Heart-leaf madder stem
Lu Hui	***Aloe vera*** var. ***chinensis***	Resina Aloidis	Lou Wui		Aloe resin

MANDARIN	SCIENTIFIC	PHARMACEUTICAL	CANTONESE	JAPANESE	ENGLISH
Lu Ji Wei	***Microsorium bancockii, M. dilatatum***	Herba Microsorii	Luk Gai Mei		Microsorium herb
Lu Jiao	***Cervus nippon*** **and spp**	Cornu Cervi	Luk Gok	Rokkaku	Mature deer antler
Lu Jiao Jiao	***Cervus nippon*** **and spp**	Colla cornu Cervi	Luk Gok Gaau	Rokkakukyo	Mature deer antler glue
Lu Jiao Shuang, Rong Mo	***Cervus nippon*** **and spp**	Cornu Cervi degelatinatum	Luk Gok Shuen	Rokkakuso	Mature deer antler powder
Lu Lu Tong	***Liquidambar taiwaniana***	Fructus Liquidambaris	Lou Lou Tung	Rorotsu	Taiwan maple fruit
Lu Rong, Rong Tou, Nen Lu Rong	***Cervus nippon*** **and spp**	Cornu cervi parvum	Luk Yan	Rokujo	Velvet deer antler
Lu Wei Ba	***Cervus nippon*** **and spp**	Cauda Cervi	Luk Mei Ba		Mature deer tail
Lu Xian Cao, Lu Ti Cao	***Pyrola rotundifolia subsp. chinensis, P. Japonica***	Radix et herba Pyrolae	Luk Haam Chou, Luk Tai Chou	Rokuteiso	Asian wintergreen root and herb
Lu Yi Zhi Qiao, Gou Yuan	***Poncirus trifoliata***	Fructus Ponciri immaturi	Luk Ji Ji Hok, Gau Yun		Immature trifoliate orange fruit
Lu Ying	***Sambucus japonicus***	Cortex Sambuci japonici		Rakutokuda	Japanese elder bark
Luo Bo Gen	***Raphanus sativus***	Radix Raphani recentis	Lo Ba Gan		Fresh radish root
Luo Bo Ye	***Raphanus sativus***	Folium Raphani	Lo Ba Yip		Radish leaf
Luo Bu Ma	***Apocynum lancifolium, A. venetum, A. hendersonii***	Radix et herba Apocyni	Lo Bou Ma		Dogbane root and herb
Luo Fu Mu	***Rauvolfia verticillata, R. yunnanensis, R. latifrons, R. serpentina*** **and spp**	Radix Rauvolfiae	Lo Fu Mou		Rauvolfia root
Luo Han Guo	***Momordica grosvenori***	Fructus Momordicae grosvenorii	Lou Haan Kwo	Rakanka	Arhat fruit
Luo Han Ye	***Momordica grosvenori***	Folium Momordicae grosvenorii	Lou Haan Yip	Rakankayo	Arhat leaf
Luo Shi Teng	***Trachelospermum jasminoides***	Caulis Trachelospermi	Lok Sek Tang	Chikusekito	Star jasmine stem
Luo Xin Fu	***Astilbe chinensis***	Rhizoma Astilbis	Lok San Fu		Astilbe root
Ma Bao	***Equus caballos***	Calculus Equi	Ma Bou		Horse bezoar
Ma Bian Cao	***Verbena officinalis***	Herba Verbenae	Ma Bin Chou		Vervain herb
Ma Bin Lang	***Capparis masaikai***	Semen Capparis	Ma Ban Long	Kuttokei	Capparis berry
Ma Bo	***Lasiosphaera fenslii*** **and spp, *Calvatia lilacina, C. fenzlii, C. gigantea***	Sclerotium Lasiosphaerae seu Calvatiae	Ma But	Babotsu	Puffball mushroom
Ma Chi Xian	***Portulacca oleracea***	Herba Portulaccae	Ma Chi Yin	Bashiken	Purslane herb
Ma Di Jin	***Dichondra repens***	Herba Dichondrae	Ma Dei Jing	Kinsenso	Dichondra herb

MANDARIN	SCIENTIFIC	PHARMACEUTICAL	CANTONESE	JAPANESE	ENGLISH
Ma Dou Ling	***Aristolochia contorta, A. debilis***	Fructus Aristolochiae	Ma Dau Ling	Batorei	Green birthwort capsule
Ma Huang	***Ephedra sinica***	Herba Ephedrae	Ma Wong	Mao	Ephedra stem
Ma Huang Gen	***Ephedra sinica***	Radix Ephedrae	Ma Wong Gan	Maokon	Ephedra root
Ma Lan	***Aster indicus* and spp**	Herba Asteris indici	Ma Laan		Indian aster herb
Ma Lan Gen	***Baphicacanthus cusia***	Radix Baphicacanthi	Ma Laam Gan	Banrankon	Assam indigo root
Ma Lan Gen	***Strobilanthes flaccidifolius***	Radix Strobilanthis	Ma Laam Gan		Strobilanthes root
Ma Lan Jin, Peng Qi Ju	***Wedelia chinensis***	Herba Wedeliae	Paang Kei Guk		Wedelia herb
Ma Lan Ye	***Baphicacanthus cusia***	Folium Baphicacanthi	Ma Laam Yip	Banranyo	Assam indigo leaf
Ma Lin Zi	***Iris pallasii* var. *chinensis***	Semen Iris pallasii	Ma Leun Ji		North China iris seed
Ma Ming Dui	***Bombyx mori***	Periostracum Bombycis	Ma Ming Teui		Silkworm slough
Ma Nao	***Agate***	Agate			Agate
Ma Qian Zi	***Strychnos pierrana, S. nux-vomica* and spp**	Semen Strychnotis preparatae	Ma Chin Ji	Basenshi	Vomit nut
Ma Sang Ye	***Coriaria sinica***	Folium Coriariae	Ma Song Yip		Coriaria leaf
Ma Zhi Hu, Feng Qi Cao	***Adenostemma lavenia***	Herba Adenostemmae	Ma Ji Wu, Fung Hei Chou		Adenostemma herb
Mai (Men) Dong	***Ophiopogon japonicus***	Radix Ophiopogonis	Mak (Mun) Dung	Bakumondo	Dwarf lilyturf root
Mai (Men) Dong, Hu Bei Mai Men Dong	***Liriope spicata***	Radix Liriopis spicatae	Mak (Mun) Dung, Wu Ba Mak Dung		Lance-leaf liriope root
Mai Men Dong	***Liriope platyphylla***	Radix Liriopis platyphyllae	Mak (Mun) Dung		Broad-leaf liriope root
Mai Ya	***Hordeum vulgare***	Fructus germinatus Hordei	San Man Nga	Bakuga	Sprouted barley grain
Man Jing Zi	***Vitex rotundifolia, V. trifolia***	Fructus Viticis rotundifoliae	Maan Ging Ji	Mankeishi	Seashore chastetree berry
Man Shan Hong	***Rhododendron dauricum, R. mariesii***	Folium Rhododendri daurici	Mun Saan Hung		Daurian rhododendron leaf
Man Shan Xiang	***Lysimachia capillipes***	Rhizoma seu herba Lysimachiae capillipis	Mun Sam Heung		Lysimachia root or herb
Man Tian Xing	***Pavetta hongkongiensis***	Herba Pavettae	Mun Tin Sing, Daai Sa Yip		Pavetta herb
Mang Guo Zi	***Mangifera indica***	Semen Mangiferae	Man Gou Wat		Mango seed
Mang Jing	***Miscanthus sinensis***	Herba Miscanthi	Mong Hong		Miscanthus herb
Mang Xiao	***Mirabilitum***	Mirabilitum	Mong Seu	Bosho	Mirabilite
Mao Dong Qing	***Ilex pubescens***	Radix Ilicis pubescentis	Mou Dung Ching	Motosei	Furry holly root
Mao Gen	***Ranunculus japonicus***	Radix et herba Ranunculi japonicae	Maau Gan		Japanese buttercup root and herb
Mao Gu Xiao	***Sambucus formosana/taiwaniana***	Caulis et folium Sambuci formosanae	Mon Gwat Siu		Taiwan elder stem and leaf
Mao Mei, Hao Tian Biao	***Rubus parvifolius***	Folium Rubi parvifolii	Mau Mui		Small-leaf raspberry leaf
Mao She Xiang	***Adenosma glutinosum***	Herba Adenosmae glutinosi	Mou Se Heung		Adenosma herb

MANDARIN	SCIENTIFIC	PHARMACEUTICAL	CANTONESE	JAPANESE	ENGLISH
Mao Xu Cao	***Clerodendranthus spicatus***	Herba Clerodendranthi	Maau Sao Chou		Orthosiphon herb
Mao Xu Kao, Hua Shi Cao	***Orthosiphon aristatus, O. grandiflorus***	Herba Orthosiphonis	Maau Sou Chou, Fa Sek Chou		Orthosiphon herb
Mao Zhao Cao, Mao Zhua Cao	***Ranunculus ternatus***	Radix Ranunculi	Maau Jau Chou		Ternate buttercup root
Mei Gui Hua	***Rosa rugosa***	Flos Rosae rugosae	Mui Gwai Fa	Maikaika	Japanese rose flower
Mei Gui Zi	***Rosa rugosa***	Fructus Rosae rugosae	Mui Gwai Ji		Japanese rosehip
Mei Ren Jiao (Gen)	***Canna indica***	Rhizoma Cannae	Mei Yan Jiu (Gan)	Dandoku	Canna lily root
Mei Ye Wei Ling Cai	***Potentilla fragarioides***	Radix Potentillae fragarioidis	Mui Yip Wai Ling Choi		Strawberry-leaf cinquefoil root
Meng Chong	***Tabanus bivittatus***	Tabanus	Mung Chung		Gadfly
Meng Shi, Jin Meng Shi	***Mica, Chloritum***	Mica, Chloritum	Mung Sek, Ching Mung Sek		Mica, Chlorite schist
Mi Die Xiang	***Rosmarinus officinalis***	Herba Rosmarini	Mai Dit Heung		Rosemary herb
Mi Hou Tao, Teng Li	***Actinidia chinensis***	Fructus Actinidiae chinensis	Nei Hau Tou		Kiwi fruit
Mi Huan Jun	***Armillaria mellea***	Sclerotium Armillariae			Honey mushroom
Mi Meng Hua	***Buddleia officinalis***	Flos Buddleiae	Mat Mung Fa	Mitsumoka	Buddleia flower and bud
Mi Tuo Seng	***Lithargyrum***	Lithagyrum	Muk Toi Sang	Mitsudaso	Litharge
Mi Zao	***Zizyphus jujuba* var. *inermis***	Fructus Zizyphi jujubae praeparatae	Mat Jou		Honey-preserved jujube berry
Mian Hua Gen	***Gossypium hirsutum, G. herbaceum***	Cortex radicis Gossypii	Min Fa Gan		Cotton root bark
Mian Hua Zi	***Gossypium hirsutum, G. herbaceum***	Semen Gossypii	Min Fa Ji		Cotton seed
Mian Zao Ren	***Zizyphus mauritiana***	Semen Zizyphi mauritianae	Mai Jou Yan		Mauritius jujube seed
Ming Dang Shen	***Changium smyrnioides***	Radix Changii	Ming Dong Sam	Mintojin	Bright changium root
Ming Fan	***Alumen***	Alumen	Ming Faan	Myoban	Alum
Mo Han Lian, Han Lian Cao	***Eclipta prostata, E. alba***	Herba Ecliptae	Hon Lin Chou	Kanrenso	Field lotus herb
Mo Li Gen	***Jasminum sambac***	Radix Jasmini sambacis	Mut Lei Gan		Jasmine sambac root
Mo Li Hua	***Jasminum sambac***	Flos Jasmini sambacis	Mut Lei Fa		Jasmine sambac flower
Mo Pan Cao, Mi Lan Cao	***Abutilon indicum***	Herba Abutilonis indici	Mo Bun Chou		Country mallow herb
Mo Shi Zi	***Quercus infectoria***	Galla Querci	Mut Sik Ji		Oak gall
Mo Yao	***Commiphora myrrha***	Resina Commiphorae	Mut Yeuk	Motsuyaku	Myrrh resin
Mu Bie Zi	***Momordica cochinchinensis***	Semen Momordicae cochinchinensis	Muk Bit Ji	Mokubesshi	Cochin bitter melon seed
Mu Dan Pi, Dan Pi	***Paeonia suffruticosa***	Cortex radicis Paeoniae suffruticosae	Maau Daan Pei, Daan Pei	Botanpi	Tree peony root bark

MANDARIN	SCIENTIFIC	PHARMACEUTICAL	CANTONESE	JAPANESE	ENGLISH
Mu Dou Hui	*Ixeris denticulata*	Herba Ixeris	Mou Tau Wui		Ixeris herb
Mu Dou Zi	*Cajanus cajan*	Semen Cajani	Muk Dau Ji		Pigeon pea seed
Mu Er	*Auricularia auricula*	Sclerotium Auriculariae	Muk Yi	Kikurage	Wood ear mushroom
Mu Fang Ji	*Cocculus trilobus*	Radix Cocculi	Muk Fong Gei		Three-leaf cocculus root
Mu Gua, Chuan Mu Gua	*Chaenomeles lagenaria*	Fructus Chaenomelis lagenariae	Muk Gwa, Chyun Muk Gwa	Mokka	Chinese quince fruit
Mu Gua, Ming Za	*Chaenomeles sinensis*	Fructus Chaenomelis sinensis	Muk Gwa		Chinese quince fruit
Mu Gua, Tie Geng Hai Tang	*Chaenomeles speciosa*	Fructus Chaenomelis speciosae	Muk Gwa, Tip Gang Hoi Teng		Flowering quince fruit
Mu Hu Die	*Oroxylum indicum*	Semen Oroxyli	Muk Wu Dip	Mokukocho	Oroxylum seed
Mu Jin Hua	*Hibiscus syriacus*	Flos Hibisci syriaci	Mut Gan Fa		Rose of Sharon flower
Mu Jin Pi	*Hibiscus syriacus*	Cortex radicis Hibisci syriacus	Mut Gan Pei		Rose of Sharon root bark
Mu Jing Ye	*Vitex negundo* var. *cannabifolia*	Folium Viticis negundonis	Maau Ging Yip		Five-leaf chastetree leaf
Mu Jing Zi	*Vitex negundo* var. *cannabifolia*	Fructus Viticis negundonis	Maau Ging Ji		Five-leaf chastetree berry
Mu Lan Ye	*Indigofera tinctoria*	Folium Indigoferae	Muuk Laam Yip		Indigo leaf
Mu Li	*Ostrea gigas* and spp	Concha Ostreae	Mou Lai	Borei	Oyster shell
Mu Mian Hua	*Gossampinus malabarica*	Flos Gossampini	Muk Min Fa		Silk cotton tree flower
Mu Tian Lian	*Actinidia polygama*	Galla fructi Actinidiae	Muk Tin Lin	Mokutenryo	Actinidia gall
Mu Tong, Bai Mu Tong	*Akebia quinata, A. trifoliata*	Caulis Akebiae	Baak Muk Tong	Mokutsu	Akebia stem
Mu Xiang, Yun Mu Xiang	*Saussurea lappa*	Radix Saussureae lappae	Muk Heung	Mokko	Wood aromatic root
Mu Zei	*Equisetum hiemale*	Herba Equiseti hiemalis	Muuk Chaak	Mokuzoku	Horsetail herb
Nan Gua Zi	*Cucurbita moschata*	Semen Cucurbitae	Naam Gwa Ji	Nankashi	Red squash seed
Nan He Zao	*Daucus carota*	Fructus Dauci	Naam Hok Sat		Wild carrot seed
Nan Sha Shen	*Adenophora stricta, A. capillaris, A. tetraphylla* and spp	Radix Adenophorae strictae	Naam Sa Sam	Nanshajin	Upright ladybell root
(Nan) Tian Zhu Gen	*Nandina domestica*	Radix et caulis Nandinae	(Naam) Tin Juk Gan		Sacred bamboo root and stem
(Nan) Tian Zhu Ye	*Nandina domestica*	Folium Nandinae	(Naam) Tin Juk Yip		Sacred bamboo leaf
(Nan) Tian Zhu Zi	*Nandina domestica*	Fructus Nandinae	(Naam) Tin Juk Ji		Sacred bamboo fruit
Nan Xing Ren	*Prunus armeniaca* and var.	Semen Pruni armeniacae dulcis	Naam Hang Yan		Sweet apricot kernel
Nan Zhu	*Lyonia ovafolia, L. neziki*	Herba Lyoniae	Naam Juk		Lyonia herb

MANDARIN	SCIENTIFIC	PHARMACEUTICAL	CANTONESE	JAPANESE	ENGLISH
Nao Sha	***Salammonitum* and *Halitum***	Salmiacum	Lou Sa		Salmiac, Sal ammoniac
Nao Yang Hua, Huang Du Juan	***Rhododendron molle***	Flos Rhododendri mollis	Naau Yeung Fa, Wong Dou Gun		Yellow azalea flower
Niao Bu Su, Bai Ma Niao	***Zanthoxylum avicennae***	Radix Zanthoxyli avicennae	Niu Bat Suk		Prickly ash root
Niu Bang Zi	***Arctium lappa***	Fructus Arctii	Ngau Pong Ji	Goboshi	Burdock seed
Niu Da Li	***Millettia philipinensis***	Radix Millettiae philipinensis	Ngao Daai Lik		Millettia root
Niu Dan	***Bos taurus domesticus, Bubalis bubalis***	Vesica fellae Bovis	Ngau Daam	Gyutan	Ox gallbladder
Niu Er Da Huang	***Rumex crispus***	Radix Rumicis crispi	Ngau Yi Daai Wong		Yellow dock root
Niu Huang	***Bos taurus domesticus, Bubalis bubalis***	Calculus Bovis	Ngau Wong	Goo	Ox gallstone
Niu Pi	***Bos taurus domesticus, Bubalis bubalis***	Corium Bovis	Ngau Pei		Ox hide
Niu Xi, Huai Niu Xi	***Achyranthes bidentata***	Radix Achyranthis	Ngau Sat, Wai Ngau Sat	Goshitsu	White oxknee Root
Nu Zhen Zi	***Ligustrum japonicum, L. lucidum***	Fructus Ligustri	Neui Jing Ji	Joteishi	Glossy privet berry
Nuo Dao Gen (Xu)	***Oryza sativa***	Radix Oryzae	No Du Gan	Jubeikon	Sweet rice root
Nuo Mi	***Oryza sativa***	Fructus Oryzae	Lo Mai		Sweet rice
Ou Dang Gui	***Ligusticum levisticum***	Radix Ligustici levistici	Au Dong Gwai		Garden lovage root
Ou Jie	***Nelumbo nucifera***	Rhizoma nodi Nelumbinis	Ngau Jit		Lotus root node
Pa Shan Hu, Di Jin	***Parthenocissus tricuspidata***	Caulis Parthenocissi	Pa San Fu, Dei Gam		Japanese creeper stem
Pan Long Shen	***Spiranthes sinensis***	Herba Spiranthis	Pun Lung Sam		Chinese pearltwist herb
Pang Da Hai	***Sterculia staphigera, S. lychnophera***	Semen Sterculiae	Bun Daai Hoi	Bantaikai	Sterculia seed
Pao Jiang	***Zingiber officinalis***	Rhizoma Zingiberis	Bou Geung	Hokyo	Quick-fried ginger root
Pao Tong Hua	***Paulownia tomentosa***	Flos Paulowniae	Pau Tung Fa		Paulownia flower
Pei Lan	***Eupatorium fortunei***	Herba Eupatorii fortunei	Pui Laan	Haikan	Orchid-grass herb
Peng Lai Cao, Ya She Huang	***Lippia nodiflora***	Herba Lippiae	Fung Loi Chou, Ngaap Sit Wong		Frogfruit herb
Peng Sha	***Borax***	Borax	Pang Sa	Hosha	Borax
Pi Jiu Hua	***Humulus lupulus***	Flos Humuli lupuli	Be Jau Fa		Hops flower
Pi Pa	***Eriobotrya japonica***	Fructus Eriobotryae	Pei Pa		Loquat fruit
Pi Pa Ye	***Eriobotrya japonica***	Folium Eriobotryae	Pei Pa Yip	Biwayo	Loquat leaf
Pi Shi, Xin Shi	***Arsenicum album***	Arsenolitum			White arsenic
Ping	***Marsilea quaddrifolia***	Folium Marsileae	Ping		European water clover leaf
Ping Er Xiao Cao	***Ophioglossum vulgatum***	Herba Ophioglossi	Ping Yi Siu Chou		Adder's tongue herb

MANDARIN	SCIENTIFIC	PHARMACEUTICAL	CANTONESE	JAPANESE	ENGLISH
Ping Peng Cao Gan	***Nuphar japonicum, N. pumilum***	Rhizoma Nupharis	Ping Fung Chou Gan	Senkotu	Yellow pond lily root
Pu Gong Ying	***Taraxacum mongolicum***	Radix et herba Taraxaci	Pou Gung Ying	Hokoei	Mongolian dandelion root and herb
Pu Huang Tan	***Typha latifolia, T. angustifolia*** and spp	Pollen Typhae carbonisatus	Pou Wong Taan		Charred cattail pollen
Pu Huang, Xiang Pu	***Typha latifolia, T. angustifolia*** and spp	Pollen Typhae	Pou Wong, Heung Pou	Hoo	Cattail pollen
Pu Jiang Gen	***Vitex quinata***	Radix Viticis quinatae	Pou Geung Gan		Quinate chasteberry root
Pu Suo	***Quercus dentata, Q. acutissima***	Ramulus et cortex Querci	Pok Sau	Bokuso	Oak twig and bark
Pu Yan Pian	***Rhus chinensis***	Radix Rhudis chinensis	Pou Yim Pin		Chinese sumac root
Qi Cao	***Holotrichia diomphalia***	Holotrichia	Chai Chou		June beetle grub (larva)
Qi Dai	***Homo sapiens***	Funis umbilici Hominis	Chi Daai		Umbilical cord
Qi Feng Teng	***Sabia japonica***	Ramulus Sabiae	Ching Fung Tang		Sabia twig
Qi Gu Cao	***Sagina japonica***	Herba Saginae	Chat Gu Chou		Japanese pearlwort herb
Qi Li Xiang	***Buddleia lindleyana***	Radix Buddleiae lindleyanae	Chat Lei Heung		Buddleia root
Qi Li Xiang	***Pittosporum pentandrum***	Radix Pittospori	Chat Lei Heung		Pittosporum root
Qi Xing Cao	***Polypodium hastatum***	Herba Polypodii	Chat Sing Chou		Polypody herb
Qi Ye Lian	***Schefflera arboricola, S. kwangsiensis, S. venulosa***	Folium et caulis Schefflerae	Chat Yip Lin		Taiwan schefflera leaf and stem
Qi Ye Yi Zhi Hua, Zao Xiu	***Paris polyphylla, P. chinensis, P. formosana*** and var.	Rhizoma Paris	Chak Yip Jek Ji Fa, Sat Yau	Kenjin	Paris root
Qian Cang Ta, Pu Di Wu Gong, Guo Jiang Long, Yu Bai	***Lycopodium serratum*** and spp	Pollen Lycopodii	Jin Jang Tap		Lycopodium pollen
Qian Cao Gen	***Rubia cordifolia***	Radix Rubiae cordifoliae	Sin Chou Gan	Seisokon	Heart-leaf madder root
Qian Cu Cai	***Lythrum salicaria***	Herba Lythri salicariae	Jin Wat Choi		Loosestrife herb
Qian Dan, Huang Dan	***Minium***	Minium	Chin Daan, Wong Daan	Entan	Red lead oxide
Qian Fen	***Cerussa***	Cerussa	Yun Fan		Cerusite
Qian Hu	***Peucedanum praeruptorum, P. decursivum***	Radix Peucedani	Chin Wu	Zenko	Asian masterwort root
Qian Jin Teng	***Stephania japonica***	Caulis Stephaniae japonicae	Chin Gam Tang		Japanese stephania stem
Qian Jin Zi	***Euphorbia lathyris***	Semen Euphorbiae lathyris	Chin Gam Ji	Zokuzuishi	Caper spurge seed
Qian Li Guang	***Senecio scandens***	Herba Senecionis scandens	Chin Lei Gwong		Climbing ragwort herb

MANDARIN	SCIENTIFIC	PHARMACEUTICAL	CANTONESE	JAPANESE	ENGLISH
Qian Nian Jian	***Homalomena occulta***	Rhizoma Homalomenae	Chin Nin Gin	Sennenken	Homalomena root
Qian Niu Zi	***Pharbitis nil, P. purpurea*** **and spp**	Semen Pharbitis	Hin Ngau Ji		Japanese morning glory seed
Qian Ri Hong	***Gomphrena globosa***	Flos Gomphrenae	Jin Yat Hung		Globe amaranth flower
Qian Shi	***Euryale ferox***	Semen Euryalis	Him Sat	Kenjitsu	Foxnut
Qiang Huo	***Notopterygium incisum, N. forbesii, N. francherii***	Rhizoma et radix Notopterigii	Geung Wut	Kyokatsu	Notoptery-gium root
Qiang Wei Gen	***Rosa polyantha*** **and spp**	Radix Rosae polyanthae			Polyanth rose root
Qie Gen	***Solanum melongena***	Radix et rhizoma Solani melongenae	Ke Gan		Eggplant root
Qin Jiao	***Gentiana macrophylla, G. tibetica, G. dahurica*** **and spp**	Radix Gentianae macrophyllae	Cheun Gau	Jingyo	Large-leaf gentian root
Qin Pi	***Fraxinus rhynchophyllae, F. bungeana, F. chinensis*** **and spp**	Cortex Fraxini	Cheun Pei		Korean ash bark
Qing Dai	***Isatis tinctoria*** **and spp,** ***Baphicacanthus cusia, Indigofera suffruticosa, Polygonum tinctorium***	Indigo pulverata levis	Ching Doi		Woad pigment
Qing Fen	***Calomelas***	Calomelas	Ching Fan	Keifun	Calomel
Qing Feng Teng	***Sinomenium acutum***	Radix Sinomenii	Ching Fung Tang		Sinomenium root
Qing Hao	***Artemisia apiacea***	Herba Artemisiae apiaceae	Ching Hou	Seiko	Celery wormwood herb
Qing Ma (Zi)	***Abutilon theophrastii***	Semen Abutili theophrasti	King Ma (Ji)		China jute seed
Qing Meng Shi	***Chloris***	Chloris	Ching Mein Sek		Chlorite schist
Qing Mu Xiang, Ma Dou Ling Gen	***Aristolochia contorta, A. debilis***	Radix Aristolochiae	Ching Muk Heung	Seimokko	Green birthwort root
Qing Pi	***Citrus reticulata, C. tangerina, C. erythrosa***	Pericarpium Citri reticulatae viride	Ching Pei	Johi	Unripe tangerine rind
Qing Tian Kui	***Nervilia fordii***	Herba Nerviliae	Ching Tin Kwai		Nervilia herb
Qing Xiang Zi	***Celosia argentea***	Semen Celosiae argenteae	Ching Seung Ji	Seisoshi	Silver quail-grass seed
Qu Mai	***Dianthus superbus, D. chinensis***	Herba Dianthi	Geui Mak	Kubaku	Proud pink herb
Qu Mai, Shi Zhu	***Dianthus chinensis***	Herba Dianthi chinensis	Geui Mak, Sek Juk		Chinese pink herb
Quan Shen	***Polygonum bistorta***	Radix Polygoni bistortae	Kyun Sam		Bistort root
Quan Xie	***Buthus Martensi***	Buthus	Chyun Kit	Zenkatsu	Scorpion
Rang He	***Zingiber mioga***	Rhizoma Zingiberis miogae	Yeung Ho		Mioga ginger root

MANDARIN	SCIENTIFIC	PHARMACEUTICAL	CANTONESE	JAPANESE	ENGLISH
Rao Hua	***Wikstroemia chamaedaphne***	Flos Wikstroaemiae chamaedaphnis	Iu Fa		Wikstroemia flower
Ren Niao	***Homo sapiens***	Urina Hominis	Yan Niu		Human urine
Ren Shen	***Panax ginseng***	Radix Panacis ginsengis	Yan Sam	Ninjin	Asian ginseng root
Ren Shen Hua	***Panax ginseng***	Flos Panacis ginsengis	Yan Sam Fa		Asian ginseng flower
Ren Shen Lu	***Panax ginseng***	Rhizoma Panacis ginsengis	Yan Sam Lu	Ninjinro	Asian ginseng neck
Ren Shen Xu, Shen Xu	***Panax ginseng***	Extremas radicis Panacis ginsengis praeparatae	(Yan) Sam Son		Rock candy cured Asian ginseng root tail
Ren Shen Ye	***Panax ginseng***	Folium Panacis ginsengis	Yan Sam Yip	Ninjinyo	Asian ginseng leaf
Ren Zhong Bai, Qiu Shi Dan	***Homo sapiens***	Sedimen urinae Hominis	Yan Jung Baak		Human urine sediment
Ren Zhong Huang	***Glycirrhiza uralensis, G. glabra*** and spp	Radix Glycirrhizae preparatae cum urino	Yan Chung Wong		Urine-prepared licorice root
Rou Cong Rong	***Cistanche salsa*** and spp	Herba Cistanchis	Yuk Chung Yung	Nikujuyo	Fleshy broomrape herb
Rou Dou Gen	***Dolichos lablab***	Radix Dolichoris	Yuk Dau Gan		Hyacinth bean root
Rou Dou Kou	***Myristica fragrans***	Semen Myristicae	Yuk Dau Kau	Nikuzuku	Nutmeg seed
Rou Gui (Pi)	***Cinnamomum cassia***	Cortex Cinnamomi cassiae	Yuk Gwai (Pei)	Nikkei	Cassia Cinnamon bark
Rou Gui Xin	***Cinnamomum cassia***	Cortex intimum Cinnamomi cassiae	Yuk Gwai San		Cassia cinnamon inner bark
Rou Gui, Xi Lan Rou Gui	***Cinnamomum zeylanicum***	Cortex Cinnamomi zeylanici	Yuk Gwai, Sek Laan Yuk Gwai		Ceylon cinnamon bark
Ru Di Jin Niu, Liang Mian Zhen	***Zanthoxylum nitidum***	Radix Zanthoxyli nitidi	Yap Dei Gam Ngau		Shiny bramble root
Ru Xiang	***Boswellia carterii*** and spp.	Resina Boswelliae	Yu Heung	Nyuko	Frankincense resin
Rui Ren (Rou)	***Prinsepia uniflora***	Semen Prinsepiae	Seui Yan (Yuk)		Prinsepia seed
Rui Xiang Hua	***Daphne odora***	Flos Daphnis odorae	Seui Heung Fa		Mezerum flower
San Bai Cao	***Saururus chinensis***	Herba Saururi	Saam Baak Chou		Chinese lizardtail herb
San Jian Shan	***Cephalotaxus fortunei***	Ramulus et folium Cephalotaxi	Saam Jim Chaam		Yew twig and leaf
San Ke Zhen	***Berberis sargentiana, B. wilsonae, B. vernae*** and spp	Radix Berberis sargentianae	Saam Gwo Jam		Three-needle barberry root
San Leng	***Sparganium simplex, S. stoloniferum, S. stenophyllum***	Rhizoma Sparganii	Saam Ling		Bur-reed root
San Qi Cao, Ju San Qi	***Gynura segetum***	Folium Gynurae	Sam Chat Chou		Canton sanchi leaf
San Qi Hua	***Panax notoginseng***	Flos Panacis notoginsengis	Saam Chat Fa	Sanshishika	Pseudoginseng flower
San Qi, Tian Qi	***Panax notoginseng***	Radix Panacis notoginsengis	Saam Chat Tin Chat	Sanshishi	Pseudoginseng root

MANDARIN	SCIENTIFIC	PHARMACEUTICAL	CANTONESE	JAPANESE	ENGLISH
San Xian Dan	***Hydragyrum chloratum***	Compositum hydragyri oxydati crudi	Sam Gong Daan		Mercury oxide (crude)
San Ya Ku (Gen)	***Evodia lepta***	Radix Evodiae leptae	Sam Nga Fu (Gan)		Bitter evodia root
San Ye Gui Zhen Cao	***Bodens pilosa***	Herba Bidentis pilosae	Sam Yip Gwai Jam Chou		
Sang Bai Pi	***Morus alba***	Cortex radicis Mori	Song Baak Pei	Sohakuhi	Mulberry root bark
Sang Ji Sheng	***Loranthus parasiticus, L. yadorici*** and spp	Ramulus Loranthi	Song Gei Sang	Sokisei	Asian mistletoe twig
Sang Piao Xiao	***Paratenodera sinensis*** and ***augustipennis, Hierodula patellifera, Mantis religiosa, Statilia maculata***	Paratenodera seu Hierodula seu Mantis seu Statilia	Song Piu Seu		Praying mantis egg case
Sang Shen (Zi)	***Morus alba***	Fructus Mori	Song Sam (Ji)	Sojin	Mulberry fruit
Sang Ye	***Morus alba***	Folium Mori	Song Yip	Soyo	Mulberry leaf
Sang Zhi	***Morus alba***	Ramulus Mori	Song Ji	Soshi	Mulberry twig
Sha Ji	***Hippophae rhamnoides***	Fructus Hippophae	Sa Jik		Sea buckthorn berry
Sha Ren Hua, (Yang) Chun Sha Hua	***Amomum villosum***	Flos Amomi villosi	Sa Yan Fa, (Yeung) Chyun Sa Fa	Saninka	Wild cardamom flower
Sha Ren Ke	***Amomum villosum***	Pericarpium Amomi villosi	Sa Yan Hok		Wild cardamom shell
Sha Ren, (Yang) Chun Sha Ren	***Amomum villosum***	Fructus Amomi villosi	Sa Yan, (Yeung) Chyun Sa Yan	Sanin	Wild cardamom pod (fruit)
Sha Ren, Hai Nan Sha Ren	***Amomum longiligulare***	Fructus Amomi longiligularis	Sai Yan, Hoi Naam Sa Yan		Hainan cardamom pod
Sha Ren, Suo Sha Mi	***Amomum xanthioides***	Fructus Amomi xanthioidis	Sa Yan, Suk Sa Mat		Cocklebur cardamom pod
Sha Tang Mu, Jiang Xiang	***Acronychia laurifolia***	Lignum Acronychiae	Sa Tong Muk		Acronychia heartwood
Sha Yuan Zi, Sha Yuan Ji Li	***Astragalus complanatus*** and spp	Semen Astragali complanati	Sa Yun Ji, Sa Yun Jek Lai	Saenshi, Toshitsuri	Flat milkvetch seed
Shan Cha Hua	***Camellia japonica***	Flos Camelliae japonicae	Saan Cha Fa		Common camellia flower
Shan Chen, Qu Tou Ji	***Melodinus suaveolens***	Fructus Melodini	Saan Chaang		Melodinus fruit
Shan Ci Gu	***Cremastra variabilis***	Rhizoma et radix Cremastrae	Saan Chi Gu		Cremastra corm
Shan Ci Gu	***Iphigenia indica***	Bulbus Iphigeniae	San Chi Gok		Iphigenia bulb
Shan Ci Gu	***Pleione bulbocodioides***	Rhizoma Pleionis	Saan Chi Gu		Pleione corm
Shan Ci Gu, Guang Ci Gu	***Tulipa edulis***	Rhizoma et radix Tulipae	San Chi Gu, Gwong Chi Gu		Chinese tulip bulb
Shan Dan	***Lilium concolor***	Bulbus Liliii concoloris	Saan Daan		Japanese red star lily bulb
Shan Diao Zhu, Xu Chang Jing	***Pycnostelma paniculatum***	Herba Pycnostelmae	Cheui Cheung Hing		Paniculate swallowwort herb
Shan Dou Gen	***Sophora subprostata***	Radix Sophorae subprostatae	Saan Dau Gan		Pigeon-pea root

MANDARIN	SCIENTIFIC	PHARMACEUTICAL	CANTONESE	JAPANESE	ENGLISH
Shan Gan Cao	***Mussaenda pubescens, M. parviflora***	Caulis et folium Mussaendae	Saan Gam Chou		Mountain licorice stem and leaf
Shan Nai, Sha Jiang	***Kaempferia galanga***	Rhizoma Kaempferiae	Saan Noi		Galanga root
Shan Ren Zi	***Rhodomyrtus tomentosa***	Semen Rhodomyrti	Saan Nam Ji		Rosemyrtle seed
Shan Shen Zi	***Glossogyne tenuifolia***	Herba Glossogyne	Saan Sam Jai		Thin-leaf glossgyne herb
Shan Teng Teng Yang	***Vitis amurensis***	Radix Vitis amurensis	Saan Tang Tang Yeung		Amur grape root
Shan Yang Jiao	***Naemorrhedis***	Cornu Naemorrhedis	San Yeung Gok	Sanyokaku	Goat horn
Shan Yao, Shu Yu	***Dioscorea opposita, D. batatas***	Rhizoma Dioscoreae oppositae	Wai Saan, Saan Yeuk	Sanyaku	Mountain yam root
Shan Zha (Rou)	***Crataegus pinnatifida, C. cuneata*** and spp	Fructus Crataegi	Saan Ja (Yuk)	Sanzashi	Asian hawthorn berry
Shan Zha Tan	***Crataegus pinnatifida, C. cuneata*** and spp	Fructus Crataegi carbonisatus	Saan Ja Tan		Charred Asian hawthorn berry
Shan Zhi Ma	***Helicteres angustifolia***	Herba Helicteres	Saan Ji Ma		Helicteres herb
Shan Zhi Zi	***Gardenia jasminoides***	Fructus Gardeniae	Saan Ji Ji	Sanshishi	Gardenia pod
Shan Zhu Yu, Shan Yu Rou	***Cornus officinalis***	Fructus Corni	San Jyu Yu, San Yu Yuk	Sanshuyu	Japanese dogwood berry
Shang Lu	***Phytolacca acinosa, P. esculenta***	Radix Phytolaccae acinosae	Seung Luk	Shoriku	Asian poke root
Shao Zi	***Nephelium lappaceum***	Fructus Nephelii	Siu Ji		Rambutan fruit
She Chuang Zi	***Cnidium monnieri***	Fructus Cnidii	Se Chong Ji	Jashoshi	Cnidium seed
She Dan	***Naja naja atra, Bungarus fasciatus, Elaphe radiata***	Fel Najae seu Bungari seu Elaphis	Se Daam		Viper gallbladder
She Gan	***Belamcanda chinensis***	Rhizoma Belamcandae	Se Gon	Yakan	Leopard flower root
She Gan Miao	***Belamcanda chinensis***	Herba Belamcandae	Se Gon Miu		Leopard flower herb
She Han Shi	***Pyritum rotundum***	Pyritum rotundum			Iron pyrite
She Mei	***Duchesnea indica***	Herba Duchesneae	Se Mui		Mock strawberry herb
She Pu Tao, Shan Pu Tao	***Ampelopsis brevipedunculata***	Radix et folium Ampelopsis brevipedunculatae	Se Pou Tou, Saan Pou Tou		Snake grape root and leaf
She Tui (Pi)	***Elephe taeniurus*** and spp, ***Dinodon rufozonatum***	Periostracum/Exuviae Elephis	Se Teui (Pei)	Dataihi	Snakeskin slough
She Xiang	***Moschus berezovskii*** and spp	Secretio Moschi	Se Heung	Jako	Musk
Shen Jin Cao	***Lycopodium clavatum***	Herba Lycopodi	Sam Gam Chou		Clubmoss herb
Shen Qu		Massa fermentata	Sam Chau	Shinkiku	Medicated leaven

MANDARIN	SCIENTIFIC	PHARMACEUTICAL	CANTONESE	JAPANESE	ENGLISH
Shen Qu Cha		Massa fermentata	Sam Chau Cha		Medicated leaven tea
Sheng Ban Xia	***Pinellia ternata***	Rhizoma pinelliae ternatae	Sang Bun Ha, So Bun Ha	Shohange	Raw pinellia corm
Sheng Di (Huang)	***Rehmannia glutinosa***	Radix Rehmanniae	Sang Dei (Wong)	Shojio	Fresh Rehmannia root
Sheng Jiang	***Zingiber officinalis***	Rhizoma Zingiberis recentis	Saang Geung	Shokyo	Fresh ginger root
Sheng Jiang Pi, Jiang Pi	***Zingiber officinalis***	Rhizoma Zingiberis	(Saang) Geung Pei		Fresh ginger root skin
Sheng Ma	***Cimicifuga foetida***	Radix Cimicifugae foetidae	Sing Ma	Shoma	Rising hemp root
Sheng Ma, Ta San Ye Sheng Ma	***Cimicifuga heracleifolia***	Radix Cimicifugae heracleifoliae	Sing Ma, Da Sam Yip Sing Ma	Shoma	Heraclean rising hemp root
Sheng Ma, Xing An Sheng Ma	***Cimicifuga dahurica***	Radix Cimicifugae dahuricae	Sing Ma, Hing On Sing Ma	Shoma	Dahurian rising hemp root
Sheng Shai Shen	***Panax ginseng***	Radix Panacis ginsengis	Sang Sai Sam		Dried Asian ginseng root
Sheng Tie Luo	***Ferrum***	Frusta Ferrum	Sang Tit Lo		Iron filing/cinder
Shi Bing Shuang	***Diospyros kaki***	Saccharum Diospyris	Chi Beng Sheung		Persimmon frost
Shi Chang Pu	***Acorus gramineus***	Rhizoma Acori graminei	Sek Cheung Pou		Rock sweetflag root
Shi Da Gong Lao Gen	***Mahonia japonica***	Radix Mahoniae japonicae	Sap Daai Gung Lou Gan		Japanese mahonia root
Shi Da Gong Lao Ye, Kuo Ye Shi Da Gong Lao Ye	***Mahonia bealei***	Folium Mahoniae bealei	Sap Daai Gung Lou Yip, Fut Yip Sap Daai Gung Lou Yip	Judaikoro	Leather-leaf mahonia leaf
Shi Da Gong Lao Ye, Xi Ye Shi Da Gong Lao Ye	***Mahonia fortunei***	Folium Mahoniae fortunei	Gung Lou Yip, Sai Yip Sap Daai Gung Lou Yip	Judaikoro	Mahonia leaf
Shi Di	***Diospyros kaki***	Calyx Diospyri	Chi Dai	Shitei	Persimmon calyx
Shi Diao Bai	***Asparagus officinalis***	Rhizoma Asparagi officinalis	Sek Diu Baak		Asparagus root
Shi Diao Lan	***Lysionotus pauciflora***	Herba Lysinoti	Sek Diu Laan		Lysionotus herb
Shi Er	***Parmelia tinctorum, P. reticulata***	Thallus Parmeliae			Parmelia thallus
Shi Er	***Umbilicaria esculenta***	Sclerotium Umbilicariae	Sek Yi		Stone ear mushroom
Shi Gao	***Gypsum fibrosum***	Gypsum	Sek Gou	Sekko	Gypsum
Shi Hu	***Dendrobium nobile, D. linawianum, D. officinale*** and spp	Herba Dendrobii	Sek Wu	Sekkoku	Stonebushel stem
Shi Hu	***Ephemerantha fimbriata***	Herba Ephemeranthae	Sek Hap	Sekkoku	Ephemerantha stem
Shi Hu, Jin Sha Shi Hu	***Dendrobium nobile***	Herba Dendrobii nobilis	Sek Wu, Gam Ja Sek Wu		Stonebushel stem
Shi Hu, Ma Bian Shi Hu	***Dendrobium fimbriatum***	Herba Dendrobii fimbriati	Sek Wu, Ma Bin Sek Wu		Stonebushel stem
Shi Hu, Shu Hua Shi Hu	***Dendrobium chrysanthum***	Herba Dendrobii chrysanthi	Sek Wu, Chuk Fa Shi Hu		Stonebushel stem
Shi Hu, Tie Pi Shi Hu	***Dendrobium officinalis***	Herba Dendrobii officinalis	Sek Wu, Tit Pei Sek Wu		Stonebushel stem

MANDARIN	SCIENTIFIC	PHARMACEUTICAL	CANTONESE	JAPANESE	ENGLISH
Shi Hu, Wan Cao Shi Hu	***Dendrobium loddigesii***	Herba Dendrobii loddigesii	Sek Wu, Waan Chou Sek Wu		Stonebushel stem
Shi Hua	***Porites nigrescens***	Os Poritis	Sek Fa		Coral skeleton
Shi Ji Sheng	***Taxillus yadoriki, T. chinensis***	Ramulus Taxilli	Chi Gei Sang		Asian mistletoe twig
Shi Jian Chuan, Chai Shen, Zi Shen	***Salvia chinensis***	Radix et herba Salviae chinensis	Sek Gin Chyun, Toi Sam, Ji Sam		Chinese sage root and herb
Shi Jue Ming	***Haliotis diversicolor, H. gigantea* and spp**	Concha Haliotis	Sek Kyut Ming	Sekketsumei	Abalone shell
Shi Jun Zi	***Quisqualis indica***	Fructus Quisqualis	Si Gwan Ji	Shikunshi	Rangoon creeper nut
Shi Liu Gen Pi	***Punica granatum***	Cortex Radicis Punicae	Sek Lau Gan Pei	Sekiryu-kombi	Pomegranate root bark
Shi Liu Pi	***Punica granatum***	Pericarpium Punicae	Sek Lau Pei	Sekiryuhi	Pomegranate husk
Shi Nan Teng	***Piper wallichii***	Ramulus Piperis wallichii	Sek Naam Tang		Wild pepper twig
Shi Nan Teng, Shi Nan Ye	***Photinia serrulata***	Caulis et folium Photiniae	Sek Naam Tang, Sek Naam Yip		Photinia stem or leaf
Shi Shang Bai	***Selaginella doederleinii, S. involvens***	Herba Selaginellae	Sek Song Paap		Spikemoss herb
Shi Shuang Bing	***Diospyros kaki***	Fructus Diospyri	Chi Shuen Bing		Persimmon frosted fruit
Shi Suan	***Lycoris radiata***	Rhizoma Lycoris	Sek Syun		Red spiderlily corm
Shi Wei	***Pyrrosia lingua, P. petiolosa* and spp**	Folium Pyrrosiae	Sek Wai		Felt fern leaf
Shi Wei, Lu Shan Shi Wei	***Pyrrosia sheareri***	Folium Pyrrosiae sheareri	Sek Wai, Lou San Sek Wai	Sekii	Shearer's felt fern leaf
Shi Xian Tao Gen	***Pholidota chinensis***	Radix Pholidotae	Sek Sin Tou Gan		Rattlesnake orchid root
Shi Ye	***Diospyros kaki***	Folium Diospyri	Chi Yip		Persimmon leaf
Shou Gong, Bi Hu	***Gecko chinensis, G. japonicus* and spp**	Gecko chinensis	Sau Gung, Bik Fu		House lizard
Shu Chi Shi	***Halloysitum rubrum***	Halloysitum	Chek Sek Ji		Roasted red kaolin
Shu Di (Huang)	***Rehmannia glutinosa***	Radix Rehmanniae preparatae	Suk Dei (Wong)	Jukujio	Prepared Rehmannia root
Shu Fu	***Armadillidium vulgare, Porcellio scaber***	Armadillidium	Syu Fu		Wood louse
Shu Liang	***Dioscorea cirrhosa***	Rhizoma Dioscoreae cirrhosae	Syu Leung		Dyer's yam root
Shu Peng Sha	***Borax***	Borax	Syu Pang Sa		Roasted borax
Shu Qi	***Dichroa febrifuga***	Folium Dichroae	Suk Chat	Shokushitsu	Feverflower leaf
Shu Qu Cao	***Gnaphalium affine***	Herba Gnaphalii	Syu Guk Chou		Cudweed herb
Shu Shi Gao	***Gypsum fibrosum***	Gypsum dehydratum	Chek Sek Gou		Dehydrated gypsum
Shu Yi Ren	***Coix lachryma-jobi* var. *Ma-yuen***	Semen Coicis preparatae	Suk Yi Mai		Dry-fried Job's-tears seed

MANDARIN	SCIENTIFIC	PHARMACEUTICAL	CANTONESE	JAPANESE	ENGLISH
Shuang Liu Huang	***Limnophila sessiliflora***	Herba Limnophilae	Seung Lan Wong		Limnophila herb
Shui Ban Xia	***Typhonium flagelliforme***	Rhizoma Typhonii flagelliformis preparata	Seui Bun Ha		Prepared flagellate typhonium root
Shui Cai Ye	***Menyanthes trifoliata***	Folium Menyanthis	Seui Choi Yip	Suisayo, Meisai	Bogbean leaf
Shui Chang Pu, Bai Chang Pu	***Acorus calamus***	Rhizoma Acori calami	Seui Cheung Pou, Baak Cheung Pou	Shobu	Sweetflag root
Shui Ding Xiang	***Ludwigia prostata***	Herba Ludwigiae	Seui Ding Heung		Water clove herb
Shui Duo Nian, Shan Nian Gen	***Rhodomyrtus tomentosa***	Radix Rhodomyrti	Seui Do Lin, San Nim Gan		Downy rosemyrtle root
Shui Fei Ji	***Silybum marianum***	Herba Silybi	Seui Fei Gai		Blessed thistle herb
Shui Hu Man	***Clerodendron inerme***	Folium Clerodendronis inermis	Seui Wu Mun		Glorybower leaf
Shui Liao	***Polygonum hydropiper***	Herba et radix Polygoni hydropiperis	Seui Liu		Water pepper herb and root
Shui Niu Jiao	***Bubalus bubalis***	Cornu Bubali	Seui Ngau Gok		Water buffalo horn
Shui Qin	***Oenanthe javanica***	Herba Oenanthis	Seui Kan		Water dropwort
Shui Song Mao	***Glyptostrobus pensilis***	Cacumen Glyptostrobi	Seui Chung Ma		Chinese water pine tip
Shui Tong Hua Cao, Hong Cao	***Polygonum orientale***	Herba Polygoni orientalis	Seui Tung Fa Chou Hung Chou		Prince's feather herb
Shui Tong Hua Zi	***Polygonum orientale***	Fructus Polygoni orientalis	Seui Tung Fa Ji		Prince's feather berry
Shui Weng Hua	***Cleistocalyx operculatus***	Gemma Cleistocalycis	Seui Yung Fa		Cleistolcalyx bud
Shui Wu Gong	***Kyllinga brevifolia***	Herba Kyllingae	Seui Ng Gung		Kyllinga herb
Shui Xian Gen	***Narcissus tazetta*** var. ***chinensis***	Bulbus Narcissi	Seui Sin Gan		Chinese sacred lily bulb
Shui Xian Zi	***Narcissus tazetta*** var. ***chinensis***	Fructus Narcissi	Seui Sin Ji		Chinese sacred lily seed
Shui Yang Mei	***Adina rubella***	Flos Adinae	Seui Yeung Mui		Red modelwood flower
Shui Yang Zhi	***Salix purpurea***	Ramulus Salicis purpureae	Seui Yeung Ji		Purple willow twig
Shui Yin	***Hydragyrum***	Hydragyrum	Seui Yin		Mercury
Shui Zhi	***Hirudo nipponia, Whitmania pigra*** and spp	Hirudo seu Whitmania	Seui Jik		Leech
Shuo Diao	***Sambucus javanica***	Caulis et folium Sambuci javanici	Sok Duk		Java elder stem and leaf
Shuo Zhuo	***Sambucus chinensis*** and spp	Caulis et folium Sambuci chinensis	Sok Dik		Chinese elder stem and leaf
Si Gua Luo	***Luffa cylindrica, L. acutangula***	Fasciculus vascularis Luffae	Si Gwa Lou	Shikaraku	Spongegourd
Si Gua Pi	***Luffa cylindrica, L. acutangula***	Pericarpium Luffae	Si Gwa Pei		Luffa skin

MANDARIN	SCIENTIFIC	PHARMACEUTICAL	CANTONESE	JAPANESE	ENGLISH
Si Ji Qing, Dong Qing Ye	***Ilex chinensis***	Folium Ilicis chinensis	Sei Gwai Ching, Dung Ching Yip		Wintergreen holly leaf
Song Hua Fen	***Pinus massoniana, P. tabulaeformis*** **and spp**	Pollen Pini	Chung Fa Fan		Pine pollen
Song Jie, You Song Jie	***Pinus tabulaeformis, P. massoniana, P. yunnanensis***	Lignum Pini nodi	Chung Jit, Yao Chung Jit	Shosetsu	Knotty pine wood shaving
Song Lan Ye	***Isatis indigotica***	Folium Isatis indigoticae	Song Laan Yip		Woad leaf
Song Luo	***Usnea diffracta*** **and spp**	Thallus Usneae	Chung Lo		Beard lichen thallus
Song Mu Bai Pi	***Aralia chinensis***	Radix Araliae chinensis	Sung Muk Baak Pei		Chinese aralia root
Song Xiang	***Pinus massoniana, P. tabulaeformis*** **and spp,** ***Larix*** **spp**	Resina Pini preparatae, Colophonium	Chung Heung		Pine resin
Song Zi	***Pinus tabulaeformis*** **and spp**	Semen Pini	Chung Ji		Pine kernel
Su He Xiang	***Liquidambar orientalis***	Resina Liquidambaris (Styrax liquidis)	Sou Hap Heung	Sogoko	Storax resin
Su Mu	***Caesalpinia sappan***	Lignum Caesalpiniae	Sou Muk	Soboku	Sappanwood
Su Tie Zi	***Cycas revoluta***	Semen Cycadis	Sou Tit Ji		Sago palm seed
Su Xin Hua	***Jasminum officinale*** **var.** ***grandiflorum***	Flos Jasmini officinalis	Sou Hing Fa		Jasmine flower
Su Ya	***Setaria italica***	Fructus germinatus Setariae	Suk Nga		Sprouted millet grain
Suan Jiang Gen	***Physalis alkakengi*** **(var.** ***franchetii)***	Rhizoma Physalis	Syun Jeung Gan		Chinese lantern root
Suan Jiang, Jing Deng Long	***Physalis alkekengi*** **(var.** ***franchetii)***	Calyx seu fructus Physalis	Syun Jeung, Ching Dang Lung		Chinese lantern calyx or fruit
Suan Zao Ren, Jin Zao Ren	***Zizyphus spinosa***	Semen Zizyphi spinosae	Syun Jou Yan	Sansonin	Sour jujube seed
Sun Tai Lang Chun	***Protohermes grandis***	Vermiculus Protohermis	Syun Taai Long Chung	Magotaro-mushi	Protohermes larva
Suo Luo Zi	***Aesculus wilsonii, A. chinensis***	Fructrus Aesculi	So Lo Ji		Chinese horse chestnut
Suo Yang	***Cynomorium songaricum***	Herba Cynomorii	Soi Yeung	Sayo	Lock yang stem
Ta Gan	***Lutra lutra***	Jecur Lutrae	Taap Gon		Otter liver
Ta Hua Xi Xin	***Asarum maximum***	Herba Asari maximi	Daai Fa Sai San		Large flower wild ginger herb
Tai Wan Ji Sheng	***Scurrula ritozanensis***	Ramulus Scurrulae	Toi Waan Ji Sang		Taiwan mistletoe twig
Tai Wu	***Lindera strychnifolia***	Radix Linderae	Toi Wu	Uyaku	Lindera root
Tai Zi Shen	***Pseudostellaria heterophylla***	Radix Pseudostellariae	Yi Sam, Taai Ji Sam	Taishijin	Prince ginseng root
Tan Gen	***Dalbergia hupeana***	Folium Dalbergiae hupeanae	Taan Gan		Hupei rosewood
Tan Xiang	***Santalum album***	Lignum Santalum	Taan Heung		Sandalwood

MANDARIN	SCIENTIFIC	PHARMACEUTICAL	CANTONESE	JAPANESE	ENGLISH
Tang Shi Song	***Commelina benghalensis***	Herba Commelinae	Tong Sek Chung		Bengal dayflower herb
Tang Song Cao	***Thalictrum foliolosum***	Herba Thalictri			Meadow rue herb
Tao Er Qi	***Podophyllum emodi***	Rhizoma Podophylli emodii	Tou Yi Chat		Emodi's podophullum root
Tao Ren	***Prunus persica*** and spp	Semen Pruni persicae	Tou Yan	Tonin	Peach kernel
Teng Huang	***Garcinia morella***	Resina Garciniae	Tang Wong		Gamboge resin
Teng Li Gen	***Actinidia chinensis***	Fructus Actinidiae chinensis	Tang Li Gan		Kiwi root
Tian (Men) Dong	***Asparagus cochinchinensis***	Rhizoma Asparagi cochinensis	Tin (Mun) Dung	Tenmondo	Shiny asparagus root
Tian Chen	***Citrus sinensis***	Fructus Citri sinensis	Tim Chaang		Sweet orange fruit
Tian Gua Di	***Cucumis melo***	Caulis Cucumis	Tim Gwa Dai	Katei	Young cantaloupe stalk
Tian Gua Zi	***Cucumis melo***	Semen Cucumis	Tim Gwa Ji		Cantaloupe seed
Tian Hu Sui	***Hydrocotyle sibthorpioides***	Herba Hydrocotylis	Tin Wu Seui		Lawn (water) pennywort herb
Tian Hua Fen	***Trichosanthes kirilowii, T. japonica, T. uniflora***	Radix Trichosanthis	Tin Fa Fun	Tenkafun	Snakegourd root
Tian Ji Huang, Di Er Cao	***Hypericum japonicum***	Herba Hyperici japonici	Tin Jik Wong, Dei Yi Chou		Japanese St. John's wort herb
Tian Kui	***Semiaquilegia adoxoides***	Radix Semiaquilegiae	Tin Kwai		Semiaquilegia root
Tian Kui	***Semiaquilegia adoxoides***	Herba Semiaquilegiae	Tin Kwai		Semiaquilegia herb
Tian Ma	***Gastrodia elata***	Rhizoma Gastrodiae	Tin Ma	Temma	Celestial hemp corm
Tian Ming Jing	***Carpesium abrotanoides***	Herba Carpesii	Tin Ming Jing		Starwort herb
Tian Nan Xing, Zhi Nan Xing	***Arisaema consanguineum, A. amurense*** and spp	Rhizoma Arisaemae preparatae	Tin Naam Sing, Jek Naam Sing		Prepared dragon arum corm
Tian Qi	***Panax notoginseng***	Radix Panacis notoginsengis	Tin Chat	Sanshishi	Pseudoginseng root
Tian Qiang Ke	***Metaplexis japonica***	Fructus Metaplexis	Tin Cheung Hok		Metaplexis fruit
Tian Xian Teng	***Aristolochia contorta, A. debilis***	Caulis Aristolochiae	Tin Sin Tang	Tensendo	Green birthwort stem
Tian Xian Zi	***Hyoscyamus niger***	Semen Hyoscyami	Tin Sin Ji		Black henbane seed
Tian Xiang Lu, Jin Shi Lu	***Osbeckia chinensis***	Herba Osbeckiae	Tin Heung Lou		Chinese osbeckia herb
Tian Xing Ren, Nan Xing Ren	***Prunus armeniaca*** and var.	Semen Pruni armeniacae dulcis	Tim Hang Yan, Naam Hang Yan		Sweet apricot kernel
Tian Yuan Zhi	***Polygala sibirica***	Radix Polygalae sibiricae	Tin Yun Ji		Siberian milkwort root
Tian Zhu Huang	***Phyllostachys nigra*** var. ***henonis*** and spp	Concretio silicea bambusae	Tin Juk Wong		Tabasheer

MANDARIN	SCIENTIFIC	PHARMACEUTICAL	CANTONESE	JAPANESE	ENGLISH
Tie Bao Jin	***Berchemia lineata***	Radix Berchemiae	Tit Bau Gam		Supplejack root
Tie Shu	***Cycas revoluta***	Folium Cycadis	Tit Syu		Sago palm leaf
Tie Xian (Cai)	***Acalypha australis***	Herba Acalyphae	Tit Yin		Annual copperleaf herb
Tie Xian Lian	***Clematis florida***	Herba Clematis floridae	Ti Chik Lin		Flowering clematis herb
Ting Li Zi	***Descurainia sophia***	Semen Descurainiae	Ting Lai Ji	Teirekishi	Tansy mustard seed
Ting Li Zi	***Lepidium apetalum, L. virginicum***	Semen Lepidii	Ting Lai Ji	Teirekishi	Wood whitlow grass seed
Tong Cao	***Tetrapanax papyrifera***	Medulla Tetrapanacis	Tong Chou, Bai Tong Chou	Toso	Rice paper pith
Tong Lu	***Malachitum***	Malachitum	Tung Luk		Copper rust
Tou Gu Cao	***Impatiens balsamina***	Herba Impatientis	Tau Gwat Chou		Garden balsam herb
Tou Gu Cao	***Speranskia tuberculata***	Herba Speranskiae	Tau Gwat Chou		Speranskia herb
Tu Bai Lian	***Melothria heterophylla***	Radix Melothriae heterolphyllae	Taou Baak Lin		Native peppervine root
Tu Bie Chong	***Eupolyphaga sinensis***	Eupolyphaga	Dei Bit Chung	Shachu	Cockroach
Tu Dang Gui	***Aralia cordata***	Radix Araliae cordatae	Tou Dong Gwai		Heart-leaf aralia root
Tu Dang Shen	***Campanumoea javanica***	Radix Campanumoeae	Tou Dong Sam		Java bellflower root
Tu Fu Ling	***Smilax glabra***	Rhizoma Smilacis glabrae	Tou Fuk Ling		Glabrous greenbrier root
Tu Jing Jie	***Chenopodium ambrosioides***	Herba Chenopodii ambrosioidis	Tou Ging Gai		Wormseed herb
Tu Jing Pi	***Pseudolarix amabilis. P. kaempferi***	Cortex radicis Pseudolaricis	Tou Ging Pei		Golden larch root bark
Tu Mu Xiang	***Inula helenium***	Radix Inula helenii	Tou Muk Heung		Elecampane root
Tu Mu Xiang, Zong Zhuang Tu Mu Xiang	***Inula racemosa***	Radix Inulae racemosae	Tou Muk Heung, Chung Ching Tou Muk Heung		Racemose elecampane root
Tu Niu Xi	***Achyranthes longifolia***	Radix Achyranthis longae	Tou Ngau Sat		Long-leaf oxknee root
Tu Ren Shen	***Talinum paniculatum***	Radix Talini	Tou Yan Sam		Fameflower root
Tu Si Zi	***Cuscuta chinensis, C. japonica***	Semen Cuscutae	Tou Si Ji	Toshishi	Asian dodder seed
Tu Xiang Fei	***Cephalotaxus sinensis***	Ramulus et folium Cephalotaxi sinensis	Tou Heung Fei		Plum yew twig and leaf
Tu Yin Chen, Tu Xiang Ru	***Origanum vulgare***	Herba Origani vulgaris	Tou Gam Chan, Tou Heung Yu		Oregano herb
Tu Yin Hua, Shan Yin Hua	***Lonicera confusa***	Flos Lonicerae confusae	Tou Ngan Fa		Wild honeysuckle flower
Wa Leng Zi	***Arca inflata*** **and spp**	Concha Arcae	Nga Ling Ji	Garyoshi	Cockle shell

MANDARIN	SCIENTIFIC	PHARMACEUTICAL	CANTONESE	JAPANESE	ENGLISH
Wa Song	***Orostachys fimbriatus***	Herba Orostachis	Nga Chung		Fimbriate orostachys herb
Wa Song	***Orostachys japonica, O. fimbriatus***	Herba Orostachis	Nga Chung		Hens-and-chickens herb
Wan Nian Xing	***Rhodea japonica***	Herba Rhodeae			Rhodea herb
Wan Shou Ju	***Tagetes erecta***	Flos Tagetis	Maan Sau Guk		African marigold flower
Wang Bu Liu Xing	***Vaccaria segetalis***	Semen Vaccariae	Wong Bat Lau Hang	Ofurugyo	Cowcockle seed
Wang Jiang Nan Zi	***Cassia occidentalis***	Semen Cassiae occidentalis	Mong Gong Naam	Banshashi	Coffee senna seed
Wang Yue Sha	***Lepus*** **spp**	Excrementum Lepi	Mong Yut Sa		Rabbit dropping
Wei Jing	***Phragmites communis***	Ramulus Phragmitis	Lou Ging		Water-reed twig
Wei Ling Cai	***Potentilla chinensis***	Herba Potentillae chinensis	Wai Ling Choi		Chinese cinquefoil herb
Wei Ling Xian	***Clematis chinensis, C. hexapetala*** **and spp**	Radix Clematis chinensis	Wai Ling Sin	Ireisen	Chinese clematis root
Wei Ling Xian, Mian Tuan Tie Xian Lian	***Clematis hexapetala***	Radix Clematis hexapetalae	Wai Ling Sin, Min Tyun Ti Chik Lin		Six-petal clematis root
Wei Niu Xi, Ju Niu Xi, Dou Kou Cao	***Achyranthes aspera***	Radix Achyranthis asperae	Wai Ngau Sat, Dou Kau Chou		Rough oxknee root
Wen Ge	***Meretrix meretrix***	Concha Metretris	Man Gap		Asian venus clam shell
Wu Bei Zi	***Rhus sinensis*** **and spp, *Schlechtendaria chinensis***	Galla Rhudis sinensis	Ng Pan Ji		Chinese sumac gallnut
Wu Gong	***Scolopendra subspinipes mutilans***	Scolopendra	Ng Gung	Gosho	Centipede
Wu Gu Chong	***Chrysomyia megacephala*** **and spp**	Larva Chrysomyiae	Ng Guk Chung		Maggot
Wu Gu Teng	***Fissistigma glaucescens***	Herba Fissistigmae	Wu Gwat Tang		Fissistigma herb
Wu Gu Teng	***Marsdenia tenacissima***	Herba Marsdeniae	Wu Gwat Tang		Marsdenia herb
Wu Hua Guo	***Ficus carica***	Flos Fici	Wu Fa Gwat		Fig flower
Wu Huan Gen, Mu Huan Gen	***Sapindus mukorossi***	Radix Sapindi	Mou Waan Gan		Soapnut tree root
Wu Huan Zi, Mu Huan Zi	***Sapindus mukorossi***	Semen Sapindi	Mou Waan Ji		Soapnut seed, Bodhi seed
Wu Jia Pi	***Acanthopanax gracilistylus, A. spinosus, A. sessiliflorus*** **and spp**	Cortex radicis Acanthopanacis	Ng Ga Pei	Gokahi	Five additions root bark
Wu Jia Pi, Bai Le	***Acanthopanax trifoliatus***	Cortex radicis Acanthopanacis trifoliati	Ng Ga Pei, Baak Lak		Three-leaf acanthopanax root bark

MANDARIN	SCIENTIFIC	PHARMACEUTICAL	CANTONESE	JAPANESE	ENGLISH
Wu Jia Pi, Xi Zhu Wu Jia	***Acanthopanax gracilistylus***	Cortex radicis Acanthopanacis gracilistylus	Ng Ga Pei, Sai Chu Ng Ga		Five additions root bark
Wu Jiu (Mu) Gen Pi	***Sapium sebiferum***	Cortex radicis Sapii sebiferi	Wu Kau Muk Gan Pei	Ukyukompi	Chinese tallow tree root bark
Wu Lian Mei	***Cayratia japonica***	Herba Cayratiae	Wu Lin Mui		Cayratia herb
Wu Ling Zhi	***Trogopterus xanthipes* and spp, *Pteromys volans* and spp**	Excrementum Trogopteri seu Pteromi	Ng Ling Ji		Flying squirrel dropping
Wu Mei (Rou)	***Prunus mume***	Fructus Pruni mumis	Wu Mui (Yuk)	Ubai	Black plum fruit
Wu Ming Yi	***Manganitum***	Manganitum	Mon Ming Yi		Manganite
Wu Ming Zi	***Pyrolusitum***	Pyrolusitum	Mou Ming Ji		Pyrolusite
Wu Se Mei	***Lantana camara***	Herba Lantanae	Ng Sik Mui		Wild sage herb
Wu Shao She	***Zaocys dhumnades***	Zaocys	U Sau Se	Ushoda	Black grass-snake
Wu Tong Zi	***Firmiana simplex***	Semen Firmianae	Ng Tung Ji		Chinese parasol tree seed
Wu Wei Zi	***Schisandra chinensis***	Fructus Schisandrae	Ng Mei Ji	Gomishi	Schisandra berry
Wu Wei Zi, Hua Zheng Wu Wei Zi	***Schizandra sphenantera***	Fructus Schisandrae sphenanterae	Ng Mei Ji, Wa Jung Ng Mei Ji	Gomishi	Central China schisandra berry
Wu Xue Teng	***Gymnema sylvestre* and spp**	Caulis et radix Gymnemae	Mou Heu Tang		Gymnema stem and root
Wu Yao, Tai Wu	***Lindera strychnifolia***	Radix Linderae	Wu Yeuk, Toi Wu	Uyaku	Lindera root
Wu Yi	***Ulmus macrocarpa***	Praeparatio fructus Ulmi	Mon Yi	Bui	Stinking elm fruit paste
Wu Zhao Long	***Ipomoea cairica***	Herba Ipomoeae cairicae	Ng Jaau Lung		Cairo morning-glory herb
Wu Zhu Yu	***Evodia rutaecarpa***	Fructus Evodiae rutecarpae	Ng Jyu Yu	Goshuyu	Evodia berry
Xi Fan Lian	***Passiflora coeruleae***	Herba Passiflorae coeruleae	Sai Faan Lin		Cerulean passionflower herb
Xi Gua	***Citrullus vulgaris***	Fructus Citrulli	Sai Gwa	Seika	Watermelon fruit
Xi Gua Pi	***Citrullus vulgaris***	Pericarpium Citrulli	Sai Pa Pei		Watermelon rind
Xi He Liu	***Tamarix chinensis***	Cacumen Tamaricis	Sei Ho Lau	Seikaryu	Chinese tamarisk tip
Xi Hong Hua, Fan Hong Hua	***Crocus sativus***	Stigma Croci	Fun Hung Fa	Bankoka	Saffron stigma
Xi Jiao	***Rhinoceros unicornis, R. bicornis***	Cornu Rhinoceri	Sai Gok		Rhinoceros horn
Xi Jing Shi Hu, Xiao Wan Chai	***Dendrobium moniliforme***	Caulis Dendrobii miniliformis	Sai Ging Sek Wu		Stonebushel stem
Xi Ming	***Thlaspi arvense***	Herba Thlaspis	Sik Ming		Boor's mustard herb
Xi Sheng Teng	***Cissampelos pareira***	Radix Cissampeli	Sak Sang Tang		Ice vine root
Xi Shu	***Camptotheca acuminata***	Cortex radicis Camptothecae	Hei Syu		Happy tree root bark
Xi Shu Guo	***Camptotheca acuminata***	Fructus Camptothecae	Hei Syu Gwo		Happy tree seed

MANDARIN	SCIENTIFIC	PHARMACEUTICAL	CANTONESE	JAPANESE	ENGLISH
Xi Shuai	***Gryllulus chinensis, G. mitratus, Gampsocleis buergeri***	Gryllulus	Sik Seut		Cricket
Xi Xian Cao	***Siegesbeckia pubescens, S. orientalis, S. glabrescens***	Herba Siegesbeckiae	Hei Lim Chou		Hairy siegesbeckia herb
Xi Xin	***Asarum sieboldii, A. heterotropoides*** and spp	Radix et herba Asari	Sai San	Saishin	Asian wild ginger root and herb
Xi Xin, Bei Xi Xin	***Asarum heterotropoides***	Herba Asari heterotropoidis	Bak Sai San		Northern wild ginger root
Xi Xin, Hua Xi Xin	***Asarum sieboldii***	Herba Asari sieboldii	Wa Sai San		Siebold's wild ginger herb
Xi Yang Shen	***Panax quinquefolius***	Radix Panacis quinquefolii	Fa Kei Sam, Sei Yang Sam	Seiyojin	American ginseng root
Xia Ku Cao	***Prunella vulgaris***	Spica Prunellae	Ha Fu Chou	Kagoso	Selfheal spike
Xia Tian Wu	***Corydalis decumbens***	Herba Corydalis decumbensis	Ha Tin Mou		Decumbent corydalis herb
Xian Cao, Liang Fen Cao	***Mesona chinensis***	Herba Mesonae	Heun Chou, Leung Fan Chou		Jellywort herb
Xian Feng Cao	***Bidens pilosa*** var. ***minor*** and spp	Herba Bidentis pilosae	Heun Fung Chou		Hairy beggartick herb
Xian He Cao	***Agrimonia pilosa*** var. ***japonica***	Herba Agrimoniae pilosae	Sin Hok Chou	Senkakuso	Furry agrimony herb
Xian Ji Gui Hua Pan	***Helianthus annuus***	Receptaculum Helianthi	Heung Yat Kwai Fa Bun		Sunflower receptacle
Xian Ling Pi	***Epimedium saggitatum, E. macranthum*** and spp	Folium Epimedii	Sin Ling Pei	Inyokaku	Horny goat weed leaf
Xian Mao	***Curculigo orchioides***	Rhizoma Curculigonis	Sin Maau	Sembo	Golden eye-grass root
Xian Ren Zhang	***Opuntia dillenii*** and spp	Rhizoma Opuntiae	Sin Yan Jeung		Prickly pear root
Xiang Fu	***Cyperus rotundus***	Rhizoma Cyperi	Heung Fu	Kobushi	Purple nutsedge root
Xiang Gu	***Lentinula edodes***	Sclerotium Lentinulae	Heung Gu	Shiitake	Shiitake mushroom
Xiang Hua Cai, Liu Lan Xiang	***Mentha spicata***	Herba Menthae spicatae	Heung Fa Choi, Lou Laan Heung		Spearmint herb
Xiang Mao	***Cymbopogon citratus***	Herba Cymbopogonis	Heung Maau		Lemongrass herb
Xiang Ru (Cao)	***Elsholtzia splendens, E. stauntonii***	Herba Elsholtziae	Heung Yu (Chou)	Koju	Aromatic madder herb
Xiang Shi	***Quercus acutissima***	Fructus Querci acutissimae	Jeung Sat		Oak fruit
Xiang Si Zi Gen	***Abrus precatorius, A. cantoniensis***	Radix Abri	Seung Si Ji Gan		Licorice bean root
Xiang Ye	***Pelargonium graveolens***	Herba Pelargonii	Heung Yip		Rose geranium herb
Xiang Yuan Pi, Gou Yuan Pi	***Citrus medica, C. wilsonii***	Pericarpium Citri medicae	Heung Yun Pei, Gau Yun Pei		Citron rind
Xiang Yuan, Gou Yuan	***Citrus medica, C. wilsonii***	Fructus Citri medicae	Heung Yun		Citron fruit

MANDARIN	SCIENTIFIC	PHARMACEUTICAL	CANTONESE	JAPANESE	ENGLISH
Xiao Guo Lu Huang	***Lysimachia congestiflora***	Herba Lysimachiae congestiflorae	Siu Gwo Lou Wong		Full-flowered lysimachia
Xiao Hui Xiang	***Foeniculum vulgare***	Fructus Foeniculi	Siu Wui Heung	Shouikyo	Fennel seed
Xiao Ji	***Cephalanoplos segetum***	Radix et herba Cephalanoplis	Siu Gai		Field thistle herb and root
Xiao Jin Ying, Hong Gen	***Rosa cymosa***	Cortex radicis Rosae cymosae	Hung Chi Teng, Siu Gam Ying		Cymose rose root bark
Xiao Mi	***Setaria italica***	Fructus Setariae	Suk Mai		Millet grain
Xiao Nie	***Berberis thunbergii***	Lignum Berberis thunbergii	Siu Maak	Megi	Barberry wood
Xiao Shi	***Niter***	Niter	Siu Sek	Shoseki	Potassium nitrate
Xie Bai	***Allium macrostemon***	Bulbus Allii macrostemonis	Se Baak	Gaihaku	Chinese chive bulb
Xie Cao	***Valeriana officinalis, V. hardwickii***	Rhizoma Valerianae	Kit Chou		Valerian root
Xin Jiang Bai Shao (Yao)	***Paeonia sinjiangensis***	Radix Paeoniae sinjiangensis	San Geung Chek Cheuk		Xinjiang peony root
Xin Yi Hua	***Magnolia liliflora, M. denudata, M. yulan*** **and spp**	Gemma Magnoliae	San Yi Fa	Shinika	Yulan magnolia bud
Xing Ren, Ku Xing Ren	***Prunus armeniaca*** **and var.**	Semen Pruni armeniacae	Baak Hang Yan	Kyonin	Bitter apricot kernel
Xiong Dan	***Ursus arctos*** **and spp**	Fel Ursi	Hung Daam	Yutan	Bear gallbladder
Xiong Huang	***Realgar***	Realgar	Song Wong	Yuo	Realgar
Xu Chang Qing, Liao Diao Zhu	***Cynanchum paniculatum***	Radix et herba Cynanchi paniculati	Cheui Cheung Hing		Panicled dogbane root and herb
Xu Duan	***Dipsacus japonica***	Radix Dipsaci japonicae	Juk Dyun	Zokudan	Japanese teasel root
Xu Duan, Chuan Duan	***Dipsacus asperoides***	Radix Dipsaci asperoides	Juk Dyun, Chyun Dyun		Sichuan teasel root
Xuan Cao (Gen)	***Hemerocallis fulva***	Radix Hemerocallis	Syun Chou Gan		Tawny day lily root
Xuan Cao Hua	***Hemerocallis fulva***	Flos Hemerocallis	Syun Chou Fa		Tawny day lily flower
Xuan Fu Hua	***Inula japonica, I. brittanica, I. linariaefolia***	Flos Inulae	Syun Fuk Fa	Sembukuka	Elecampane flower
Xuan Jing Shi	***Selenitum***	Selenitum	San Ching Sek		Selenite
Xuan Ming Fan	***Mirabilitum***	Mirabilitum purum	San Ming Fun	Bosho	Glauber's salt, Pure mirabilite
Xuan Shen, Yuan Shen	***Scrophularia ningpoensis, S. buergeriana***	Radix Scrophulariae ningpoensis	Yun Sam, Yun Sam	Genjin	Black figwort root
Xue Dan	***Hemsleya amabilis, H. macrosperma*** **and spp.**	Radix Hemsleyae	Hat Daam		Hemsleya tuber
Xue Feng Teng, Qing Pi Mao	***Ventilago leiocarpa***	Radix et rhizoma Ventilaginis	Hyut Fung Tang		Ventilago root and stem
Xue Jie	***Daemonorops draco***	Resina Daemonoropsis (Sanguis draconis)	Hyut Kit	Kekketsu	Dragon's-blood resin

MANDARIN	SCIENTIFIC	PHARMACEUTICAL	CANTONESE	JAPANESE	ENGLISH
Xue Lian Gen	***Saussurea laniceps, S. involucrata*** and spp	Radix Saussureae lanicepsis	Hat Ling Gan		Snow lotus root
Xue Lian Hua	***Saussurea laniceps, S. involucrata*** and spp	Herba Saussureae lanicepsis	Hat Ling Fa		Snow lotus herb
Xue Shang Yi Zhi Yao	***Aconitum brachypodum*** and spp	Radix Aconiti brachypodi	Syu Seung Yat Ji Hou		Brachypode aconite root
Xue Yu Tan	***Homo sapiens***	Crinis carbonisatus Hominis	Hyut Yu Taan		Charred human hair
Xun Gu Feng, Mian Mao Ma Dou Ling	***Aristolochia mollissima***	Herba Aristolochiae mollissimae	Cham Gwat Fung, Min Mou Ma Dou Ling		Soft birthwort herb
Ya Dan Zi	***Brucea javanica***	Fructus Bruceae	Nga Daan Ji	Atanshi	Brucea berry
Ya Jiao Mu Pi	***Schefflera octophylla***	Cortex Scheffierae octophyllae	Ngaap Geuk Muk Pei		Umbrella tree bark
Ya Ma Zi	***Linum usitatissimum***	Semen Lini	A Ma Ji		Flax seed
Ya Zhi Cao	***Commelina communis***	Herba Commelinae	Ngaap Jek Chou		Common dayflower herb
Yan Fu Mu	***Rhus chinensis***	Cortex Rhudis chinensis	Yim Fo Muk	Gobaishi	Chinese sumac bark
Yan Hu Suo, Chi Ban Yan Hu Suo	***Corydalis turtschaninovii***	Rhizoma Corydalis	Yin Wu Sok, Chi Faan Yin Wu Sok	Engosaku	Dentate-leaf corydalis corm
Yan Hu Suo, Dong Bei Yan Hu Suo	***Corydalis ambigua*** var. ***amurensis***	Rhizoma Corydalis ambiguae	Yin Wu Sok, Dung Bak Yin Wu Sok		Amur corydalis corm
Yan Hu Suo, Yuan Hu	***Corydalis yanhusuo***	Rizoma Corydalis yanhusuoidis	Yin Wu Sok, Yun Wu	Engosaku	Asian corydalis corm
Yan Shu Shuang	***Mogera robusta*** and spp., ***Scaptochirus moschatus***	Mogera carbonisatus	Yim Syu Seung	Ensosu	Carbonized mogera
Yan Sui Zi	***Coriandrum sativum***	Fructus Coriandri	Yun Sai Ji		Coriander seed
Yang Jiao Yao	***Strophanthus divaricatus***	Semen Strophanthi	Yeung Gok Aau		Strophanthus seed
Yang Jin Hua	***Datura metel***	Flos Daturae	Yeung Gam Fa		Jimsonweed flower
Yang Ju, Shi Ye Shen	***Codonopsis lanceolata***	Radix Codonopsis lanceolatae	Yang Guk, Sei Yip Sam	Yonyu, Shiyojin	Goat's-tit bellflower root
Yang Mei Pi	***Myrica rubra***	Cortex Myricae rubrae	Yeung Miu Pei		Red bayberry bark
Yang Qi Shi	***Actinolitum***	Actinolitum	Yeung Hei Sek		Actinolite
Yang Tao	***Averrhoa carambola***	Fructus Averrhoae	Yeung Tou		Carambola fruit
Yang Tao Hua	***Averrhoa carambola***	Flos Averrhoae	Yeung Tou Fa		Carambola flower
Yang Ti	***Rumex japonicus, R. nepalensis***	Radix Rumicis japonici	Yeung Tai		Japanese dock root
Yang Ti Cao	***Emilia sonchifolia***	Herba Emiliae	Yeung Tai Chou		Red tasselflower herb
Ye Bai He	***Crotalaria sessiliflora***	Herba Crotalariae	Ye Baak Hap		Thin-leaf rattlebox herb

MANDARIN	SCIENTIFIC	PHARMACEUTICAL	CANTONESE	JAPANESE	ENGLISH
Ye Dian Jie	***Solanum surratense***	Herba Solani surattensis	Ye Din Ke		Soda-apple nightshade herb
Ye Gan Cao, Zhu Cai Cao Gen	***Scoparia dulcis***	Radix Scopariae	Ye Gam Chou, Chu Jai Chou Gan		Scoparia root
Ye Guan Men	***Lespedeza cuneata***	Herba Lespedezae	Ye Gwaan Mun		Perennial lespedeza herb
Ye Hua Jiao	***Zanthoxylum simulans***	Fructus Zanthoxyli simulansis	Ye Fa Jiu		Sichuan peppercorn
Ye Jiao Teng	***Polygonum multiflorum***	Caulis Polygoni multiflori	Ye Gou Tang	Yakoto	Flowery knotweed stem
Ye Ju Hua	***Chrysanthemum indicum***	Flos Chrysanthemi indici	Gam Guk Fa, Ye Guk Fa	Nogikuka	Wild chrysanthe-mum flower
Ye Ma Zhui, Jian Pei Lan	***Eupatorium lindleyanum*** var. ***tripartum***	Herba Eupatorii	Ye Ma Jeui, Jim Pui Laan		Lindley's eupatorium herb
Ye Ming Cao	***Isodon japonicus***	Herba Isodonis	Yin Ming Chou	Enmeiso	Isodon herb
Ye Ming Sha	***Vespertilium murinum***	Excrementum Vespertilii	Ye Ming Sa	Yamyosha	Bat dropping
Ye Mu Dan	***Melastoma candidum***	Herba Melastomae candidae	Ye Maau Daan		Melastoma herb
Ye Pu Tao	***Vitis thunbergii*** and spp	Radix Vitis	Ye Pou Tou		Wild grape root
Ye Qiang Wei Gen	***Rosa multiflora***	Radix Rosae multiflorae	Ye Cheung Mei Gan		Wild rose root
Ye Shan Shen	***Panax ginseng***	Radix Panacis ginsengis	Gam San Sam		Wild Asian ginseng
Ye Shan Zha	***Crataegus cuneata***	Fructus Crataegus cuneatae	Ye Saan Ja		Wild hawthorn berry
Ye Yan Ye Gen, Tu Yen Tou	***Solanum verbascifolium***	Radix Solani verbascifolii	Ye Yin Yip Gan, Tou Yin Tau		Tobacco nightshade root
Yi Bei Mu	***Fritillaria pallidiflora***	Bulbus Fritillariae pallidiflorae	Yi Bui Mou		Pale-flower fritillary bulb
Yi Bei Mu, Tuo Li Bei Mu	***Fritillaria tortifolia***	Bulbus Fritillariae tortifoliae	Yi Bui Mou, Tok Lei Bui Mou		Twist-leaf fritillary bulb
Yi Bei Mu, Yu Min Bei Mu	***Fritillaria yuminensis***	Bulbus Fritillariae yuminensis	Yi Bui Mou, Yu Man Bui Mou		Yumin fritillary bulb
Yi Dian Hong	***Cypripedium formosanum***	Herba Cypripedii	Yut Dim Hung		Formosa lady' slipper herb
Yi Mu Cao, Chong Wei	***Leonorus heterophyllus, L. japonicus, L. sibiricus*** and spp	Herba Leonori	Yik Mou Chou, Chong Wai	Yakumoso	Asian motherwort herb
Yi Tang, Jiao Yi	***Hordeum vulgare***	Saccharum Hordei	Yi Tong		Barley malt sugar
Yi Tiao Gen	***Moghania macrophylla, M. philippinensis***	Radix Moghaniae	Yat Tiu Gan		Moghania root
Yi Wu Gen	***Eleagnus oldhamii***	Radix Eleagni oldhamii	Yi Ng Gan		Oldham's eleagnus root
Yi Ye Qiu	***Securinega suffruticosa***	Gemma et radix Securinegae	Yat Yip Chau		Securinega shoot and root
Yi Yi Gen	***Coix lachryma-jobi*** var. ***Ma-yuen***	Radix Coicis	Yi Yi Gan		Job's-tears root

MANDARIN	SCIENTIFIC	PHARMACEUTICAL	CANTONESE	JAPANESE	ENGLISH
Yi Yi Ren	***Coix lachryma-jobi*** var. ***Ma-yuen***	Semen Coicis	San Yi Mai, Yi Yi Yan	Yokuinin	Job's-tears seed
Yi Zhi Huang Hua, Liu Zhi Huang	***Solidago virgaurea, S. derurrens***	Herba Solidaginis	Yat Ji Wong Fa, Lau Ji Wong		Goldenrod herb
Yi Zhi Ren	***Alpinia oxyphylla***	Fructus Alpiniae oxyphyllae	Yik Ji Yan	Yakuchinin	Sharp-leaf galangal berry
Yi Zhi Xiang	***Vernonia cinerea***	Herba Vernoniae	Yat Ji Heung		Vernonia herb
Yin Chai Hu	***Gypsophyla oldhamiana***	Radix Gypsophylae	Ngan Chaai Wu		Gypsophyla root
Yin Chai Hu	***Stellaria dichotoma*** var. ***lanceolata***	Radix Stellariae	Ngan Chaai Wu	Ginsaiko	Stellaria root
Yin Chen (Hao), Mian Yin Chen	***Artemisia capillaris, A. scoparia***	Herba Artemisiae capillaris	Yan Chan (Hou), Min Yan Chan	Inchinko	Downy wormwood herb
Yin Xing Ye, Bai Guo Ye	***Ginkgo biloba***	Folium Ginkgoidis	Ngan Hang Yip, Baak Gwo Yip	Ginkyoyo	Ginkgo leaf
Yin Yang Huo, Xian Ling Pi	***Epimedium saggitatum, E. macranthum*** and spp	Folium Epimedii	Yam Yeung Fok, Sin Ling Pei	Inyokaku	Horny goat weed leaf
Yin Yu	***Skimmia reevesiana, S. japonica***	Caulis et folium Skimmiae	Yan Wu		Skimmia stem and leaf
Ying Pi	***Prunus jamasakura, P. yedoensis***	Cortex Pruni	Ying Pei	Ouhi	Plum tree bark
Ying Su Ke	***Papaver somniferum***	Pericarpium Papaveris	Ngang Suk Hok	Ozokukoku	Opium poppy husk
You He	***Citrus grandis***	Semen Citri grandi immaturi	Yau Hat		Pomelo seed
You Pi (Ju Hong), Hua Ju Hong	***Citrus grandis***	Pericarpium Citri grandi immaturi	Yau Pei (Gwat Hung), Fa Gwat Hung		Pomelo rind
You Tong Zi	***Aleurites fordii***	Semen Aleuritis	Yau Tung Ji		Tung seed
You Ye	***Citrus grandis***	Folium Citri grandi immaturi	Yau Yip		Pomelo leaf
Yu Biao Jiao	***Acipenser sinensis, Miichthys*** spp	Colla piscis	Yu Biu Gaau		Fish airbladder
Yu Jin	***Curcuma longa, C. aromatica***	Tuber Curcumae	Yuk Gam	Ukon	Turmeric tuber
Yu Li Ren	***Prunus japonica***	Semen Pruni japonicae	Yuk Lei Yan	Ikurinin	Bush cherry kernel
Yu Li Ren, Ou Li	***Prunus humilis***	Semen Pruni humili	Yuk Lei Yan, Ngao Lei		Dwarf cherry kernel
Yu Liang Shi	***Limonitum***	Limonitum	Yu Leung Sek	Uyoryo	Clay ironstone
Yu Mi Xin	***Zea mays***	Medulla Zeae	Yuk Mai Sam		Corn cob
Yu Mi Xu, Yu Mi Rui	***Zea mays***	Stylus Zeae	Yuk Mai So, Yuk Mai Yeui	Gyokuma-ishu	Cornsilk style
Yu Nao Shi	***Pseudosciaena crocea, P. polyactis, Sciaena schlegeli***	Otozithum Sciaenae	Yu Nou Sek		Fish otolith
Yu Qian	***Ulmus pumila***	Cortex Ulmi pumilae	Yu Chin		White elm bark
Yu Shu Shu	***Zea mays***	Fructus Zeae	Yuk Suk Syu		Corn grain
Yu Tou Gen	***Colocasia esculenta***	Radix Colocasiae	Wu Tau Gan		Taro root
Yu Xing Cao	***Houttuynia cordata***	Herba Houttuyniae	Yu Seng Chou	Juyakuso	Fishwort herb

MANDARIN	SCIENTIFIC	PHARMACEUTICAL	CANTONESE	JAPANESE	ENGLISH
Yu Zhu	***Polygonatum odoratum*** var. ***pluriflorum, P. plurifolium***	Rhizoma Polygonati odorati	Yuk Juk	Gyokuchiku	Fragrant Solomon's seal root
Yuan Bao Cao	***Hypericum sampsonii***	Herba Hyperici sampsonii	Yun Bou Chou		South China St. John's wort herb
Yuan Hu	***Corydalis yanhusuo***	Rizoma Corydalis yanhusuoidis	Yun Wu	Engosaku	Asian corydalis corm
Yuan Hua	***Daphne genkwa***	Flos Daphnis genkwae	Yun Fa	Genka	Lilac daphne flower
Yuan Shen	***Scrophularia ningpoensis, S. buergeriana***	Radix Scrophulariae ningpoensis	Yun Sam	Genjin	Black figwort root
Yuan Wei	***Iris tectorum***	Rhizoma Iris tectoris	Yun Mei		Kite-tail iris root
Yuan Zhi	***Polygala tenuifolia***	Radix Polygalae	Yun Ji	Onji	Thin-leaf milkwort root
Yue Ji Gen	***Rosa chinensis***	Radix Rosae chinensis	Yut Gwai Gan		Moonseason rose root
Yue Ji Hua	***Rosa chinensis***	Gemma Rosae chinensis	Yut Gwai Fa	Gekkika	Moonseason rose bud
Yun Mu Shi	***Muscovitum***	Muscovitum	Wan Mou Sek		Muscovite
Yun Xiang Cao	***Cymbopogon distans***	Herba Cymbopogonis distansis	Yun Heung Chou		Distant lemongrass herb
Yun Zhi	***Coriolus versicolor*** (syn. ***Trametes versicolor)***	Sclerotium Corioli versicolori	Wan Ji		Turkey tail mushroom
Zang Qie	***Anisodus tanguticus***	Redix seu semen Anisodi	Jong Ke		Anisodus root or seed
Zao Fan, Lu Fan	***Melanteritum***	Melanteritum	Jou Faan		Green vitriol
Zao Jiao Ci	***Gleditsia sinensis* and spp**	Spina Gleditsiae	Jou Gok Chi	Sokakushi	Honeylocust spine
Zao Jiao Zi	***Gleditsia sinensis* and spp.**	Semen Gleditsiae	Jou Gok Ji		Honeylocust fruit
Zao Jiao, Zao Jia	***Gleditsia sinensis* and spp**	Fructus Gleditsiae	Jou Gok, Jou Gaap	Sokaku	Honeylocust pod
Ze Lan	***Lycopus lucidus***	Herba Lycopi	Jaak Laan	Takuran	Bright bugleweed herb
Ze Qi	***Euphorbia helioscopia***	Herba Euphorbiaeheliosc opiae	Jaak Chat	Takushitsu	Sunspurge herb
Ze Xie	***Alisma orientalis***	Rhizoma Alismae	Jaak Se	Takusha	Water plantain root
Zhang Mu	***Cinnamomum camphora***	Lignum Cinnamomi camphorae	Jeung Muk		Camphor wood
Zhang Nao	***Cinnamomum camphora***	Camphora	Jeung Naau	Shono	Camphor flake
Zhang Ye Ban Xia, Wu Zhang Nan Xing	***Pinellia pedatisecta***	Rhizoma Pinelliae pedatisectae	Jeung Yip Bun Ha, Fu Jeung Lam Sing		Pedatisect pinellia corm
Zhe Bei Mu	***Fritillaria thunbergii***	Bulbus Fritillariae thunbergii	Chit Bui Mou	Setsubaimo	Zhejiang fritillary bulb
Zhe Tong Pi	***Zanthoxylum ailanthoides***	Cortex Zanthoxyli ailanthoidis	Jit Tung Pei		Zhejiang prickly ash bark
Zhen Zhu	***Pteria margaritiferae***	Fructus conchae Pteriae	Chan Ju	Shinju	Pearl

MANDARIN	SCIENTIFIC	PHARMACEUTICAL	CANTONESE	JAPANESE	ENGLISH
Zhen Zhu Mu	***Pteria margaritifera*** and spp	Concha Pteriae	Chan Ju Mou		Mother of pearl shell
Zhi Gan Cao	***Glycirrhiza uralensis, G. glabra*** and spp	Radix Glycirrhizae preparatae	Jek Gam Chou	Shakanzo	Honey-fried licorice root
Zhi Ju Zi	***Hovenia dulcis***	Semen et fructus Hoveniae	Ji Gwat Ji		Hovenia seed and fruit
Zhi Ke, Zhi Qiao, Dai Dai Hua Zhi Qiao	***Citrus aurantium*** var. ***amara***	Fructus Citri aurantii amarae	Ji Hok, Doi Doi Fa Ji Hok	Kikoku	Ripe bitter orange fruit
Zhi Ma Qian Zi	***Strychnos pierrana, S. nux-vomica*** and spp	Semen Strychnotis preparatae	Ma Chin Ji	Basenshi	Prepared vomit nut
Zhi Mu	***Anemarrhena asphodeloides***	Radix Anemarrhenae	Ji Mou	Chimo	Know mother root
Zhi Pao	***Thladiantha dubia***	Fructus Thladianthae	Chek Pau		Thladiantha fruit
Zhi Shi	***Catalpa ovata***	Fructus Catalpae	San Sat	Kisasage	Catalpa fruit
Zhi Shi	***Citrus aurantium, C. wilsonii***	Fructus Citri aurantii immaturi	Ji Sat	Kijitsu	Unripe bitter orange fruit
Zhi Xie Mu Pi	***Holarrhenia antidysenterica***	Cortex Holarrheniae	Ji Se Muk Pei		Conessi bark
Zhi Zi, Shan Zhi Zi	***Gardenia jasminoides***	Fructus Gardeniae	Ji Ji, Saan Ji Ji	Sanshishi	Gardenia pod
Zhong Lou, Qi Ye Yi Zhi Hua	***Paris chinensis***	Rhizoma Paris chinensis	Jung Lau, Chat Yip Yat Ji Pa		Chinese paris root
Zhong Lou, Yun Nan Zhong Lou	***Paris yunnanensis***	Rhizoma Paris yunnanensis	Jung Lau, Wan Laam Jung Lau		Yunnan paris root
Zhu Dan	***Sus scrofa domestica***	Fel Suidis	Ju Daam		Pig gallbladder
Zhu Er Shen	***Panax major, P. repens***	Radix Panacis majoris	Ju Yi Sam		Pearl ginseng root
Zhu Jie (Ren) Shen	***Panax japonicus***	Radix Panacis japonici	Juk Jit (Yan) Sam	Tikusetu-ninjin	Japanese ginseng root
Zhu Li	***Phyllostachys nigra*** var. ***henonis*** and spp	Succus Phyllostachis	Juk Lai	Chikureki	Black bamboo sap
Zhu Ling	***Polyporus umbellatus***	Sclerotium Polypori	Ju Ling	Chorei	Umbel polypore mushroom
Zhu Long Cao	***Nepenthes mirabilis***	Herba Nepenthis	Jyu Lung Chou		Pitcher plant herb
Zhu Ma Gen	***Boehmeria nivea***	Radix Boehmeriae	Chyu Ma Gan		Ramie root
Zhu Mao Cai	***Salsola collina, S. ruthenica, S. richteri***	Radix et herba Salsolae	Jyu Mou Choi		Salsola root and herb
Zhu Ru	***Phyllostachys nigra*** var. ***henonis*** and spp	Caulis Phyllostachis in taeniis	Juk Yu	Chikujo	Black bamboo shaving
Zhu Sha	***Cinnabarum***	Cinnabarum	Ju Sa	Shusha	Cinnabar
Zhu Ye	***Phyllostachys nigra*** var. ***henonis*** and spp	Folium Phyllostachis	Juk Yip		Black bamboo leaf
Zhu Ye Jiao	***Zanthoxylum planispinum***	Fructus Zanthoxyli planispini	Juk Yip Jiu		Prickly ash berry
Zhu Zi Ye	***Quercus salicina, Q. myrsinae-folium***	Folium Querci	Jyu Ji	Urajirokashi	Oak leaf
Zi Bai Pi, Qiu Mu Pi	***Catalpa bungei***	Cortex Catalpae	San Baak Pei, Chau Muk Pei		Catalpa bark

MANDARIN	SCIENTIFIC	PHARMACEUTICAL	CANTONESE	JAPANESE	ENGLISH
Zi Bei Tian Kuei, Hong Tian Kui	***Begonia fimbristipula***	Herba Begoniae fimbristipulae	Ji Mai Tin Kwai, Hung Tin Kwai		Begonia herb
Zi Cai	***Porphyra tenera***	Herba Porphyrae	Ji Choi		Porphyra herb
Zi Cao	***Lithospermum erythrorhizon***	Radix Lithospermi	Ji Chou	Shikon	Purple groomwell root
Zi Cao	***Macrotomia euchroma***	Radix Macrotomiae	Ji Chou	Shikon	Macrotomia root
Zi Cao	***Onosma paniculatum***	Radix Onosmae	Ji Chou		Onosma root
Zi Cao Rong	***Lithospermum erythrorhizon***	Flos Lithospermi	Ji Chou Yan		Purple groomwell flower
Zi Cao, Xin Jiang Zi Cao	***Arnebia euchroma, A. guttata***	Radix Arnebiae	Ji Chou, San Geung Ji Chou	Shikon	Arnebia root
Zi He Che	***Homo sapiens***	Placenta Hominis	Ji Ho Je	Shikasha	Human placenta
Zi Hua Di Ding	***Viola yedoensis, V. japonica***	Radix et herba Violae yedoensis	Ji Fa Dei Ding	Shikajicho	Asian violet root and herb
Zi Jin Niu, Jin Niu Cao	***Ardisia japonica***	Radix et herba Ardisiae japonicae	Ji Gam Ngau		Marlberry root and herb
Zi Jing Pi	***Cercis chinensis***	Cortex Cercis	Ji Ging Pei		Chinese redbud bark
Zi Jing Pi	***Kadsura peltigera***	Cortex Kadsurae peltigerae	Ji Ging Pei		Chinese redbud bark
Zi Ran Tong	***Pyritum***	Pyritum	Ji Yin Tung	Shizendo	Pyrite
Zi Shi Ying	***Fluoritum***	Fluoritum	Ji Sek Ying		Purple fluorite
Zi Su Geng	***Perilla frutescens***	Ramulus Perillae	Sou Gan		Perilla stem
Zi Su Ye	***Perilla frutescens***	Folium Perillae	Sou Yip	Shisoyo	Perilla leaf
Zi Su Zi	***Perilla frutescens***	Fructus Perillae	Sou Ji	Soshi	Perilla seed
Zi Tan	***Pterocarpus indicus***	Lignum Pterocarpi	Ji Taan		Malay padauk wood, Burma rosewood
Zi Teng Zi, Teng Liu	***Wisteria sinensis, W. floribunda***	Galla Wisteriae	Ji Tang Ji, Tang Lau	Figikobu	Asian wisteria gall
Zi Wan	***Aster tataricus***	Radix Asteris tatarici	Ji Yun	Shion	Tartary aster root
Zi Zhu Gen	***Phyllostachys nigra*** **var.** ***henonis*** **and spp**	Radix Phyllostachis	Ji Juk Gan		Black bamboo root
Zi Zhu Ye	***Callicarpa pedunculata***	Folium Callicarpae pedunculatae	Ji Jyu Yip	Jijuso	Callicarpa leaf
Zi Zhu Ye, Ta Ye Zi Zhu	***Callicarpa macrophylla***	Folium Callicarpae macrophyllae	Ji Jyu Yip, Daai Yip Ji Jyu		Large-leaf Callicarpa leaf
Zong Lu Pi Tan	***Trachycarpus excelsa, T. fortunei***	Fibra Stipulae Trachycarpi carbonisata	Jung Leui Pei Daan		Charred windmill palm petiole
Zong Lu Zi	***Trachycarpus excelsa, T. fortunei***	Fructus Trachycarpi	Jung Leui Ji		Windmill palm seed
Zou Ma Tai	***Ardisia gigantifolia***	Rhizoma Ardisiae gigantifoliae	Jau Ma Toi		Ardisia root
Zu Shi Ma	***Daphne giraldii, D. tangutica, D. retusa***	Cortex Daphnis giraldii	Jou Si Ma		Giraldi's daphne bark
Zuan Di Feng	***Schizophragma integrifolium***	Cortex radicis Schizophragmae	Jyun Dei Fung		Schizophrag-ma root bark

Cross Index of Cantonese Remedy Names

CANTONESE	SCIENTIFIC	PHARMACEUTICAL	MANDARIN	JAPANESE	ENGLISH
	Agate	Agate	Ma Nao		Agate
	Androsaca umbellata	Herba Androsacae	Dian Di Mei		Androsaca herb
	Armillaria mellea	Sclerotium Armillariae	Mi Huan Jun		Honey mushroom
	Arsenicum album	Arsenolitum	Pi Shi, Xin Shi		White arsenic
	Bauhinia paraglauca	Herba Bauhiniae paraglaucae	Hu Die Cao		Green bauhinia herb
	Gallus gallus domesticus	Membrana follicularis ovi	Feng Huang Yi		Chicken egg membrane
	Grifola frondosa	Sclerotium Grifolae frondosae		Maitake	Hen of the woods mushroom
	Hericium erinaceus	Sclerotium Hericii	Hou Gu		Hedgehog fungus
	Hypericum chinense	Herba Hyperici Chinensis	Jin Si Tao		Chinese St. John's wort herb
	Oryza sativa	Saccharum Oryzae		Koi	Rice malt (syrup)
	Panthera	Os Leopardis	Bao Gu		Leopard bone
	Prunus persica, P. davidiana	Fructus persicae immaturi	Bi Tao Gan		Unripe peach fruit
	Pyritum rotundum	Pyritum rotundum	She Han Shi		Iron pyrite
	Raphanus sativus	Radix Raphani	Di Gu Luo		Radish root
	Rhodea japonica	Herba Rhodeae	Wan Nian Xing		Rhodea herb
	Rosa polyantha and spp.	Radix Rosae polyanthae	Qiang Wei Gen		Polyanth rose root
	Sambucus japonicus	Cortex Sambuci japonici	Lu Ying	Rakutokuda	Japanese elder bark
	Syringa manchuriensis	Cortex Syringae	Bao Ma Zi		Manchurian lilac bark
	Terminalia chebula and var.	Fructus Terminaliae immaturi	Cang Qing Guo		Unripe myrobalan fruit
	Thalictrum foliolosum	Herba Thalictri	Tang Song Cao		Meadow rue herb
	Tilia cordata	Flos Tiliae	Duan Shu Hua		Linden flower
A Ma Ji	*Linum usitatissimum*	Semen Lini	Ya Ma Zi		Flax seed
A Ngai	*Ferula foetida*	Resina Ferulae (Asafoetidae)	A Wei	Agi	Asafoetida resin
Am Leui Ji	*Artemisia keiskeana*	Fructus Artemisiae keiskeanae	An Lu Zi		Keiskeana mugwort seed
Au Dong Gwai	*Ligusticum levisticum*	Radix Ligustici levistici	Ou Dang Gui		Garden lovage root
Au Man	*Gelsemium elegans*	Radix Gelsemii	Gou Wen		Chinese gelsemium
Ba Dau	*Croton tiglium*	Semen Crotonis	Ba Dou		Croton seed
Ba Gik Tin	*Morinda officinalis*	Radix Morindae	Ba Ji Tian	Hagekiten	Morinda root
Ba Gok Lin	*Podophyllum pleianthum*	Rhizoma Podophylli pleianthi	Ba Jiao Lian		Pleianth podophyllum root

CANTONESE	SCIENTIFIC	PHARMACEUTICAL	MANDARIN	JAPANESE	ENGLISH
Ba Jiu Gan	*Musa basjoo*	Caudex Musae	Ba Jiao Gen		Ryukyu banana root
Baai Jeung Chou	*Patrinia scabiosaefolia, P. villosa*	Herba et rhizoma Patriniae	Bai Jiang Cao	Haishoso	Patrinia herb and root
Baak Bin Dau	*Dolichos lablab*	Semen Dolichis	Bai Bian Dou	Hakuhenzu	Hyacinth bean
Baak Bou, Chek Lap Baak Bou	*Stemona sessilifolia*	Radix Stemonae sessilifoliae	Bai Bu, Zhi Li Bai Bu		Sessile stemona root
Baak Bou, Deui Yip Baak Bou	*Stemona tuberosa*	Radix Stemonae tuberosae	Bai Bu, Dui Ye Bai Bu		Tuberous stemona root
Baak Bou, Maan Sang Baak Bou	*Stemona japonia*	Radix Stemonae japonicae	Bai Bu, Man Sheng Bai Bu	Hyakubu	Japanese stemona root
Baak Cheuk (Yeuk)	*Paeonia lactiflora*	Radix Paeoniae lactiflorae	Bai Shao (Yao)	Byakushaku-(yaku)	White peony root
Baak Chin	*Cynanchum stauntoni, C. glaucescens*	Radix et rhizoma Cynanchi stauntoni	Bai Qian	Byakuzen	Prime white root
Baak Chin Chang	*Melaleuca leucadendron*	Folium Melaleucae leucadendronis	Bai Qian Ceng		Cajeput leaf
Baak Chou Sheung		Pulvus fumi carbonisati	Bai Cao Shuang		Boiler or chimney soot
Baak Dau Kau	*Amomum cardamomum*	Fructus Amomi cardamomi	Bai Dou Kou	Byakuzuku	Cluster cardamom pod
Baak Dau Kau Fa, Dau Kau Fa	*Amomum cardamomum*	Flos Amomi cardamomi	(Bai) Dou Kou Hua	Byakuzu-kuka	Cluster cardamom flower
Baak Fa Daan	*Plumbago zeylanicum*	Herba Plumbaginis	Hei Mian Ma, Bai Hua Dan		Ceylon leadwort
Baak Fa Ji Chou, Fu Ngao Wong	*Leucas mollissima*	Herba Leuci	Bai Hua Zi Cao, Hu Yao Huang		Leucas herb
Baak Fa Se	*Agkistrodon acutus* and *Bungarus multicinctus*	Agkistrodon seu Bungarus	Bai Hua She	Hakkada	Multibanded krait
Baak Fa Se Sit Chou	*Oldenlandia diffusa*	Herba Oldenlandiae	Bai Hua She She Cao	Byakkaja-zesso	Snaketongue grass herb
Baak Fu Ji	*Typhonium giganteum*	Rhizoma Typhonii gigantei preparata	Bai Fu Zi, Yu Bai Fu	Byakubushi	Prepared giant typhonium root
Baak Fu Ji, Gwan Baak Fu Ji	*Aconitum coreanum*	Rhizoma Aconiti coreani	Bai Fu Zi, Guan Bai Fu		Prepared Korean aconite root
Baak Gaai Ji	*Sinapis alba*	Semen Sinapis albae	Bai Jie Zi		White mustard seed
Baak Gaau Heung	*Liquidambar taiwaniana*	Resina Liquidambaris taiwaninanae	Bai Jiao Xiang		Taiwan maple fruit resin
Baak Gap	*Bletilla striata*	Rhizoma Bletillae	Bai Ji	Byakukyu	Amethyst orchid root
Baak Geung Daan	*Hydragyrum chloratum*	Compositum hydragyri chlorati	Bai Jiang Dan		Mercury chloride
Baak Gwo, Ngan Hang Wat	*Ginkgo biloba*	Fructus Ginkgoidis	Bai Guo, Yin Xing He	Ginkyo	Ginkgo nut
Baak Hang Yan	*Prunus armeniaca* and var.	Semen Pruni armeniacae	Xing Ren, Ku Xing Ren	Kyonin	Bitter apricot kernel
Baak Hap	*Lilium brownii* var. *colchesteri*	Bulbus Lilii	Bai He	Hyakugo	Brown's lily bulb
Baak Hap Fa	*Lilium brownii* var. *colchesteri*	Flos Lilii	Bai He Hua		Brown's lily flower

CANTONESE	SCIENTIFIC	PHARMACEUTICAL	MANDARIN	JAPANESE	ENGLISH
Baak Hap Gan	*Lilium brownii* var. *colchesteri*	Radix Lilii	Bai He Gen		Brown's lily root
Baak Hap, Gyun Daan	*Lilium lancifolium*	Bulbus Liliii lancifolii	Bai He, Juan Duan		Lance-leaf lily bulb
Baak Jat Lai	*Tribulus terrestris*	Fructus Tribuli	Bai Ji Li	Byakishitsuri	Caltrop fruit
Baak Ji	*Angelica dahurica, A. anomala, A. taiwaniana*	Radix Angelicae dahuricae	Bai Zhi	Byakushi	White angelica Root
Baak Ji Yan	*Biota orientalis*	Semen Biotae orientalis	Bai Zi Ren	Hakushinin	Oriental arborvitae berry
Baak Laan Fa	*Michelia alba*	Flos Micheliae	Bai Lan Hua		White champac flower
Baak Leung Gam	*Ardisia crispa*	Herba Ardisiae crispae	Bai Liang Jin		Crisp ardisia herb
Baak Lim	*Ampelopsis japonica*	Radix Ampelopsis	Bai Lian	Byakuran	Japanese peppervine root
Baak Lin Fa	*Nelumbo nucifera*	Flos Nelumbinis	Bai Lian Hua		Lotus flower
(Baak) Long Duk	*Euphorbia pallasii, E. abracteolatae, E. fischerianae*	Radix Euphorbiae pallasii seu ebracteolatae	(Bai) Lang Du		White spurge root
Baak Lung Chyun Gan	*Clerodendron paniculatum*	Radix Clerodendronis paniculati	Bai Long Chuan Gen		Panicled clerodendron root
Baak Maau Fa	*Imperata cylindrica* var. *major*	Flos Imperatae	Bai Mao Hua		Woolly grass flower
Baak Maau Gan	*Imperata cylindrica* var. *major*	Rhizoma Imperatae	Bai Mao Gen	Bokon	Woolly grass root
Baak Mei	*Cynanchum atratum, C. versicolor*	Radix Cynanchi atrati	Bai Wei	Byakubi	Swallow-wort root
Baak Ming Fung	*Trichosporum acuminatum*	Herba Trichospori	Bai Mian Feng		Trichosporum herb
Baak Mou Ha Fu Chou, Gan Gwat Chou	*Ajuga decumbens*	Herba Ajugae	Bai Mao Xia Ku Cao, Jing Gu Cao		Bugleweed herb
Baak Mui	*Prunus mume*	Fructus Mumis immaturis preparatae	Bai Mei		Unripe prepared black plum fruit
Baak Muk Tong	*Akebia quinata, A. trifoliata*	Caulis Akebiae	Mu Tong, Bai Mu Tong	Mokutsu	Akebia stem
Baak Muk Yi	*Tremella fuciformis*	Sclerotium Tremellae fucimormis	Bai Mu Er	Hakumokuji	Silver ear mushroom
Baak Ngao Sat	*Cuccubala baccifer*	Radix Cuccubalae bacciferis	Bai Niu Xi		White oxknee root
Baak Ngau Daam	*Inula cappa*	Herba Inulae cappae	Bai Niu Dan, Bai Mian Feng		Goatear herb
Baak Pou Geung	*Buddleia asiatica*	Radix Buddleiae asiaticae	Bai Pu Jiang		Asian Buddleia root
Baak Sam	*Panax ginseng*	Radix Panacis ginsengis praeparatae	Bai Shen	Hakujin	Rock candy cured Asian ginseng root
Baak Sau Wu, Ngau Pei Siu	*Cynanchum auriculatum*	Radix Cynanchi auriculati	Bai Shou Wu, Niu Pi Xiao		Auricle dogbane root
Baak Sek Ji	*Halloysitum album*	Halloysitum album	Bai Shi Zhi		White kaolin

CANTONESE	SCIENTIFIC	PHARMACEUTICAL	MANDARIN	JAPANESE	ENGLISH
Baak Seut	*Atractylodes macrocephala*	Rhizoma Atractylodis macrocephalae	Bai Zhu	Byakujutsu	White atractylodes root
Baak Sin Pei	*Dictamnus dasycarpus*	Cortex radicis Dictamni	Bai Xian Pi	Hakusempi	Asian dittany root bark
Baak Tau Yung	*Pulsatilla chinensis, P. cernua, P. turczaninovii, P. ambigua* and spp	Radix Pulsatillae	Bai Tou Weng	Hakutoo	Asian pasqueflower root
Baak Tau Yung, Ing On Baak Tau Yung	*Pulsatilla dahurica*	Radix Pulsatillae dahuricae	Bai Tou Weng, Xing An Bai Tou Weng		Dahurian pasqueflower root
Baak Wat Choi	*Chelidonium majus* var. *asiaticum*	Herba Chelidonii	Bai Qu Cai	Hakkutusai	Asian celandine herb
Baak Ying, Baak Mou Tang	*Solanum lyratum*	Herba Solani lyrati	Bai Ying, Shu Yang Quan, Bai Mao Teng		Climbing nightshade herb
Baan Laam Gan	*Isatis tinctoria, I. indigotica*	Radix Isatis tinctoriae	Ban Lan Gen		Woad root
Baat Gok Fung	*Alangium chinense*	Radix Alangii	Ba Jiao Feng		Alangium root
Baat Gok Lin	*Dysosma pleiantha*	Rhizoma Dysosmae pleianthae	Ba Jiao Lian		Pleianth dysosma root
Baat Gok Wui Heung	*Illicium verum*	Fructus Illicii	Ba Jiao Hui Xiang		Star anise fruit
Baat Lei Ma	*Rhododendron molle*	Fructus Rhododendris mollis	Ba Li Ma		Yellow azalea fruit
Baat Sin Chou	*Galium aparine*	Herba Galii aparinis	Ba Xian Cao, Zhu Yang Yang		Cleavers herb
Baat Sin Fa	*Hydrangea macrophylla*	Flos Hydrangeae	Ba Xian Hua		French hydrangea flower
Baat Yut Jaat, Yu Ji Ji	*Akebia quinata*	Fructus Akebiae	Ba Yue Zha, Yu Zhi Zi		Akebia fruit
Bai La	*Ficus pumila*	Fructus Fici pumilae	Bi Li, Mu Man Tou		Creeping fig fruit
Bak Sai San	*Asarum heterotropoides*	Herba Asari heterotropoidis	Xi Xin, Bei Xi Xin		Northern wild ginger root
Bak Yan Chan	*Artemisia scoparia*	Herba Artemisiae scopariae	Bei Yin Chen		Northern wormwood herb
Ban Long	*Areca catechu, A. dicksonii*	Semen Arecae catechu	Bing Lang	Binroji	Betel nut
Ban Long Fa	*Areca catechu, A. dicksonii*	Flos Arecae catechu	Bing Lang Hua	Binroka	Betel nut flower
Ban Mou	*Cantharis vesicatoria*	Cantharis	Ban Mao	Hanmyo	Cantharides
Ban Mou	*Mylabris*	Mylabris	Ban Mao	Hanmyo	Asian cantharides
Bat Ching Ke	*Litsea cubeba*	Fructus Litseae	Bi Cheng Qie		Cubeb peppercorn
Bat Jai Chou	*Pogonatherum crinitum*	Herba Pogonatheri	Bi Zi Cao		Golden Hair grass
Bat Pa	*Piper longum*	Fructus Piperis longis	Bi Ba	Hihatsu	Long pepper fruit spike
Bat Tung Chou	*Equisetum ramosissimum*	Herba Equiseti ramosissimi	Bi Tong Cao		Ramose horsetail herb
Bau Bin Ling	*Lobelia chinensis*	Herba et radix Lobeliae chinensis	Ban Bian Lian	Hanbanren	Rooting lobelia herb and root
Be Jau Fa	*Humulus lupulus*	Flos Humuli lupuli	Pi Jiu Hua		Hops flower

CANTONESE	SCIENTIFIC	PHARMACEUTICAL	MANDARIN	JAPANESE	ENGLISH
Bei Gaai, Fan Bei Gaai	*Dioscorea hypoglauca*	Rhizoma Dioscoreae hypoglaucae	Bi Xie, Fen Bi Xie, Bei Xie	Hikai	Long yam root
Bei Gaai, Min Bei Gaai	*Dioscorea septemloba*	Rhizoma Dioscoreae septemlobae	Bi Xie, Mian Bi Xie		Seven-lobe yam root
Bei Ma Ji	*Ricinus communis*	Semen Ricini	Bi Ma Zi		Castor bean
Bin Chuk	*Polygonum aviculare*	Herba Polygoni avicularis	Bian Xu	Henchiku	Knotgrass herb
Bin Dau Fa	*Dolichos lablab*	Gemma Dolichis	Bian Dou Hua	Henzuka	Hyacinth bean bud
Bin Dau Yi	*Dolichos lablab*	Testa Dolichoris	Bian Dou Yi		Hyacinth bean capsule
Bin Gei Sang	*Viscum liquidambaricum*	Ramulus Visci liquidambarici	Bian Ji Sheng		Asian mistletoe twig
Bing Pin	*Dryobalanops camphora*	Borneolum	Bing Pian	Ryuno	Borneo camphor
Bit Gaap	*Amyda sinensis, Trionix sinensis*	Carapax Amydae seu Trionis	Bie Jia	Bekko	Asian soft-shell turtle shell
Bok Gwat Daam	*Gendarussa vulgaris*	Herba Gendarussae	Bo Gu Dan		Gendarussa herb
Bok Ho	*Mentha arvensis*	Herba Menthae arvensis	Bo He	Hakka	Asian fieldmint herb
Bok Lok Wui	*Macleaya cordata*	Herba Macleayae	Bo Luo Hui		Plum poppy herb
Bou Geung	*Zingiber officinalis*	Rhizoma Zingiberis	Pao Jiang	Hokyo	Quick-fried ginger root
Bou Gwat Ji	*Psoralea corylifolia*	Fructus Psoraleae	Bu Gu Zhi	Hokotsushi	Scurf pea berry
Bou Jai Yip	*Microcos paniculata*	Folium Microcotis	Bu Zha Ye		Microcos leaf
Bun Daai Hoi	*Sterculia staphigera, S. lychnophera*	Semen Sterculiae	Pang Da Hai	Bantaikai	Sterculia seed
Bun Fung Ho Gan	*Pterospermum heterophyllum*	Radix Pterospermi	Ban Feng He Gen		Pterospermum root
Bun Ha Chau	*Pinellia ternata*	Rhizoma Pinelliae fermentatae	Ban Xia Qu		Fermented Pinellia corm
Bun Ha, Faat Bun Ha	*Pinellia ternata*	Rhizoma Pinelliae ternatae preparatae	Ban Xia Fa Ban Xia	Hange, Kohange	Prepared pinellia corm
Bun Ji Lin	*Scutellaria barbata, B. rivularis*	Radix et herba Scutellariae barbatae	Ban Zhi Lian		Barbed skullcap root and herb
But Chai	*Heleocharis plantaginea*	Herba Heleocharis	Bi Qi	Bossai	Water chestnut herb
Cha Si Wong	*Stellaria aquatica*	Herba Stellariae aquaticae	Cha Chi Huang		Water chickweed herb
Cha Yip	*Camellia sinensis*	Folium Camelliae sinensis	Cha Ye	Fujucha, Chayo	Tea leaf
Chaai Wu	*Bupleurum chinense, B. falcatum, B. longiradiatum* and spp	Radix Bupleuri	Chai Hu	Saiko	Asian buplever root
Chaai Wu, Hap Yip Chaai Wu	*Bupleurum scorzonerifolium*	Radix Bupleuri scorzonerifolii	Chai Hu, Xia Ye Chai Hu		Thin-leaf buplever root
Chaam Sa	*Bombyx mori*	Excrementum Bombicis	Can Sha	Sansha	Silkworm dropping
Chai Choi	*Capsella bursa-pastoris*	Herba Capsellae	Ji Cai	Seisai	Shepherd's purse herb

CANTONESE	SCIENTIFIC	PHARMACEUTICAL	MANDARIN	JAPANESE	ENGLISH
Chai Chou	*Holotrichia diomphalia*	Holotrichia	Qi Cao		June beetle grub (larva)
Chai Ni	*Adenophora trachelioides, A. remotifolia*	Radix Adenophorae trachelioidis	Ji Ni		Common harebell root
Chai Pan Chou	*Sedum sarmentosum*	Radix et herba Sedi sarmentosi	Chui Pen Cao		Stringy stonecrop root and herb
Chak Yip Jek Ji Fa, Sat Yau	*Paris polyphylla, P. chinensis, P. formosana* and var.	Rhizoma Paris	Qi Ye Yi Zhi Hua, Zao Xiu	Kenjin	Paris root
Cham Gwat Fung, Min Mou Ma Dou Ling	*Aristolochia mollissima*	Herba Aristolochiae mollissimae	Xun Gu Feng, Mian Mao Ma Dou Ling		Soft birthwort herb
Cham Heung	*Aquilaria agallocha, A. sinensis*	Lignum Aquilariae	Chen Xiang	Jinko	Aloeswood
Chan (Baak) Pei	*Ailanthus altissima*	Cortex Ailanthi	Chun (Bai) Pi		Tree of heaven bark
Chan Bu Chi	*Cypraea moneta, C. macula* and spp	Concha Cypraeae	Bei Zi		Cowrie shell
Chan Gan Pei	*Ailanthus altissima*	Cortex radicis Ailanthi	Chun Gen Pi		Tree of heaven root bark
Chan Ju	*Pteria margaritiferae*	Fructus conchae Pteriae	Zhen Zhu	Shinju	Pearl
Chan Ju Mou	*Pteria margaritifera* and spp	Concha Pteriae	Zhen Zhu Mu		Mother of pearl shell
Chan Pei, Gwat Pei	*Citrus reticulata, C. tangerina, C. erythrosa*	Pericarpium Citri reticulatae	Chen Pi, Ju Pi	Chimpi	Ripe tangerine rind
Chan Sa	*Ferrum*	Pulvis ferri	Chen Sha		Black iron oxide
Chan Sek Wei	*Calcaria*	Calcaria	Chen Shi Hui		Calcium hydroxide
Chat Gu Chou	*Sagina japonica*	Herba Saginae	Qi Gu Cao		Japanese pearlwort herb
Chat Lei Heung	*Buddleia lindleyana*	Radix Buddleiae lindleyanae	Qi Li Xiang		Buddleia root
Chat Lei Heung	*Pittosporum pentandrum*	Radix Pittospori	Qi Li Xiang		Pittosporum root
Chat Sing Chou	*Polypodium hastatum*	Herba Polypodii	Qi Xing Cao		Polypody herb
Chat Yip Lin	*Schefflera arboricola, S. kwangsiensis, S. venulosa*	Folium et caulis Schefflerae	Qi Ye Lian		Taiwan schefflera leaf and stem
Chau Chou	*Ruta graveolens*	Herba Rutae	Chou Cao		Rue herb
Chau Maau Daan	*Clerodendron bungei*	Folium Clerodendronis bungeis	Chou Mu Dan		Bung's Clerodendron leaf
Chau Ng Tung (Yip)	*Clerodendron trichotomum*	Folium Clerodendronis trichotomi	Chou Wu Tong (Ye)		Forked glorybower leaf
Che Chin Chou	*Plantago asiatica, P. depressa* and spp	Folium Plantaginis	Che Qian Cao	Shazenso	Asian plantain leaf
Che Chin Ji	*Plantago asiatica, P. depressa* and spp	Semen Plantaginis	Che Qian Zi	Shazenshi	Asian plantain seed

CANTONESE	SCIENTIFIC	PHARMACEUTICAL	MANDARIN	JAPANESE	ENGLISH
Chek Cheuk (Yeuk)	*Paeonia lactiflora, P. obovata, P. veitchii*	Radix Paeoniae rubrae	Chi Shao (Yao)	Sekishaku-(yaku)	Red peony root
Chek Fuk Ling	*Poria cocos*	Sclerotium Poriae rubrae	Chi Fu Ling	Sekibikuryo	Red hoelen
Chek Pau	*Thladiantha dubia*	Fructus Thladianthae	Zhi Pao		Thladiantha fruit
Chek Sek Chi	*Halloysitum rubrum*	Halloysitum	Chi Shi Zhi	Shakusekishi	Red kaolin
Chek Sek Gou	*Gypsum fibrosum*	Gypsum dehydratum	Shu Shi Gao		Dehydrated gypsum
Chek Sek Ji	*Halloysitum rubrum*	Halloysitum	Shu Chi Shi		Roasted red kaolin
Chek Siu Dau	*Phaseolus calcaratus, P. angularis*	Semen Phaseoli calcarati	Chi Xiao Dou	Sekishozu	Aduki bean
Cheui Cheung Hing	*Cynanchum paniculatum*	Radix et herba Cynanchi paniculati	Xu Chang Qing, Liao Diao Zhu		Panicled dogbane root and herb
Cheui Cheung Hing	*Pycnostelma paniculatum*	Herba Pycnostelmae	Shan Diao Zhu, Xu Chang Jing		Paniculate swallowwort herb
Cheui Chung Guk	*Pyrethrum cinerariifolium*	Flos Pyrethri	Chu Chong Ju		Dalmatia pellitory flower
Cheun Gau	*Gentiana macrophylla, G. tibetica, G. daburica* and spp	Radix Gentianae macrophyllae	Qin Jiao	Jingyo	Large-leaf gentian root
Cheun Pei	*Fraxinus rhynchophyllae, F. bungeana, F. chinensis* and spp	Cortex Fraxini	Qin Pi		Korean ash bark
Cheung Cheun Fa	*Catharanthus roseus*	Radix et herba Catharanthi	Chang Chun Hua		Madagascar periwinkle root and herb
Chi Beng Sheung	*Diospyros kaki*	Saccharum Diospyris	Shi Bing Shuang		Persimmon frost
Chi Daai	*Homo sapiens*	Funis umbilici Hominis	Qi Dai		Umbilical cord
Chi Dai	*Diospyros kaki*	Calyx Diospyri	Shi Di	Shitei	Persimmon calyx
Chi Fung Fa	*Euphorbia milii*	Herba Euphorbiae milii	Ci Peng Hua		Prickly spurge herb
Chi Gei Sang	*Taxillus yadoriki, T. chinensis*	Ramulus Taxilli	Shi Ji Sheng		Asian mistletoe twig
Chi Ng Ga (Gan Pei)	*Eleutherococcus senticosus*	Radix seu cortex radicis Eleutherococci senticosi	Ci Wu Jia (Gen Pi)		Eleuthero ginseng root
Chi Sek	*Magnetitum*	Magnetitum	Ci Shi		Magnetite
Chi Shuen Bing	*Diospyros kaki*	Fructus Diospyri	Shi Shuang Bing		Persimmon frosted fruit
Chi Wai Pei	*Erinaceaus europoeus, Hemichianum dauricus*	Corium Erinacei	Ci Wei Pi		Hedgehog hide
Chi Wong	*Orpimentum*	Orpimentum	Ci Huang, Xiong Huang		Orpiment
Chi Yip	*Diospyros kaki*	Folium Diospyri	Shi Ye		Persimmon leaf

CANTONESE	SCIENTIFIC	PHARMACEUTICAL	MANDARIN	JAPANESE	ENGLISH
Chin Daan, Wong Daan	*Minium*	Minium	Qian Dan, Huang Dan	Entan	Red lead oxide
Chin Gam Ji	*Euphorbia lathyris*	Semen Euphorbiae lathyris	Qian Jin Zi	Zokuzuishi	Caper spurge seed
Chin Gam Tang	*Stephania japonica*	Caulis Stephaniae japonicae	Qian Jin Teng		Japanese stephania stem
Chin Lei Gwong	*Senecio scandens*	Herba Senecionis scandens	Qian Li Guang		Climbing ragwort herb
Chin Nin Gin	*Homalomena occulta*	Rhizoma Homalomenae	Qian Nian Jian	Sennenken	Homalomena root
Chin Wu	*Peucedanum praeruptorum, P. decursivum*	Radix Peucedani	Qian Hu	Zenko	Asian masterwort root
Ching Doi	*Isatis tinctoria* and spp, *Baphicacanthus cusia, Indigofera suffruticosa, Polygonum tinctorium*	Indigo pulverata levis	Qing Dai		Woad pigment
Ching Fan	*Calomelas*	Calomelas	Qing Fen	Keifun	Calomel
Ching Fung Tang	*Sabia japonica*	Ramulus Sabiae	Qi Feng Teng		Sabia twig
Ching Fung Tang	*Sinomenium acutum*	Radix Sinomenii	Qing Feng Teng		Sinomenium root
Ching Hou	*Artemisia apiacea*	Herba Artemisiae apiaceae	Qing Hao	Seiko	Celery wormwood herb
Ching Mein Sek	*Chloris*	Chloris	Qing Meng Shi		Chlorite schist
Ching Muk Heung	*Aristolochia contorta, A. debilis*	Radix Aristolochiae	Qing Mu Xiang, Ma Dou Ling Gen	Seimokko	Green birthwort root
Ching Pei	*Citrus reticulata, C. tangerina, C. erythrosa*	Pericarpium Citri reticulatae viride	Qing Pi	Johi	Unripe tangerine rind
Ching Seung Ji	*Celosia argentea*	Semen Celosiae argenteae	Qing Xiang Zi	Seisoshi	Silver quail-grass seed
Ching Tin Kwai	*Nervilia fordii*	Herba Nerviliae	Qing Tian Kui		Nervilia herb
Chit Bui Mou	*Fritillaria thunbergii*	Bulbus Fritillariae thunbergii	Zhe Bei Mu	Setsubaimo	Zhejiang fritillary bulb
Chong Seut, Gwan Chong Seut	*Atractylodes japonica*	Rhizoma Atractylodis japonicae	Cang Zhu, Guan Cang Zhu		Japanese black Atractylodes root
Chong Seut, Mau Chong Seut	*Atractylodes lancea, A. sinensis* and spp	Rhizoma Atractylodis lanceae	Cang Zhu, Mao Cang Zhu	Sojutsu	Black atractylodes root
Chong Wai Ji	*Leonorus heterophyllus* and spp	Semen Leonori	Chong Wei Zi		Asian motherwort seed
Chong Yi Ji	*Xanthium sibiricum, X. strumarium*	Fructus Xanthii	Cang Er Zi	Sojishi	Siberian cocklebur
Chou Dau Kau	*Alpinia katsumadai*	Semen Alpiniae katsumadis	Cao Dou Kou	Sozuku	Katsumada's galangal seed
Chou Gwat (Yan)	*Amomum tsao-ko*	Fructus Amomi tsao-konis	Cao Guo (Ren)	Soka	Cochin cardamom fruit
Chou Jeung Chou	*Oxalis corniculata*	Herba Oxalis	Cu Jiang Cao		Indian sorrel herb

CANTONESE	SCIENTIFIC	PHARMACEUTICAL	MANDARIN	JAPANESE	ENGLISH
Chou Wu, Mai Wu Tau	*Aconitum chinense, A. kusnezoffii* and spp	Radix Aconiti chinensis	Cao Wu, Bei Wu Tou	So-u	Prepared wild aconite root tuber
Chu Lou Nga	*Aralia elata, A. elata* var. *suninermis*	Cortex Araliae elatate	Ci Lao Ya Pi	Taranoki	Aralia bark
Chung Baak	*Allium fistulosum*	Bulbus Allii fistulosi	Cong Bai		Fresh scallion bulb
Chung Baak Laap	*Ericerus pela*	Ericerus	Chong Bai La		Ericerus worm
Chung Fa Fan	*Pinus massoniana, P. tabulaeformis* and spp	Pollen Pini	Song Hua Fen		Pine pollen
Chung Heung	*Pinus massoniana, P. tabulaeformis* and spp, *Larix* spp	Resina Pini preparatae, Colophonium	Song Xiang		Pine resin
Chung Ji	*Allium fistulosum*	Semen Allii fistulosi	Cong Zi	Sohaku	Scallion seed
Chung Ji	*Pinus tabulaeformis* and spp	Semen Pini	Song Zi		Pine kernel
Chung Jit, Yao Chung Jit	*Pinus tabulaeformis, P. massoniana, P. yunnannensis*	Lignum Pini nodi	Song Jie, You Song Jie	Shosetsu	Knotty pine wood shaving
Chung Lo	*Usnea diffracta* and spp	Thallus Usneae	Song Luo		Beard lichen thallus
Chyu Ma Gan	*Boehmeria nivea*	Radix Boehmeriae	Zhu Ma Gen		Ramie root
Chyu Sat Ji	*Broussonetia papyrifera*	Fructus Broussonetiae	Chu Shi Zi		Paper mulberry fruit
Chyun Bui Mou	*Fritillaria cirrhosa*	Bulbus Fritillariae cirrhosae	Chuan Bei Mu	Senbaimo	Sichuan fritillary bulb
Chyun Bui Mou, Am Ji Bui Mou	*Fritillaria unibracteata*	Bulbus Fritillariae unibracteatae	Chuan Bei Mu, An Zi Bei Mu		Single-bract fritillary bulb
Chyun Bui Mou, Taai Baak Bui Mou	*Fritillaria taipaiensis*	Bulbus Fritillariae taipaiensis	Chuan Bei Mu, Tai Bai Bei Mu		Taipei fritillary bulb
Chyun Dong Sam	*Codonopsis tangshen*	Radix Codonopsis tangshenis	Dang Shen, Chuan Dang Shen		Sichuan bellflower root
Chyun Gen Tang	*Psychotria serpens*	Herba Psychotriae serpentis	Chuan Gen Teng, Bo Gu Cao		Twining psychotria herb
Chyun Gung	*Ligusticum walichii*	Radix Ligustici walichii	Chuan Xiong, Xiong Qiong	Senkyu	Sichuan lovage root
Chyun Jiu, Fa Jiu	*Zanthoxylum bungeanum*	Fructus Zanthoxyli bungeani	Chuan Jiao, Hua Jiao	Shokusho	Sichuan peppercorn
Chyun Kit	*Buthus Martensi*	Buthus	Quan Xie	Zenkatsu	Scorpion
Chyun Lin Ji	*Melia toosendan*	Fructus Meliae toosendanis	Chuan Lian Zi		Sichuan bead tree berry
Chyun Muk Heung	*Dolomiaea souliei*	Radix Dolomiaeae souliei	Chuan Mu Xiang		Sichuan Dolomiaea root
Chyun Muk Tong	*Clematis montana, C. armandii*	Caulis Clematis montanae	Chuan Mu Tong		Mountain clematis stem
Chyun Ngau Sat	*Cyathula officinalis,. C. officinalis*	Radix Cyathulae	Chuan Niu Xi		Hookweed root

CANTONESE	SCIENTIFIC	PHARMACEUTICAL	MANDARIN	JAPANESE	ENGLISH
Chyun Po Sek	*Cudrania cochinchinensis*	Radix Cudraniae cochinchinensis	Chuan Po Shi		Cochin cudrania root
Chyun Saan Lung	*Dioscorea nipponica*	Rhizoma Dioscoreae nipponicae	Chuan Shan Long		Nippon yam root
Chyun Sam Lin	*Andrographis paniculata*	Folium Andrographis	Chuan Xin Lian	Senshinren	Heart-thread lotus leaf
Chyun San Gaap	*Manis pentadactyla*	Squama manis	Chuan Shan Jia	Senzanko	Pangolin scale
Chyun Tung Pei	*Kalopanax septemlobus*	Cortex Septemlobi	Chuan Tong Pi		Kalopanax bark
Chyun Wu, Wu Tau	*Aconitum carmichaeli*	Radix Aconiti carmichaeli	Chuan Wu Wu Tou	Uzu	Prepared Sichuan aconite root tuber
Da Po Wun Fa Fa	*Anemone hupehensis*	Herba Anemonis hupehensis	Da Po Wan Hua Hua		Hubei anemone herb
Daai Cheng Yip	*Clerodendron cyrtophyllum*	Folium Clerodendronis cyrtophylli	Da Qing Ye		Green-white clerodendron leaf
Daai Ching Yim	*Halitum*	Halitum	Da Qing Yan		Rock salt
Daai Ching Yip	*Isatis tinctoria*	Folium Isatis tinctoriae	Da Qing Ye		Woad leaf
Daai Chou Kau	*Alpinia zerumbet*	Fructus Alpiniae zerumbetsis	Da Cao Kou		Beautiful galangal berry
Daai Fa Sai San	*Asarum maximum*	Herba Asari maximi	Ta Hua Xi Xin		Large flower wild ginger herb
Daai Fuk Pei	*Areca catechu, A. dicksonii*	Pericarpium Arecae	Da Fu Pi	Daifukuhi	Betel husk
Daai Fung Ji	*Hydnocarpus anthelmintica, H. hainanensis*	Semen Hydnocarpi	Da Feng Zi	Daifushi	Chaulmoogra seed
Daai Gai	*Cirsium japonicum*	Herba Cirsii japonici	Da Ji	Taikei	Japanese thistle herb
Daai Hyut Tang	*Sargentodoxa cuneata*	Caulis Sargentodoxae	Da Xue Teng		Sargentodoxa stem
Daai Jou	*Zizyphus jujuba* var. *inermis*	Fructus Zizyphi jujubae	Da Zao	Taiso	Black jujube berry
Daai Ju Si Dau	*Crotalaria assamica*	Semen seu herba Crotalariae assamicae	Da Zhu Shi Dou, Zi Xiao Rong		Assam crotalaria seed or herb
Daai Leung Geung	*Alpinia galanga*	Radix Alpiniae galangae	Da Liang Jiang		Greater galangal root
Daai Mei Yiu	*Heliotropium indicum*	Herba Heliotropi	Da Wei Yao, Er Gou Cao		Heliotrope herb
Daai Syun	*Allium sativum*	Bulbus Allii sativi	Da Suan	Taisan	Garlic bulb
Daai Wong	*Rheum palmatum, R. tanguticum, R. officinale*	Rhizoma Rhei	Da Huang	Daio	Rhubarb root
Daam Choi	*Mytilus crassitesta* and spp	Mytilus	Dan Cai		Mussel
Daam Juk Gan	*Lopatherum gracile*	Radix Lopatheri	Dan Zhu Gen		Bamboo grass root
Daam Juk Yip	*Lopatherum gracile*	Folium Lopatheri	Dan Zhu Ye	Tanchikuyo	Bamboo grass leaf
Daam Naam Sing	*Arisaema consanguineum, A. amurense* and spp	Pulvis Arisaemae cum felle Bovis	Dan Nan Xing	Tannansho	Powdered dragon arum corm with ox bile

CANTONESE	SCIENTIFIC	PHARMACEUTICAL	MANDARIN	JAPANESE	ENGLISH
Daan Faan	*Chalcanthitum*	Chalcanthitum	Dan Fan, Shi Dan	Tanban	Crystallized blue vitriol
Daan Sam	*Salvia miltiorrhiza*	Radix Salviae miltiorrhizae	Dan Shen	Tanjin	Cinnabar sage root
Daan Sam, Gam Sai Syu Mei	*Salvia przelwalskii*	Radix	Dan Shen, Gan Xi Shu Wei		Gan Xi cinnabar sage root
Daan Sam, Naam Dam Sam	*Salvia bowleyana*	Radix Salviae bowleyanae	Dan Shen, Nan Dan Shen		Southern cinnabar sage root
Daan Tiu Chou	*Lysimachia candida*	Herba Lysimachiae candidae	Dan Tian Cao		White lysimachia herb
Dang Lung Chou	*Physalis peruviana*	Herba Physalis peruvianae	Deng Long Cao		Peru lantern herb
Dang Sam Chou	*Juncus effusus*	Medulla Junci	Deng Xin Cao	Toshinso	Bulrush pith
Dau (Wong) Geun	*Glycene max*	Semen Glycinis germinati	Dou (Huang) Juan		Sprouting soybean
Dau Chek Geung	*Litsea cubeba*	Radix et caulis Litseae	Dou Chi Jiang	Toshikyo	Cubeb root and stem
Dei Baak Chou	*Viola diffusa*	Radix et herba Violae diffusae	Di Bai Cao		Spreading violet root and herb
Dei Bit Chung	*Eupolyphaga sinensis*	Eupolyphaga	Tu Bie Chong	Shachu	Cockroach
Dei Fu Ji	*Kochia scoparia*	Semen Kochiae	Di Fu Zi	Jibushi	Kochia seed
Dei Gam Chou	*Euphorbia humifusa*	Herba Euphorbiae humifusae	Di Jin Cao		Wolf'smilk herb
Dei Gwat Pei	*Lycium chinense*	Cortex radicis Lycii	Di Gu Pi	Jikoppi	Wolfberry root bark
Dei Hat Tou	*Viola collina*	Radix et herba Violae collinae	Di He Tao		Collina violet root and herb
Dei Jiu	*Thymus mongolicus*	Herba Thymi mongolici	Di Jiao		Mongolian thyme herb
Dei Lung	*Pheretima aspergillum, Allolobophora caliginosa*	Pheretima seu Allolobophora	Di Long	Jiryu	Earthworm
Dei Ng Gung	*Helminthostachys zeylanica*	Rhizoma Helminthostachys	Di Wu Song		Helmintho-stachys root
Dei Seun	*Lycopus lucidus*	Rhizoma Lycopi lucidi	Di Sun		Bright bugleweed root
Dei Yu	*Sanguisorba officinalis*	Radix Sanguisorbae	Di Yu	Jiyu	Great burnet root
Deui Yip Dau Yip	*Cassia alata*	Folium Cassiae alatae	Dui Ye Dou Ye		Ringworm bush leaf
Ding Ging Chou	*Lindernia anagallis*	Herba Linderniae	Ding Jing Cao		Lindernia herb
Ding Gung Tang	*Erycibes obtusifolia*	Radix et caulis Erycibis	Ding Gong Teng		Erycibe root and stem
Ding Heung	*Eugenia caryophyllata*	Gemma Eugeniae	Ding Xiang	Choko	Clove bud
Ding Sam Fa	*Juncus effusus*	Flos Junci	Deng Xin Hua		Bulrush flower
Diu Gam Jung	*Melothria mederospatana*	Radix Melothriae mederospatanae	Diao Jin Zhong		Melothria root
Doi Jyu Sek	*Haematitum*	Haematitum	Dai Zhe Shi	Taishaseki	Hematite
Doi Mou	*Eretmochelys imbricata*	Plastrum Eretmochelis	Dai Mao	Taimai	Hawksbill turtle shell
Dong Gwa Yan	*Benincasa hispida*	Semen Benincasae	Dong Gua Ren	Tokanin	Waxgourd seed

CANTONESE	SCIENTIFIC	PHARMACEUTICAL	MANDARIN	JAPANESE	ENGLISH
Dong Gwai	*Angelica acutiloba*	Radix Angelicae acutilobae	Dang Gui		Dong quai root
Dong Gwai	*Angelica sinensis*	Radix Angelicae sinensis	Dang Gui	Toki	Dong quai root
Dong Gwai Mai	*Angelica sinensis, A. acutiloba*	Extremas radicis Angelicae sinensis	Dang Gui Wei	Tokio	Dong quai tail
Dong Gwai Tou	*Angelica sinensis, A. acutiloba*	Caput Angelicae sinensis	Dang Gui Tou	Tokito	Dong quai head
Dong Sam, Kau Fa Dong Sam	*Codonopsis subglobosa*	Radix Codonopsis subglobosae	Dang Shen, Qiu Hua Dang Shen		Subglobular bellflower root
Dong Yeuk	*Swertia pseudochinensis* and spp	Radix Swertiae	Dang Yao		Asian green gentian root
Dong Yeuk Chou	*Swertia japonica, S. pseudochinensis*	Herba Swertiae	Dang Yao Cao	Toyaku	Japanese green gentian herb
Dou Dau	*Canavalia gladiata, C. ensiformis*	Semen Canavaliae	Dao Dou		Swordbean seed
Dou Hang	*Asarum forbesii*	Rhizoma Asari forbesii	Du Heng		Forbes' wild ginger root
Dou Jung	*Eucommia ulmoides*	Cortex Eucommiae	Du Zhong	Tochu	Eucommia bark
Dou Jung Yip	*Eucommia ulmoides*	Folium Eucommiae	Du Zhong Ye		Eucommia leaf
Dou Sang Gan	*Rubus coreanus*	Fructus Rubi coreani	Dao Sheng Gen		Korean raspberry fruit
Duk Geuk Gam	*Striga asiatica*	Herba Strigae	Du Jiao Gan		Witchweed herb
Duk Gok Lin	*Typhonium giganteum*	Radix Typhonii	Du Jiao Lan		Typhonium root
Duk Wut	*Angelica pubescens, A. laxiflora* and spp	Radix Angelicae pubescentis	Du Huo	Dokkatsu	Hairy angelica Root
Duk Wut	*Heracleum candicans*	Radix Heraclei candicantis	Du Huo		White cow parsnip root
Dun Ling Chou	*Rabdosia rubescens* and spp	Herba Rabdosiae	Dong Ling Cao		Rabdosia herb
Dung Chung Ha Chou	*Cordyceps sinensis* and host larvae *Hepialus armoricanus* or *Holotrichia koraiensis*	Sclerotium Cordycepsis	Dong Chong Xia Cao	Tochukaso	Chinese caterpillar mushroom
Dung Fung Gwat Gan	*Atalantia buxifolia*	Radix Atalantiae	Dong Feng Ju Gen	Tofukitsu	Atalantia root
Dung Gwa Pei	*Benincasa hispida*	Epicarpium Benincasae	Dong Gua Pi	Tokahi	Waxgourd fruit rind
Dung Kwai Ji	*Malva verticillata*	Semen Malvae	Dong Kui Zi		Musk mallow seed
Fa Kei Sam, Sei Yang Sam	*Panax quinquefolius*	Radix Panacis quinquefolii	Xi Yang Shen	Seiyojin	American ginseng root
Fa Luk Sam	*Cervus nippon* and spp	Testes et penis Cervi	Hua Lu Shen		Male deer genitals
Fa Sang Pei	*Arachis hypogaea*	Pericarpium Arachis	Hua Sheng Pi	Kashohi	Peanut skin
Fa Yeui Sek	*Ophicalcitum*	Ophicalcitum	Hua Rui Shi	Kazuiseki	Dolomite
Faan Baak Chou	*Potentilla discolor*	Herba Potentillae discoloris	Fan Bai Cao		Discolored cinquefoil herb
Faan Bei	*Agkistrodon halys*	Agkistrodon	Fan Bi		Viper
Faan Haang	*Tetragonia tatragonoides*	Herba Tetragoniae	Fan Xing	Bankyo, Mantsai	Tetragonia herb

CANTONESE	SCIENTIFIC	PHARMACEUTICAL	MANDARIN	JAPANESE	ENGLISH
Faan Sek Lau Gon Yip	*Psidium guajava*	Folium Psidii	Fan Shi Liu Gan Ye		Guava leaf
Faan Sie Yip	*Senna acutifolia, S. angustifolia*	Folium Sennae	Fan Xie Ye		Senna leaf
Faan Tyun Tang	*Kadsura coccinea*	Caulis Kadsurae coccineae	Fan Tuan Teng		Scarlet kadsura stem
Fau Hoi Sek	*Pumus*	Lapis Pumicis	Fu Hai Shi	Kaifuseki	Pumice
Fau Ping	*Lemna minor*	Herba Lemnae	Fu Ping		Duckweed herb
Fau Ping	*Spirodela polyrrhiza*	Herba Spirodelae	Fu Ping		Duckweed herb
Fau Siu Mak	*Triticum aestivum*	Fructus Tritici	Fu Xiao Mai	Fushobaku	Wheat berry
Fei Ji	*Torreya grandis, T. nucifera*	Semen Torreyae	Fei Zi		Japanese torreya nut
Fei Jou Choi	*Gymnocladus chinensis*	Fructus Gymnocladi	Fei Zao Jia		Chinese gymnocladus berry
Fei Lung Jeung Hyut	*Toddalia asiatica*	Radix Toddaliae	Fei Long Zhang Xue		Asian toddalia root
Fo Hyut Lin	*Coniogramme japonica*	Herba Coniogrammis	Huo Xue Lian		Bamboo fern herb
Fo Ma Yan	*Cannabis sativa*	Semen Cannabis	Huo Ma Ren	Mashinin	Cannabis seed
Fo Tan Mou (Chou)	*Polygonum chinense*	Herba Polygoni chinensis	Huo Tan Mu (Cao), Qing Fan Teng		Chinese knotweed herb
Fok Heung	*Agastache rugosa*	Herba Agastachis	Huo Xiang	Kakko	Rugose giant hyssop herb
Fong Dong Sam	*Codonopsis pilosula, C. tangshen, C. nervosa*	Radix Codonopsis	Dang Shen	Tojin	Downy bellflower root
Fong Fung	*Ledebouriella divaricata, L. seseloides*	Radix Ledebouriellae	Fang Feng	Bofu	Wind-protector root
Fong Gei, Gwong Fong Gei	*Aristolochia fangchi, A. westlandii*	Radix Aristolochiae fangchis	Fang Ji, Guang Fang Ji		Fangchi birthwort root
Fong Kwai	*Peucedanum japonicum*	Radix Peucedani japonici	Fang Gui		Japanese masterwort root
Fu (Syu) Muk	*Picrasma quassioides*	Ramulus et folium Picrasmae	Ku (Shu) Mu		Quassiawood twig and leaf
Fu Choi	*Sonchus oleraceus*	Herba Sonchi	Ku Cai		Annual sowthistle herb
Fu Dei Daam	*Elephantopus scaber*	Herba Elephantopi	Di Dan Tou, Ku Di Dan, Tu Gong Ying		Rough elephant's foot herb
Fu Ding Cha	*Ilex latifolia*	Folium Ilicis latifoliae	Ku Ding Cha		Broadleaf holly leaf
Fu Gwa (Gam)	*Momordica charantia*	Fructus Momordicae charantiae	Ku Gua (Gan)		Bitter melon fruit
Fu Gwat	*Panthera*	Os tigris	Hu Gu	Kokotsu	Tiger bone
Fu Jeung	*Polygonum cuspidatum*	Radix et folium Polygoni cuspidati	Hu Zhang		Japanese Knotweed root and leaf
Fu Ji	*Aconitum carmichaeli*	Radix lateralis Aconiti carmichaeli praeparatae	Fu Zi	Bushi	Prepared Sichuan aconite root
Fu Juk Yip	*Pleioblastus amarus*	Folium Pleioblasti	Ku Zhu Ye		Bitter bamboo leaf

CANTONESE	SCIENTIFIC	PHARMACEUTICAL	MANDARIN	JAPANESE	ENGLISH
Fu Ke	*Solanum dulcamara*	Caulis Solani dulcamari	Ku Qie		Bittersweet stem
Fu Lin (Gan) Pei	*Melia azedarach, M. toosendan*	Cortex radicis Meliae	Ku Lian (Gen) Pi	Kurenkombi	Bead tree root bark
Fu Po	*Pinus succinifera*	Resina Pini succiniferae (Succinum)	Hu Po		Amber resin
Fu Sam	*Sophora flavescens*	Radix Sophorae flavescentis	Ku Shen		Yellow pagoda tree root
Fu Sam Ji	*Sophora flavescens*	Fructus Sophorae flavescentis	Ku Shen Zi		Yellow pagoda tree berry
Fu Sek Lin (Ji)	*Caesalpinia minax*	Semen Caesalpiniae minacis	Ku Shi Lian (Zi)		Caesalpinia seed
Fu Song Fa	*Hibiscus rosa-sinensis*	Flos Hibisci rosa-sinensis	Fu Sang Hua		Shoe flower
Fu Syu Pei	*Picrasma quassioides*	Cortex Picrassiae	Ku Shu Pi		Quassiawood bark
Fu Yi Chou	*Saxifraga stolonifera*	Herba Saxifragae stoloniferae	Hu Er Cao		Saxifrage herb
Fu Yung	*Crossostephium chinense*	Herba Crossostephii	Fu Rong		Crossosteph-ium herb
Fu Yung Fa	*Hibiscus mutabilis*	Flos Hibisci mutabili	Fu Rong Hua		Cotton rose flower
Fu Yung Yip	*Hibiscus mutabilis*	Folium Hibisci mutabilis	Fu Rong Ye		Cotton rose leaf
Fuk Ling, Waan Ling	*Poria cocos*	Sclerotium Poriae	Fu Ling	Bukuryo	Hoelen fungus
Fuk Ling Pei	*Poria cocos*	Cortex Poriae	Fu Ling Pi	Bukuryoshi	Hoelen skin
Fuk Lung Gon		Terra flava usta, Bolus usta	Fu Long Gan	Bukuryukan	Wood stove clay
Fuk Pun Ji	*Rubus chingii*	Fructus Rubi chingii	Fu Pen Zi	Fukubonshi	Chinese raspberry fruit
Fuk Sau Chou	*Adonis amurensis*	Herba Adonis	Fu Shou Cao		Amur adonis herb
Fun Dung Fa	*Tussilago farfara*	Flos Tussilaginis	Kuan Dong Hua	Kantoka	Coltsfoot flower
Fun Hung Fa	*Crocus sativus*	Stigma Croci	Xi Hong Hua, Fan Hong Hua	Bankoka	Saffron stigma
Fung Che Yi	*Dioscorea japonica*	Rhizoma Dioscoreae japonicae	Feng Che Er		Japanese yam root
Fung Dau Choi	*Petasites japonicus*	Flos Petasitis	Feng Dou Cai		Japanese butterbur flower
Fung Fa Fan	*Pollen*	Granum floris pollinis	Feng Hua Fen		Flower (bee) pollen
Fung Laap	*Apis cerana* and spp	Cera flava	Feng La		Beeswax
Fung Loi Chou, Ngaap Sit Wong	*Lippia nodiflora*	Herba Lippiae	Peng Lai Cao, Ya She Huang		Frogfruit herb
Fung Mat	*Apis cerana* and spp	Mel	Feng Mi		Honey
Fung Mei Chou	*Pteris multifida* and spp	Herba Pterii	Feng Wei Cao		Phoenix-tail fern
Fung Ngaan Chou	*Ailanthus altissima*	Fructus Ailanthi	Feng Yen Cao		Tree of heaven fruit
Fut Sao Fa	*Citrus medica* var. *sarctodactylus*	Flos Citri sarctodactylis	Fo Shou (Gan) Hua	Bushukan	Finger lemon flower
Fut Sau (Gam)	*Citrus medica* var. *sarcodactylis*	Fructus Citri medicae	Fo Shou (Gan)		Finger lemon fruit

CANTONESE	SCIENTIFIC	PHARMACEUTICAL	MANDARIN	JAPANESE	ENGLISH
Gaam Laam	*Canarium album*	Fructus Canarii	Gan Lan, Jing Guo		Asian olive fruit
Gaan Geung	*Zingiber officinalis*	Rhizoma Zingiberis	Gan Jiang	Kankyo	Dried ginger root
Gaan Gu Laam	*Gynostemma pentaphyllum*	Herba Gynostemmae	Jiao Gu Lan		Gynostemma herb
Gaau Lung Tang, Lung Sou Tang	*Bauhinia championi*	Caulis bauhiniae championi	Jiu Long Teng, Wu Teng		Bauhinia stem
Gaau Nga Fa	*Ervatamia divaricata, E. hainaensis*	Herba Ervatamiae	Gou Ya Hua		Crepe jasmine herb
Gai Daan Fa	*Plumeria rubra* var. *acutifolia*	Flos Plumeriae	Ji Dan Hua		Frangipani flower
Gai Fa	*Loropetalum chinense*	Flos Loropetali	Ji Hua		Strap flower
Gai Gun Fa	*Celosia cristata*	Herba Celosiae cristatae	Ji Guan Hua		Cock'scomb herb
Gai Gwat Chou	*Abrus precatorius, A. cantoniensis*	Herba Abri	Ji Gu Cao		Licorice bean herb
Gai Gwat Heung	*Croton crassifolius*	Radix Crotonis crassifolii	Ji Gu Xiang		Thick-leaf croton root
Gai Ji Wong	*Gallus gallus domesticus*	Vitellus Galli	Ji Zi Huang		Egg yolk
Gai Muk	*Loropetalum chinense*	Cortex Loropetali	Ji Mu		Strap flower bark
Gai Na Gam	*Gallus gallus domesticus*	Endothelium corneum gigeriae Galli	Ji Nei Jin	Keinaikin	Chicken gizzard lining
Gai Niu Tang	*Paederia scandens*	Radix et caulis Paederiae	Ji Shi Teng	Hakumokeis hito	Chicken dung vine root and stem
Gai Yut Tang	*Millettia dielsiana, M. reticulata, M. nitida*	Radix et caulis Millettiae dielsianae	Ji Xue Teng	Keiketto	Millettia root and stem
Gai Yut Tang Gaau	*Spatholobus suberectus*	Gelatinum Spatholobi	Ji Xue Teng Jiao		Spatholobus gel
Gai Yut Tang, Mat Fa Dau	*Spatholobus suberectus*	Caulis Spatholobi	Ji Xue Teng, Mi Hua Dou		Spatholobus stem
Gam Bat Wun	*Lycopodium serratum* and *varieties*	Herba Lycopodii serrati	Jin Bu Huan		Serrated clubmoss
Gam Bat Wun	*Stephania sinica*	Caulis Stephaniae sinicae	Jin Bu Huan		Chinese stephania stem
Gam Bin Lung Sit Laan	*Agave americana*	Folium Agavis americanae	Jin Bian Long She Lan		Agave leaf
Gam Bok	*Aurum*	Folium Auri	Jin Bo		Gold foil
Gam Cha	*Hydrangea serrata* var. *thunbergii*	Folium Hydrangeae	Gan Cha	Amatya, Dochouzan	Sweet tea leaf
Gam Chin Chou, Gwo Lou Wong	*Lysimachia christinae, L. hemsleyana*	Herba Lysimachiae	Jin Qian Cao, Guo Lu Huang	Kinsenso	Asian moneywort herb
Gam Chou	*Glycirrhiza uralensis, G. glabra* and spp	Radix Glycirrhizae	Gan Cao	Kanzo	Ural licorice root
Gam Chung	*Nardostachys jatamansi, N. chinensis*	Radix Nardostachis	Gan Song		Indian spikenard root
Gam Dei Lo	*Drosera burmanni*	Herba Droserae	Jin Di Luo		Sundew herb

CANTONESE	SCIENTIFIC	PHARMACEUTICAL	MANDARIN	JAPANESE	ENGLISH
Gam Fai Chou	*Inula japonica, I. brittanica, I. linariaefolia*	Herba Inulae	Jin Fei Cao	Kinfutsuso	Elecampane herb
Gam Gaat Gan, Ai Ji Sam	*Adenophora trachelioides*	Radix Adenophorae trachelioidis	Gan Jie Geng		Sweet ladybell root
Gam Gai Laak	*Cinchona succiruba* and spp	Cortex Cinchonae	Jin Ji Le, Jin Ji Na Pi		Cinchona bark
Gam Gong Tang, Bat Kai	*Smilax china*	Rhizoma Smilacis chinensis	Jin Gang Teng, Ba Qi		Chinese greenbrier root, China root
Gam Guk Fa, Ye Guk Fa	*Chrysanthemum indicum*	Flos Chrysanthemi indici	Ye Ju Hua	Nogikuka	Wild chrysanthe-mum flower
Gam Gwo Laam	*Tinospora sagittata, T. capillipes*	Radix Tinosporae	Jin Guo Lan	Kinkaran	Tinospora root
Gam Jeuk Fa	*Caragana sinica* and spp	Flos Caraganae	Jin Que Hua		Caragana flower
Gam Jik Yi	*Caragana sinica, C., microphylla* and spp	Radix Caraganae	Jin Ji Er		Caragana root
Gam Kiu Mak Gan	*Fagopyrum cymosum*	Rhizoma Fagopyri	Jin Qiao Mai Gen		Buckwheat root
Gam Mein Sek	*Chloris*	Chloris	Jin Meng Shi		Mica schist
Gam Mung Sek	*Phlogopitum*	Phlogopitum	Jin Meng Shi		Phlogopite, Red mica
Gam Ngan Fa Yan Dung Fa	*Lonicera japonica*	Flos Lonicerae japonicae	Jin Yin Hua, Ren Dong Hua	Kinginka	Japanese honeysuckle flower
Gam Ngan Tang, Yan Dung Tang	*Lonicera japonica*	Ramus et folium Lonicerae japonicae	Jin Yin Teng, Ren Dong Teng		Japanese honeysuckle stem and leaf
Gam San Sam	*Panax ginseng*	Radix Panacis ginsengis	Ye Shan Shen		Wild Asian ginseng
Gam Seui	*Euphorbia kansui*	Radix Euphorbiae kansui	Gan Sui	Kansui	Sweet spurge root
Gam Ying Ji	*Rosa laevigata*	Fructus Rosae laevigatae	Jin Ying Zi	Kinoshi	Cherokee rosehip
Gang Mai	*Oryza sativa*	Fructus Oryzae	Jing Mi		Rice grain
Gap Gaai	*Gecko gecko, G. verticilatus*	Gecko	Ge Jie	Gokai	Toad-headed lizard
Gap Juk Tou Yip	*Nerium indicum*	Folium Nerii	Jiao Zhu Tao Ye		Indian oleander leaf
Gat Gan	*Platycodon grandiflorum*	Radix Platycodonis	Jie Geng, Ku Jie Geng	Kikyo	Balloonflower root
Gau Bit Ying	*Ilex rotunda*	Folium Ilicis rotundis	Jiu Bi Ying		Round-leaf holly leaf
Gau Choi Ji	*Allium tuberosum*	Semen Alii tuberosi	Jiu Cai Zi	Kyushi	Asian leek seed
Gau Gei Ji, Gei Ji	*Lycium chinense, L. barbarum*	Fructus Lycii	Gou Qi Zi	Kukoshi	Wolfberry
Gau Gwat	*Poncirus trifoliata*	Fructus Ponciri	Gou Ju		Trifoliate orange fruit
Gau Gwat Yip	*Ilex cornuta*	Folium Ilicis cornutae	Gou Gu Ye		Cat thorn holly leaf
Gau Heung Chung	*Aspongopus*	Aspongopus	Jiu Xiang Chong		Stinkbug
Gau Jek	*Cibotium barometz*	Rhizoma Cibotii	Gou Ji	Kuseki	Dogspine root
Gau Ji Yip	*Lycium chinense, L. barbarum*	Folium Lycii chinensis	Gou Qi Ye		Wolfberry leaf

CANTONESE	SCIENTIFIC	PHARMACEUTICAL	MANDARIN	JAPANESE	ENGLISH
Gau Jit Cheung Pou	*Anemone altaica*	Rhizoma Anemoni altaicae	Jiu Jie Chang Pu	Arutai ginrenkon	Altai anemone root
Gau Jit Fung	*Sarcandra glabra*	Herba Sarcandrae	Jiu Jie Feng		Smooth sarcandra herb
Gau Lei Heung	*Murraya paniculata*	Ramulus et folium Murrayae	Jiu Li Xiang		Burma boxwood twig and leaf
Gau Sit Chou	*Senecio kirilowii*	Herba Senecionis kirilowii	Kou She Cao		Kirilow's ragwort herb
Gei Hat Tang, Seung Cheun Yao Ma Tang	*Mucuna birdwoodiana, M. sempervirens*	Radix et caulis Mucunae	Ji Xue Teng, Chang Chun You Ma Teng		Mucuna root and stem
Geui Jeung Yip	*Piper betle*	Folium Piperis betlis	Ju Jiang Ye, Qing Lou Ye		Betel pepper leaf
Geui Mak	*Dianthus superbus, D. chinensis*	Herba Dianthi	Qu Mai	Kubaku	Proud pink herb
Geui Mak, Sek Juk	*Dianthus chinensis*	Herba Dianthi chinensis	Qu Mai, Shi Zhu		Chinese pink herb
Geui Sing Ji	*Dipsacus chinensis* and spp	Fructus Dipsaci	Ju Sheng Zi		Chinese teasel fruit
Geui Yeuk	*Amorphophallus rivieri, A. sinensis, A. knojac*	Rhizoma Amorphophalli	Ju Ruo		Amorphop-hallus root
Geung Chaam	*Bombyx mori* infected with *Beauveria bassiana*	Bombyx beauveriatus	Jiang Can		Silkworm larva
Geung Heung	*Dalbergia odorifera*	Lignum Dalbergiae odoriferae	Jiang Xiang		Asian rosewood
Geung Wong	*Curcuma longa. C. aromatica*	Rhizoma Curcumae	Jiang Huang	Kyoo	Turmeric root
Geung Wut	*Notopterygium incisum, N. forbesii, N. francherii*	Rhizoma et radix Notopterigii	Qiang Huo	Kyokatsu	Notoptery-gium root
Geung Yung	*Bombyx mori artificially* infected with *Beauveria bassiana*	Bombyx beauveriatus	Jiang Yong		Silkworm larva
Gim Fa	*Hylocereus undatus*	Flos Hylocerei	Jian Hua, Ba Wang Hua		Cereus flower
Gin Fung Hung	*Anagallis arvensis*	Herba Anagallis	Jian Feng Hong		Scarlet pimpernel herb
Gin Laan Fa	*Cymbidium ensifolium*	Herba et radix Cymbidii	Jian Lan Hua		Cymbidium orchid herb and root
Gin Laan Gan	*Cymbidium ensifolium*	Radix Cymbidii	Jian Lan Gen		Cymbidium orchid root
Gin Laan Yip	*Cymbidium ensifolium*	Folium Cymbidii	Jian Lan Ye		Cymbidium orchid leaf
Ging Daai Gik	*Euphorbia pekinensis*	Radix Euphorbiae pekinensis	Jing Da Ji	Taigeki	Peking spurge root
Ging Gaai	*Schizonepeta tenuifolia*	Herba Schizonepetae	Jing Jie	Keigai	Japanese catnip herb
Ging Tin	*Sedum erythrostictum*	Herba Sedi erythrosticti	Jing Tian (San Qi)		Red stonecrop herb
Ging Tin Saam Chat	*Sedum aizoon*	Herba Sedi aizoonis	Jing Tian San Qi		Aizoon stonecrop herb

CANTONESE	SCIENTIFIC	PHARMACEUTICAL	MANDARIN	JAPANESE	ENGLISH
Ging Ting Fa	*Sedum erythrosticum*	Flos Sedi erythrostici	Jing Tian Hua		Red stonecrop flower
Git Heung Fa, Mung Fa	*Edgeworthiae chrysantha*	Flos Edgeworthiae chrysanthae	Jie Xiang Hua, Meng Hua		Oriental paperbush flower
Gon Chat	*Rhus verniciflua*	Succus exsiccatus Rhudis	Gan Qi		Lacquer
Gong Bun Gwai, Gwan Yip Lou	*Polygonum perfoliatum*	Herba Polygoni perfoliati	Gang Ban Gui, Guan Ye Liao		Perfoliate knotweed herb
Gong Lau Pei , Heung Lau Pei	*Periploca sepium*	Cortex radicis Periplocae	Gang Liu Pi, Xiang Liu Pi		Silk vine root bark
Gong Mui Gan, Maan Dim Gam	*Ilex asprella*	Folium et radix Ilicis asprellae	Gang Mei (Gen), Wang Dian Jing		Rough holly leaf and root
Gong Naam Kyun Paap	*Selaginella moellendorfii*	Herba Selaginella moellendorfii	Jiang Nan Juan Bai		Moellendorf's spikemoss herb
Got Fa	*Pueraria lobata, P. omeiensis* and spp	Flos Puerariae	Ge Hua		Kudzu flower
Got Gan	*Pueraria lobata, P. omeiensis* and spp	Radix Puerariae	Ge Gen	Kakkon	Kudzu root
Got Leui Jap Gan	*Vitis flexuosa*	Radix Vitis flexuosis	Ge Lei Zhi Gen		Flexuose grape root
Gou Bun	*Ligusticum sinense, L. jebolense*	Radix Ligustici sinensis	Gao Ben	Kohon	Chinese lovage root
Gou Leung Geung	*Alpinia officinarum*	Rhizoma Alpiniae officinari	Gao Liang Jiang	Koryokyo	Galangal root
Gu Faan	*Alumen*	Alumen praeparatum	Ku Fan		Prepared alum
Gu Nga	*Oryza sativa*	Fructus Oryzae germinatus	Gu Ya	Kokuga	Sprouted rice grain
Gu Sou Fa	*Desmodium umbellatum*	Flos Desmodii umbellati	Gu Su Hua		Umbel desmodium flower
Guk Fa	*Chrysanthemum* x *morifolium*	Flos Chrysanthemi	Ju Hua, Gan Ju Hua		Chrysanthe-mum flower
Guk Jing Chou	*Eriocaulon buergerianum, E. sieboldianum*	Herba Eriocaulonis	Gu Jing Cao	Kokuseiso	Pipewort herb
Guk Jing Ji	*Eriocaulon buergerianum, E. sieboldianum*	Fructus Eriocaulonis	Gu Jing Zi		Pipewort seed
Gung Lou Yip, Sai Yip Sap Daai Gung Lou Yip	*Mahonia fortunei*	Folium Mahoniae fortunei	Shi Da Gong Lao Ye, Xi Ye Shi Da Gong Lao Ye	Judaikoro	Mahonia leaf
Gwa Ji Gam	*Polygala japonica*	Herba Polygalae japonicae	Gua Zi Jin		Japanese milkwort herb
Gwaan Muk Tung	*Aristolochia manshuriensis, A. moupinensis*	Caulis Aristolochiae manshuriensis	Guan Mu Tong		Manchurian birthwort stem
Gwai Baan	*Chinemys reevesii*	Plastrum Chinemis	Gui Ban	Kiban	Tortoise shell
Gwai Baan Gaau	*Chinemys reevesii*	Gelatinum carapaxis Chinemis	Gui Ban Jiao		Tortoise shell gel
Gwai Fa Pei	*Osmanthus fragrans*	Cortex ramuli Osmanthi	Gui Hua Pi		Osmanthus twig bark
Gwai Jam Chou	*Bidens bipinnata*	Herba Bidentis bipinnatae	Gui Zhen Cao		Beggartick herb

CANTONESE	SCIENTIFIC	PHARMACEUTICAL	MANDARIN	JAPANESE	ENGLISH
Gwai Ji	*Cinnamomum cassia*	Ramulus Cinnamomi cassiae	Gui Zhi , Rou Gui Zhi	Keishi	Cassia cinnamon twig
Gwai Jin Yu	*Euonymus alata*	Ramulus Eunymi alati	Gui Jian Yu		Winged spindletree twig
Gwai Kau	*Dysosma versipellis*	Rhizoma Dysosmae versipellis	Gui Jiu		Common dysosma root
Gwai Pei	*Cinnamomum japonicum, C. zeylanicum, C. obtusifolium*	Cortex Cinnamomi japonici	Gui Pi		Cinnamon bark
Gwai Yu Jin	*Buchnera cruciata*	Herba Buchnerae	Gui Yu Jian		Cruciate bluehart herb
Gwan Bou	*Laminaria japonica* and spp	Thallus Laminariae	Kun Bu	Kombu	Kelp seaweed
Gwan Gam Tang	*Cissus pteroclada*	Caulis Cissi	Kuan Jin Teng		Cissus stem
Gwan Gam Tang	*Tinospora sinensis*	Caulis Tinosporae sinensis	Kuan Jin Teng	Kankinto	Chinese tinospora stem
Gwat Hat	*Citrus reticulata, C. tangerina, C. erythrosa*	Semen Citri reticulatae	Ju He		Tangerine seed
Gwat Heung	*Citrus grandis* and spp.	Fructus Citri grandi immaturi	Ju Hong Zhu		Unripe citrus fruit
Gwat Heung (Pei), Fa Gwat Pei	*Citrus grandis* and spp	Exocarpium rubrum Citri	Ju Hong (Pi), Hua Ju Pi		Red citrus outer rind
Gwat Heung Fa	*Citrus grandis* and spp	Flos Citri grandi	Ju Hong Hua		Citrus flower
Gwat Kut	*Limax agrestic*	Limax	Guo Yu		Slug
Gwat Lok	*Citrus* spp	Fasciculus vascularis Citri, Endocarpium Citri	Ju Luo, Ju Bai		Citrus fibre
Gwat Seui Bou	*Davallia divaricata*	Rhizoma Davalliae	Gu Sui Bu	Kotsusaiho	Boneknit root
Gwat Seui Bou	*Drynaria fortunei* and spp	Rhizoma Drynariae	Gu Sui Bu	Kotsusaiho	Boneknit root
Gwat Seui Bou	*Pseudodrynaria fortunei, D. baronii*	Rhizoma Pseudodrynariae	Gu Sui Bu	Kotsusaiho	Boneknit root
Gwat Yip	*Citrus* spp.	Folium Aurantium	Ju Ye		Citrus leaf
Gwo Tong Se	*Jussiaea repens*	Herba Jussiaeae	Kuo Tang She		Clove strip herb
Gwon Jam Wong, Ye Gu	*Aeginetia indica*	Herba Aeginetiae	Guan Zhen Huang, Ye Gu		Aeginetia herb
Gwong Dung (Gam) Chin Chou	*Desmodium styracifolium*	Herba Desmodii	Guang Dong (Jin) Qian Cao	Kinsenso	Coin-leaf desmodium herb
Gwong Dung Jing Ma	*Serratula chinensis*	Radix Serratulae	Guang Dong Sheng Ma		Serratula root
Gwong Fok Heung	*Pogostemon cablin*	Herba Pogostemis	Guang Huo Xiang		Patchouli herb
Gwong Gau Sam	*Canis*	Testes et penis canis	Guang Gou Shen	Kujin	Male dog genitals
Gwong Ming Ji	*Ocimum Basilicum*	Fructus Ocimi	Guang Ming Zi		Basil seed
Gwong Sa Yan	*Amomum villosum*	Semen Amomi villosi	Guang Sha Ren		Wild cardamom seed
Gwun Jung	*Cyathea spinulosa*	Rhizoma Cyatheae	Guan Zhong		Cyathea root
Gwun Jung	*Lunathyrum vegetius, L. giraldii*	Rhizoma Lunathyri	Guan Zhong		Lunathyrum fern root

CANTONESE	SCIENTIFIC	PHARMACEUTICAL	MANDARIN	JAPANESE	ENGLISH
Gwun Jung, Dung Fong Wu Mou Kyut Yip	*Blechnum orientale*	Rhizoma Blechni	Guan Zhong, Wu Mao Jue Guan Zhong, Dong Fang Wu Mao Jue Ye	Kanju	Oriental hammock fern root
Gwun Jung, Fan Gai Tau	*Cyrtomium fortunei*	Rhizoma Cyrtomi	Guan Zhong, Hun Ji Tou,		Boss fern root
Gwun Jung, Gau Jek Gun Jung	*Woodwardia japonica, W. unigemmata*	Rhizoma Woodwardiae	Guan Zhong, Gou Ji Guan Zhong		Chain-fern root
Gwun Jung, Ji Kei Gwun Jung	*Osmunda japonica*	Rhizoma Osmundae	Guan Zhong, Zi Qi Guan Zhong	Tohoku-kanju	Japanese flowering fern root
Gwun Jung, Min Ma Gwun Jung	*Dryopteris crassirhizoma*	Rhizoma Dryopteris	Guan Zhong, Mian Ma Guan Zhong	Tohoku-kanju	Shield fern root
Gwun Jung, Ying Gwo Kyut Gwun Jung	*Matteucia struthiopteris*	Rhizoma Matteuciae	Guan Zhong, Jia Guo Jue Guan Zhong		Ostrich-feather fern root
Ha Fu Chou	*Prunella vulgaris*	Spica Prunellae	Xia Ku Cao	Kagoso	Selfheal spike
Ha Tin Mou	*Corydalis decumbens*	Herba Corydalis decumbensis	Xia Tian Wu		Decumbent corydalis herb
Haai Yi Chou	*Rungia pectinata*	Herba Rungiae	Hai Er Cao		Rungia herb
Haak Dau Yi	*Glycine max*	Pericarpium Glycinis	Hei Dou Yi		Soybean husk
Haak Min Yip	*Breynia fruticosa*	Cacumen Breyniae	Hei Mian Ye		Breynia tip
Haan Fong Gei Fong Gei	*Stephania tetrandra*	Radix Stephaniae tetrandrae	Han Fang Ji, Fang Ji	Kamboi	Stephania root
Hak Ji Ma	*Sesamum indicum*	Fructus Sesami	Hei Zhi Ma Hu Ma Ren		Black sesame seed
Ham Sau Chou	*Mimosa pudica*	Herba mimosae pudicae	Han Xiu Cao		Mimosa herb
Hao Gaau	*Macaca mulatta*	Gelatinum Macacae	Hou Jiao		Macaque gel
Hap Fun Fa	*Albizzia julibrissin, A. lebbek* and spp	Flos Albizziae	He Huan Hua	Gokanka	Mimosa flower
Hap Fun Pei	*Albizzia julibrissin, A. lebbak* and spp	Cortex Albizziae	He Huan Pi	Gokanhi	Mimosa bark
Hap Ji Chou	*Actinostemma lobata*	Folium at semen Actinostemmae	He Zi Cao		Actinostemma leaf and seed
Hat Daam	*Hemsleya amabilis, H. macrosperma* and spp.	Radix Hemsleyae	Xue Dan		Hemsleya tuber
Hat Ling Fa	*Saussurea laniceps, S. involucrata* and spp	Herba Saussureae lanicepsis	Xue Lian Hua		Snow lotus herb
Hat Ling Gan	*Saussurea laniceps, S. involucrata* and spp	Radix Saussureae lanicepsis	Xue Lian Gen		Snow lotus root
Hau Jou	*Macaca mulatta*	Calculus Macacae	Hou Zao	Koso	Macaque bezoar
Hau Pok Fa	*Magnolia officinalis, M. biloba, M. obovata*	Flos Magnoliae officinalis	Hou Po Hua	Koboka, Kobokuka	Magnolia flower
Hau Pok, Chyun Pok	*Magnolia officinalis, M. biloba, M. obovata*	Cortex Magnoliae officinalis	Hou Po Chuan Po	Koboku	Magnolia bark

CANTONESE	SCIENTIFIC	PHARMACEUTICAL	MANDARIN	JAPANESE	ENGLISH
Hau Yip Chyun Muk Heung	*Dolomiaea berardioidea*	Radix Dolomiaea berardioidea	Hou Ye Chuan Mu Xiang		Thick-leaf Dolomiaea root
Hei Lim Chou	*Siegesbeckia pubescens, S. orientalis, S. glabrescens*	Herba Siegesbeckiae	Xi Xian Cao		Hairy siegesbeckia herb
Hei Syu	*Camptotheca acuminata*	Cortex radicis Camptothecae	Xi Shu		Happy tree root bark
Hei Syu Gwo	*Camptotheca acuminata*	Fructus Camptothecae	Xi Shu Guo		Happy tree seed
Heun Chou, Leung Fan Chou	*Mesona chinensis*	Herba Mesonae	Xian Cao, Liang Fen Cao		Jellywort herb
Heun Fung Chou	*Bidens pilosa* var. *minor* and spp	Herba Bidentis pilosae	Xian Feng Cao		Hairy beggartick herb
Heung Fa Choi, Lou Laan Heung	*Mentha spicata*	Herba Menthae spicatae	Xiang Hua Cai, Liu Lan Xiang		Spearmint herb
Heung Fu	*Cyperus rotundus*	Rhizoma Cyperi	Xiang Fu	Kobushi	Purple nutsedge root
Heung Gu	*Lentinula edodes*	Sclerotium Lentinulae	Xiang Gu	Shiitake	Shiitake mushroom
Heung Maau	*Cymbopogon citratus*	Herba Cymbopogonis	Xiang Mao		Lemongrass herb
Heung Yat Kwai Fa Bun	*Helianthus annuus*	Receptaculum Helianthi	Xian Ji Gui Hua Pan		Sunflower receptacle
Heung Yip	*Pelargonium graveolens*	Herba Pelargonii	Xiang Ye		Rose geranium herb
Heung Yu (Chou)	*Elsholtzia splendens, E. stauntonii*	Herba Elsholtziae	Xiang Ru (Cao)	Koju	Aromatic madder herb
Heung Yun	*Citrus medica, C. wilsonii*	Fructus Citri medicae	Xiang Yuan, Gou Yuan		Citron fruit
Heung Yun Pei, Gau Yun Pei	*Citrus medica, C. wilsonii*	Pericarpium Citri medicae	Xiang Yuan Pi, Gou Yuan Pi		Citron rind
Him Sat	*Euryale ferox*	Semen Euryalis	Qian Shi	Kenjitsu	Foxnut
Hin Ngau Ji	*Pharbitis nil, P. purpurea* and spp	Semen Pharbitis	Qian Niu Zi		Japanese morning glory seed
Ho Ji (Yuk)	*Terminalia chebula* and var.	Fructus Terminaliae	He Zi (Rou)	Kashi	Myrobalan fruit
Ho Sau Wu	*Polygonum multiflorum*	Radix Polygoni multiflori	He Shou Wu	Kashuu	Flowery knotweed root
Ho Yip	*Nelumbo nucifera*	Folium Nelumbinis	He Ye, Lian Lie	Kayo	Lotus leaf
Hoi Chou	*Sargassum fusiforme* and spp	Herba Sargassi	Hai Zao	Kaiso	Sargassum seaweed
Hoi Daai	*Laminaria* spp	Herba Laminariae	Hai Dai		Algae
Hoi Fung Tang	*Kadsura heteroclita*	Caulis Kadsurae heteroclitae	Hai Feng Teng		Heteroclite kadsura stem
Hoi Fung Tang	*Piper hancei*	Caulis Piperis hanceis	Hai Feng Teng		Kadsura pepper stem
Hoi Fung Tang	*Piper hancei* var. *squamiglandiferu m*	Caulis Piperis squamiglandiferi	Hai Feng Teng, Xian Lin Ju		Fujian kadsura pepper stem
Hoi Gam Sa	*Lygodium japonicum*	Spora Lygodii	Hai Jin Sha	Kaikinsha	Japanese climbing fern spore
Hoi Gam Sa Tang	*Lygodium japonicum*	Herba Lygodii	Hai Jin Sha Teng	Kaikinshato	Japanese climbing fern herb

CANTONESE	SCIENTIFIC	PHARMACEUTICAL	MANDARIN	JAPANESE	ENGLISH
Hoi Gam So	*Polygonum cymosum*	Radix et rhizoma Polygoni cymosi	Kai Jin Suo		Cymose knotweed Root
Hoi Gap Hok	*Cyclina sinensis*	Concha Cyclinae	Hai Ge Ke, Ke Li	Kaigokaku	Clam shell
Hoi Gau Sam	*Callorhinus ursinus, Phoca vitulina*	Testes et penis Callorhini seu Phocae	Hai Gou Shen	Kaikujin	Seal genitals
Hoi Jit	*Rhopilema esculenta*	Tentaculum Rhopilema	Hai Zhe		Jellyfish tentacle
Hoi Lung	*Solenognathus* spp., *Syngnathoides biaculeatus*	Solenognathus	Hai Long		Pipefish
Hoi Ma	*Hippocampus kelloggiand* spp	Hippocampus	Hai Ma	Kaiba	Sea horse
Hoi Piu Seui	*Sepia esculenta, Sepiella maindroni*	Os Sepiae seu Sapiellae	Hai Piao Xiao, Wu Zei Gu		Cuttlefish bone
Hoi Sam	*Stichopus japonicus*	Stichopus	Hai Shen		Sea cucumber
Hoi Tung Pei	*Erythrina variegata* var. *orientalis*	Cortex Erythrinae	Hai Tong Pi	Kaitohi	Asian coral tree bark
Hoi Wu	*Alocasia odora*	Rhizoma Alocasiae	Guang Lang Du, Hai Yu		Alocasia root
Hok	*Mactra sulcataria*	Concha Mactrae	Ge	Jiseki	Mactra shell
Hok Chou Nga	*Agrimonia pilosa* var. *japonica*	Gemma Agrimoniae pilosae	He Cao Ya		Furry agrimony winter bud
Hok Sat	*Carpesium abrotanoides*	Fructus seu semen Carpesii	He Shi	Kakushitsu	Starwort fuit or seed
Hon Choi	*Rorippa montana, R. indica*	Herba Rorippae	Han Cai		Nasturtium herb
Hon Lin Chou	*Eclipta prostata, E. alba*	Herba Ecliptae	Han Lian Cao, Mo Han Lian	Kanrenso	Field lotus herb
Hon Sam Chou	*Scutellaria indica*	Herba Scutellariae indicae	Han Xin Cao		India skullcap herb
Hon Seui Sek	*Calcitum*	Calcitum	Han Shui Shi, Fang Jie Shi	Kansuiseki	Calcite
Hon Seui Sek, Hung Sek Gau	*Gypsum rubrum*	Gypsum rubrum	Han Shui Shi, Hong Shi Gao		Red gypsum
Hung Bun Bin Lin	*Begonia crassirostris*	Herba Begoniae crassirostris	Hong Ban Bian Lian		Begonia herb
Hung Chi Teng, Siu Gam Ying	*Rosa cymosa*	Cortex radicis Rosae cymosae	Hong Ci Teng, Hong Gen, Xiao Jin Ying		Cymose rose root bark
Hung Daai Gik	*Knoxia valerianoides*	Radix Knoxiae	Hong Da Ji	Kogataigeki	Knoxia root
Hung Daam	*Ursus arctos* and spp	Fel Ursi	Xiong Dan	Yutan	Bear gallbladder
Hung Dau Kau	*Alpinia galanga*	Fructus Alpiniae Galangae	Hong Dou Kou		Greater galangal berry
Hung Fa	*Carthamus tinctorius*	Flos Carthami tinctorii	Hong Hua	Koka	Safflower
Hung Hon Lin	*Hypericum ascyron*	Herba Hyperici ascyronis	Hong Han Lian		St. John's wort
Hung Jou	*Zizyphus jujuba* var. *inermis*	Fructus Zizyphi jujubae	Hong Zao	Koso	Red jujube berry
Hung Ju Mai	*Oryza sativa* and *Monascus purpureus*	Fructus Oryzae fermentatus cum Monasco	Hong Qu Mi		Fermented rice with red yeast

CANTONESE	SCIENTIFIC	PHARMACEUTICAL	MANDARIN	JAPANESE	ENGLISH
Hung Leung Ji	*Huechys sanguinea, H, philaemata*	Huechys	Hong Niang Zi		Red cicada
Hung Long Duk, Long Duk	*Stellera chamaejasme*	Radix Stellerae	Hong Lang Du, Lang Du		Stellara root
Hung Maau Cha	*Statice sinensis*	Radix Staticis	Hong Mao Cha		Statice root
Hung Mou Chat	*Leontice robustum*	Radix Leonticis	Hong Mao Qi		Leontice root
Hung Muk Heung	*Kadsura longipedunculata*	Radix Kadsurae longipedunculatae	Hong Mu Xiang		Long-stalk kadsura root
Hung Sam Lin Ji Chou	*Alternanthera philoxeroides*	Herba Alternantherae	Kong Xiu Lian Zi Cao		Alligator Alternanthera herb
Hung Yan Sam	*Panax ginseng*	Radix Panacis ginsengis praeparatae	Hong Ren Shen	Koninjin	Red cured Asian ginseng root
Hyut Fung Tang	*Ventilago leiocarpa*	Radix et rhizoma Ventilaginis	Xue Feng Teng, Qing Pi Mao		Ventilago root and stem
Hyut Kit	*Daemonorops draco*	Resina Daemonoropsis (Sanguis draconis)	Xue Jie	Kekketsu	Dragon's-blood resin
Hyut Yu Taan	*Homo sapiens*	Crinis carbonisatus Hominis	Xue Yu Tan		Charred human hair
Iu Fa	*Wikstroemia chamaedaphne*	Flos Wikstroaemiae chamaedaphnis	Rao Hua		Wikstroemia flower
Jaak Chat	*Euphorbia helioscopia*	Herba Euphorbiaeheliosc opiae	Ze Qi	Takushitsu	Sunspurge herb
Jaak Laan	*Lycopus lucidus*	Herba Lycopi	Ze Lan	Takuran	Bright bugleweed herb
Jaak Se	*Alisma orientalis*	Rhizoma Alismae	Ze Xie	Takusha	Water plantain root
Jak Paak Yip	*Biota orientalis*	Cacumen Biotae orientalis	Ce Bai Ye	Sokuhakuyo	Oriental arborvitae tip
Jau Ma Toi	*Ardisia gigantifolia*	Rhizoma Ardisiae gigantifoliae	Zou Ma Tai		Ardisia root
Je Muk	*Cudrania tricuspidata*	Lignum Cudraniae tricuspidatae	Da Ding Huang, Zhe Mu		Cudrania heartwood
Jek Chin Fa	*Impatiens balsamina*	Flos Impatiensis	Ji Xing Hua		Garden balsam flower
Jek Chin Ji	*Impatiens balsamina*	Semen Impatiensis	Ji Xing Zi	Kyuseishi	Garden balsam seed
Jek Gam Chou	*Glycirrhiza uralensis, G. glabra* and spp	Radix Glycirrhizae preparatae	Zhi Gan Cao	Shakanzo	Honey-fried licorice root
Jeuk Chong	*Rostellulariae procumbens*	Herba Rostellulariae	Jue Chuang		Creeping rostellularia herb
Jeuk Chong, Syu Mei Wong	*Justicia procumbens*	Herba Justiciae	Jue Chuang Cao, Shu Wei Huang		Justicia herb
Jeun Haai	*Eriocheir sinensis, E. japonicus*	Eriocheir	Jin Xie	Zukani	Tianjin crab
Jeung Long Chung	*Catharsius molossus, Xylotrupes dichotomus*	Catharsius seu Xylotrupes	Jiang Lan Chong		Dung beetle
Jeung Muk	*Cinnamomum camphora*	Lignum Cinnamomi camphorae	Zhang Mu		Camphor wood

CANTONESE	SCIENTIFIC	PHARMACEUTICAL	MANDARIN	JAPANESE	ENGLISH
Jeung Naau	*Cinnamomum camphora*	Camphora	Zhang Nao	Shono	Camphor flake
Jeung Sat	*Quercus acutissima*	Fructus Querci acutissimae	Xiang Shi		Oak fruit
Jeung Yip Bun Ha, Fu Jeung Lam Sing	*Pinellia pedatisecta*	Rhizoma Pinelliae pedatisectae	Zhang Ye Ban Xia, Wu Zhang Nan Xing		Pedatisect pinellia corm
Ji Choi	*Porphyra tenera*	Herba Porphyrae	Zi Cai		Porphyra herb
Ji Chou	*Lithospermum erythrorhizon*	Radix Lithospermi	Zi Cao	Shikon	Purple groomwell root
Ji Chou	*Macrotomia euchroma*	Radix Macrotomiae	Zi Cao	Shikon	Macrotomia root
Ji Chou	*Onosma paniculatum*	Radix Onosmae	Zi Cao		Onosma root
Ji Chou Yan	*Lithospermum erythrorhizon*	Flos Lithospermi	Zi Cao Rong		Purple groomwell flower
Ji Chou, San Geung Ji Chou	*Arnebia euchroma, A. guttata*	Radix Arnebiae	Zi Cao, Xin Jiang Zi Cao	Shikon	Arnebia root
Ji Fa Dei Ding	*Viola yedoensis, V. japonica*	Radix et herba Violae yedoensis	Zi Hua Di Ding	Shikajicho	Asian violet root and herb
Ji Gam Ngau	*Ardisia japonica*	Radix et herba Ardisiae japonicae	Zi Jin Niu, Jin Niu Cao		Marlberry root and herb
Ji Ging Pei	*Cercis chinensis*	Cortex Cercis	Zi Jing Pi		Chinese redbud bark
Ji Ging Pei	*Kadsura peltigera*	Cortex Kadsurae peltigerae	Zi Jing Pi		Chinese redbud bark
Ji Gwat Ji	*Hovenia dulcis*	Semen et fructus Hoveniae	Zhi Ju Zi		Hovenia seed and fruit
Ji Ho Je	*Homo sapiens*	Placenta Hominis	Zi He Che	Shikasha	Human placenta
Ji Hok, Doi Doi Fa Ji Hok	*Citrus aurantium* var. *amara*	Fructus Citri aurantii amarae	Zhi Ke, Zhi Qiao, Dai Dai Hua Zhi Qiao	Kikoku	Ripe bitter orange fruit
Ji Ji, Saan Ji Ji	*Gardenia jasminoides*	Fructus Gardeniae	Zhi Zi Shan Zhi Zi	Sanshishi	Gardenia pod
Ji Juk Gan	*Phyllostachys nigra* var. *henonis* and spp	Radix Phyllostachis	Zi Zhu Gen		Black bamboo root
Ji Jyu Yip	*Callicarpa pedunculata*	Folium Callicarpae pedunculatae	Zi Zhu Ye	Jijuso	Callicarpa leaf
Ji Jyu Yip, Daai Yip Ji Jyu	*Callicarpa macrophylla*	Folium Callicarpae macrophyllae	Zi Zhu Ye, Ta Ye Zi Zhu		Large-leaf Callicarpa leaf
Ji Mai Tin Kwai, Hung Tin Kwai	*Begonia fimbristipula*	Herba Begoniae fimbristipulae	Zi Bei Tian Kuei Hong Tian Kui		Begonia herb
Ji Mou	*Anemarrhena asphodeloides*	Radix Anemarrhenae	Zhi Mu	Chimo	Know mother root
Ji Sat	*Citrus aurantium, C. wilsonii*	Fructus Citri aurantii immaturi	Zhi Shi	Kijitsu	Unripe bitter orange fruit
Ji Se Muk Pei	*Holarrhenia antidysenterica*	Cortex Holarrheniae	Zhi Xie Mu Pi		Conessi bark
Ji Sek Ying	*Fluoritum*	Fluoritum	Zi Shi Ying		Purple fluorite
Ji Taan	*Pterocarpus indicus*	Lignum Pterocarpi	Zi Tan		Malay padauk wood, Burma rosewood
Ji Tang Ji, Tang Lau	*Wisteria sinensis, W. floribunda*	Galla Wisteriae	Zi Teng Zi, Teng Liu	Figikobu	Asian wisteria gall
Ji Yan	*Biota orientalis*	Semen Biotae orientalis	Bai Zi Ren	Hakushinin	Oriental arborvitae berry

CANTONESE	SCIENTIFIC	PHARMACEUTICAL	MANDARIN	JAPANESE	ENGLISH
Ji Yin Tung	*Pyritum*	Pyritum	Zi Ran Tong	Shizendo	Pyrite
Ji Yun	*Aster tataricus*	Radix Asteris tatarici	Zi Wan	Shion	Tartary aster root
Jik Cheung Pou	*Acorus tatarinowii*	Rhizoma Acori tatarinowii	Jie Chang Pu		Tatarinow's sweetflag root
Jik Syut Chou, Pang Daai Yan	*Centella asiatica*	Folium Centellae	Ji Xue Cao, Peng Da Wan		Gotu kola leaf
Jin Dou Chou	*Clinopodium confine*	Herba Clinopodii	Jian Dao Cao		Clinopodium herb
Jin Jang Tap	*Lycopodium serratum* and spp	Pollen Lycopodii	Qian Cang Ta, Pu Di Wu Gong, Guo Jiang Long, Yu Bai		Lycopodium pollen
Jin Wat Choi	*Lythrum salicaria*	Herba Lythri salicariae	Qian Cu Cai		Loosestrife herb
Jin Yat Hung	*Gomphrena globosa*	Flos Gomphrenae	Qian Ri Hong		Globe amaranth flower
Jip Gwat Sin Tou	*Veronica peregrina*	Herba et radix Veronicae	Jie Gu Xian Tao		Peregrine speedwell herb and root
Jit Tung Pei	*Zanthoxylum ailanthoides*	Cortex Zanthoxyli ailanthoidis	Zhe Tong Pi		Zhejiang prickly ash bark
Jong Ke	*Anisodus tanguticus*	Redix seu semen Anisodi	Zang Qie		Anisodus root or seed
Jou Faan	*Melanteritum*	Melanteritum	Zao Fan, Lu Fan		Green vitriol
Jou Gok Chi	*Gleditsia sinensis* and spp	Spina Gleditsiae	Zao Jiao Ci	Sokakushi	Honeylocust spine
Jou Gok Ji	*Gleditsia sinensis* and spp.	Semen Gleditsiae	Zao Jiao Zi		Honeylocust fruit
Jou Gok, Jou Gaap	*Gleditsia sinensis* and spp	Fructus Gleditsiae	Zao Jiao, Zao Jia	Sokaku	Honeylocust pod
Jou Si Ma	*Daphne giraldii, D. tangutica, D. retusa*	Cortex Daphnis giraldii	Zu Shi Ma		Giraldi's daphne bark
Ju Daam	*Sus scrofa domestica*	Fel Suidis	Zhu Dan		Pig gallbladder
Ju Ling	*Polyporus umbellatus*	Sclerotium Polypori	Zhu Ling	Chorei	Umbel polypore mushroom
Ju Sa	*Cinnabarum*	Cinnabarum	Zhu Sha	Shusha	Cinnabar
Ju Yi Sam	*Panax major, P. repens*	Radix Panacis majoris	Zhu Er Shen		Pearl ginseng root
Juk Dyun	*Dipsacus japonica*	Radix Dipsaci japonicae	Xu Duan	Zokudan	Japanese teasel root
Juk Dyun, Chyun Dyun	*Dipsacus asperoides*	Radix Dipsaci asperoides	Xu Duan, Chuan Duan		Sichuan teasel root
Juk Jit (Yan) Sam	*Panax japonicus*	Radix Panacis japonici	Zhu Jie (Ren) Shen	Tikusetu-ninjin	Japanese ginseng root
Juk Lai	*Phyllostachys nigra* var. *henonis* and spp	Succus Phyllostachis	Zhu Li	Chikureki	Black bamboo sap
Juk Yip	*Phyllostachys nigra* var. *henonis* and spp	Folium Phyllostachis	Zhu Ye		Black bamboo leaf
Juk Yip Jiu	*Zanthoxylum planispinum*	Fructus Zanthoxyli planispini	Zhu Ye Jiao		Prickly ash berry
Juk Yu	*Phyllostachys nigra* var. *henonis* and spp	Caulis Phyllostachis in taeniis	Zhu Ru	Chikujo	Black bamboo shaving

CANTONESE	SCIENTIFIC	PHARMACEUTICAL	MANDARIN	JAPANESE	ENGLISH
Jung Gan Baak Pei	*Cedrela sinensis*	Cortex radicis Cedrelae	Chun Gen Bai Pi		Cedrela root bark
Jung Lau, Chat Yip Yat Ji Pa	*Paris chinensis*	Rhizoma Paris chinensis	Zhong Lou, Qi Ye Yi Zhi Hua		Chinese paris root
Jung Lau, Wan Laam Jung Lau	*Paris yunnanensis*	Rhizoma Paris yunnanensis	Zhong Lou, Yun Nan Zhong Lou		Yunnan paris root
Jung Leui Ji	*Trachycarpus excelsa, T. fortunei*	Fructus Trachycarpi	Zong Lu Zi		Windmill palm seed
Jung Leui Pei Daan	*Trachycarpus excelsa, T. fortunei*	Fibra Stipulae Trachycarpi carbonisata	Zong Lu Pi Tan		Charred windmill palm petiole
Jyu Ji	*Quercus salicina, Q. myrsinaefolium*	Folium Querci	Zhu Zi Ye	Urajirokashi	Oak leaf
Jyu Lung Chou	*Nepenthes mirabilis*	Herba Nepenthis	Zhu Long Cao		Pitcher plant herb
Jyu Mou Choi	*Salsola collina, S. ruthenica, S. richteri*	Radix et herba Salsolae	Zhu Mao Cai		Salsola root and herb
Jyu Sa Gan	*Ardisia crenata, A. bicolor*	Radix Ardisiae crenatae	Da Lo San, Zhu Sha Gen	Shushakon	Coralberry root
Jyun Dei Fung	*Schizophragma integrifolium*	Cortex radicis Schizophragmae	Zuan Di Feng		Schizophrag-ma root bark
Kap Gei	*Chloranthus serratus*	Radix Chloranthi	Ji Ji		Serrate-leaf chloranthus
Ke Gan	*Solanum melongena*	Radix et rhizoma Solani melongenae	Qie Gen		Eggplant root
King Ma (Ji)	*Abutilon theophrastii*	Semen Abutili theophrasti	Qing Ma (Zi)		China jute seed
Kit Chou	*Valeriana officinalis, V. hardwickii*	Rhizoma Valerianae	Xie Cao		Valerian root
Kwai Sat Ji	*Livistona chinensis*	Semen Livistonae	Kui Shu Zi		Fan palm seed
Kwan Ming Gai Yut Tang	*Millettia reticulata*	Radix et caulis Millettiae reticulatae	Ji Xue Teng, Kun Ming Ji Xue Teng		Millettia root and stem
Kwan Ming Saan Hoi Tong	*Tripterygium hypoglaucum*	Radix Tripterygii hypoglauci decorticati	Kun Ming Shan Hai Tang, Diao Mao Cao		Peeled Tripterygium root
Kwut Lau	*Trichosanthes kirilowii, T. japonica, T. uniflora*	Fructus Tricosanthis	Gua Lou (Shi)	Karo	Snakegourd fruit
Kwut Lau Pei	*Trichosanthes kirilowii, T. japonica, T. uniflora*	Pericarpium Tricosanthis	Gua Lou Pi	Karohi	Snakegourd rind
Kwut Lau Yan	*Trichosanthes kirilowii, T. japonica, T. uniflora*	Semen Trichosanthis	Gua Lou Ren	Karonin	Snakegourd seed
Kyun Paap	*Selaginella tamariscina*	Herba Selaginellae tamariscinae	Juan Bai		Resurrection plant herb
Kyun Sam	*Polygonum bistorta*	Radix Polygoni bistortae	Quan Shen		Bistort root
Kyut Ming Ji, Chou Kyut Ming	*Cassia tora, C. obtusifolia* and spp	Semen Cassiae torae	Jue Ming Zi, Cao Jue Ming	Ketsumeishi	Sickle senna seed
La Lou Chou	*Polygonum lapathifolium*	Herba Polygoni lapathifolii	La Liao Cao		Knotweed herb

CANTONESE	SCIENTIFIC	PHARMACEUTICAL	MANDARIN	JAPANESE	ENGLISH
Laam Sat	*Polygonum tinctorium*	Herba Polygoni tinctorii	Lan Shi		Chinese indigo herb
Laap Mui Fa	*Chimonanthus praecox*	Flos Chimonanthi	La Mei Hua	Sakubaika	Wintersweet flower
Lai Ji Ho	*Litchi chinensis*	Semen Litchis	Li Zhi He		Lychee seed
Lai Ji Hok	*Litchi chinensis*	Pericarpium Litchis	Li Zhi Ke		Lychee rind
Lai Jik Chou	*Salvia plebeia*	Herba et radix Salviae plebeiae	Li Zhi Cao		Plebeian sage herb and root
Lai Lou	*Hemerocallis thunbergii*	Rhizoma et radix Hemerocallis thunbergii	Li Lu		Day lily root
Lai Lou	*Veratrum nigrum* and spp	Radix et rhizoma Veratri	Li Lu	Riro	False hellebore root
Lai Tau Chou	*Viola japonica*	Radix et herba Violae japonicae	Li Tou Cao		Japanese violet root and herb
Lai Tau Jim	*Typhonium divaricatum*	Rhizoma Typhonii divaricatii	Li Tou Jian		Divaricate typhonium root
Lat Mui Fa	*Prunus mume*	Flos Pruni mumis	Lu Er Mei, Lu Mei Hua		Black plum flower
Lau Gei Nou	*Artemisia anomala*	Herba Artemisiae anomalae	Liu Ji Niu	Ryukido	Anomalous wormwood herb
Lau Ji	*Salix babylonica, S. gracilistyla*	Ramulus Salicis	Liu Zhi		Weeping willow twig
Lau Lou	*Echinops latifolius, E. gmelinii*	Radix Echinopsis	Lou Lu		Globe thistle root
Lau Lou	*Rhaponticum uniflorum*	Radix Rhapontici	Lou Lu	Roro	Swiss centaury root
Lau Sam Fa	*Spilanthes acmella* var. *oleracea*	Flos Spilanthis	Liu Shen Hua		Six god flower
Lau Wong, Sek Lau Wong	*Sulphurum*	Sulphurum	Liu Huang, Shi Liu Huang	Io	Sulphur
Lau Yip	*Salix babylonica, S. gracilistyla*	Folium Salicis	Liu Ye		Weeping willow twig
Lei Gan Baak Pei	*Prunus salicina*	Cortex radicis Pruni salicinae	Li Gen Bai Pi		Willow plum root bark
Lei Pei	*Pyrus betulaefolia*	Pericarpium Pyri	Li Pi		Chinese pear rind
Lei Yu	*Cyprinus carpio*	Cyprinus	Li Yu		Carp
Leui Gung Tang	*Tripterygium wilfordii*	Medulla radicis Tripterygii	Lei Gong Teng		Yellow vine root pith
Leui Yun	*Mylitta lapidescens*	Sclerotium Mylittae	Lei Wan		Thunder ball fungus
Leung Tau Jim	*Anemone raddeana*	Rhizoma Anemonis raddeanae	Liang Tou Jian		Anemone root
Leut Chou	*Humulus scandens*	Herba Humuli scandentis	Lu Cao		Climbing hops flower
Leut Ji	*Castanea mollissima*	Fructus Castaneae	Li Zi, Feng Li Gu	Furitsukaku	Chinese chestnut
Lim Yan Fa	*Desmodium sinnatum*	Herba Desmodii sinnati	Guo Lu Huang, Nian Ren Hua		Sinnate desmodium herb
Lin Fong	*Nelumbo nucifera*	Receptaculum Nelumbinis	Lian Fang	Renshin	Lotus receptacle
Lin Gang	*Nelumbo nucifera*	Ramulus Nelumbinis	Lian Geng		Lotus stem
Lin Ji	*Nelumbo nucifera*	Semen Nelumbinis	Lian Zi	Renshi	Lotus seed
Lin Ji Sam	*Nelumbo nucifera*	Epicentrum seminis Nelumbinis	Lian Zi Xin		Lotus seed heart

CANTONESE	SCIENTIFIC	PHARMACEUTICAL	MANDARIN	JAPANESE	ENGLISH
Lin Kiu	*Forsythia suspensa*	Fructus Forsythiae	Lian Qiao	Rengyo	Forsythia valve
Lin Sam	*Nelumbo nucifera*	Plumula Nelumbinis	Lian Xin		Lotus plumule
Lin Sou	*Nelumbo nucifera*	Stamen Nelumbinis	Lian Xu	Renshu	Lotus stamen
Ling Chin Chou	*Glechoma hederacea, G. longituba*	Herba Glechomae	Lian Qian Cao		Ground ivy herb
Ling Gok	*Trapa bispinosa, T. bicornis*	Fructus Trapae	Ling Qiao		Water caltrop fruit
Ling Ji (Chou)	*Ganoderma lucidum, G. sinense, G applanatum* and spp	Sclerotium Ganodermae	Ling Zhi (Cao)	Reishi	Reishi mushroom
Ling Ling Heung	*Lysimachia sikokiana*	Herba Lysimachiae sikokianae	Ling Ling Xiang		Lysimachia herb
Ling Siu Fa	*Campsis grandiflora*	Flos Campsis grandiflorae	Ling Xiao Hua		Asian trumpetcree-per flower
Ling Siu Fa, Mei Jau Ling Siu	*Campsis radicans*	Flos Campsis radicantis	Ling Xiao Hua, Mei Jou Ling Xiao		Common trumpetcree-per flower
Ling Siu Gan	*Campsis grandiflora*	Radix Campsis grandiflorae	Ling Xiao Gen	Ryoshoka	Asian trumpetcree-per root
Ling Yeung Gok	*Saiga tatarica*	Cornu Saigae	Ling Yang Jiao	Reiyokaku	Antelope horn
Lit Dong	*Orobanche caerulescens* and spp	Herba Orobanchis	Lie Dang		Orobanche herb
Liu Go Wong	*Wickstroemia indica*	Radix Wickstroemiae	Liao Ge Wang (Gen)	Ryokao	Wikstroemia root
Lo Ba Gan	*Raphanus sativus*	Radix Raphani recentis	Luo Bo Gen		Fresh radish root
Lo Ba Yip	*Raphanus sativus*	Folium Raphani	Luo Bo Ye		Radish leaf
Lo Bou Ma	*Apocynum lancifolium, A. venetum, A. hendersonii*	Radix et herba Apocyni	Luo Bu Ma		Dogbane root and herb
Lo Fu Mou	*Rauvolfia verticillata, R. yunnanensis, R. latifrons, R. serpentina* and spp	Radix Rauvolfiae	Luo Fu Mu		Rauvolfia root
Lo Lak	*Ocimum basilicum*	Herba Ocimi	Jiu Ceng Ta, Luo Le		Basil herb
Lo Mai	*Oryza sativa*	Fructus Oryzae	Nuo Mi		Sweet rice
Lo Mo	*Metaplexis japonica*	Herba Metaplexis	Guo Lu Huang, Luo Mo		Metaplexis herb
Loi Fuk Ji	*Raphanus sativus*	Semen Raphani	Lai Fu Zi		Radish seed
Lok San Fu	*Astilbe chinensis*	Rhizoma Astilbis	Luo Xin Fu		Astilbe root
Lok Sek Tang	*Trachelospermum jasminoides*	Caulis Trachelospermi	Luo Shi Teng	Chikusekito	Star jasmine stem
Long Duk, Daai Long Duk	*Euphorbia nematocypha*	Radix Euphorbiae nematocyphae	Lang Du, Da Lang Du		Gigantic spurge root
Long Duk, Gai Cheung Long Duk	*Euphorbia prolifera*	Radix Euphorbiae proliferae	Lang Du, Ji Chang Lang Du		Prolific spurge root
Long Duk, Long Duk Daai Gik	*Euphorbia fischeriana*	Radix Euphorbiae fischerianae	Lang Du, Lang Du Da Ji		Fischer's spurge root

CANTONESE	SCIENTIFIC	PHARMACEUTICAL	MANDARIN	JAPANESE	ENGLISH
Long Duk, Yu Sin Daai Gik	*Euphorbia ebracteolata*	Radix Euphorbiae ebracteolatae	Lang Du, Yue Xian Da Ji		Bractless spurge root
Long Yu Pei	*Ulmus parvifolia*	Cortex Ulmi parvifoliae	Lang Yu Pi		Chinese elm bark
Lou Baak Fa Pei	*Bauhinia variegata*	Cortex Bauhiniae variegatae	Lao Bai Hua Pi		Orchid tree bark
Lou Fun Fong	*Polistes mandarinus, Parapolybia varia*	Nidus Polistis seu Parapolybiae	Lu Feng Fang		Hornet nest
Lou Gam Sek	*Calamina, Smithsonitum*	Calamina, Smithsonitum	Lu Gan Shi	Rokanseki	Calamine
Lou Gan	*Phragmites communis*	Radix Phragmitis	Lu Gen	Rokon	Water-reed root
Lou Ging	*Phragmites communis*	Ramulus Phragmitis	Wei Jing		Water-reed twig
Lou Gung Chuk	*Ficus microcarpa, F. retusa*	Radix Fici microcarpae seu retusae	Lao Gong Xu, Rong Shu Xu		Aerial fig root
Lou Gwun Chou	*Erodium stephaniarum, Geranium* spp	Herba Erodii seu Geranii	Lao Guan Cao		Storksbill or cranesbill herb
Lou Haan Kwo	*Momordica grosvenori*	Fructus Momordicae grosvenorii	Luo Han Guo	Rakanka	Arhat fruit
Lou Haan Yip	*Momordica grosvenori*	Folium Momordicae grosvenorii	Luo Han Ye	Rakankayo	Arhat leaf
Lou Hap Chou	*Geranium wilfordii, G. thunbergii*	Herba Geranii	Lao He Cao	Gennoshio-uko	Geranium herb
Lou Lou Tung	*Liquidambar taiwaniana*	Fructus Liquidambaris	Lu Lu Tong	Rorotsu	Taiwan maple fruit
Lou Sa	*Salammonitum* and *Halitum*	Salmiacum	Nao Sha		Salmiac, Sal ammoniac
Lou Sek	*Polygonum hydropiper*	Fructus Polygoni hydropiperis	Liao Shi		Water pepper fruit
Lou Syu Laak	*Acanthus ilicifolius*	Radix Acanthi ilicifolii	Lao Shu Le		Holly-leaf acanthus root
Lou Wui	*Aloe vera* var. *chinensis*	Resina Aloidis	Lu Hui		Aloe resin
Lu Gwat Daan	*Rubia cordifolia*	Caulis Rubiae cordifoliae	Lu Gu Dan		Heart-leaf madder stem
Luk Dau	*Phaseolus radiatum*	Semen Phaseoli radiati	Lu Dou	Ryokuzu	Mung bean
Luk Dau Fa	*Phaseolus mungo*	Flos Phaseoli	Lu Dou Hua		Mung bean flower
Luk Dau Yip	*Phaseolus radiatum*	Testa Phaseoli radiatae	Lu Dou Yi		Mung bean husk
Luk Gai Mei	*Microsorium bancockii, M. dilatatum*	Herba Microsorii	Lu Ji Wei		Microsorium herb
Luk Gok	*Cervus nippon* and spp	Cornu Cervi	Lu Jiao	Rokkaku	Mature deer antler
Luk Gok Gaau	*Cervus nippon* and spp	Colla cornu Cervi	Lu Jiao Jiao	Rokkakukyo	Mature deer antler glue
Luk Gok Shuen	*Cervus nippon* and spp	Cornu Cervi degelatinatum	Lu Jiao Shuang, Rong Mo	Rokkakuso	Mature deer antler powder
Luk Haam Chou, Luk Tai Chou	*Pyrola rotundifolia subsp. chinensis, P. Japonica*	Radix et herba Pyrolae	Lu Xian Cao, Lu Ti Cao	Rokuteiso	Asian wintergreen root and herb

CANTONESE	SCIENTIFIC	PHARMACEUTICAL	MANDARIN	JAPANESE	ENGLISH
Luk Ji Ji Hok, Gau Yun	*Poncirus trifoliata*	Fructus Ponciri immaturi	Lu Yi Zhi Qiao, Gou Yuan		Immature trifoliate orange fruit
Luk Mei Ba	*Cervus nippon* and spp	Cauda Cervi	Lu Wei Ba		Mature deer tail
Luk Yan	*Cervus nippon* and spp	Cornu cervi parvum	Lu Rong, Rong Tou, Nen Lu Rong	Rokujo	Velvet deer antler
Lung Daam Chou	*Gentiana scabra, G. triflora, G. manshurica*	Radix Gentianae scabrae	Long Dan Cao	Ryutan	Scabrous gentian root
Lung Gwat	*Stegodon orientalis, S. rhinocerus sinensis, Hipparion*	Os Stegodontis	Long Gu	Ryukotsu	Dragon bone
Lung Ji	*Stegodon orientalis et al.*	Dens Stegodontis	Long Chi		Dragon tooth
Lung Kwai	*Solanum nigrum*	Herba Solani nigri	Long Kui		Winter cherry herb
Lung Lei Yip	*Sauropus rostratus, S. changianus*	Folium Sauropi	Long Li Ye		Lizardtail leaf
Lung Ngaan Fa	*Euphoria longan*	Flos Euphoriae	Long Yan Hua		Longan flower
Lung Ngaan Ho	*Euphoria longan*	Semen Euphoriae	Long Yan He		Longan seed
Lung Ngaan Yuk	*Euphoria longan*	Arillus Euphoriae	Long Yan Rou	Ryuganniku	Longan fruit pulp
Lung Ngan Gu	*Fomes applanatus* and host fruit *Euphoria longana*	Sclerotium Fomis	Long Yan Gu		Longan fungus
Lung Sek Wong	*Desmodium pseudotriquetrum , D. triquetrum*	Herba Desmodii pseudotriquetrii	Long Shi Huang		Bottlegourd herb
Lung Syun Fa Gan	*Ixora chinensis*	Radox Ixorae	Long Chuan Hua Gen		Ixora root
Ma Ban Long	*Capparis masaikai*	Semen Capparis	Ma Bin Lang	Kuttokei	Capparis berry
Ma Bin Chou	*Verbena officinalis*	Herba Verbenae	Ma Bian Cao		Vervain herb
Ma Bou	*Equus caballos*	Calculus Equi	Ma Bao		Horse bezoar
Ma But	*Lasiosphaera fenslii* and spp, *Calvatia lilacina, C. fenzlii, C. gigantea*	Sclerotium Lasiosphaerae seu Calvatiae	Ma Bo	Babotsu	Puffball mushroom
Ma Chi Yin	*Portulacca oleracea*	Herba Portulaccae	Ma Chi Xian	Bashiken	Purslane herb
Ma Chin Ji	*Strychnos pierrana, S. nux-vomica* and spp	Semen Strychnotis preparatae	(Zhi) Ma Qian Zi	Basenshi	Prepared vomit nut
Ma Dau Ling	*Aristolochia contorta, A. debilis*	Fructus Aristolochiae	Ma Dou Ling	Batorei	Green birthwort capsule
Ma Dei Jing	*Dichondra repens*	Herba Dichondrae	Ma Di Jin	Kinsenso	Dichondra herb
Ma Ji Wu, Fung Hei Chou	*Adenostemma lavenia*	Herba Adenostemmae	Ma Zhi Hu, Feng Qi Cao		Adenostemma herb
Ma Laam Gan	*Baphicacanthus cusia*	Radix Baphicacanthi	Ma Lan Gen	Banrankon	Assam indigo root
Ma Laam Gan	*Strobilanthes flaccidifolius*	Radix Strobilanthis	Ma Lan Gen		Strobilanthes root
Ma Laam Yip	*Baphicacanthus cusia*	Folium Baphicacanthi	Ma Lan Ye	Banranyo	Assam indigo leaf

CANTONESE	SCIENTIFIC	PHARMACEUTICAL	MANDARIN	JAPANESE	ENGLISH
Ma Laan	*Aster indicus* and spp	Herba Asteris indici	Ma Lan		Indian aster herb
Ma Leun Ji	*Iris pallasii* var. *chinensis*	Semen Iris pallasii	Ma Lin Zi		North China iris seed
Ma Ming Teui	*Bombyx mori*	Periostracum Bombycis	Ma Ming Dui		Silkworm slough
Ma Song Yip	*Coriaria sinica*	Folium Coriariae	Ma Sang Ye		Coriaria leaf
Ma Wong	*Ephedra sinica*	Herba Ephedrae	Ma Huang	Mao	Ephedra stem
Ma Wong Gan	*Ephedra sinica*	Radix Ephedrae	Ma Huang Gen	Maokon	Ephedra root
Maan Ging Ji	*Vitex rotundifolia, V. trifolia*	Fructus Viticis rotundifoliae	Man Jing Zi	Mankeishi	Seashore chastetree berry
Maan Sau Guk	*Tagetes erecta*	Flos Tagetis	Wan Shou Ju		African marigold flower
Maau Daan Pei, Daan Pei	*Paeonia suffruticosa*	Cortex radicis Paeoniae suffruticosae	Mu Dan Pi, Dan Pi	Botanpi	Tree peony root bark
Maau Gan	*Ranunculus japonicus*	Radix et herba Ranunculi japonicae	Mao Gen		Japanese buttercup root and herb
Maau Ging Ji	*Vitex negundo* var. *cannabifolia*	Fructus Viticis negundonis	Mu Jing Zi		Five-leaf chastetree berry
Maau Ging Yip	*Vitex negundo* var. *cannabifolia*	Folium Viticis negundonis	Mu Jing Ye		Five-leaf chastetree leaf
Maau Jau Chou	*Ranunculus ternatus*	Radix Ranunculi	Mao Zhao Cao, Mao Zhua Cao		Ternate buttercup root
Maau Sao Chou	*Clerodendranthus spicatus*	Herba Clerodendranthi	Mao Xu Cao		Orthosiphon herb
Maau Sou Chou, Fa Sek Chou	*Orthosiphon aristatus, O. grandiflorus*	Herba Orthosiphonis	Mao Xu Kao, Hua Shi Cao		Orthosiphon herb
Mai Dit Heung	*Rosmarinus officinalis*	Herba Rosmarini	Mi Die Xiang		Rosemary herb
Mai Jou Yan	*Zizyphus mauritiana*	Semen Zizyphi mauritianae	Mian Zao Ren		Mauritius jujube seed
Mai Sa Sam	*Glehnia littoralis*	Radix Glehniae	Bei Sha Shen	Shajin	Northern sandroot
Mak (Mun) Dung	*Liriope platyphylla*	Radix Liriopis platyphyllae	Mai Men Dong		Broad-leaf liriope root
Mak (Mun) Dung	*Ophiopogon japonicus*	Radix Ophiopogonis	Mai (Men) Dong	Bakumondo	Dwarf lilyturf root
Mak (Mun) Dung, Wu Ba Mak Dung	*Liriope spicata*	Radix Liriopis spicatae	Mai (Men) Dong, Hu Bei Mai Men Dong		Lance-leaf liriope root
Man Gap	*Meretrix meretrix*	Concha Metretris	Wen Ge		Asian venus clam shell
Man Gou Wat	*Mangifera indica*	Semen Mangiferae	Mang Guo Zi		Mango seed
Mat Jou	*Zizyphus jujuba* var. *inermis*	Fructus Zizyphi jujubae praeparatae	Mi Zao		Honey-preserved jujube berry
Mat Mung Fa	*Buddleia officinalis*	Flos Buddleiae	Mi Meng Hua	Mitsumoka	Buddleia flower and bud
Mau Mui	*Rubus parvifolius*	Folium Rubi parvifolii	Mao Mei, Hao Tian Biao		Small-leaf raspberry leaf
Mei Yan Jiu (Gan)	*Canna indica*	Rhizoma Cannae	Mei Ren Jiao (Gen)	Dandoku	Canna lily root
Min Fa Gan	*Gossypium hirsutum, G. herbaceum*	Cortex radicis Gossypii	Mian Hua Gen		Cotton root bark

CANTONESE	SCIENTIFIC	PHARMACEUTICAL	MANDARIN	JAPANESE	ENGLISH
Min Fa Ji	*Gossypium hirsutum, G. herbaceum*	Semen Gossypii	Mian Hua Zi		Cotton seed
Ming Dong Sam	*Changium smyrnioides*	Radix Changii	Ming Dang Shen	Mintojin	Bright changium root
Ming Faan	*Alumen*	Alumen	Ming Fan	Myoban	Alum
Mo Bun Chou	*Abutilon indicum*	Herba Abutilonis indici	Mo Pan Cao, Mi Lan Cao		Country mallow herb
Mon Gwat Siu	*Sambucus formosana/taiwaniana*	Caulis et folium Sambuci formosanae	Mao Gu Xiao		Taiwan elder stem and leaf
Mon Ming Yi	*Manganitum*	Manganitum	Wu Ming Yi		Manganite
Mon Yi	*Ulmus macrocarpa*	Praeparatio fructus Ulmi	Wu Yi	Bui	Stinking elm fruit paste
Mong Gong Naam	*Cassia occidentalis*	Semen Cassiae occidentalis	Wang Jiang Nan Zi	Banshashi	Coffee senna seed
Mong Hong	*Miscanthus sinensis*	Herba Miscanthi	Mang Jing		Miscanthus herb
Mong Seu	*Mirabilitum*	Mirabilitum	Mang Xiao	Bosho	Mirabilite
Mong Yut Sa	*Lepus* spp	Excrementum Lepi	Wang Yue Sha		Rabbit dropping
Mou Dung Ching	*Ilex pubescens*	Radix Ilicis pubescentis	Mao Dong Qing	Motosei	Furry holly root
Mou Heu Tang	*Gymnema sylvestre* and spp	Caulis et radix Gymnemae	Wu Xue Teng		Gymnema stem and root
Mou Lai	*Ostrea gigas* and spp	Concha Ostreae	Mu Li	Borei	Oyster shell
Mou Ming Ji	*Pyrolusitum*	Pyrolusitum	Wu Ming Zi		Pyrolusite
Mou Se Heung	*Adenosma glutinosum*	Herba Adenosmae glutinosi	Mao She Xiang		Adenosma herb
Mou Tau Wui	*Ixeris denticulata*	Herba Ixeris	Mu Dou Hui		Ixeris herb
Mou Waan Gan	*Sapindus mukorossi*	Radix Sapindi	Wu Huan Gen, Mu Huan Gen		Soapnut tree root
Mou Waan Ji	*Sapindus mukorossi*	Semen Sapindi	Wu Huan Zi, Mu Huan Zi		Soapnut seed, Bodhi seed
Mui Gwai Fa	*Rosa rugosa*	Flos Rosae rugosae	Mei Gui Hua	Maikaika	Japanese rose flower
Mui Gwai Ji	*Rosa rugosa*	Fructus Rosae rugosae	Mei Gui Zi		Japanese rosehip
Mui Yip Wai Ling Choi	*Potentilla fragarioides*	Radix Potentillae fragarioidis	Mei Ye Wei Ling Cai		Strawberry-leaf cinquefoil root
Muk Bit Ji	*Momordica cochinchinensis*	Semen Momordicae cochinchinensis	Mu Bie Zi	Mokubesshi	Cochin bitter melon seed
Muk Dau Ji	*Cajanus cajan*	Semen Cajani	Mu Dou Zi		Pigeon pea seed
Muk Fong Gei	*Cocculus trilobus*	Radix Cocculi	Mu Fang Ji		Three-leaf cocculus root
Muk Gwa	*Chaenomeles sinensis*	Fructus Chaenomelis sinensis	Mu Gua, Ming Za		Chinese quince fruit
Muk Gwa, Chyun Muk Gwa	*Chaenomeles lagenaria*	Fructus Chaenomelis lagenariae	Mu Gua, Chuan Mu Gua	Mokka	Chinese quince fruit
Muk Gwa, Tip Gang Hoi Teng	*Chaenomeles speciosa*	Fructus Chaenomelis speciosae	Mu Gua, Tie Geng Hai Tang		Flowering quince fruit
Muk Heung	*Saussurea lappa*	Radix Saussureae lappae	Mu Xiang, Yun Mu Xiang	Mokko	Wood aromatic root
Muk Min Fa	*Gossampinus malabarica*	Flos Gossampini	Mu Mian Hua		Silk cotton tree flower
Muk Tin Lin	*Actinidia polygama*	Galla fructi Actinidiae	Mu Tian Lian	Mokutenryo	Actinidia gall
Muk Toi Sang	*Lithargyrum*	Lithagyrum	Mi Tuo Seng	Mitsudaso	Litharge

CANTONESE	SCIENTIFIC	PHARMACEUTICAL	MANDARIN	JAPANESE	ENGLISH
Muk Wu Dip	*Oroxylum indicum*	Semen Oroxyli	Mu Hu Die	Mokukocho	Oroxylum seed
Muk Yi	*Auricularia auricula*	Sclerotium Auriculariae	Mu Er	Kikurage	Wood ear mushroom
Mun Saan Hung	*Rhododendron dauricum, R. mariesii*	Folium Rhododendri daurici	Man Shan Hong		Daurian rhododendron leaf
Mun Sam Heung	*Lysimachia capillipes*	Rhizoma seu herba Lysimachiae capillipis	Man Shan Xiang		Lysimachia root or herb
Mun Tin Sing, Daai Sa Yip	*Pavetta hongkongiensis*	Herba Pavettae	Man Tian Xing		Pavetta herb
Mung Chung	*Tabanus bivittatus*	Tabanus	Meng Chong		Gadfly
Mung Sek, Ching Mung Sek	*Mica, Chloritum*	Mica, Chloritum	Meng Shi, Jin Meng Shi		Mica, Chlorite schist
Mut Gan Fa	*Hibiscus syriacus*	Flos Hibisci syriaci	Mu Jin Hua		Rose of Sharon flower
Mut Gan Pei	*Hibiscus syriacus*	Cortex radicis Hibisci syriacus	Mu Jin Pi		Rose of Sharon root bark
Mut Lei Fa	*Jasminum sambac*	Flos Jasmini sambacis	Mo Li Hua		Jasmine sambac flower
Mut Lei Gan	*Jasminum sambac*	Radix Jasmini sambacis	Mo Li Gen		Jasmine sambac root
Mut Sik Ji	*Quercus infectoria*	Galla Querci	Mo Shi Zi		Oak gall
Mut Yeuk	*Commiphora myrrha*	Resina Commiphorae	Mo Yao	Motsuyaku	Myrrh resin
Muuk Chaak	*Equisetum hiemale*	Herba Equiseti hiemalis	Mu Zei	Mokuzoku	Horsetail herb
Muuk Laam Yip	*Indigofera tinctoria*	Folium Indigoferae	Mu Lan Ye		Indigo leaf
Naam Gwa Ji	*Cucurbita moschata*	Semen Cucurbitae	Nan Gua Zi	Nankashi	Red squash seed
Naam Hok Sat	*Daucus carota*	Fructus Dauci	Nan He Zao		Wild carrot seed
Naam Juk	*Lyonia ovafolia, L. neziki*	Herba Lyoniae	Nan Zhu		Lyonia herb
Naam Sa Sam	*Adenophora stricta, A. capillaris, A. tetraphylla* and spp	Radix Adenophorae strictae	Nan Sha Shen	Nanshajin	Upright ladybell root
Naam Tin Juk Gan, Tin Juk Gan	*Nandina domestica*	Radix et caulis Nandinae	(Nan) Tian Zhu Gen		Sacred bamboo root and stem
Naam Tin Juk Ji, Tin Juk Ji	*Nandina domestica*	Fructus Nandinae	(Nan) Tian Zhu Zi		Sacred bamboo fruit
Naam Tin Juk Yip, Tin Juk Yip	*Nandina domestica*	Folium Nandinae	(Nan) Tian Zhu Ye		Sacred bamboo leaf
Naau Yeung Fa, Wong Dou Gun	*Rhododendron molle*	Flos Rhododendri mollis	Nao Yang Hua, Huang Du Juan		Yellow azalea flower
Nei Hau Tou	*Actinidia chinensis*	Fructus Actinidiae chinensis	Mi Hou Tao, Teng Li		Kiwi fruit
Neui Jing Ji	*Ligustrum japonicum, L. lucidum*	Fructus Ligustri	Nu Zhen Zi	Joteishi	Glossy privet berry

CANTONESE	SCIENTIFIC	PHARMACEUTICAL	MANDARIN	JAPANESE	ENGLISH
Ng Ga Pei	*Acanthopanax gracilistylus, A. spinosus, A. sessiliflorus* and spp	Cortex radicis Acanthopanacis	Wu Jia Pi	Gokahi	Five additions root bark
Ng Ga Pei, Baak Lak	*Acanthopanax trifoliatus*	Cortex radicis Acanthopanacis trifoliati	Wu Jia Pi, Bai Le		Three-leaf acanthopanax root bark
Ng Ga Pei, Sai Chu Ng Ga	*Acanthopanax gracilistylus*	Cortex radicis Acanthopanacis gracilistylus	Wu Jia Pi, Xi Zhu Wu Jia		Five additions root bark
Ng Guk Chung	*Chrysomyia megacephala* and spp	Larva Chrysomyiae	Wu Gu Chong		Maggot
Ng Gung	*Scolopendra subspinipes mutilans*	Scolopendra	Wu Gong	Gosho	Centipede
Ng Jaau Lung	*Ipomoea cairica*	Herba Ipomoeae cairicae	Wu Zhao Long		Cairo morning-glory herb
Ng Jyu Yu	*Evodia rutaecarpa*	Fructus Evodiae rutecarpae	Wu Zhu Yu	Goshuyu	Evodia berry
Ng Ling Ji	*Trogopterus xanthipes* and spp, *Pteromys volans* and spp	Excrementum Trogopteri seu Pteromi	Wu Ling Zhi		Flying squirrel dropping
Ng Mei Ji	*Schisandra chinensis*	Fructus Schisandrae	Wu Wei Zi	Gomishi	Schisandra berry
Ng Mei Ji, Wa Jung Ng Mei Ji	*Schizandra sphenantera*	Fructus Schisandrae sphenanterae	Wu Wei Zi, Hua Zheng Wu Wei Zi	Gomishi	Central China schisandra berry
Ng Pan Ji	*Rhus sinensis* and spp, *Schlechtendaria chinensis*	Galla Rhudis sinensis	Wu Bei Zi		Chinese sumac gallnut
Ng Sik Mui	*Lantana camara*	Herba Lantanae	Wu Se Mei		Wild sage herb
Ng Tung Ji	*Firmiana simplex*	Semen Firmianae	Wu Tong Zi		Chinese parasol tree seed
Ng Tung Leui	*Calophyllum inophyllum*	Resina Calophylli	Hu Tong Lei		Foraha resin
Nga Chung	*Orostachys fimbriatus*	Herba Orostachis fimbriati	Wa Song		Fimbriate orostachys herb
Nga Chung	*Orostachys japonica, O. fimbriatus*	Herba Orostachis	Wa Song		Hens-and-chickens herb
Nga Daan Ji	*Brucea javanica*	Fructus Bruceae	Ya Dan Zi	Atanshi	Brucea berry
Nga Ling Ji	*Arca inflata* and spp	Concha Arcae	Wa Leng Zi	Garyoshi	Cockle shell
Ngaai Naap Heung	*Blumea balsamifera*	Herba Blumeae balsamiferae	Ai Na Xiang, Da Feng Cao	Daifuso	Camphor plant
Ngaai Yang, Ngaai Yip	*Artemisia argyi*	Folium Artemisiae argyi	Ai Ye	Gaiyo	Asian mugwort leaf
Ngaap Geuk Muk Pei	*Schefflera octophylla*	Cortex Schefflerae octophyllae	Ya Jiao Mu Pi		Umbrella tree bark
Ngaap Jek Chou	*Commelina communis*	Herba Commelinae	Ya Zhi Cao		Common dayflower herb
Ngan Chaai Wu	*Gypsophyla oldhamiana*	Radix Gypsophylae	Yin Chai Hu		Gypsophyla root
Ngan Chaai Wu	*Stellaria dichotoma* var. *lanceolata*	Radix Stellariae	Yin Chai Hu	Ginsaiko	Stellaria root

CANTONESE	SCIENTIFIC	PHARMACEUTICAL	MANDARIN	JAPANESE	ENGLISH
Ngan Hang Yip, Baak Gwo Yip	*Ginkgo biloba*	Folium Ginkgoidis	Yin Xing Ye, Bai Guo Ye	Ginkyoyo	Ginkgo leaf
Ngang Suk Hok	*Papaver somniferum*	Pericarpium Papaveris	Ying Su Ke	Ozokukoku	Opium poppy husk
Ngao Daai Lik	*Millettia philipinensis*	Radix Millettiae philipinensis	Niu Da Li		Millettia root
Ngau Daam	*Bos taurus domesticus, Bubalis bubalis*	Vesica fellae Bovis	Niu Dan	Gyutan	Ox gallbladder
Ngau Jit	*Nelumbo nucifera*	Rhizoma nodi Nelumbinis	Ou Jie		Lotus root node
Ngau Pei	*Bos taurus domesticus, Bubalis bubalis*	Corium Bovis	Niu Pi		Ox hide
Ngau Pong Ji	*Arctium lappa*	Fructus Arctii	Niu Bang Zi	Goboshi	Burdock seed
Ngau Sat, Wai Ngau Sat	*Achyranthes bidentata*	Radix Achyranthis	Niu Xi, Huai Niu Xi	Goshitsu	White oxknee Root
Ngau Tang, Sheung Ngau (Tang)	*Uncaria rhynchophylla, U. hirsuta, U. macrophylla* and spp	Ramulus et uncus Uncariae	Gou Teng	Choto	Gambir vine twig
Ngau Wong	*Bos taurus domesticus, Bubalis bubalis*	Calculus Bovis	Niu Huang	Goo	Ox gallstone
Ngau Yi Daai Wong	*Rumex crispus*	Radix Rumicis crispi	Niu Er Da Huang		Yellow dock root
Ngo Bat Sik Chou	*Centipeda minima*	Herba Centipedae	E Bu Shi Cao	Sekikozui, Gabusho-kuso	Centipeda herb
Ngo Gun Sek	*Stalactitum, Balanophylla* spp.	Stalactitum	E Guan Shi, Shi Zhong Ru		Stalactite tip
Ngo Seut, Fung Ngo Seut	*Curcuma zedoaria, C. aeruginosa* and spp	Rhizoma Curcumae zedoariae	E Zhu, Peng Er Zhu	Gajutsu	Zedoary root
Ngo Seut, Gwong Sai Ngo Seut	*Curcuma kwangsiensis*	Rhizoma Curcumae kwangsiensis	E Zhu, Guang Xi Er Zhu		Guangxi turmeric root
Ngon Sik Heung	*Styrax benzoin*	Benzoinum	An Xi Xiang	Ansokuko	Benzoin
Ngon Yip	*Eucalyptus globulus*	Folium Eucalypti globuli	An Ye		Eucalyptus leaf
Niu Bat Suk	*Zanthoxylum avicennae*	Radix Zanthoxyli avicennae	Niao Bu Su, Bai Ma Niao		Prickly ash root
No Du Gan	*Oryza sativa*	Radix Oryzae	Nuo Dao Gen (Xu)	Jubeikon	Sweet rice root
O Gaau	*Equus asinus* and spp	Gelatinum corii Equi asini	E Jiao	Akyo	Ass hide glue
Pa San Fu, Dei Gam	*Parthenocissus tricuspidata*	Caulis Parthenocissi	Pa Shan Hu, Di Jin		Japanese creeper stem
Paang Kei Guk	*Wedelia chinensis*	Herba Wedeliae	Ma Lan Jin, Peng Qi Ju		Wedelia herb
Pan Dau Gan	*Menispermum dauricum*	Radix Menispermi	Bei Dou Gen		Siberian moonseed root
Pang Sa	*Borax*	Borax	Peng Sha	Hosha	Borax
Pau Tung Fa	*Paulownia tomentosa*	Flos Paulowniae	Pao Tong Hua		Paulownia flower
Pei Pa	*Eriobotrya japonica*	Fructus Eriobotryae	Pi Pa		Loquat fruit
Pei Pa Yip	*Eriobotrya japonica*	Folium Eriobotryae	Pi Pa Ye	Biwayo	Loquat leaf

CANTONESE	SCIENTIFIC	PHARMACEUTICAL	MANDARIN	JAPANESE	ENGLISH
Ping	*Marsilea quaddrifolia*	Folium Marsileae	Ping		European water clover leaf
Ping Fung Chou Gan	*Nuphar japonicum, N. pumilum*	Rhizoma Nupharis	Ping Peng Cao Gan	Senkotu	Yellow pond lily root
Ping Gon Sing Ma	*Eupatorium lindleyanum*	Herba Eupatorii lindleyani	Cheng Gan Sheng Ma		Lindley's eupatorium herb
Ping Yi Siu Chou	*Ophioglossum vulgatum*	Herba Ophioglossi	Ping Er Xiao Cao		Adder's tongue herb
Pok Sau	*Quercus dentata, Q. acutissima*	Ramulus et cortex Querci	Pu Suo	Bokuso	Oak twig and bark
Pou Fuk Sam	*Poria cocos*	Sclerotium Poriae paradicis	Fu Shen	Bukushin	Hoelen spirit
Pou Geung Gan	*Vitex quinata*	Radix Viticis quinatae	Pu Jiang Gen		Quinate chasteberry root
Pou Gung Ying	*Taraxacum mongolicum*	Radix et herba Taraxaci	Pu Gong Ying	Hokoei	Mongolian dandelion root and herb
Pou Wong Taan	*Typha latifolia, T. angustifolia* and spp	Pollen Typhae carbonisatus	Pu Huang Tan		Charred cattail pollen
Pou Wong, Heung Pou	*Typha latifolia, T. angustifolia* and spp	Pollen Typhae	Pu Huang, Xiang Pu	Hoo	Cattail pollen
Pou Yim Pin	*Rhus chinensis*	Radix Rhudis chinensis	Pu Yan Pian		Chinese sumac root
Pui Laan	*Eupatorium fortunei*	Herba Eupatorii fortunei	Pei Lan	Haikan	Orchid-grass herb
Pun Lung Sam	*Spiranthes sinensis*	Herba Spiranthis	Pan Long Shen		Chinese pearltwist herb
Sa Jik	*Hippophae rhamnoides*	Fructus Hippophae	Sha Ji		Sea buckthorn berry
Sa Tong Muk	*Acronychia laurifolia*	Lignum Acronychiae	Sha Tang Mu, Jiang Xiang		Acronychia heartwood
Sa Yan Fa, (Yeung) Chyun Sa Fa	*Amomum villosum*	Flos Amomi villosi	Sha Ren Hua, (Yang) Chun Sha Hua	Saninka	Wild cardamom flower
Sa Yan Hok	*Amomum villosum*	Pericarpium Amomi villosi	Sha Ren Ke		Wild cardamom shell
Sa Yan, (Yeung) Chyun Sa Yan	*Amomum villosum*	Fructus Amomi villosi	Sha Ren, (Yang) Chun Sha Ren	Sanin	Wild cardamom pod (fruit)
Sa Yan, Suk Sa Mat	*Amomum xanthioides*	Fructus Amomi xanthioidis	Sha Ren, Suo Sha Mi		Cocklebur cardamom pod
Sa Yun Ji, Sa Yun Jek Lai	*Astragalus complanatus* and spp	Semen Astragali complanati	Sha Yuan Zi, Sha Yuan Ji Li	Saenshi, Toshitsuri	Flat milkvetch seed
Saam Baak Chou	*Saururus chinensis*	Herba Saururi	San Bai Cao		Chinese lizardtail herb
Saam Chat Tin Chat	*Panax notoginseng*	Radix Panacis notoginsengis	San Qi Tian Qi	Sanshishi	Pseudoginseng root
Saam Chat Fa	*Panax notoginseng*	Flos Panacis notoginsengis	San Qi Hua	Sanshishika	Pseudoginseng flower
Saam Gwo Jam	*Berberis sargentiana, B. wilsonae, B. vernae* and spp	Radix Berberis sargentianae	San Ke Zhen		Three-needle barberry root

CANTONESE	SCIENTIFIC	PHARMACEUTICAL	MANDARIN	JAPANESE	ENGLISH
Saam Jim Chaam	*Cephalotaxus fortunei*	Ramulus et folium Cephalotaxi	San Jian Shan		Yew twig and leaf
Saam Ling	*Sparganium simplex, S. stoloniferum, S. stenophyllum*	Rhizoma Sparganii	San Leng		Bur-reed root
Saan Cha Fa	*Camellia japonica*	Flos Camelliae japonicae	Shan Cha Hua		Common camellia flower
Saan Chaang	*Melodinus suaveolens*	Fructus Melodini	Shan Chen, Qu Tou Ji		Melodinus fruit
Saan Chi Gu	*Cremastra variabilis*	Rhizoma et radix Cremastrae	Shan Ci Gu		Cremastra corm
Saan Chi Gu	*Pleione bulbocodioides*	Rhizoma Pleionis	Shan Ci Gu		Pleione corm
Saan Daan	*Lilium concolor*	Bulbus Liliii concoloris	Shan Dan		Japanese red star lily bulb
Saan Dau Gan	*Sophora subprostata*	Radix Sophorae subprostatae	Shan Dou Gen		Pigeon-pea root
Saan Gam Chou	*Mussaenda pubescens, M. parviflora*	Caulis et folium Mussaendae	Shan Gan Cao		Mountain licorice stem and leaf
Saan Ja (Yuk)	*Crataegus pinnatifida, C. cuneata* and spp	Fructus Crataegi	Shan Zha (Rou)	Sanzashi	Asian hawthorn berry
Saan Ja Tan	*Crataegus pinnatifida, C. cuneata* and spp	Fructus Crataegi carbonisatus	Shan Zha Tan		Charred Asian hawthorn berry
Saan Ji Ma	*Helicteres angustifolia*	Herba Helicteres	Shan Zhi Ma		Helicteres herb
Saan Nam Ji	*Rhodomyrtus tomentosa*	Semen Rhodomyrti	Shan Ren Zi		Rosemyrtle seed
Saan Noi	*Kaempferia galanga*	Rhizoma Kaempferiae	Shan Nai, Sha Jiang		Galanga root
Saan Sam Jai	*Glossogyne tenuifolia*	Herba Glossogyne	Shan Shen Zi		Thin-leaf glossgyne herb
Saan Tang Tang Yeung	*Vitis amurensis*	Radix Vitis amurensis	Shan Teng Teng Yang		Amur grape root
Saang Geung	*Zingiber officinalis*	Rhizoma Zingiberis recentis	Sheng Jiang	Shokyo	Fresh ginger root
Saang Geung Pei	*Zingiber officinalis*	Rhizoma Zingiberis	(Sheng) Jiang Pi		Fresh ginger root skin
Sai Faan Lin	*Passiflora coeruleae*	Herba Passiflorae coeruleae	Xi Fan Lian		Cerulean passionflower herb
Sai Ging Sek Wu	*Dendrobium moniliforme*	Caulis Dendrobii miniliformis	Xi Jing Shi Hu, Xiao Wan Chai		Stonebushel stem
Sai Gok	*Rhinoceros unicornis, R. bicornis*	Cornu Rhinoceri	Xi Jiao		Rhinoceros horn
Sai Gwa	*Citrullus vulgaris*	Fructus Citrulli	Xi Gua	Seika	Watermelon fruit
Sai Pa Pei	*Citrullus vulgaris*	Pericarpium Citrulli	Xi Gua Pi		Watermelon rind
Sai San	*Asarum sieboldii, A. heterotropoides* and spp	Radix et herba Asari	Xi Xin	Saishin	Asian wild ginger root and herb
Sai Yan, Hoi Naam Sa Yan	*Amomum longiligulare*	Fructus Amomi longiligularis	Sha Ren, Hai Nan Sha Ren		Hainan cardamom pod
Sak Sang Tang	*Cissampelos pareira*	Radix Cissampeli	Xi Sheng Teng		Ice vine root
Sam Chat Chou	*Gynura segetum*	Folium Gynurae	San Qi Cao, Ju San Qi		Canton sanchi leaf

CANTONESE	SCIENTIFIC	PHARMACEUTICAL	MANDARIN	JAPANESE	ENGLISH
Sam Chau		Massa fermentata	Shen Qu	Shinkiku	Medicated leaven
Sam Chau Cha		Massa fermentata	Shen Qu Cha		Medicated leaven tea
Sam Gam Chou	*Lycopodium clavatum*	Herba Lycopodi	Shen Jin Cao		Clubmoss herb
Sam Gong Daan	*Hydragyrum chloratum*	Compositum hydragyri oxydati crudi	San Xian Dan		Mercury oxide (crude)
Sam Nga Fu (Gan)	*Evodia lepta*	Radix Evodiae leptae	San Ya Ku (Gen)		Bitter evodia root
Sam Yip Gwai Jam Chou	*Bodens pilosa*	Herba Bidentis pilosae	San Ye Gui Zhen Cao		
San Baak Pei, Chau Muk Pei	*Catalpa bungei*	Cortex Catalpae	Zi Bai Pi, Qiu Mu Pi		Catalpa bark
San Chi Gok	*Iphigenia indica*	Bulbus Iphigeniae	Shan Ci Gu		Iphigenia bulb
San Chi Gu, Gwong Chi Gu	*Tulipa edulis*	Rhizoma et radix Tulipae	Shan Ci Gu, Guang Ci Gu		Chinese tulip bulb
San Ching Sek	*Selenitum*	Selenitum	Xuan Jing Shi		Selenite
San Geung Baak Cheuk	*Paeonia sinjiangensis*	Radix Paeoniae sinjiangensis	Xin Jiang Bai Shao (Yao)		Xinjiang peony root
San Jyu Yu, San Yu Yuk	*Cornus officinalis*	Fructus Corni	Shan Zhu Yu, Shan Yu Rou	Sanshuyu	Japanese dogwood berry
San Man Nga	*Hordeum vulgare*	Fructus germinatus Hordei	Mai Ya	Bakuga	Sprouted barley grain
San Ming Fun	*Mirabilitum*	Mirabilitum purum	Xuan Ming Fan	Bosho	Glauber's salt, Pure mirabilite
San Sa	*Ferrum*	Pulvis ferri	Chen Sha		Black ferric oxide
San Sat	*Catalpa ovata*	Fructus Catalpae	Zhi Shi	Kisasage	Catalpa fruit
San Yeung Gok	*Naemorrhedis*	Cornu Naemorrhedis	Shan Yang Jiao	Sanyokaku	Goat horn
San Yi Fa	*Magnolia liliflora, M. denudata, M. yulan* and spp	Gemma Magnoliae	Xin Yi Hua	Shinika	Yulan magnolia bud
San Yi Mai, Yi Yi Yan	*Coix lachryma-jobi* var. *Ma-yuen*	Semen Coicis	Yi Yi Ren	Yokuinin	Job's-tears seed
Sang Bun Ha, So Bun Ha	*Pinellia ternata*	Rhizoma pinelliae ternatae	Sheng Ban Xia	Shohange	Raw pinellia corm
Sang Dei (Wong)	*Rehmannia glutinosa*	Radix Rehmanniae	Sheng Di (Huang)	Shojio	Fresh Rehmannia root
Sang Sai Sam	*Panax ginseng*	Radix Panacis ginsengis	Sheng Shai Shen		Dried Asian ginseng root
Sang Tit Lo	*Ferrum*	Frusta Ferrum	Sheng Tie Luo		Iron filing/cinder
Sap Daai Gung Lou Gan	*Mahonia japonica*	Radix Mahoniae japonicae	Shi Da Gong Lao Gen		Japanese mahonia root
Sap Daai Gung Lou Yip, Fut Yip Sap Daai Gung Lou Yip	*Mahonia bealei*	Folium Mahoniae bealei	Shi Da Gong Lao Ye, Kuo Ye Shi Da Gong Lao Ye	Judaikoro	Leather-leaf mahonia leaf
Sau Gung, Bik Fu	*Gecko chinensis, G. japonicus* and spp	Gecko chinensis	Shou Gong, Bi Hu		House lizard
Se Baak	*Allium macrostemon*	Bulbus Allii macrostemonis	Xie Bai	Gaihaku	Chinese chive bulb
Se Chong Ji	*Cnidium monnieri*	Fructus Cnidii	She Chuang Zi	Jashoshi	Cnidium seed

CANTONESE	SCIENTIFIC	PHARMACEUTICAL	MANDARIN	JAPANESE	ENGLISH
Se Daam	*Naja naja atra, Bungarus fasciatus, Elaphe radiata*	Fel Najae seu Bungari seu Elaphis	She Dan		Viper gallbladder
Se Gon	*Belamcanda chinensis*	Rhizoma Belamcandae	She Gan	Yakan	Leopard flower root
Se Gon Miu	*Belamcanda chinensis*	Herba Belamcandae	She Gan Miao		Leopard flower herb
Se Heung	*Moschus berezovskii* and spp	Secretio Moschi	She Xiang	Jako	Musk
Se Mui	*Duchesnea indica*	Herba Duchesneae	She Mei		Mock strawberry herb
Se Pou Tou, Saan Pou Tou	*Ampelopsis brevipedunculata*	Radix et folium Ampelopsis brevipedunculatae	She Pu Tao, Shan Pu Tao		Snake grape root and leaf
Se Teui (Pei)	*Elephe taeniurus* and spp, *Dinodon rufozonatum*	Periostracum/Exuviae Elephis	She Tui (Pi)	Dataihi	Snakeskin slough
Sei Gwai Ching, Dung Ching Yip	*Ilex chinensis*	Folium Ilicis chinensis	Si Ji Qing, Dong Qing Ye		Wintergreen holly leaf
Sei Ho Lau	*Tamarix chinensis*	Cacumen Tamaricis	Xi He Liu	Seikaryu	Chinese tamarisk tip
Sei Yang Sam , Fa Kei Sam	*Panax quinquefolius*	Radix Panacis quinquefolii	Xi Yang Shen	Seiyojin	American ginseng root
Sek Cheung Pou	*Acorus gramineus*	Rhizoma Acori graminei	Shi Chang Pu		Rock sweetflag root
Sek Diu Baak	*Asparagus officinalis*	Rhizoma Asparagi officinalis	Shi Diao Bai		Asparagus root
Sek Diu Laan	*Lysionotus pauciflora*	Herba Lysinoti	Shi Diao Lan		Lysionotus herb
Sek Fa	*Porites nigrescens*	Os Poritis	Shi Hua		Coral skeleton
Sek Gin Chyun, Toi Sam, Ji Sam	*Salvia chinensis*	Radix et herba Salviae chinensis	Shi Jian Chuan, Chai Shen, Zi Shen		Chinese sage root and herb
Sek Gou	*Gypsum fibrosum*	Gypsum	Shi Gao	Sekko	Gypsum
Sek Hap	*Ephemerantha fimbriata*	Herba Ephemeranthae	Shi Hu	Sekkoku	Ephemerantha stem
Sek Kyut Ming	*Haliotis diversicolor, H. gigantea* and spp	Concha Haliotis	Shi Jue Ming	Sekketsumei	Abalone shell
Sek Lau Gan Pei	*Punica granatum*	Cortex Radicis Punicae	Shi Liu Gen Pi	Sekiryu-kombi	Pomegranate root bark
Sek Lau Pei	*Punica granatum*	Pericarpium Punicae	Shi Liu Pi	Sekiryuhi	Pomegranate husk
Sek Naam Tang	*Piper wallichii*	Ramulus Piperis wallichii	Shi Nan Teng		Wild pepper twig
Sek Naam Tang, Sek Naam Yip	*Photinia serrulata*	Caulis et folium Photiniae	Shi Nan Teng, Shi Nan Ye		Photinia stem or leaf
Sek Sin Tou Gan	*Pholidota chinensis*	Radix Pholidotae	Shi Xian Tao Gen		Rattlesnake orchid root
Sek Song Paap	*Selaginella doederleinii, S. involvens*	Herba Selaginellae	Shi Shang Bai		Spikemoss herb
Sek Syun	*Lycoris radiata*	Rhizoma Lycoris	Shi Suan		Red spiderlily corm
Sek Wai	*Pyrrosia lingua, P. petiolosa* and spp	Folium Pyrrosiae	Shi Wei		Felt fern leaf

CANTONESE	SCIENTIFIC	PHARMACEUTICAL	MANDARIN	JAPANESE	ENGLISH
Sek Wai, Lou San Sek Wai	*Pyrrosia sheareri*	Folium Pyrrosiae sheareri	Shi Wei, Lu Shan Shi Wei	Sekii	Shearer's felt fern leaf
Sek Wu	*Dendrobium nobile, D. linawianum, D. officinale* and spp	Herba Dendrobii	Shi Hu	Sekkoku	Stonebushel stem
Sek Wu, Chuk Fa Shi Hu	*Dendrobium chrysanthum*	Herba Dendrobii chrysanthi	Shi Hu, Shu Hua Shi Hu		Stonebushel stem
Sek Wu, Gam Ja Sek Wu	*Dendrobium nobile*	Herba Dendrobii nobilis	Shi Hu, Jin Sha Shi Hu		Stonebushel stem
Sek Wu, Ma Bin Sek Wu	*Dendrobium fimbriatum*	Herba Dendrobii fimbriati	Shi Hu, Ma Bian Shi Hu		Stonebushel stem
Sek Wu, Tit Pei Sek Wu	*Dendrobium officinalis*	Herba Dendrobii officinalis	Shi Hu, Tie Pi Shi Hu		Stonebushel stem
Sek Wu, Waan Chou Sek Wu	*Dendrobium loddigesii*	Herba Dendrobii loddigesii	Shi Hu, Wan Cao Shi Hu		Stonebushel stem
Sek Yi	*Parmelia tinctorum, P. reticulata*	Thallus Parmeliae	Shi Er		Parmelia thallus
Sek Yi	*Umbilicaria esculenta*	Sclerotium Umbilicariae	Shi Er		Stone ear mushroom
Seui Bun Ha	*Typhonium flagelliforme*	Rhizoma Typhonii flagelliformis preparata	Shui Ban Xia		Prepared flagellate typhonium root
Seui Cheung Pou, Baak Cheung Pou	*Acorus calamus*	Rhizoma Acori calami	Shui Chang Pu, Bai Chang Pu	Shobu	Sweetflag root
Seui Choi Yip	*Menyanthes trifoliata*	Folium Menyanthis	Shui Cai Ye	Suisayo, Meisai	Bogbean leaf
Seui Chung Ma	*Glyptostrobus pensilis*	Cacumen Glyptostrobi	Shui Song Mao		Chinese water pine tip
Seui Ding Heung	*Ludwigia prostata*	Herba Ludwigiae	Shui Ding Xiang		Water clove herb
Seui Do Lin, San Nim Gan	*Rhodomyrtus tomentosa*	Radix Rhodomyrti	Shui Duo Nian, Shan Nian Gen		Downy rosemyrtle root
Seui Fei Gai	*Silybum marianum*	Herba Silybi	Shui Fei Ji		Blessed thistle herb
Seui Heung Fa	*Daphne odora*	Flos Daphnis odorae	Rui Xiang Hua		Mezerum flower
Seui Jik	*Hirudo nipponia, Whitmania pigra* and spp	Hirudo seu Whitmania	Shui Zhi		Leech
Seui Kan	*Oenanthe javanica*	Herba Oenanthis	Shui Qin		Water dropwort
Seui Liu	*Polygonum hydropiper*	Herba et radix Polygoni hydropiperis	Shui Liao		Water pepper herb and root
Seui Ng Gung	*Kyllinga brevifolia*	Herba Kyllingae	Shui Wu Gong		Kyllinga herb
Seui Ngau Gok	*Bubalus bubalis*	Cornu Bubali	Shui Niu Jiao		Water buffalo horn
Seui Sin Gan	*Narcissus tazetta* var. *chinensis*	Bulbus Narcissi	Shui Xian Gen		Chinese sacred lily bulb
Seui Sin Ji	*Narcissus tazetta* var. *chinensis*	Fructus Narcissi	Shui Xian Zi		Chinese sacred lily seed
Seui Tung Fa Chou Hung Chou	*Polygonum orientale*	Herba Polygoni orientalis	Shui Tong Hua Cao Hong Cao		Prince's feather herb
Seui Tung Fa Ji	*Polygonum orientale*	Fructus Polygoni orientalis	Shui Tong Hua Zi		Prince's feather berry

CANTONESE	SCIENTIFIC	PHARMACEUTICAL	MANDARIN	JAPANESE	ENGLISH
Seui Wu Mun	*Clerodendron inerme*	Folium Clerodendronis inermis	Shui Hu Man		Glorybower leaf
Seui Yan (Yuk)	*Prinsepia uniflora*	Semen Prinsepiae	Rui Ren (Rou)		Prinsepia seed
Seui Yeung Ji	*Salix purpurea*	Ramulus Salicis purpureae	Shui Yang Zhi		Purple willow twig
Seui Yeung Mui	*Adina rubella*	Flos Adinae	Shui Yang Mei		Red modelwood flower
Seui Yin	*Hydragyrum*	Hydragyrum	Shui Yin		Mercury
Seui Yung Fa	*Cleistocalyx operculatus*	Gemma Cleistocalycis	Shui Weng Hua		Cleistolcalyx bud
Seung Cheun Tang	*Hedera nepalensis* var. *sinensis*	Herba Hederae nepalensis	Chang Chun Teng		Nepalese ivy leaf
Seung Lan Wong	*Limnophila sessiliflora*	Herba Limnophilae	Shuang Liu Huang		Limnophila herb
Seung Luk	*Phytolacca acinosa, P. esculenta*	Radix Phytolaccae acinosae	Shang Lu	Shoriku	Asian poke root
Seung Saan	*Dichroa febrifuga*	Radix Dichroae	Chang Shan	Joszan	Feverflower root
Seung Si Ji Gan	*Abrus precatorius, A. cantoniensis*	Radix Abri	Xiang Si Zi Gen		Licorice bean root
Si Gwa Lou	*Luffa cylindrica, L. acutangula*	Fasciculus vascularis Luffae	Si Gua Luo	Shikaraku	Spongegourd
Si Gwa Pei	*Luffa cylindrica, L. acutangula*	Pericarpium Luffae	Si Gua Pi		Luffa skin
Si Gwan Ji	*Quisqualis indica*	Fructus Quisqualis	Shi Jun Zi	Shikunshi	Rangoon creeper nut
Sik Ming	*Thlaspi arvense*	Herba Thlaspis	Xi Ming		Boor's mustard herb
Sik Seut	*Gryllulus chinensis, G. mitratus, Gampsocleis buergeri*	Gryllulus	Xi Shuai		Cricket
Sim Fa, Gam Sim Fa	*Cordyceps scotianus* and *host Cryptotympana atrata* and spp	Sclerotium Cordycepsis scotianus	Chan Hua, Jin Chan Hua		Cicada fungus
Sim Sou	*Bufo gargarizans, B. melanostictus*	Secretio Bufonis	Chan Su	Senjo	Toad venom
Sim Teui, Sim Tyut	*Cryptotympana atrata* and spp	Periostracum Cryptotympanae	Chan Tui	Sentai	Cicada slough
Sin Chou Gan	*Rubia cordifolia*	Radix Rubiae cordifoliae	Qian Cao Gen	Seisokon	Heart-leaf madder root
Sin Hok Chou	*Agrimonia pilosa* var. *japonica*	Herba Agrimoniae pilosae	Xian He Cao	Senkakuso	Furry agrimony herb
Sin Maau	*Curculigo orchioides*	Rhizoma Curculigonis	Xian Mao	Sembo	Golden eye-grass root
Sin Yan Jeung	*Opuntia dillenii* and spp	Rhizoma Opuntiae	Xian Ren Zhang		Prickly pear root
Sing Ma	*Cimicifuga foetida*	Radix Cimicifugae foetidae	Sheng Ma	Shoma	Rising hemp root
Sing Ma, Da Sam Yip Sing Ma	*Cimicifuga heracleifolia*	Radix Cimicifugae heracleifoliae	Sheng Ma, Ta San Ye Sheng Ma	Shoma	Heraclean rising hemp root
Sing Ma, Hing On Sing Ma	*Cimicifuga dahurica*	Radix Cimicifugae dahuricae	Sheng Ma, Xing An Sheng Ma	Shoma	Dahurian rising hemp root
Siu Gai	*Cephalanoplos segetum*	Radix et herba Cephalanoplis	Xiao Ji		Field thistle herb and root

CANTONESE	SCIENTIFIC	PHARMACEUTICAL	MANDARIN	JAPANESE	ENGLISH
Siu Gwo Lou Wong	*Lysimachia congestiflora*	Herba Lysimachiae congestiflorae	Xiao Guo Lu Huang		Full-flowered lysimachia
Siu Ji	*Nephelium lappaceum*	Fructus Nephelii	Shao Zi		Rambutan fruit
Siu Maak	*Berberis thunbergii*	Lignum Berberis thunbergii	Xiao Nie	Megi	Barberry wood
Siu Sek	*Niter*	Niter	Xiao Shi	Shoseki	Potassium nitrate
Siu Wui Heung	*Foeniculum vulgare*	Fructus Foeniculi	Xiao Hui Xiang	Shouikyo	Fennel seed
So Lo Ji	*Aesculus wilsonii, A. chinensis*	Fructrus Aesculi	Suo Luo Zi		Chinese horse chestnut
Soi Yeung	*Cynomorium songaricum*	Herba Cynomorii	Suo Yang	Sayo	Lock yang stem
Sok Dik	*Sambucus chinensis* and spp	Caulis et folium Sambuci chinensis	Shuo Zhuo		Chinese elder stem and leaf
Sok Duk	*Sambucus javanica*	Caulis et folium Sambuci javanici	Shuo Diao		Java elder stem and leaf
Song Baak Pei	*Morus alba*	Cortex radicis Mori	Sang Bai Pi	Sohakuhi	Mulberry root bark
Song Gei Sang	*Loranthus parasiticus, L. yadorici* and spp	Ramulus Loranthi	Sang Ji Sheng	Sokisei	Asian mistletoe twig
Song Ji	*Morus alba*	Ramulus Mori	Sang Zhi	Soshi	Mulberry twig
Song Laan Yip	*Isatis indigotica*	Folium Isatis indigoticae	Song Lan Ye		Woad leaf
Song Piu Seu	*Paratenodera sinensis* and *augustipennis, Hierodula patellifera, Mantis religiosa, Statilia maculata*	Paratenodera seu Hierodula seu Mantis seu Statilia	Sang Piao Xiao		Praying mantis egg case
Song Sam (Ji)	*Morus alba*	Fructus Mori	Sang Shen (Zi)	Sojin	Mulberry fruit
Song Wong	*Realgar*	Realgar	Xiong Huang	Yuo	Realgar
Song Yip	*Morus alba*	Folium Mori	Sang Ye	Soyo	Mulberry leaf
Sou Gan	*Perilla frutescens*	Ramulus Perillae	Zi Su Geng		Perilla stem
Sou Hap Heung	*Liquidambar orientalis*	Resina Liquidambaris (Styrax liquidis)	Su He Xiang	Sogoko	Storax resin
Sou Hing Fa	*Jasminum officinale* var. *grandiflorum*	Flos Jasmini officinalis	Su Xin Hua		Jasmine flower
Sou Ji	*Perilla frutescens*	Fructus Perillae	Zi Su Zi	Soshi	Perilla seed
Sou Muk	*Caesalpinia sappan*	Lignum Caesalpiniae	Su Mu	Soboku	Sappanwood
Sou Tit Ji	*Cycas revoluta*	Semen Cycadis	Su Tie Zi		Sago palm seed
Sou Yip	*Perilla frutescens*	Folium Perillae	Zi Su Ye	Shisoyo	Perilla leaf
Suk Chat	*Dichroa febrifuga*	Folium Dichroae	Shu Qi	Shokushitsu	Feverflower leaf
Suk Dei (Wong)	*Rehmannia glutinosa*	Radix Rehmanniae preparatae	Shu Di (Huang)	Jukujio	Prepared Rehmannia root
Suk Mai	*Setaria italica*	Fructus Setariae	Xiao Mi		Millet grain
Suk Nga	*Setaria italica*	Fructus germinatus Setariae	Su Ya		Sprouted millet grain
Suk Yi Mai	*Coix lachryma-jobi* var. *Ma-yuen*	Semen Coicis preparatae	Shu Yi Ren		Dry-fried Job's-tears seed
Sung Muk Baak Pei	*Aralia chinensis*	Radix Araliae chinensis	Song Mu Bai Pi		Chinese aralia root

CANTONESE	SCIENTIFIC	PHARMACEUTICAL	MANDARIN	JAPANESE	ENGLISH
Syu Fu	*Armadillidium vulgare, Porcellio scaber*	Armadillidium	Shu Fu		Wood louse
Syu Guk Chou	*Gnaphalium affine*	Herba Gnaphalii	Shu Qu Cao		Cudweed herb
Syu Jou Yan	*Zizyphus spinosa*	Semen Zizyphi spinosae preparatae	Chao Suan Zao Ren		Roasted sour jujube seed
Syu Leung	*Dioscorea cirrhosa*	Rhizoma Dioscoreae cirrhosae	Shu Liang		Dyer's yam root
Syu Pang Sa	*Borax*	Borax	Shu Peng Sha		Roasted borax
Syu Seung Yat Ji Hou	*Aconitum brachypodum* and spp	Radix Aconiti brachypodi	Xue Shang Yi Zhi Yao		Brachypode aconite root
Syun Chou Fa	*Hemerocallis fulva*	Flos Hemerocallis	Xuan Cao Hua		Tawny day lily flower
Syun Chou Gan	*Hemerocallis fulva*	Radix Hemerocallis	Xuan Cao (Gen)		Tawny day lily root
Syun Fuk Fa	*Inula japonica, I. brittanica, I. linariaefolia*	Flos Inulae	Xuan Fu Hua	Sembukuka	Elecampane flower
Syun Jeung Gan	*Physalis alkakengi* (var. *franchetii)*	Rhizoma Physalis	Suan Jiang Gen		Chinese lantern root
Syun Jeung, Ching Dang Lung	*Physalis alkekengi* (var. *franchetii)*	Calyx seu fructus Physalis	Suan Jiang, Jing Deng Long		Chinese lantern calyx or fruit
Syun Jou Yan	*Zizyphus spinosa*	Semen Zizyphi spinosae	Suan Zao Ren, Jin Zao Ren	Sansonin	Sour jujube seed
Syun Taai Long Chung	*Protohermes grandis*	Vermiculus Protohermis	Sun Tai Lang Chun	Magotaro-mushi	Protohermes larva
Taam Dau Si	*Glycine max*	Semen Glycinis preparatum	Dan Dou Chi	Tantoshi	Fermented soybean
Taan Gan	*Dalbergia hupeana*	Folium Dalbergiae hupeanae	Tan Gen		Hupei rosewood
Taan Heung	*Santalum album*	Lignum Santalum	Tan Xiang		Sandalwood
Taan Lung Gwat	*Stegodon orientalis et al.*	Os Stegodontis calcinatum	Duan Long Gu, Shu Long Gu		Calcined dragon bone
Taan Mou Lai	*Ostrea gigas*	Concha Ostreae calcinati	Duan Mu Li		Calcined oyster shell
Taap Gon	*Lutra lutra*	Jecur Lutrae	Ta Gan		Otter liver
Tang Li Gan	*Actinidia chinensis*	Fructus Actinidiae chinensis	Teng Li Gen		Kiwi root
Tang Wong	*Garcinia morella*	Resina Garciniae	Teng Huang		Gamboge resin
Taou Baak Lin	*Melothria heterophylla*	Radix Melothriae heterophyllae	Tu Bai Lian		Native peppervine root
Tau Gwat Chou	*Impatiens balsamina*	Herba Impatientis	Tou Gu Cao		Garden balsam herb
Tau Gwat Chou	*Speranskia tuberculata*	Herba Speranskiae	Tou Gu Cao		Speranskia herb
Teun Yip Syu Yu	*Dioscorea zingiberensis*	Rhizoma Dioscoreae zingiberis	Dun Ye Shu Yu		Shield-leaf yam root
Ti Chik Lin	*Clematis florida*	Herba Clematis floridae	Tie Xian Lian		Flowering clematis herb
Tim Chaang	*Citrus sinensis*	Fructus Citri sinensis	Tian Chen		Sweet orange fruit
Tim Gwa Dai	*Cucumis melo*	Caulis Cucumis	Tian Gua Di	Katei	Young cantaloupe stalk

CANTONESE	SCIENTIFIC	PHARMACEUTICAL	MANDARIN	JAPANESE	ENGLISH
Tim Gwa Ji	*Cucumis melo*	Semen Cucumis	Tian Gua Zi		Cantaloupe seed
Tim Hang Yan, Naam Hang Yan	*Prunus armeniaca* and var.	Semen Pruni armeniacae dulcis	Tian Xing Ren, Nan Xing Ren		Sweet apricot kernel
Tin (Mun) Dung	*Asparagus cochinchinensis*	Rhizoma Asparagi cochinensis	Tian (Men) Dong	Tenmondo	Shiny asparagus root
Tin Cheung Hok	*Metaplexis japonica*	Fructus Metaplexis	Tian Qiang Ke		Metaplexis fruit
Tin Fa Fun	*Trichosanthes kirilowii, T. japonica, T. uniflora*	Radix Trichosanthis	Tian Hua Fen	Tenkafun	Snakegourd root
Tin Heung Lou	*Osbeckia chinensis*	Herba Osbeckiae	Tian Xiang Lu, Jin Shi Lu		Chinese osbeckia herb
Tin Jik Wong, Dei Yi Chou	*Hypericum japonicum*	Herba Hyperici japonici	Tian Ji Huang, Di Er Cao		Japanese St. John's wort herb
Tin Juk Wong	*Phyllostachys nigra* var. *henonis* and spp	Concretio silicea bambusae	Tian Zhu Huang		Tabasheer
Tin Kwai	*Semiaquilegia adoxoides*	Radix Semiaquilegiae	Tian Kui		Semiaquilegia root
Tin Kwai	*Semiaquilegia adoxoides*	Herba Semiaquilegiae	Tian Kui		Semiaquilegia herb
Tin Ma	*Gastrodia elata*	Rhizoma Gastrodiae	Tian Ma	Temma	Celestial hemp corm
Tin Ming Jing	*Carpesium abrotanoides*	Herba Carpesii	Tian Ming Jing		Starwort herb
Tin Naam Sing, Jek Naam Sing	*Arisaema consanguineum, A. amurense* and spp	Rhizoma Arisaemae preparatae	Tian Nan Xing, Zhi Nan Xing		Prepared dragon arum corm
Tin Sin Ji	*Hyoscyamus niger*	Semen Hyoscyami	Tian Xian Zi		Black henbane seed
Tin Sin Tang	*Aristolochia contorta, A. debilis*	Caulis Aristolochiae	Tian Xian Teng	Tensendo	Green birthwort stem
Tin Wu Seui	*Hydrocotyle sibthorpioides*	Herba Hydrocotylis	Tian Hu Sui		Lawn (water) pennywort herb
Tin Yun Ji	*Polygala sibirica*	Radix Polygalae sibiricae	Tian Yuan Zhi		Siberian milkwort root
Ting Lai Ji	*Descurainia sophia*	Semen Descurainiae	Ting Li Zi	Teirekishi	Tansy mustard seed
Ting Lai Ji	*Lepidium apetalum, L. virginicum*	Semen Lepidii	Ting Li Zi	Teirekishi	Wood whitlow grass seed
Tit Bau Gam	*Berchemia lineata*	Radix Berchemiae	Tie Bao Jin		Supplejack root
Tit Syu	*Cycas revoluta*	Folium Cycadis	Tie Shu		Sago palm leaf
Tit Yin	*Acalypha australis*	Herba Acalyphae	Tie Xian (Cai)		Annual copperleaf herb
Toi Waan Ji Sang	*Scurrula ritozanensis*	Ramulus Scurrulae	Tai Wan Ji Sheng		Taiwan mistletoe twig
Tong Chou, Bai Tong Chou	*Tetrapanax papyrifera*	Medulla Tetrapanacis	Tong Cao	Toso	Rice paper pith
Tong Sek Chung	*Commelina benghalensis*	Herba Commelinae	Tang Shi Song		Bengal dayflower herb
Tou Dong Gwai	*Aralia cordata*	Radix Araliae cordatae	Tu Dang Gui		Heart-leaf aralia root

CANTONESE	SCIENTIFIC	PHARMACEUTICAL	MANDARIN	JAPANESE	ENGLISH
Tou Dong Sam	*Campanumoea javanica*	Radix Campanumoeae	Tu Dang Shen		Java bellflower root
Tou Fuk Ling	*Smilax glabra*	Rhizoma Smilacis glabrae	Tu Fu Ling		Glabrous greenbrier root
Tou Gam Chan, Tou Heung Yu	*Origanum vulgare*	Herba Origani vulgaris	Tu Yin Chen, Tu Xiang Ru		Oregano herb
Tou Ging Gai	*Chenopodium ambrosioides*	Herba Chenopodii ambrosioidis	Tu Jing Jie		Wormseed herb
Tou Ging Pei	*Pseudolarix amabilis. P. kaempferi*	Cortex radicis Pseudolaricis	Tu Jing Pi		Golden larch root bark
Tou Heung Fei	*Cephalotaxus sinensis*	Ramulus et folium Cephalotaxi sinensis	Tu Xiang Fei		Plum yew twig and leaf
Tou Muk Heung	*Inula helenium*	Radix Inula helenii	Tu Mu Xiang		Elecampane root
Tou Muk Heung, Chung Ching Tou Muk Heung	*Inula racemosa*	Radix Inulae racemosae	Tu Mu Xiang, Zong Zhuang Tu Mu Xiang		Racemose elecampane root
Tou Ngan Fa	*Lonicera confusa*	Flos Lonicerae confusae	Tu Yin Hua, Shan Yin Hua		Wild honeysuckle flower
Tou Ngau Sat	*Achyranthes longifolia*	Radix Achyranthis longae	Tu Niu Xi		Long-leaf oxknee root
Tou Si Ji	*Cuscuta chinensis , C. japonica*	Semen Cuscutae	Tu Si Zi	Toshishi	Asian dodder seed
Tou Yan	*Prunus persica* and spp	Semen Pruni persicae	Tao Ren	Tonin	Peach kernel
Tou Yan Sam	*Talinum paniculatum*	Radix Talini	Tu Ren Shen		Fameflower root
Tou Yi Chat	*Podophyllum emodi*	Rhizoma Podophylli emodii	Tao Er Qi		Emodi's podophyllum root
Tung Luk	*Malachitum*	Malachitum	Tong Lu		Copper rust
Tung Tin Chou	*Uraria lagopodioides*	Herba Urariae	Hu Li Wei, Tong Tian Cao		Uraria herb
U Sau Se	*Zaocys dhumnades*	Zaocys	Wu Shao She	Ushoda	Black grass-snake
Wa Muk Pei	*Betula platyphylla*	Cortex Betulae	Hua Mu Pi		Asian birch bark
Wa Sai San	*Asarum sieboldii*	Herba Asari sieboldii	Xi Xin, Hua Xi Xin		Siebold's wild ginger herb
Wa Tau Chou	*Viola patrinii*	Herba Violae patriniae	Hua Tou Cao		Patrinium violet herb
Waai (Fa) Mai	*Sophora japonica*	Gemma Sophorae japonicae	Huai (Hua) Mi		Japanese pagoda tree bud
Waai Fa	*Sophora japonica*	Flos Sophorae japonicae	Huai Hua		Japanese pagoda tree flower
Waai Tung	*Aristolochia moupiensis*	Radix seu caulis Aristolochiae moupiensis	Huai Tong		Birthwort root or stem
Wai Jiu (Ji)	*Sophora japonica*	Fructus Sophorae japonicae	Huai Jiao (Zi)		Japanese pagoda tree fruit
Wai Ling Choi	*Potentilla chinensis*	Herba Potentillae chinensis	Wei Ling Cai		Chinese cinquefoil herb

CANTONESE	SCIENTIFIC	PHARMACEUTICAL	MANDARIN	JAPANESE	ENGLISH
Wai Ling Sin	*Clematis chinensis, C. hexapetala* and spp	Radix Clematis chinensis	Wei Ling Xian	Ireisen	Chinese clematis root
Wai Ling Sin, Min Tyun Ti Chik Lin	*Clematis hexapetala*	Radix Clematis hexapetalae	Wei Ling Xian, Mian Tuan Tie Xian Lian		Six-petal clematis root
Wai Ngau Sat, Dou Kau Chou	*Achyranthes aspera*	Radix Achyranthis asperae	Wei Niu Xi, Ju Niu Xi, Dou Kou Cao		Rough oxknee root
Wai Saan, Saan Yeuk	*Dioscorea opposita, D. batatas*	Rhizoma Dioscoreae oppositae	Shan Yao Shu Yu	Sanyaku	Mountain yam root
Wan Ji	*Coriolus versicolor (syn. Trametes versicolor)*	Sclerotium Corioli versicolori	Yun Zhi		Turkey tail mushroom
Wan Mou Sek	*Muscovitum*	Muscovitum	Yun Mu Shi		Muscovite
Wat Sek	*Talcum*	Talcum	Hua Shi	Kasseki	Talc
Wo Ngau	*Eulota peliomphala*	Eulota	Gua Niu		Snail
Wong Bat Lau Hang	*Vaccaria segetalis*	Semen Vaccariae	Wang Bu Liu Xing	Ofurugyo	Cowcockle seed
Wong Fa Gaap Juk Tou (Yip)	*Thevetia peruviana*	Folium et semen Thevetiae	Huang Hua Jia Zhu Tao (Ye)		Peruvian thevetia leaf and seed
Wong Fa Hou, Ching Hou	*Artemisia annua*	Herba Artemisiae annuae	Huang Hua Hao Qing Hao		Annual wormwood herb
Wong Fuk Ling, Waan Ling	*Poria cocos*	Sclerotium Poriae	Fu Ling	Bukuryo	Hoelen fungus
Wong Ging Ji	*Vitex negundo*	Fructus Viticis negundonis	Huang Jing Zi		Negundo chastetree berry
Wong Jin Kwai	*Vanieria cochinchinensis*	Caulis Vanieriae	Huang Jin Kui, Chuan Po Shi		Vanieria stem
Wong Jing	*Polygonatum sibiricum, P. cyrtonema, P. kingianum*	Rhizoma Polygonati	Huang Jing	Osei	Siberian Solomon's-seal root
Wong Kei, Hung Kei	*Hedysarum polybotrys* and spp	Radix Hedysari polybotris	Huang Qi, Hong Qi		Hedysarum root
Wong Kei, Paak Kei	*Astragalus membranaceus, A. mongholicus* and spp	Radix Astragali	Huang Qi	Ogi	Astragalus root
Wong Lin Nga	*Pistacia chinensis*	Folium Pistaciae	Huang Lian Ya		Pistachio leaf
Wong Lin, Chyun Wong Lin	*Coptis chinensis, C. omeiensis* and spp	Rhizoma Coptis	Huang Lian, Chuan Lian	Oren	Goldthread root
Wong Ling Pei, Fuk Ling Pei	*Poria cocos*	Cortex Poriae	Fu Ling Pi	Bukuryoshi	Hoelen skin
Wong Muk Yi	*Tremella mesenterica*	Sclerotium Tremellae mesentericae	Huang Mu Er		Yellow ear mushroom
Wong Ngau Cha	*Cratoxylon ligustrinum*	Folium Cratoxyli	Huang Niu Cha		Cratoxylon leaf
Wong Paak, Chyun Paak	*Phellodendron amurense, P. chinense*	Cortex Phellodendris	Huang Bai Chuan Bai	Obaku	Siberian cork tree bark
Wong Pei Gwo	*Clausenia lansium*	Pericarpium Clauseniae	Huang Pi Guo		Wampi fruit

CANTONESE	SCIENTIFIC	PHARMACEUTICAL	MANDARIN	JAPANESE	ENGLISH
Wong Pei Ho	*Clausenia lansium*	Semen Clauseniae	Huang Pi He		Wampi seed
Wong Pei Yip	*Clausenia lansium*	Folium Clauseniae	Huang Pi Ye		Wampi leaf
Wong Sam	*Scutellaria baicalensis, S. viscidula, S. amoena*	Radix Scutellariae baicalensis	Huang Qin	Ogon	Baikal skullcap root
Wong Seui Ke	*Solanum xanthocarpum*	Herba Solani xanthocarpi	Huang Shui Qie		Prickly nightshade fruit
Wong Tang Gan	*Daemonorops margaritae*	Radix Daemonoropsis	Huang Teng Gen		Daemonorops root
Wong Yeuk Ji	*Dioscorea bulbifera*	Rhizoma Dioscoreae bulbiferae	Huang Yao Zi	Oyakushi	Potato yam tuber
Wu Bak Bui Mou	*Fritillaria hupehensis*	Bulbus Fritillariae hupehensis	Hu Bei Bei Mu		Hubei fritillary bulb
Wu Bak Bui Mou, Pou Kei Bui Mou	*Fritillaria puqiensis*	Bulbus Fritillariae puqiensis	Hu Bei Bei Mu, Pu Qi Bei Mu		Puqi fritillary bulb
Wu Fa Gwat	*Ficus carica*	Flos Fici	Wu Hua Guo		Fig flower
Wu Gei Sang	*Viscum coloratum, V. album*	Herba Visci	Hu Ji Sheng		Western mistletoe herb
Wu Gwat Tang	*Fissistigma glaucescens*	Herba Fissistigmae	Wu Gu Teng		Fissistigma herb
Wu Gwat Tang	*Marsdenia tenacissima*	Herba Marsdeniae	Wu Gu Teng		Marsdenia herb
Wu Jiu Gan	*Piper nigrum*	Radix Piperis nigri	Hu Jiao Gen		Black pepper root
Wu Jiu, Mai Wu Jiu	*Piper nigrum*	Fructus Piperis nigri	Hu Jiao, Hei Hu Jiao	Kosho	Black pepper corn
Wu Kau Muk Gan Pei	*Sapium sebiferum*	Cortex radicis Sapii sebiferi	Wu Jiu (Mu) Gen Pi	Ukyukompi	Chinese tallow tree root bark
Wu Lin Mui	*Cayratia japonica*	Herba Cayratiae	Wu Lian Mei		Cayratia herb
Wu Lok Hok	*Lagenaria siceraria*	Fructus Lagenariae	Hu Lu Ke		Bottle gourd fruit
Wu Lou Ba	*Trigonella foenum-graecum*	Semen Trigonellae	Hu Lu Ba		Fenugreek seed
Wu Mui (Yuk)	*Prunus mume*	Fructus Pruni mumis	Wu Mei (Rou)	Ubai	Black plum fruit
Wu Sai	*Coriandrum sativum*	Herba Coriandri	Hu Sui		Coriander herb
Wu Tau Gan	*Colocasia esculenta*	Radix Colocasiae	Yu Tou Gen		Taro root
Wu Teui (Ji) Yip	*Eleagnus pungens*	Folium Eleagni pungensis	Hu Tui (Zi) Ye		Thorny eleagnus leaf
Wu Tou Ji	*Juglans regia*	Ramulus Juglandis	Hu Tao Zhi		Walnut twig
Wu Tou Yan	*Juglans regia*	Semen Juglandis	Hu Tao Ren	Kotoniku	Walnut meat
Wu Tou Yip	*Juglans regia*	Folium Juglandis	Hu Tao Ye		Walnut leaf
Wu Tung Leui	*Populus euphratica* and spp	Resina Populi	Hu Tong Lei		Poplar resin
Wu Wong Lin	*Picrorrhiza kurroa*	Radix Picrorrhizae	Hu Huang Lian	Kooren	Picrorrhiza root
Wu Yeuk, Toi Wu	*Lindera strychnifolia*	Radix Linderae	Wu Yao, Tai Wu	Uyaku	Lindera root
Yam Yeung Fok, Sin Ling Pei	*Epimedium saggitatum, E. macranthum* and spp	Folium Epimedii	Yin Yang Huo, Xian Ling Pi	Inyokaku	Horny goat weed leaf

CANTONESE	SCIENTIFIC	PHARMACEUTICAL	MANDARIN	JAPANESE	ENGLISH
Yan Chan (Hou), Min Yan Chan	*Artemisia capillaris, A. scoparia*	Herba Artemisiae capillaris	Yin Chen (Hao), Mian Yin Chen	Inchinko	Downy wormwood herb
Yan Chung Wong	*Glycirrhiza uralensis, G. glabra* and spp	Radix Glycirrhizae preparatae cum urino	Ren Zhong Huang		Urine-prepared licorice root
Yan Jung Baak	*Homo sapiens*	Sedimen urinae Hominis	Ren Zhong Bai, Qiu Shi Dan		Human urine sediment
Yan Niu	*Homo sapiens*	Urina Hominis	Ren Niao		Human urine
Yan Sam	*Panax ginseng*	Radix Panacis ginsengis	Ren Shen	Ninjin	Asian ginseng root
Yan Sam Fa	*Panax ginseng*	Flos Panacis ginsengis	Ren Shen Hua		Asian ginseng flower
Yan Sam Lu	*Panax ginseng*	Rhizoma Panacis ginsengis	Ren Shen Lu	Ninjinro	Asian ginseng neck
Yan Sam Son, Sam Son	*Panax ginseng*	Extremas radicis Panacis ginsengis praeparatae	(Ren) Shen Xu		Rock candy cured Asian ginseng root tail
Yan Sam Yip	*Panax ginseng*	Folium Panacis ginsengis	Ren Shen Ye	Ninjinyo	Asian ginseng leaf
Yan Wu	*Skimmia reevesiana, S. japonica*	Caulis et folium Skimmiae	Yin Yu		Skimmia stem and leaf
Yang Guk, Sei Yip Sam	*Codonopsis lanceolata*	Radix Codonopsis lanceolatae	Yang Ju, Shi Ye Shen	Yonyu, Shiyojin	Goat's-tit bellflower root
Yap Dei Gam Ngau	*Zanthoxylum nitidum*	Radix Zanthoxyli nitidi	Ru Di Jin Niu, Liang Mian Zhen		Shiny bramble root
Yat Ji Heung	*Vernonia cinerea*	Herba Vernoniae	Yi Zhi Xiang		Vernonia herb
Yat Ji Wong Fa, Lau Ji Wong	*Solidago virgaurea, S. derurrens*	Herba Solidaginis	Yi Zhi Huang Hua, Liu Zhi Huang		Goldenrod herb
Yat Tiu Gan	*Moghania macrophylla, M. philippinensis*	Radix Moghaniae	Yi Tiao Gen		Moghania root
Yat Yip Chau	*Securinega suffruticosa*	Gemma et radix Securinegae	Yi Ye Qiu		Securinega shoot and root
Yau Hat	*Citrus grandis*	Semen Citri grandi immaturi	You He		Pomelo seed
Yau Pei (Gwat Hung), Fa Gwat Hung	*Citrus grandis*	Pericarpium Citri grandi immaturi	You Pi (Ju Hong), Hua Ju Hong		Pomelo rind
Yau Tung Ji	*Aleurites fordii*	Semen Aleuritis	You Tong Zi		Tung seed
Yau Yip	*Citrus grandis*	Folium Citri grandi immaturi	You Ye		Pomelo leaf
Ye Baak Hap	*Crotalaria sessiliflora*	Herba Crotalariae	Ye Bai He		Thin-leaf rattlebox herb
Ye Cheung Mei Gan	*Rosa multiflora*	Radix Rosae multiflorae	Ye Qiang Wei Gen		Wild rose root
Ye Din Ke	*Solanum surratense*	Herba Solani surattensis	Ye Dian Jie		Soda-apple nightshade herb
Ye Fa Jiu	*Zanthoxylum simulans*	Fructus Zanthoxyli simulansis	Ye Hua Jiao		Sichuan peppercorn
Ye Gam Chou, Chu Jai Chou Gan	*Scoparia dulcis*	Radix Scopariae	Ye Gan Cao, Zhu Cai Cao Gen		Scoparia root
Ye Gou Tang	*Polygonum multiflorum*	Caulis Polygoni multiflori	Ye Jiao Teng	Yakoto	Flowery knotweed stem
Ye Gwaan Mun	*Lespedeza cuneata*	Herba Lespedezae	Ye Guan Men		Perennial lespedeza herb

CANTONESE	SCIENTIFIC	PHARMACEUTICAL	MANDARIN	JAPANESE	ENGLISH
Ye Ma Jeui, Jim Pui Laan	*Eupatorium lindleyanum* var. *tripartum*	Herba Eupatorii	Ye Ma Zhui, Jian Pei Lan		Lindley's eupatorium herb
Ye Maau Daan	*Melastoma candidum*	Herba Melastomae candidae	Ye Mu Dan		Melastoma herb
Ye Ming Sa	*Vespertilium murinum*	Excrementum Vespertilii	Ye Ming Sha	Yamyosha	Bat dropping
Ye Pou Tou	*Vitis thunbergii* and spp	Radix Vitis	Ye Pu Tao		Wild grape root
Ye Saan Ja	*Crataegus cuneata*	Fructus Crataegus cuneatae	Ye Shan Zha		Wild hawthorn berry
Ye Yin Yip Gan, Tou Yin Tau	*Solanum verbascifolium*	Radix Solani verbascifolii	Ye Yan Ye Gen, Tu Yen Tou		Tobacco nightshade root
Yeung Gam Fa	*Datura metel*	Flos Daturae	Yang Jin Hua		Jimsonweed flower
Yeung Gok Aau	*Strophanthus divaricatus*	Semen Strophanthi	Yang Jiao Yao		Strophanthus seed
Yeung Hei Sek	*Actinolitum*	Actinolitum	Yang Qi Shi		Actinolite
Yeung Ho	*Zingiber mioga*	Rhizoma Zingiberis miogae	Rang He		Mioga ginger root
Yeung Miu Pei	*Myrica rubra*	Cortex Myricae rubrae	Yang Mei Pi		Red bayberry bark
Yeung Tai	*Rumex japonicus, R. nepalensis*	Radix Rumicis japonici	Yang Ti		Japanese dock root
Yeung Tai Chou	*Emilia sonchifolia*	Herba Emiliae	Yang Ti Cao		Red tasselflower herb
Yeung Tou	*Averrhoa carambola*	Fructus Averrhoae	Yang Tao		Carambola fruit
Yeung Tou Fa	*Averrhoa carambola*	Flos Averrhoae	Yang Tao Hua		Carambola flower
Yi Bui Mou	*Fritillaria pallidiflora*	Bulbus Fritillariae pallidiflorae	Yi Bei Mu		Pale-flower fritillary bulb
Yi Bui Mou, Tok Lei Bui Mou	*Fritillaria tortifolia*	Bulbus Fritillariae tortifoliae	Yi Bei Mu, Tuo Li Bei Mu		Twist-leaf fritillary bulb
Yi Bui Mou, Yu Man Bui Mou	*Fritillaria yuminensis*	Bulbus Fritillariae yuminensis	Yi Bei Mu, Yu Min Bei Mu		Yumin fritillary bulb
Yi Cha	*Acacia catechu*	Pasta Acaciae seu Uncariae	Er Cha	Asenyaku	Catechu paste
Yi Cha	*Uncaria gambir* and spp	Pasta Uncaria seu Acaciae	Er Cha		Catechu paste
Yi Ng Gan	*Eleagnus oldhamii*	Radix Eleagni oldhamii	Yi Wu Gen		Oldham's eleagnus root
Yi Ngau Chou	*Heliotropium indicum*	Herba Heliotropi	Er Gou Cao		Indian heliotrope herb
Yi Sam, Taai Ji Sam	*Pseudostellaria heterophylla*	Radix Pseudostellariae	Tai Zi Shen	Taishijin	Prince ginseng root
Yi Tong	*Hordeum vulgare*	Saccharum Hordei	Yi Tang, Jiao Yi		Barley malt sugar
Yi Yi Gan	*Coix lachryma-jobi* var. *Ma-yuen*	Radix Coicis	Yi Yi Gen		Job's-tears root
Yik Ji Yan	*Alpinia oxyphylla*	Fructus Alpiniae oxyphyllae	Yi Zhi Ren	Yakuchinin	Sharp-leaf galangal berry
Yik Mou Chou, Chong Wai	*Leonorus heterophyllus, L. japonicus, L. sibiricus* and spp	Herba Leonori	Yi Mu Cao, Chong Wei	Yakumoso	Asian motherwort herb
Yim Fo Muk	*Rhus chinensis*	Cortex Rhudis chinensis	Yan Fu Mu	Gobaishi	Chinese sumac bark

CANTONESE	SCIENTIFIC	PHARMACEUTICAL	MANDARIN	JAPANESE	ENGLISH
Yim Syu Seung	*Mogera robusta* and spp., *Scaptochirus moschatus*	Mogera carbonisatus	Yan Shu Shuang	Ensosu	Carbonized mogera
Yin Ming Chou	*Isodon japonicus*	Herba Isodonis	Ye Ming Cao	Enmeiso	Isodon herb
Yin Wu Sok, Chi Faan Yin Wu Sok	*Corydalis turtschaninovii*	Rhizoma Corydalis	Yan Hu Suo, Chi Ban Yan Hu Suo	Engosaku	Dentate-leaf corydalis corm
Yin Wu Sok, Dung Bak Yin Wu Sok	*Corydalis ambigua* var. *amurensis*	Rhizoma Corydalis ambiguae	Yan Hu Suo, Dong Bei Yan Hu Suo		Amur corydalis corm
Yin Wu Sok, Yun Wu	*Corydalis yanhusuo*	Rizoma Corydalis yanhusuoidis	Yan Hu Suo, Yuan Hu	Engosaku	Asian corydalis corm
Ying Pei	*Prunus jamasakura, P. yedoensis*	Cortex Pruni	Ying Pi	Ouhi	Plum tree bark
Yu Biu Gaau	*Acipenser sinensis, Miichthys* spp	Colla piscis	Yu Biao Jiao		Fish airbladder
Yu Chin	*Ulmus pumila*	Cortex Ulmi pumilae	Yu Qian		White elm bark
Yu Heung	*Boswellia carterii* and spp.	Resina Boswelliae	Ru Xiang	Nyuko	Frankincense resin
Yu Leung Sek	*Limonitum*	Limonitum	Yu Liang Shi	Uyoryo	Clay ironstone
Yu Nou Sek	*Pseudosciaena crocea, P. polyactis, Sciaena schlegeli*	Otozithum Sciaenae	Yu Nao Shi		Fish otolith
Yu Seng Chou	*Houttuynia cordata*	Herba Houttuyniae	Yu Xing Cao	Juyakuso	Fishwort herb
Yuk Chung Yung	*Cistanche salsa* and spp	Herba Cistanchis	Rou Cong Rong	Nikujuyo	Fleshy broomrape herb
Yuk Dau Gan	*Dolichos lablab*	Radix Dolichoris	Rou Dou Gen		Hyacinth bean root
Yuk Dau Kau	*Myristica fragrans*	Semen Myristicae	Rou Dou Kou	Nikuzuku	Nutmeg seed
Yuk Gam	*Curcuma longa, C. aromatica*	Tuber Curcumae	Yu Jin	Ukon	Turmeric tuber
Yuk Gwai (Pei)	*Cinnamomum cassia*	Cortex Cinnamomi cassiae	Rou Gui (Pi)	Nikkei	Cassia Cinnamon bark
Yuk Gwai San	*Cinnamomum cassia*	Cortex intimum Cinnamomi cassiae	Rou Gui Xin		Cassia cinnamon inner bark
Yuk Gwai, Sek Laan Yuk Gwai	*Cinnamomum zeylanicum*	Cortex Cinnamomi zeylanici	Rou Gui, Xi Lan Rou Gui		Ceylon cinnamon bark
Yuk Juk	*Polygonatum odoratum* var. *pluriflorum, P. plurifolium*	Rhizoma Polygonati odorati	Yu Zhu	Gyokuchiku	Fragrant Solomon's seal root
Yuk Lei Yan	*Prunus japonica*	Semen Pruni japonicae	Yu Li Ren	Ikurinin	Bush cherry kernel
Yuk Lei Yan, Ngao Lei	*Prunus humilis*	Semen Pruni humili	Yu Li Ren, Ou Li		Dwarf cherry kernel
Yuk Mai Sam	*Zea mays*	Medulla Zeae	Yu Mi Xin		Corn cob
Yuk Mai So, Yuk Mai Yeui	*Zea mays*	Stylus Zeae	Yu Mi Xu, Yu Mi Rui	Gyokuma-ishu	Cornsilk style
Yuk Suk Syu	*Zea mays*	Fructus Zeae	Yu Shu Shu		Corn grain
Yun Bou Chou	*Hypericum sampsonii*	Herba Hyperici sampsonii	Yuan Bao Cao		South China St. John's wort herb
Yun Fa	*Daphne genkwa*	Flos Daphnis genkwae	Yuan Hua	Genka	Lilac daphne flower
Yun Fan	*Cerussa*	Cerussa	Qian Fen		Cerusite

CANTONESE	SCIENTIFIC	PHARMACEUTICAL	MANDARIN	JAPANESE	ENGLISH
Yun Heung Chou	*Cymbopogon distans*	Herba Cymbopogonis distansis	Yun Xiang Cao		Distant lemongrass herb
Yun Ji	*Polygala tenuifolia*	Radix Polygalae	Yuan Zhi	Onji	Thin-leaf milkwort root
Yun Mei	*Iris tectorum*	Rhizoma Iris tectoris	Yuan Wei		Kite-tail iris root
Yun Sai Ji	*Coriandrum sativum*	Fructus Coriandri	Yan Sui Zi		Coriander seed
Yun Sam, Yun Sam	*Scrophularia ningpoensis, S. buergeriana*	Radix Scrophulariae ningpoensis	Xuan Shen, Yuan Shen	Genjin	Black figwort root
Yut Dim Hung	*Cypripedium formosanum*	Herba Cypripedii	Yi Dian Hong		Formosa lady' slipper herb
Yut Gwai Fa	*Rosa chinensis*	Gemma Rosae chinensis	Yue Ji Hua	Gekkika	Moonseason rose bud
Yut Gwai Gan	*Rosa chinensis*	Radix Rosae chinensis	Yue Ji Gen		Moonseason rose root

Cross Index of Japanese Remedy Names

JAPANESE	SCIENTIFIC	PHARMACEUTICAL	MANDARIN	CANTONESE	ENGLISH
Agi	*Ferula foetida*	Resina Ferulae (Asafoetidae)	A Wei	A Ngai	Asafoetida resin
Akyo	*Equus asinus* and spp	Gelatinum corii Equi asini	E Jiao	O Gaau	Ass hide glue
Amatya, Dochouzan	*Hydrangea serrata* var. *thunbergii*	Folium Hydrangeae	Gan Cha	Gam Cha	Sweet tea leaf
Ansokuko	*Styrax benzoin*	Benzoinum	An Xi Xiang	Ngon Sik Heung	Benzoin
Arutai ginrenkon	*Anemone altaica*	Rhizoma Anemoni altaicae	Jiu Jie Chang Pu	Gau Jit Cheung Pou	Altai anemone root
Asenyaku	*Acacia catechu*	Pasta Acaciae seu Uncariae	Er Cha	Yi Cha	Catechu paste
Atanshi	*Brucea javanica*	Fructus Bruceae	Ya Dan Zi	Nga Daan Ji	Brucea berry
Babotsu	*Lasiosphaera fenslii* and spp, *Calvatia lilacina, C. fenzlii, C. gigantea*	Sclerotium Lasiosphaerae seu Calvatiae	Ma Bo	Ma But	Puffball mushroom
Bakuga	*Hordeum vulgare*	Fructus germinatus Hordei	Mai Ya	San Man Nga	Sprouted barley grain
Bakumondo	*Ophiopogon japonicus*	Radix Ophiopogonis	Mai (Men) Dong	Mak (Mun) Dung	Dwarf lilyturf root
Bankoka	*Crocus sativus*	Stigma Croci	Xi Hong Hua, Fan Hong Hua	Fun Hung Fa	Saffron stigma
Bankyo, Mantsai	*Tetragonia tatragonoides*	Herba Tetragoniae	Fan Xing	Faan Haang	Tetragonia herb
Banrankon	*Baphicacanthus cusia*	Radix Baphicacanthi	Ma Lan Gen	Ma Laam Gan	Assam indigo root
Banranyo	*Baphicacanthus cusia*	Folium Baphicacanthi	Ma Lan Ye	Ma Laam Yip	Assam indigo leaf
Banshashi	*Cassia occidentalis*	Semen Cassiae occidentalis	Wang Jiang Nan Zi	Mong Gong Naam	Coffee senna seed
Bantaikai	*Sterculia staphigera, S. lychnophera*	Semen Sterculiae	Pang Da Hai	Bun Daai Hoi	Sterculia seed
Basenshi	*Strychnos pierrana, S. nux-vomica* and spp	Semen Strychnotis preparatae	(Zhi) Ma Qian Zi	Ma Chin Ji	Prepared vomit nut
Bashiken	*Portulacca oleracea*	Herba Portulaccae	Ma Chi Xian	Ma Chi Yin	Purslane herb
Batorei	*Aristolochia contorta, A. debilis*	Fructus Aristolochiae	Ma Dou Ling	Ma Dau Ling	Green birthwort capsule
Bekko	*Amyda sinensis, Trionix sinensis*	Carapax Amydae seu Trionis	Bie Jia	Bit Gaap	Asian soft-shell turtle shell
Binroji	*Areca catechu, A. dicksonii*	Semen Arecae catechu	Bing Lang	Ban Long	Betel nut
Binroka	*Areca catechu, A. dicksonii*	Flos Arecae catechu	Bing Lang Hua	Ban Long Fa	Betel nut flower
Biwayo	*Eriobotrya japonica*	Folium Eriobotryae	Pi Pa Ye	Pei Pa Yip	Loquat leaf
Bofu	*Ledebouriella divaricata, L. seseloides*	Radix Ledebouriellae	Fang Feng	Fong Fung	Wind-protector root

JAPANESE	SCIENTIFIC	PHARMACEUTICAL	MANDARIN	CANTONESE	ENGLISH
Bokon	*Imperata cylindrica* var. *major*	Rhizoma Imperatae	Bai Mao Gen	Baak Maau Gan	Woolly grass root
Bokuso	*Quercus dentata, Q. acutissima*	Ramulus et cortex Querci	Pu Suo	Pok Sau	Oak twig and bark
Borei	*Ostrea gigas* and spp	Concha Ostreae	Mu Li	Mou Lai	Oyster shell
Bosho	*Mirabilitum*	Mirabilitum	Mang Xiao	Mong Seu	Mirabilite
Bosho	*Mirabilitum*	Mirabilitum purum	Xuan Ming Fan	San Ming Fun	Glauber's salt, Pure mirabilite
Bossai	*Heleocharis plantaginea*	Herba Heleocharis	Bi Qi	But Chai	Water chestnut herb
Botanpi	*Paeonia suffruticosa*	Cortex radicis Paeoniae suffruticosae	Mu Dan Pi, Dan Pi	Maau Daan Pei, Daan Pei	Tree peony root bark
Bui	*Ulmus macrocarpa*	Praeparatio fructus Ulmi	Wu Yi	Mon Yi	Stinking elm fruit paste
Bukuryo	*Poria cocos*	Sclerotium Poriae	Fu Ling	(Wong) Fuk Ling, Waan Ling	Hoelen fungus
Bukuryoshi	*Poria cocos*	Cortex Poriae	Fu Ling Pi	Wong Ling Pei, Fuk Ling Pei	Hoelen skin
Bukuryukan		Terra flava usta, Bolus usta	Fu Long Gan	Fuk Lung Gon	Wood stove clay
Bukushin	*Poria cocos*	Sclerotium Poriae paradicis	Fu Shen	Pou Fuk Sam	Hoelen spirit
Bushi	*Aconitum carmichaeli*	Radix lateralis Aconiti carmichaeli praeparatae	Fu Zi	Fu Ji	Prepared Sichuan aconite root
Bushukan	*Citrus medica* var. *sarctodactylus*	Flos Citri sarctodactylis	Fo Shou (Gan) Hua	Fut Sao Fa	Finger lemon flower
Byakishitsuri	*Tribulus terrestris*	Fructus Tribuli	Bai Ji Li	Baak Jat Lai	Caltrop fruit
Byakkaja-zesso	*Oldenlandia diffusa*	Herba Oldenlandiae	Bai Hua She She Cao	Baak Fa Se Sit Chou	Snaketongue grass herb
Byakubi	*Cynanchum atratum, C. versicolor*	Radix Cynanchi atrati	Bai Wei	Baak Mei	Swallow-wort root
Byakubushi	*Typhonium giganteum*	Rhizoma Typhonii gigantei preparata	Bai Fu Zi, Yu Bai Fu	Baak Fu Ji	Prepared giant typhonium root
Byakujutsu	*Atractylodes macrocephala*	Rhizoma Atractylodis macrocephalae	Bai Zhu	Baak Seut	White atractylodes root
Byakukyu	*Bletilla striata*	Rhizoma Bletillae	Bai Ji	Baak Gap	Amethyst orchid root
Byakuran	*Ampelopsis japonica*	Radix Ampelopsis	Bai Lian	Baak Lim	Japanese peppervine root
Byakushaku-(yaku)	*Paeonia lactiflora*	Radix Paeoniae lactiflorae	Bai Shao (Yao)	Baak Cheuk (Yeuk)	White peony root
Byakushi	*Angelica dahurica, A. anomala, A. taiwaniana*	Radix Angelicae dahuricae	Bai Zhi	Baak Ji	White angelica Root
Byakuzen	*Cynanchum stauntoni, C. glaucescens*	Radix et rhizoma Cynanchi stauntoni	Bai Qian	Baak Chin	Prime white root
Byakuzuku	*Amomum cardamomum*	Fructus Amomi cardamomi	Bai Dou Kou	Baak Dau Kau	Cluster cardamom pod
Byakuzu-kuka	*Amomum cardamomum*	Flos Amomi cardamomi	(Bai) Dou Kou Hua	(Baak) Dau Kau Fa	Cluster cardamom flower

JAPANESE	SCIENTIFIC	PHARMACEUTICAL	MANDARIN	CANTONESE	ENGLISH
Chikujo	*Phyllostachys nigra* var. *henonis* and spp	Caulis Phyllostachis in taeniis	Zhu Ru	Juk Yu	Black bamboo shaving
Chikureki	*Phyllostachys nigra* var. *henonis* and spp	Succus Phyllostachis	Zhu Li	Juk Lai	Black bamboo sap
Chikusekito	*Trachelospermum jasminoides*	Caulis Trachelospermi	Luo Shi Teng	Lok Sek Tang	Star jasmine stem
Chimo	*Anemarrhena asphodeloides*	Radix Anemarrhenae	Zhi Mu	Ji Mou	Know mother root
Chimpi	*Citrus reticulata, C. tangerina, C. erythrosa*	Pericarpium Citri reticulatae	Chen Pi, Ju Pi	Chan Pei, Gwat Pei	Ripe tangerine rind
Choko	*Eugenia caryophyllata*	Gemma Eugeniae	Ding Xiang	Ding Heung	Clove bud
Chorei	*Polyporus umbellatus*	Sclerotium Polypori	Zhu Ling	Ju Ling	Umbel polypore mushroom
Choto	*Uncaria rhynchophylla, U. hirsuta, U. macrophylla* and spp	Ramulus et uncus Uncariae	Gou Teng	Ngau Tang, Sheung Ngau (Tang)	Gambir vine twig
Daifukuhi	*Areca catechu, A. dicksonii*	Pericarpium Arecae	Da Fu Pi	Daai Fuk Pei	Betel husk
Daifushi	*Hydnocarpus anthelmintica, H. hainanensis*	Semen Hydnocarpi	Da Feng Zi	Daai Fung Ji	Chaulmoogra seed
Daifuso	*Blumea balsamifera*	Herba Blumeae balsamiferae	Ai Na Xiang, Da Feng Cao	Ngaai Naap Heung	Camphor plant
Daio	*Rheum palmatum, R. tanguticum, R. officinale*	Rhizoma Rhei	Da Huang	Daai Wong	Rhubarb root
Dandoku	*Canna indica*	Rhizoma Cannae	Mei Ren Jiao (Gen)	Mei Yan Jiu (Gan)	Canna lily root
Dataihi	*Elephe taeniurus* and spp, *Dinodon rufozonatum*	Periostracum/Exuviae Elephis	She Tui (Pi)	Se Teui (Pei)	Snakeskin slough
Dokkatsu	*Angelica pubescens, A. laxiflora* and spp	Radix Angelicae pubescentis	Du Huo	Duk Wut	Hairy angelica Root
Engosaku	*Corydalis turtschaninovii*	Rhizoma Corydalis	Yan Hu Suo, Chi Ban Yan Hu Suo	Yin Wu Sok, Chi Faan Yin Wu Sok	Dentate-leaf corydalis corm
Engosaku	*Corydalis yanhusuo*	Rizoma Corydalis yanhusuoidis	Yan Hu Suo, Yuan Hu	Yin Wu Sok, Yun Wu	Asian corydalis corm
Enmeiso	*Isodon japonicus*	Herba Isodonis	Ye Ming Cao	Yin Ming Chou	Isodon herb
Ensosu	*Mogera robusta* and spp., *Scaptochirus moschatus*	Mogera carbonisatus	Yan Shu Shuang	Yim Syu Seung	Carbonized mogera
Entan	*Minium*	Minium	Qian Dan, Huang Dan	Chin Daan, Wong Daan	Red lead oxide
Figikobu	*Wisteria sinensis, W. floribunda*	Galla Wisteriae	Zi Teng Zi, Teng Liu	Ji Tang Ji, Tang Lau	Asian wisteria gall
Fujucha, Chayo	*Camellia sinensis*	Folium Camelliae sinensis	Cha Ye	Cha Yip	Tea leaf
Fukubonshi	*Rubus chingii*	Fructus Rubi chingii	Fu Pen Zi	Fuk Pun Ji	Chinese raspberry fruit
Furitsukaku	*Castanea mollissima*	Fructus Castaneae	Li Zi, Feng Li Gu	Leut Ji	Chinese chestnut

JAPANESE	SCIENTIFIC	PHARMACEUTICAL	MANDARIN	CANTONESE	ENGLISH
Fushobaku	*Triticum aestivum*	Fructus Tritici	Fu Xiao Mai	Fau Siu Mak	Wheat berry
Gaihaku	*Allium macrostemon*	Bulbus Allii macrostemonis	Xie Bai	Se Baak	Chinese chive bulb
Gaiyo	*Artemisia argyi*	Folium Artemisiae argyi	Ai Ye	Ngaai Yang, Ngaai Yip	Asian mugwort leaf
Gajutsu	*Curcuma zedoaria, C. aeruginosa* and spp	Rhizoma Curcumae zedoariae	E Zhu, Peng Er Zhu	Ngo Seut, Fung Ngo Seut	Zedoary root
Garyoshi	*Arca inflata* and spp	Concha Arcae	Wa Leng Zi	Nga Ling Ji	Cockle shell
Gekkika	*Rosa chinensis*	Gemma Rosae chinensis	Yue Ji Hua	Yut Gwai Fa	Moonseason rose bud
Genjin	*Scrophularia ningpoensis, S. buergeriana*	Radix Scrophulariae ningpoensis	Xuan Shen, Yuan Shen	Yun Sam, Yun Sam	Black figwort root
Genka	*Daphne genkwa*	Flos Daphnis genkwae	Yuan Hua	Yun Fa	Lilac daphne flower
Gennoshio-uko	*Geranium wilfordii, G. thunbergii*	Herba Geranii	Lao He Cao	Lou Hap Chou	Geranium herb
Ginkyo	*Ginkgo biloba*	Fructus Ginkgoidis	Bai Guo, Yin Xing He	Baak Gwo, Ngan Hang Wat	Ginkgo nut
Ginkyoyo	*Ginkgo biloba*	Folium Ginkgoidis	Yin Xing Ye, Bai Guo Ye	Ngan Hang Yip, Baak Gwo Yip	Ginkgo leaf
Ginsaiko	*Stellaria dichotoma* var. *lanceolata*	Radix Stellariae	Yin Chai Hu	Ngan Chaai Wu	Stellaria root
Gobaishi	*Rhus chinensis*	Cortex Rhudis chinensis	Yan Fu Mu	Yim Fo Muk	Chinese sumac bark
Goboshi	*Arctium lappa*	Fructus Arctii	Niu Bang Zi	Ngau Pong Ji	Burdock seed
Gokahi	*Acanthopanax gracilistylus, A. spinosus, A. sessiliflorus* and spp	Cortex radicis Acanthopanacis	Wu Jia Pi	Ng Ga Pei	Five additions root bark
Gokai	*Gecko gecko, G. verticilatus*	Gecko	Ge Jie	Gap Gaai	Toad-headed lizard
Gokanhi	*Albizzia julibrissin, A. lebbak* and spp	Cortex Albizziae	He Huan Pi	Hap Fun Pei	Mimosa bark
Gokanka	*Albizzia julibrissin, A. lebbek* and spp	Flos Albizziae	He Huan Hua	Hap Fun Fa	Mimosa flower
Gomishi	*Schisandra chinensis*	Fructus Schisandrae	Wu Wei Zi	Ng Mei Ji	Schisandra berry
Gomishi	*Schizandra sphenantera*	Fructus Schisandrae sphenanterae	Wu Wei Zi, Hua Zheng Wu Wei Zi	Ng Mei Ji, Wa Jung Ng Mei Ji	Central China schisandra berry
Goo	*Bos taurus domesticus, Bubalis bubalis*	Calculus Bovis	Niu Huang	Ngau Wong	Ox gallstone
Goshitsu	*Achyranthes bidentata*	Radix Achyranthis	Niu Xi, Huai Niu Xi	Ngau Sat, Wai Ngau Sat	White oxknee Root
Gosho	*Scolopendra subspinipes mutilans*	Scolopendra	Wu Gong	Ng Gung	Centipede
Goshuyu	*Evodia rutaecarpa*	Fructus Evodiae rutecarpae	Wu Zhu Yu	Ng Jyu Yu	Evodia berry

JAPANESE	SCIENTIFIC	PHARMACEUTICAL	MANDARIN	CANTONESE	ENGLISH
Gyokuchiku	*Polygonatum odoratum* var. *pluriflorum, P. plurifolium*	Rhizoma Polygonati odorati	Yu Zhu	Yuk Juk	Fragrant Solomon's seal root
Gyokuma-ishu	*Zea mays*	Stylus Zeae	Yu Mi Xu, Yu Mi Rui	Yuk Mai So, Yuk Mai Yeui	Cornsilk style
Gyutan	*Bos taurus domesticus, Bubalis bubalis*	Vesica fellae Bovis	Niu Dan	Ngau Daam	Ox gallbladder
Hagekiten	*Morinda officinalis*	Radix Morindae	Ba Ji Tian	Ba Gik Tin	Morinda root
Haikan	*Eupatorium fortunei*	Herba Eupatorii fortunei	Pei Lan	Pui Laan	Orchid-grass herb
Haishoso	*Patrinia scabiosaefolia, P. villosa*	Herba et rhizoma Patriniae	Bai Jiang Cao	Baai Jeung Chou	Patrinia herb and root
Hakka	*Mentha arvensis*	Herba Menthae arvensis	Bo He	Bok Ho	Asian fieldmint herb
Hakkada	*Agkistrodon acutus* and *Bungarus multicinctus*	Agkistrodon seu Bungarus	Bai Hua She	Baak Fa Se	Multibanded krait
Hakkutusai	*Chelidonium majus* var. *asiaticum*	Herba Chelidonii	Bai Qu Cai	Baak Wat Choi	Asian celandine herb
Hakuhenzu	*Dolichos lablab*	Semen Dolichis	Bai Bian Dou	Baak Bin Dau	Hyacinth bean
Hakujin	*Panax ginseng*	Radix Panacis ginsengis praeparatae	Bai Shen	Baak Sam	Rock candy cured Asian ginseng root
Hakumo-keishito	*Paederia scandens*	Radix et caulis Paederiae	Ji Shi Teng	Gai Niu Tang	Chicken dung vine root and stem
Hakumokuji	*Tremella fuciformis*	Sclerotium Tremellae fucimormis	Bai Mu Er	Baak Muk Yi	Silver ear mushroom
Hakusempi	*Dictamnus dasycarpus*	Cortex radicis Dictamni	Bai Xian Pi	Baak Sin Pei	Asian dittany root bark
Hakushinin	*Biota orientalis*	Semen Biotae orientalis	Bai Zi Ren	(Baak) Ji Yan	Oriental arborvitae berry
Hakutoo	*Pulsatilla chinensis, P. cernua, P. turczaninovii, P. ambigua* and spp	Radix Pulsatillae	Bai Tou Weng	Baak Tau Yung	Asian pasqueflower root
Hanbanren	*Lobelia chinensis*	Herba et radix Lobeliae chinensis	Ban Bian Lian	Bau Bin Ling	Rooting lobelia herb and root
Hange, Kohange	*Pinellia ternata*	Rhizoma Pinelliae ternatae preparatae	Ban Xia Fa Ban Xia	Bun Ha, Faat Bun Ha	Prepared pinellia corm
Hanmyo	*Cantharis vesicatoria*	Cantharis	Ban Mao	Ban Mou	Cantharides
Hanmyo	*Mylabris*	Mylabris	Ban Mao	Ban Mou	Asian cantharides
Henchiku	*Polygonum aviculare*	Herba Polygoni avicularis	Bian Xu	Bin Chuk	Knotgrass herb
Henzuka	*Dolichos lablab*	Gemma Dolichis	Bian Dou Hua	Bin Dau Fa	Hyacinth bean bud
Hihatsu	*Piper longum*	Fructus Piperis longis	Bi Ba	Bat Pa	Long pepper fruit spike
Hikai	*Dioscorea hypoglauca*	Rhizoma Dioscoreae hypoglaucae	Bi Xie, Fen Bi Xie, Bei Xie	Bei Gaai, Fan Bei Gaai	Long yam root

JAPANESE	SCIENTIFIC	PHARMACEUTICAL	MANDARIN	CANTONESE	ENGLISH
Hokoei	*Taraxacum mongolicum*	Radix et herba Taraxaci	Pu Gong Ying	Pou Gung Ying	Mongolian dandelion root and herb
Hokotsushi	*Psoralea corylifolia*	Fructus Psoraleae	Bu Gu Zhi	Bou Gwat Ji	Scurf pea berry
Hokyo	*Zingiber officinalis*	Rhizoma Zingiberis	Pao Jiang	Bou Geung	Quick-fried ginger root
Hoo	*Typha latifolia, T. angustifolia* and spp	Pollen Typhae	Pu Huang, Xiang Pu	Pou Wong, Heung Pou	Cattail pollen
Hosha	*Borax*	Borax	Peng Sha	Pang Sa	Borax
Hyakubu	*Stemona japonia*	Radix Stemonae japonicae	Bai Bu, Man Sheng Bai Bu	Baak Bou, Maan Sang Baak Bou	Japanese stemona root
Hyakugo	*Lilium brownii* var. *colchesteri*	Bulbus Lilii	Bai He	Baak Hap	Brown's lily bulb
Ikurinin	*Prunus japonica*	Semen Pruni japonicae	Yu Li Ren	Yuk Lei Yan	Bush cherry kernel
Inchinko	*Artemisia capillaris, A. scoparia*	Herba Artemisiae capillaris	Yin Chen (Hao), Mian Yin Chen	Yan Chan (Hou), Min Yan Chan	Downy wormwood herb
Inyokaku	*Epimedium saggitatum, E. macranthum* and spp	Folium Epimedii	Yin Yang Huo, Xian Ling Pi	Yam Yeung Fok, Sin Ling Pei	Horny goat weed leaf
Io	*Sulphurum*	Sulphurum	Liu Huang, Shi Liu Huang	Lau Wong, Sek Lau Wong	Sulphur
Ireisen	*Clematis chinensis, C. hexapetala* and spp	Radix Clematis chinensis	Wei Ling Xian	Wai Ling Sin	Chinese clematis root
Jako	*Moschus berezovskii* and spp	Secretio Moschi	She Xiang	Se Heung	Musk
Jashoshi	*Cnidium monnieri*	Fructus Cnidii	She Chuang Zi	Se Chong Ji	Cnidium seed
Jibushi	*Kochia scoparia*	Semen Kochiae	Di Fu Zi	Dei Fu Ji	Kochia seed
Jijuso	*Callicarpa pedunculata*	Folium Callicarpae pedunculatae	Zi Zhu Ye	Ji Jyu Yip	Callicarpa leaf
Jikoppi	*Lycium chinense*	Cortex radicis Lycii	Di Gu Pi	Dei Gwat Pei	Wolfberry root bark
Jingyo	*Gentiana macrophylla, G. tibetica, G. dahurica* and spp	Radix Gentianae macrophyllae	Qin Jiao	Cheun Gau	Large-leaf gentian root
Jinko	*Aquilaria agallocha, A. sinensis*	Lignum Aquilariae	Chen Xiang	Cham Heung	Aloeswood
Jiryu	*Pheretima aspergillum, Allolobophora caliginosa*	Pheretima seu Allolobophora	Di Long	Dei Lung	Earthworm
Jiseki	*Mactra sulcataria*	Concha Mactrae	Ge	Hok	Mactra shell
Jiyu	*Sanguisorba officinalis*	Radix Sanguisorbae	Di Yu	Dei Yu	Great burnet root
Johi	*Citrus reticulata, C. tangerina, C. erythrosa*	Pericarpium Citri reticulatae viride	Qing Pi	Ching Pei	Unripe tangerine rind
Joszan	*Dichroa febrifuga*	Radix Dichroae	Chang Shan	Seung Saan	Feverflower root
Joteishi	*Ligustrum japonicum, L. lucidum*	Fructus Ligustri	Nu Zhen Zi	Neui Jing Ji	Glossy privet berry

JAPANESE	SCIENTIFIC	PHARMACEUTICAL	MANDARIN	CANTONESE	ENGLISH
Jubeikon	*Oryza sativa*	Radix Oryzae	Nuo Dao Gen (Xu)	No Du Gan	Sweet rice root
Judaikoro	*Mahonia bealei*	Folium Mahoniae bealei	Shi Da Gong Lao Ye, Kuo Ye Shi Da Gong Lao Ye	Sap Daai Gung Lou Yip, Fut Yip Sap Daai Gung Lou Yip	Leather-leaf mahonia leaf
Judaikoro	*Mahonia fortunei*	Folium Mahoniae fortunei	Shi Da Gong Lao Ye, Xi Ye Shi Da Gong Lao Ye	Gung Lou Yip, Sai Yip Sap Daai Gung Lou Yip	Mahonia leaf
Jukujio	*Rehmannia glutinosa*	Radix Rehmanniae preparatae	Shu Di (Huang)	Suk Dei (Wong)	Prepared Rehmannia root
Juyakuso	*Houttuynia cordata*	Herba Houttuyniae	Yu Xing Cao	Yu Seng Chou	Fishwort herb
Kagoso	*Prunella vulgaris*	Spica Prunellae	Xia Ku Cao	Ha Fu Chou	Selfheal spike
Kaiba	*Hippocampus kelloggiand* spp	Hippocampus	Hai Ma	Hoi Ma	Sea horse
Kaifuseki	*Pumus*	Lapis Pumicis	Fu Hai Shi	Fau Hoi Sek	Pumice
Kaigokaku	*Cyclina sinensis*	Concha Cyclinae	Hai Ge Ke, Ke Li	Hoi Gap Hok	Clam shell
Kaikinsha	*Lygodium japonicum*	Spora Lygodii	Hai Jin Sha	Hoi Gam Sa	Japanese climbing fern spore
Kaikinshato	*Lygodium japonicum*	Herba Lygodii	Hai Jin Sha Teng	Hoi Gam Sa Tang	Japanese climbing fern herb
Kaikujin	*Callorhinus ursinus, Phoca vitulina*	Testes et penis Callorhini seu Phocae	Hai Gou Shen	Hoi Gau Sam	Seal genitals
Kaiso	*Sargassum fusiforme* and spp	Herba Sargassi	Hai Zao	Hoi Chou	Sargassum seaweed
Kaitohi	*Erythrina variegata* var. *orientalis*	Cortex Erythrinae	Hai Tong Pi	Hoi Tung Pei	Asian coral tree bark
Kakko	*Agastache rugosa*	Herba Agastachis	Huo Xiang	Fok Heung	Rugose giant hyssop herb
Kakkon	*Pueraria lobata, P. omeiensis* and spp	Radix Puerariae	Ge Gen	Got Gan	Kudzu root
Kakushitsu	*Carpesium abrotanoides*	Fructus seu semen Carpesii	He Shi	Hok Sat	Starwort fuit or seed
Kamboi	*Stephania tetrandra*	Radix Stephaniae tetrandrae	Han Fang Ji, Fang Ji	Haan Fong Gei Fong Gei	Stephania root
Kanju	*Blechnum orientale*	Rhizoma Blechni	Guan Zhong, Wu Mao Jue Guan Zhong, Dong Fang Wu Mao Jue Ye	Gwun Jung, Dung Fong Wu Mou Kyut Yip	Oriental hammock fern root
Kankinto	*Tinospora sinensis*	Caulis Tinosporae sinensis	Kuan Jin Teng	Gwan Gam Tang	Chinese tinospora stem
Kankyo	*Zingiber officinalis*	Rhizoma Zingiberis	Gan Jiang	Gaan Geung	Dried ginger root
Kanrenso	*Eclipta prostata, E. alba*	Herba Ecliptae	Han Lian Cao, Mo Han Lian	Hon Lin Chou	Field lotus herb
Kansui	*Euphorbia kansui*	Radix Euphorbiae kansui	Gan Sui	Gam Seui	Sweet spurge root
Kansuiseki	*Calcitum*	Calcitum	Han Shui Shi, Fang Jie Shi	Hon Seui Sek	Calcite
Kantoka	*Tussilago farfara*	Flos Tussilaginis	Kuan Dong Hua	Fun Dung Fa	Coltsfoot flower

JAPANESE	SCIENTIFIC	PHARMACEUTICAL	MANDARIN	CANTONESE	ENGLISH
Kanzo	*Glycirrhiza uralensis, G. glabra* and spp	Radix Glycirrhizae	Gan Cao	Gam Chou	Ural licorice root
Karo	*Trichosanthes kirilowii, T. japonica, T. uniflora*	Fructus Tricosanthis	Gua Lou (Shi)	Kwut Lau	Snakegourd fruit
Karohi	*Trichosanthes kirilowii, T. japonica, T. uniflora*	Pericarpium Tricosanthis	Gua Lou Pi	Kwut Lau Pei	Snakegourd rind
Karonin	*Trichosanthes kirilowii, T. japonica, T. uniflora*	Semen Trichosanthis	Gua Lou Ren	Kwut Lau Yan	Snakegourd seed
Kashi	*Terminalia chebula* and var.	Fructus Terminaliae	He Zi (Rou)	Ho Ji (Yuk)	Myrobalan fruit
Kashohi	*Arachis hypogaea*	Pericarpium Arachis	Hua Sheng Pi	Fa Sang Pei	Peanut skin
Kashuu	*Polygonum multiflorum*	Radix Polygoni multiflori	He Shou Wu	Ho Sau Wu	Flowery knotweed root
Kasseki	*Talcum*	Talcum	Hua Shi	Wat Sek	Talc
Katei	*Cucumis melo*	Caulis Cucumis	Tian Gua Di	Tim Gwa Dai	Young cantaloupe stalk
Kayo	*Nelumbo nucifera*	Folium Nelumbinis	He Ye, Lian Lie	Ho Yip	Lotus leaf
Kazuiseki	*Ophicalcitum*	Ophicalcitum	Hua Rui Shi	Fa Yeui Sek	Dolomite
Keifun	*Calomelas*	Calomelas	Qing Fen	Ching Fan	Calomel
Keigai	*Schizonepeta tenuifolia*	Herba Schizonepetae	Jing Jie	Ging Gaai	Japanese catnip herb
Keiketto	*Millettia dielsiana, M. reticulata, M. nitida*	Radix et caulis Millettiae dielsianae	Ji Xue Teng	Gai Yut Tang	Millettia root and stem
Keinaikin	*Gallus gallus domesticus*	Endothelium corneum gigeriae Galli	Ji Nei Jin	Gai Na Gam	Chicken gizzard lining
Keishi	*Cinnamomum cassia*	Ramulus Cinnamomi cassiae	Gui Zhi , Rou Gui Zhi	Gwai Ji	Cassia cinnamon twig
Kekketsu	*Daemonorops draco*	Resina Daemonoropsis (Sanguis draconis)	Xue Jie	Hyut Kit	Dragon's-blood resin
Kenjin	*Paris polyphylla, P. chinensis, P. formosana* and var.	Rhizoma Paris	Qi Ye Yi Zhi Hua, Zao Xiu	Chak Yip Jek Ji Fa, Sat Yau	Paris root
Kenjitsu	*Euryale ferox*	Semen Euryalis	Qian Shi	Him Sat	Foxnut
Ketsumeishi	*Cassia tora, C. obtusifolia* and spp	Semen Cassiae torae	Jue Ming Zi, Cao Jue Ming	Kyut Ming Ji, Chou Kyut Ming	Sickle senna seed
Kiban	*Chinemys reevesii*	Plastrum Chinemis	Gui Ban	Gwai Baan	Tortoise shell
Kijitsu	*Citrus aurantium, C. wilsonii*	Fructus Citri aurantii immaturi	Zhi Shi	Ji Sat	Unripe bitter orange fruit
Kikoku	*Citrus aurantium* var. *amara*	Fructus Citri aurantii amarae	Zhi Ke, Zhi Qiao, Dai Dai Hua Zhi Qiao	Ji Hok, Doi Doi Fa Ji Hok	Ripe bitter orange fruit
Kikurage	*Auricularia auricula*	Sclerotium Auriculariae	Mu Er	Muk Yi	Wood ear mushroom
Kikyo	*Platycodon grandiflorum*	Radix Platycodonis	Jie Geng, Ku Jie Geng	Gat Gan	Balloonflower root
Kinfutsuso	*Inula japonica, I. brittanica, I. linariaefolia*	Herba Inulae	Jin Fei Cao	Gam Fai Chou	Elecampane herb

JAPANESE	SCIENTIFIC	PHARMACEUTICAL	MANDARIN	CANTONESE	ENGLISH
Kinginka	*Lonicera japonica*	Flos Lonicerae japonicae	Jin Yin Hua, Ren Dong Hua	Gam Ngan Fa Yan Dung Fa	Japanese honeysuckle flower
Kinkaran	*Tinospora sagittata, T. capillipes*	Radix Tinosporae	Jin Guo Lan	Gam Gwo Laam	Tinospora root
Kinoshi	*Rosa laevigata*	Fructus Rosae laevigatae	Jin Ying Zi	Gam Ying Ji	Cherokee rosehip
Kinsenso	*Desmodium styracifolium*	Herba Desmodii	Guang Dong (Jin) Qian Cao	Gwong Dung (Gam) Chin Chou	Coin-leaf desmodium herb
Kinsenso	*Dichondra repens*	Herba Dichondrae	Ma Di Jin	Ma Dei Jing	Dichondra herb
Kinsenso	*Lysimachia christinae, L. hemsleyana*	Herba Lysimachiae	Jin Qian Cao, Guo Lu Huang	Gam Chin Chou, Gwo Lou Wong	Asian moneywort herb
Kisasage	*Catalpa ovata*	Fructus Catalpae	Zhi Shi	San Sat	Catalpa fruit
Koboka, Kobokuka	*Magnolia officinalis, M. biloba, M. obovata*	Flos Magnoliae officinalis	Hou Po Hua	Hau Pok Fa	Magnolia flower
Koboku	*Magnolia officinalis, M. biloba, M. obovata*	Cortex Magnoliae officinalis	Hou Po Chuan Po	Hau Pok, Chyun Pok	Magnolia bark
Kobushi	*Cyperus rotundus*	Rhizoma Cyperi	Xiang Fu	Heung Fu	Purple nutsedge root
Kogataigeki	*Knoxia valerianoides*	Radix Knoxiae	Hong Da Ji	Hung Daai Gik	Knoxia root
Kohon	*Ligusticum sinense, L. jeholense*	Radix Ligustici sinensis	Gao Ben	Gou Bun	Chinese lovage root
Koi	*Oryza sativa*	Saccharum Oryzae			Rice malt (syrup)
Koju	*Elsholtzia splendens, E. stauntonii*	Herba Elsholtziae	Xiang Ru (Cao)	Heung Yu (Chou)	Aromatic madder herb
Koka	*Carthamus tinctorius*	Flos Carthami tinctorii	Hong Hua	Hung Fa	Safflower
Kokotsu	*Panthera*	Os tigris	Hu Gu	Fu Gwat	Tiger bone
Kokuga	*Oryza sativa*	Fructus Oryzae germinatus	Gu Ya	Gu Nga	Sprouted rice grain
Kokuseiso	*Eriocaulon buergerianum, E. sieboldianum*	Herba Eriocaulonis	Gu Jing Cao	Guk Jing Chou	Pipewort herb
Kombu	*Laminaria japonica* and spp	Thallus Laminariae	Kun Bu	Gwan Bou	Kelp seaweed
Koninjin	*Panax ginseng*	Radix Panacis ginsengis praeparatae	Hong Ren Shen	Hung Yan Sam	Red cured Asian ginseng root
Kooren	*Picrorrhiza kurroa*	Radix Picrorrhizae	Hu Huang Lian	Wu Wong Lin	Picrorrhiza root
Koryokyo	*Alpinia officinarum*	Rhizoma Alpiniae officinari	Gao Liang Jiang	Gou Leung Geung	Galangal root
Kosho	*Piper nigrum*	Fructus Piperis nigri	Hu Jiao, Hei Hu Jiao	Wu Jiu, Mai Wu Jiu	Black pepper corn
Koso	*Macaca mulatta*	Calculus Macacae	Hou Zao	Hau Jou	Macaque bezoar
Koso	*Zizyphus jujuba* var. *inermis*	Fructus Zizyphi jujubae	Hong Zao	Hung Jou	Red jujube berry
Kotoniku	*Juglans regia*	Semen Juglandis	Hu Tao Ren	Wu Tou Yan	Walnut meat
Kotsusaiho	*Davallia divaricata*	Rhizoma Davalliae	Gu Sui Bu	Gwat Seui Bou	Boneknit root
Kotsusaiho	*Drynaria fortunei* and spp	Rhizoma Drynariae	Gu Sui Bu	Gwat Seui Bou	Boneknit root

JAPANESE	SCIENTIFIC	PHARMACEUTICAL	MANDARIN	CANTONESE	ENGLISH
Kotsusaiho	*Pseudodrynaria fortunei, D. baronii*	Rhizoma Pseudodrynariae	Gu Sui Bu	Gwat Seui Bou	Boneknit root
Kubaku	*Dianthus superbus, D. chinensis*	Herba Dianthi	Qu Mai	Geui Mak	Proud pink herb
Kujin	*Canis*	Testes et penis canis	Guang Gou Shen	Gwong Gau Sam	Male dog genitals
Kukoshi	*Lycium chinense, L. barbarum*	Fructus Lycii	Gou Qi Zi	Gau Gei Ji, Gei Ji	Wolfberry
Kurenkombi	*Melia azedarach, M. toosendan*	Cortex radicis Meliae	Ku Lian (Gen) Pi	Fu Lin (Gan) Pei	Bead tree root bark
Kuseki	*Cibotium barometz*	Rhizoma Cibotii	Gou Ji	Gau Jek	Dogspine root
Kuttokei	*Capparis masaikai*	Semen Capparis	Ma Bin Lang	Ma Ban Long	Capparis berry
Kyokatsu	*Notopterygium incisum, N. forbesii, N. francherii*	Rhizoma et radix Notopterigii	Qiang Huo	Geung Wut	Notoptery-gium root
Kyonin	*Prunus armeniaca* and var.	Semen Pruni armeniacae	Xing Ren, Ku Xing Ren	Baak Hang Yan	Bitter apricot kernel
Kyoo	*Curcuma longa. C. aromatica*	Rhizoma Curcumae	Jiang Huang	Geung Wong	Turmeric root
Kyuseishi	*Impatiens balsamina*	Semen Impatiensis	Ji Xing Zi	Jek Chin Ji	Garden balsam seed
Kyushi	*Allium tuberosum*	Semen Alii tuberosi	Jiu Cai Zi	Gau Choi Ji	Asian leek seed
Magotaro-mushi	*Protohermes grandis*	Vermiculus Protohermis	Sun Tai Lang Chun	Syun Taai Long Chung	Protohermes larva
Maikaika	*Rosa rugosa*	Flos Rosae rugosae	Mei Gui Hua	Mui Gwai Fa	Japanese rose flower
Maitake	*Grifola frondosa*	Sclerotium Grifolae frondosae			Maitake, Hen of the woods mushroom
Mankeishi	*Vitex rotundifolia, V. trifolia*	Fructus Viticis rotundifoliae	Man Jing Zi	Maan Ging Ji	Seashore chastetree berry
Mao	*Ephedra sinica*	Herba Ephedrae	Ma Huang	Ma Wong	Ephedra stem
Maokon	*Ephedra sinica*	Radix Ephedrae	Ma Huang Gen	Ma Wong Gan	Ephedra root
Mashinin	*Cannabis sativa*	Semen Cannabis	Huo Ma Ren	Fo Ma Yan	Cannabis seed
Megi	*Berberis thunbergii*	Lignum Berberis thunbergii	Xiao Nie	Siu Maak	Barberry wood
Mintojin	*Changium smyrnioides*	Radix Changii	Ming Dang Shen	Ming Dong Sam	Bright changium root
Mitsudaso	*Lithargyrum*	Lithagyrum	Mi Tuo Seng	Muk Toi Sang	Litharge
Mitsumoka	*Buddleia officinalis*	Flos Buddleiae	Mi Meng Hua	Mat Mung Fa	Buddleia flower and bud
Mokka	*Chaenomeles lagenaria*	Fructus Chaenomelis lagenariae	Mu Gua, Chuan Mu Gua	Muk Gwa, Chyun Muk Gwa	Chinese quince fruit
Mokko	*Saussurea lappa*	Radix Saussureae lappae	Mu Xiang, Yun Mu Xiang	Muk Heung	Wood aromatic root
Mokubesshi	*Momordica cochinchinensis*	Semen Momordicae cochinchinensis	Mu Bie Zi	Muk Bit Ji	Cochin bitter melon seed
Mokukocho	*Oroxylum indicum*	Semen Oroxyli	Mu Hu Die	Muk Wu Dip	Oroxylum seed
Mokutenryo	*Actinidia polygama*	Galla fructi Actinidiae	Mu Tian Lian	Muk Tin Lin	Actinidia gall

JAPANESE	SCIENTIFIC	PHARMACEUTICAL	MANDARIN	CANTONESE	ENGLISH
Mokutsu	*Akebia quinata, A. trifoliata*	Caulis Akebiae	Mu Tong, Bai Mu Tong	Baak Muk Tong	Akebia stem
Mokuzoku	*Equisetum hiemale*	Herba Equiseti hiemalis	Mu Zei	Muuk Chaak	Horsetail herb
Motosei	*Ilex pubescens*	Radix Ilicis pubescentis	Mao Dong Qing	Mou Dung Ching	Furry holly root
Motsuyaku	*Commiphora myrrha*	Resina Commiphorae	Mo Yao	Mut Yeuk	Myrrh resin
Myoban	*Alumen*	Alumen	Ming Fan	Ming Faan	Alum
Nankashi	*Cucurbita moschata*	Semen Cucurbitae	Nan Gua Zi	Naam Gwa Ji	Red squash seed
Nanshajin	*Adenophora stricta, A. capillaris, A. tetraphylla* and spp	Radix Adenophorae strictae	Nan Sha Shen	Naam Sa Sam	Upright ladybell root
Nikkei	*Cinnamomum cassia*	Cortex Cinnamomi cassiae	Rou Gui (Pi)	Yuk Gwai (Pei)	Cassia Cinnamon bark
Nikujuyo	*Cistanche salsa* and spp	Herba Cistanchis	Rou Cong Rong	Yuk Chung Yung	Fleshy broomrape herb
Nikuzuku	*Myristica fragrans*	Semen Myristicae	Rou Dou Kou	Yuk Dau Kau	Nutmeg seed
Ninjin	*Panax ginseng*	Radix Panacis ginsengis	Ren Shen	Yan Sam	Asian ginseng root
Ninjinro	*Panax ginseng*	Rhizoma Panacis ginsengis	Ren Shen Lu	Yan Sam Lu	Asian ginseng neck
Ninjinyo	*Panax ginseng*	Folium Panacis ginsengis	Ren Shen Ye	Yan Sam Yip	Asian ginseng leaf
Nogikuka	*Chrysanthemum indicum*	Flos Chrysanthemi indici	Ye Ju Hua	Gam Guk Fa, Ye Guk Fa	Wild chrysanthe-mum flower
Nyuko	*Boswellia carterii* and spp.	Resina Boswelliae	Ru Xiang	Yu Heung	Frankincense resin
Obaku	*Phellodendron amurense, P. chinense*	Cortex Phellodendris	Huang Bai Chuan Bai	Wong Paak Chyun Paak	Siberian cork tree bark
Ofurugyo	*Vaccaria segetalis*	Semen Vaccariae	Wang Bu Liu Xing	Wong Bat Lau Hang	Cowcockle seed
Ogi	*Astragalus membranaceus, A. mongholicus* and spp	Radix Astragali	Huang Qi	Wong Kei, Paak Kei	Astragalus root
Ogon	*Scutellaria baicalensis, S. viscidula, S. amoena*	Radix Scutellariae baicalensis	Huang Qin	Wong Sam	Baikal skullcap root
Onji	*Polygala tenuifolia*	Radix Polygalae	Yuan Zhi	Yun Ji	Thin-leaf milkwort root
Oren	*Coptis chinensis, C. omeiensis* and spp	Rhizoma Coptis	Huang Lian, Chuan Lian	Wong Lin, Chyun Wong Lin	Goldthread root
Osei	*Polygonatum sibiricum, P. cyrtonema, P. kingianum*	Rhizoma Polygonati	Huang Jing	Wong Jing	Siberian Solomon's-seal root
Ouhi	*Prunus jamasakura, P. yedoensis*	Cortex Pruni	Ying Pi	Ying Pei	Plum tree bark
Oyakushi	*Dioscorea bulbifera*	Rhizoma Dioscoreae bulbiferae	Huang Yao Zi	Wong Yeuk Ji	Potato yam tuber

JAPANESE	SCIENTIFIC	PHARMACEUTICAL	MANDARIN	CANTONESE	ENGLISH
Ozokukoku	*Papaver somniferum*	Pericarpium Papaveris	Ying Su Ke	Ngang Suk Hok	Opium poppy husk
Rakanka	*Momordica grosvenori*	Fructus Momordicae grosvenorii	Luo Han Guo	Lou Haan Kwo	Arhat fruit
Rakankayo	*Momordica grosvenori*	Folium Momordicae grosvenorii	Luo Han Ye	Lou Haan Yip	Arhat leaf
Rakutokuda	*Sambucus japonicus*	Cortex Sambuci japonici	Lu Ying		Japanese elder bark
Reishi	*Ganoderma lucidum, G. sinense, G applanatum* and spp	Sclerotium Ganodermae	Ling Zhi (Cao)	Ling Ji (Chou)	Reishi mushroom
Reiyokaku	*Saiga tatarica*	Cornu Saigae	Ling Yang Jiao	Ling Yeung Gok	Antelope horn
Rengyo	*Forsythia suspensa*	Fructus Forsythiae	Lian Qiao	Lin Kiu	Forsythia valve
Renshi	*Nelumbo nucifera*	Semen Nelumbinis	Lian Zi	Lin Ji	Lotus seed
Renshin	*Nelumbo nucifera*	Receptaculum Nelumbinis	Lian Fang	Lin Fong	Lotus receptacle
Renshu	*Nelumbo nucifera*	Stamen Nelumbinis	Lian Xu	Lin Sou	Lotus stamen
Riro	*Veratrum nigrum* and spp	Radix et rhizoma Veratri	Li Lu	Lai Lou	False hellebore root
Rokanseki	*Calamina, Smithsonitum*	Calamina, Smithsonitum	Lu Gan Shi	Lou Gam Sek	Calamine
Rokkaku	*Cervus nippon* and spp	Cornu Cervi	Lu Jiao	Luk Gok	Mature deer antler
Rokkakukyo	*Cervus nippon* and spp	Colla cornu Cervi	Lu Jiao Jiao	Luk Gok Gaau	Mature deer antler glue
Rokkakuso	*Cervus nippon* and spp	Cornu Cervi degelatinatum	Lu Jiao Shuang, Rong Mo	Luk Gok Shuen	Mature deer antler powder
Rokon	*Phragmites communis*	Radix Phragmitis	Lu Gen	Lou Gan	Water-reed root
Rokujo	*Cervus nippon* and spp	Cornu cervi parvum	Lu Rong, Rong Tou, Nen Lu Rong	Luk Yan	Velvet deer antler
Rokuteiso	*Pyrola rotundifolia subsp. chinensis, P. Japonica*	Radix et herba Pyrolae	Lu Xian Cao, Lu Ti Cao	Luk Haam Chou, Luk Tai Chou	Asian wintergreen root and herb
Roro	*Rhaponticum uniflorum*	Radix Rhapontici	Lou Lu	Lau Lou	Swiss centaury root
Rorotsu	*Liquidambar taiwaniana*	Fructus Liquidambaris	Lu Lu Tong	Lou Lou Tung	Taiwan maple fruit
Ryokao	*Wickstroemia indica*	Radix Wickstroemiae	Liao Ge Wang (Gen)	Liu Go Wong	Wikstroemia root
Ryokuzu	*Phaseolus radiatum*	Semen Phaseoli radiati	Lu Dou	Luk Dau	Mung bean
Ryoshoka	*Campsis grandiflora*	Radix Campsis grandiflorae	Ling Xiao Gen	Ling Siu Gan	Asian trumpetcree-per root
Ryuganniku	*Euphoria longan*	Arillus Euphoriae	Long Yan Rou	Lung Ngaan Yuk	Longan fruit pulp
Ryukido	*Artemisia anomala*	Herba Artemisiae anomalae	Liu Ji Niu	Lau Gei Nou	Anomalous wormwood herb
Ryukotsu	*Stegodon orientalis, S. rhinocerus sinensis, Hipparion*	Os Stegodontis	Long Gu	Lung Gwat	Dragon bone

JAPANESE	SCIENTIFIC	PHARMACEUTICAL	MANDARIN	CANTONESE	ENGLISH
Ryuno	*Dryobalanops camphora*	Borneolum	Bing Pian	Bing Pin	Borneo camphor
Ryutan	*Gentiana scabra, G. triflora, G. manshurica*	Radix Gentianae scabrae	Long Dan Cao	Lung Daam Chou	Scabrous gentian root
Saenshi, Toshitsuri	*Astragalus complanatus* and spp	Semen Astragali complanati	Sha Yuan Zi, Sha Yuan Ji Li	Sa Yun Ji, Sa Yun Jek Lai	Flat milkvetch seed
Saiko	*Bupleurum chinense, B. falcatum, B. longiradiatum* and spp	Radix Bupleuri	Chai Hu	Chaai Wu	Asian buplever root
Saishin	*Asarum sieboldii, A. heterotropoides* and spp	Radix et herba Asari	Xi Xin	Sai San	Asian wild ginger root and herb
Sakubaika	*Chimonanthus praecox*	Flos Chimonanthi	La Mei Hua	Laap Mui Fa	Wintersweet flower
Sanin	*Amomum villosum*	Fructus Amomi villosi	Sha Ren, (Yang) Chun Sha Ren	Sa Yan, (Yeung) Chyun Sa Yan	Wild cardamom pod (fruit)
Saninka	*Amomum villosum*	Flos Amomi villosi	Sha Ren Hua, (Yang) Chun Sha Hua	Sa Yan Fa, (Yeung) Chyun Sa Fa	Wild cardamom flower
Sansha	*Bombyx mori*	Excrementum Bombicis	Can Sha	Chaam Sa	Silkworm dropping
Sanshishi	*Gardenia jasminoides*	Fructus Gardeniae	Zhi Zi Shan Zhi Zi	Ji Ji, Saan Ji Ji	Gardenia pod
Sanshishi	*Panax notoginseng*	Radix Panacis notoginsengis	San Qi Tian Qi	Saam Chat Tin Chat	Pseudoginseng root
Sanshishika	*Panax notoginseng*	Flos Panacis notoginsengis	San Qi Hua	Saam Chat Fa	Pseudoginseng flower
Sanshuyu	*Cornus officinalis*	Fructus Corni	Shan Zhu Yu, Shan Yu Rou	San Jyu Yu, San Yu Yuk	Japanese dogwood berry
Sansonin	*Zizyphus spinosa*	Semen Zizyphi spinosae	Suan Zao Ren, Jin Zao Ren	Syun Jou Yan	Sour jujube seed
Sanyaku	*Dioscorea opposita, D. batatas*	Rhizoma Dioscoreae oppositae	Shan Yao Shu Yu	Wai Saan, Saan Yeuk	Mountain yam root
Sanyokaku	*Naemorrhedis*	Cornu Naemorrhedis	Shan Yang Jiao	San Yeung Gok	Goat horn
Sanzashi	*Crataegus pinnatifida, C. cuneata* and spp	Fructus Crataegi	Shan Zha (Rou)	Saan Ja (Yuk)	Asian hawthorn berry
Sayo	*Cynomorium songaricum*	Herba Cynomorii	Suo Yang	Soi Yeung	Lock yang stem
Seika	*Citrullus vulgaris*	Fructus Citrulli	Xi Gua	Sai Gwa	Watermelon fruit
Seikaryu	*Tamarix chinensis*	Cacumen Tamaricis	Xi He Liu	Sei Ho Lau	Chinese tamarisk tip
Seiko	*Artemisia apiacea*	Herba Artemisiae apiaceae	Qing Hao	Ching Hou	Celery wormwood herb
Seimokko	*Aristolochia contorta, A. debilis*	Radix Aristolochiae	Qing Mu Xiang, Ma Dou Ling Gen	Ching Muk Heung	Green birthwort root
Seisai	*Capsella bursa-pastoris*	Herba Capsellae	Ji Cai	Chai Choi	Shepherd's purse herb
Seisokon	*Rubia cordifolia*	Radix Rubiae cordifoliae	Qian Cao Gen	Sin Chou Gan	Heart-leaf madder root

JAPANESE	SCIENTIFIC	PHARMACEUTICAL	MANDARIN	CANTONESE	ENGLISH
Seisoshi	*Celosia argentea*	Semen Celosiae argenteae	Qing Xiang Zi	Ching Seung Ji	Silver quail-grass seed
Seiyojin	*Panax quinquefolius*	Radix Panacis quinquefolii	Xi Yang Shen	Fa Kei Sam, Sei Yang Sam	American ginseng root
Sekibukuryo	*Poria cocos*	Sclerotium Poriae rubrae	Chi Fu Ling	Chek Fuk Ling	Red hoelen
Sekii	*Pyrrosia sheareri*	Folium Pyrrosiae sheareri	Shi Wei, Lu Shan Shi Wei	Sek Wai, Lou San Sek Wai	Shearer's felt fern leaf
Sekikozui, Gabusho-kuso	*Centipeda minima*	Herba Centipedae	E Bu Shi Cao	Ngo Bat Sik Chou	Centipeda herb
Sekiryuhi	*Punica granatum*	Pericarpium Punicae	Shi Liu Pi	Sek Lau Pei	Pomegranate husk
Sekiryu-kombi	*Punica granatum*	Cortex Radicis Punicae	Shi Liu Gen Pi	Sek Lau Gan Pei	Pomegranate root bark
Sekishaku-(yaku)	*Paeonia lactiflora, P. obovata, P. veitchii*	Radix Paeoniae rubrae	Chi Shao (Yao)	Chek Cheuk (Yeuk)	Red peony root
Sekishozu	*Phaseolus calcaratus, P. angularis*	Semen Phaseoli calcarati	Chi Xiao Dou	Chek Siu Dau	Aduki bean
Sekketsumei	*Haliotis diversicolor, H. gigantea* and spp	Concha Haliotis	Shi Jue Ming	Sek Kyut Ming	Abalone shell
Sekko	*Gypsum fibrosum*	Gypsum	Shi Gao	Sek Gou	Gypsum
Sekkoku	*Dendrobium nobile, D. linawianum, D. officinale* and spp	Herba Dendrobii	Shi Hu	Sek Wu	Stonebushel stem
Sekkoku	*Ephemerantha fimbriata*	Herba Ephemeranthae	Shi Hu	Sek Hap	Ephemerantha stem
Sembo	*Curculigo orchioides*	Rhizoma Curculigonis	Xian Mao	Sin Maau	Golden eye-grass root
Sembukuka	*Inula japonica, I. brittanica, I. linariaefolia*	Flos Inulae	Xuan Fu Hua	Syun Fuk Fa	Elecampane flower
Senbaimo	*Fritillaria cirrhosa*	Bulbus Fritillariae cirrhosae	Chuan Bei Mu	Chyun Bui Mou	Sichuan fritillary bulb
Senjo	*Bufo gargarizans, B. melanostictus*	Secretio Bufonis	Chan Su	Sim Sou	Toad venom
Senkakuso	*Agrimonia pilosa* var. *japonica*	Herba Agrimoniae pilosae	Xian He Cao	Sin Hok Chou	Furry agrimony herb
Senkotu	*Nuphar japonicum, N. pumilum*	Rhizoma Nupharis	Ping Peng Cao Gan	Ping Fung Chou Gan	Yellow pond lily root
Senkyu	*Ligusticum walichii*	Radix Ligustici walichii	Chuan Xiong, Xiong Qiong	Chyun Gung	Sichuan lovage root
Sennenken	*Homalomena occulta*	Rhizoma Homalomenae	Qian Nian Jian	Chin Nin Gin	Homalomena root
Senshinren	*Andrographis paniculata*	Folium Andrographis	Chuan Xin Lian	Chyun Sam Lin	Heart-thread lotus leaf
Sentai	*Cryptotympana atrata* and spp	Periostracum Cryptotympanae	Chan Tui	Sim Teui, Sim Tyut	Cicada slough
Senzanko	*Manis pentadactyla*	Squama manis	Chuan Shan Jia	Chyun San Gaap	Pangolin scale
Setsubaimo	*Fritillaria thunbergii*	Bulbus Fritillariae thunbergii	Zhe Bei Mu	Chit Bui Mou	Zhejiang fritillary bulb
Shachu	*Eupolyphaga sinensis*	Eupolyphaga	Tu Bie Chong	Dei Bit Chung	Cockroach
Shajin	*Glehnia littoralis*	Radix Glehniae	Bei Sha Shen	Mai Sa Sam	Northern sandroot

JAPANESE	SCIENTIFIC	PHARMACEUTICAL	MANDARIN	CANTONESE	ENGLISH
Shakanzo	*Glycirrhiza uralensis, G. glabra* and spp	Radix Glycirrhizae preparatae	Zhi Gan Cao	Jek Gam Chou	Honey-fried licorice root
Shakusekishi	*Halloysitum rubrum*	Halloysitum	Chi Shi Zhi	Chek Sek Chi	Red kaolin
Shazenshi	*Plantago asiatica, P. depressa* and spp	Semen Plantaginis	Che Qian Zi	Che Chin Ji	Asian plantain seed
Shazenso	*Plantago asiatica, P. depressa* and spp	Folium Plantaginis	Che Qian Cao	Che Chin Chou	Asian plantain leaf
Shiitake	*Lentinula edodes*	Sclerotium Lentinulae	Xiang Gu	Heung Gu	Shiitake mushroom
Shikajicho	*Viola yedoensis, V. japonica*	Radix et herba Violae yedoensis	Zi Hua Di Ding	Ji Fa Dei Ding	Asian violet root and herb
Shikaraku	*Luffa cylindrica, L. acutangula*	Fasciculus vascularis Luffae	Si Gua Luo	Si Gwa Lou	Spongegourd
Shikasha	*Homo sapiens*	Placenta Hominis	Zi He Che	Ji Ho Je	Human placenta
Shikon	*Arnebia euchroma, A. guttata*	Radix Arnebiae	Zi Cao, Xin Jiang Zi Cao	Ji Chou, San Geung Ji Chou	Arnebia root
Shikon	*Lithospermum erythrorhizon*	Radix Lithospermi	Zi Cao	Ji Chou	Purple groomwell root
Shikon	*Macrotomia euchroma*	Radix Macrotomiae	Zi Cao	Ji Chou	Macrotomia root
Shikunshi	*Quisqualis indica*	Fructus Quisqualis	Shi Jun Zi	Si Gwan Ji	Rangoon creeper nut
Shinika	*Magnolia liliflora, M. denudata, M. yulan* and spp	Gemma Magnoliae	Xin Yi Hua	San Yi Fa	Yulan magnolia bud
Shinju	*Pteria margaritiferae*	Fructus conchae Pteriae	Zhen Zhu	Chan Ju	Pearl
Shinkiku		Massa fermentata	Shen Qu	Sam Chau	Medicated leaven
Shion	*Aster tataricus*	Radix Asteris tatarici	Zi Wan	Ji Yun	Tartary aster root
Shisoyo	*Perilla frutescens*	Folium Perillae	Zi Su Ye	Sou Yip	Perilla leaf
Shitei	*Diospyros kaki*	Calyx Diospyri	Shi Di	Chi Dai	Persimmon calyx
Shizendo	*Pyritum*	Pyritum	Zi Ran Tong	Ji Yin Tung	Pyrite
Shobu	*Acorus calamus*	Rhizoma Acori calami	Shui Chang Pu, Bai Chang Pu	Seui Cheung Pou, Baak Cheung Pou	Sweetflag root
Shohange	*Pinellia ternata*	Rhizoma pinelliae ternatae	Sheng Ban Xia	Sang Bun Ha, So Bun Ha	Raw pinellia corm
Shojio	*Rehmannia glutinosa*	Radix Rehmanniae	Sheng Di (Huang)	Sang Dei (Wong)	Fresh Rehmannia root
Shokushitsu	*Dichroa febrifuga*	Folium Dichroae	Shu Qi	Suk Chat	Feverflower leaf
Shokusho	*Zanthoxylum bungeanum*	Fructus Zanthoxyli bungeani	Chuan Jiao, Hua Jiao	Chyun Jiu, Fa Jiu	Sichuan peppercorn
Shokyo	*Zingiber officinalis*	Rhizoma Zingiberis recentis	Sheng Jiang	Saang Geung	Fresh ginger root
Shoma	*Cimicifuga dahurica*	Radix Cimicifugae dahuricae	Sheng Ma, Xing An Sheng Ma	Sing Ma, Hing On Sing Ma	Dahurian rising hemp root
Shoma	*Cimicifuga foetida*	Radix Cimicifugae foetidae	Sheng Ma	Sing Ma	Rising hemp root

JAPANESE	SCIENTIFIC	PHARMACEUTICAL	MANDARIN	CANTONESE	ENGLISH
Shoma	*Cimicifuga heracleifolia*	Radix Cimicifugae heracleifoliae	Sheng Ma, Ta San Ye Sheng Ma	Sing Ma, Da Sam Yip Sing Ma	Heraclean rising hemp root
Shono	*Cinnamomum camphora*	Camphora	Zhang Nao	Jeung Naau	Camphor flake
Shoriku	*Phytolacca acinosa, P. esculenta*	Radix Phytolaccae acinosae	Shang Lu	Seung Luk	Asian poke root
Shoseki	*Niter*	Niter	Xiao Shi	Siu Sek	Potassium nitrate
Shosetsu	*Pinus tabulaeformis, P. massoniana, P. yunnannensis*	Lignum Pini nodi	Song Jie, You Song Jie	Chung Jit, Yao Chung Jit	Knotty pine wood shaving
Shouikyo	*Foeniculum vulgare*	Fructus Foeniculi	Xiao Hui Xiang	Siu Wui Heung	Fennel seed
Shusha	*Cinnabarum*	Cinnabarum	Zhu Sha	Ju Sa	Cinnabar
Shushakon	*Ardisia crenata, A. bicolor*	Radix Ardisiae crenatae	Da Lo San, Zhu Sha Gen	Jyu Sa Gan	Coralberry root
So-u	*Aconitum chinense, A. kusnezoffii* and spp	Radix Aconiti chinensis	Cao Wu, Bei Wu Tou	Chou Wu, Mai Wu Tau	Prepared wild aconite root tuber
Soboku	*Caesalpinia sappan*	Lignum Caesalpiniae	Su Mu	Sou Muk	Sappanwood
Sogoko	*Liquidambar orientalis*	Resina Liquidambaris (Styrax liquidis)	Su He Xiang	Sou Hap Heung	Storax resin
Sohaku	*Allium fistulosum*	Semen Allii fistulosi	Cong Zi	Chung Ji	Scallion seed
Sohakuhi	*Morus alba*	Cortex radicis Mori	Sang Bai Pi	Song Baak Pei	Mulberry root bark
Sojin	*Morus alba*	Fructus Mori	Sang Shen (Zi)	Song Sam (Ji)	Mulberry fruit
Sojishi	*Xanthium sibiricum, X. strumarium*	Fructus Xanthii	Cang Er Zi	Chong Yi Ji	Siberian cocklebur
Sojutsu	*Atractylodes lancea, A. sinensis* and spp	Rhizoma Atractylodis lanceae	Cang Zhu, Mao Cang Zhu	Chong Seut, Mau Chong Seut	Black atractylodes root
Soka	*Amomum tsao-ko*	Fructus Amomi tsao-konis	Cao Guo (Ren)	Chou Gwat (Yan)	Cochin cardamom fruit
Sokaku	*Gleditsia sinensis* and spp	Fructus Gleditsiae	Zao Jiao, Zao Jia	Jou Gok, Jou Gaap	Honeylocust pod
Sokakushi	*Gleditsia sinensis* and spp	Spina Gleditsiae	Zao Jiao Ci	Jou Gok Chi	Honeylocust spine
Sokisei	*Loranthus parasiticus, L. yadorici* and spp	Ramulus Loranthi	Sang Ji Sheng	Song Gei Sang	Asian mistletoe twig
Sokuhakuyo	*Biota orientalis*	Cacumen Biotae orientalis	Ce Bai Ye	Jak Paak Yip	Oriental arborvitae tip
Soshi	*Morus alba*	Ramulus Mori	Sang Zhi	Song Ji	Mulberry twig
Soshi	*Perilla frutescens*	Fructus Perillae	Zi Su Zi	Sou Ji	Perilla seed
Soyo	*Morus alba*	Folium Mori	Sang Ye	Song Yip	Mulberry leaf
Sozuku	*Alpinia katsumadai*	Semen Alpiniae katsumadis	Cao Dou Kou	Chou Dau Kau	Katsumada's galangal seed
Suisayo, Meisai	*Menyanthes trifoliata*	Folium Menyanthis	Shui Cai Ye	Seui Choi Yip	Bogbean leaf
Taigeki	*Euphorbia pekinensis*	Radix Euphorbiae pekinensis	Jing Da Ji	Ging Daai Gik	Peking spurge root
Taikei	*Cirsium japonicum*	Herba Cirsii japonici	Da Ji	Daai Gai	Japanese thistle herb

JAPANESE	SCIENTIFIC	PHARMACEUTICAL	MANDARIN	CANTONESE	ENGLISH
Taimai	*Eretmochelys imbricata*	Plastrum Eretmochelis	Dai Mao	Doi Mou	Hawksbill turtle shell
Taisan	*Allium sativum*	Bulbus Allii sativi	Da Suan	Daai Syun	Garlic bulb
Taishaseki	*Haematitum*	Haematitum	Dai Zhe Shi	Doi Jyu Sek	Hematite
Taishijin	*Pseudostellaria heterophylla*	Radix Pseudostellariae	Tai Zi Shen	Yi Sam, Taai Ji Sam	Prince ginseng root
Taiso	*Zizyphus jujuba* var. *inermis*	Fructus Zizyphi jujubae	Da Zao	Daai Jou	Black jujube berry
Takuran	*Lycopus lucidus*	Herba Lycopi	Ze Lan	Jaak Laan	Bright bugleweed herb
Takusha	*Alisma orientalis*	Rhizoma Alismae	Ze Xie	Jaak Se	Water plantain root
Takushitsu	*Euphorbia helioscopia*	Herba Euphorbiaeheliosc opiae	Ze Qi	Jaak Chat	Sunspurge herb
Tanban	*Chalcanthitum*	Chalcanthitum	Dan Fan, Shi Dan	Daan Faan	Crystallized blue vitriol
Tanchikuyo	*Lopatherum gracile*	Folium Lopatheri	Dan Zhu Ye	Daam Juk Yip	Bamboo grass leaf
Tanjin	*Salvia miltiorrhiza*	Radix Salviae miltiorrhizae	Dan Shen	Daan Sam	Cinnabar sage root
Tannansho	*Arisaema consanguineum, A. amurense* and spp	Pulvis Arisaemae cum felle Bovis	Dan Nan Xing	Daam Naam Sing	Powdered dragon arum corm with ox bile
Tantoshi	*Glycine max*	Semen Glycinis preparatum	Dan Dou Chi	Taam Dau Si	Fermented soybean
Taranoki	*Aralia elata, A. elata* var. *suninermis*	Cortex Araliae elatate	Ci Lao Ya Pi	Chu Lou Nga	Aralia bark
Teirekishi	*Lepidium apetalum, L. virginicum*	Semen Lepidii	Ting Li Zi	Ting Lai Ji	Wood whitlow grass seed
Temma	*Gastrodia elata*	Rhizoma Gastrodiae	Tian Ma	Tin Ma	Celestial hemp corm
Tenkafun	*Trichosanthes kirilowii, T. japonica, T. uniflora*	Radix Trichosanthis	Tian Hua Fen	Tin Fa Fun	Snakegourd root
Tenmondo	*Asparagus cochinchinensis*	Rhizoma Asparagi cochinensis	Tian (Men) Dong	Tin (Mun) Dung	Shiny asparagus root
Tensendo	*Aristolochia contorta, A. debilis*	Caulis Aristolochiae	Tian Xian Teng	Tin Sin Tang	Green birthwort stem
Tikusetu-ninjin	*Panax japonicus*	Radix Panacis japonici	Zhu Jie (Ren) Shen	Juk Jit (Yan) Sam	Japanese ginseng root
Tochu	*Eucommia ulmoides*	Cortex Eucommiae	Du Zhong	Dou Jung	Eucommia bark
Tochukaso	*Cordyceps sinensis* and host larvae *Hepialus armoricanus or Holotrichia koraiensis*	Sclerotium Cordycepsis	Dong Chong Xia Cao	Dung Chung Ha Chou	Chinese caterpillar mushroom
Tofukitsu	*Atalantia buxifolia*	Radix Atalantiae	Dong Feng Ju Gen	Dung Fung Gwat Gan	Atalantia root
Tohoku-kanju	*Dryopteris crassirhizoma*	Rhizoma Dryopteris	Guan Zhong, Mian Ma Guan Zhong	Gwun Jung, Min Ma Gwun Jung	Shield fern root
Tohoku-kanju	*Osmunda japonica*	Rhizoma Osmundae	Guan Zhong, Zi Qi Guan Zhong	Gwun Jung, Ji Kei Gwun Jung	Japanese flowering fern root

JAPANESE	SCIENTIFIC	PHARMACEUTICAL	MANDARIN	CANTONESE	ENGLISH
Tojin	*Codonopsis pilosula, C. tangshen, C. nervosa*	Radix Codonopsis	Dang Shen	Fong Dong Sam	Downy bellflower root
Tokahi	*Benincasa hispida*	Epicarpium Benincasae	Dong Gua Pi	Dung Gwa Pei	Waxgourd fruit rind
Tokanin	*Benincasa hispida*	Semen Benincasae	Dong Gua Ren	Dong Gwa Yan	Waxgourd seed
Toki	*Angelica sinensis*	Radix Angelicae sinensis	Dang Gui	Dong Gwai	Dong quai root
Tokio	*Angelica sinensis, A. acutiloba*	Extremas radicis Angelicae sinensis	Dang Gui Wei	Dong Gwai Mai	Dong quai tail
Tokito	*Angelica sinensis, A. acutiloba*	Caput Angelicae sinensis	Dang Gui Tou	Dong Gwai Tou	Dong quai head
Tonin	*Prunus persica* and spp	Semen Pruni persicae	Tao Ren	Tou Yan	Peach kernel
Toshikyo	*Litsea cubeba*	Radix et caulis Litseae	Dou Chi Jiang	Dau Chek Geung	Cubeb root and stem
Toshinso	*Juncus effusus*	Medulla Junci	Deng Xin Cao	Dang Sam Chou	Bulrush pith
Toshishi	*Cuscuta chinensis , C. japonica*	Semen Cuscutae	Tu Si Zi	Tou Si Ji	Asian dodder seed
Toso	*Tetrapanax papyrifera*	Medulla Tetrapanacis	Tong Cao	Tong Chou, Bai Tong Chou	Rice paper pith
Toyaku	*Swertia japonica, S. pseudochinensis*	Herba Swertiae	Dang Yao Cao	Dong Yeuk Chou	Japanese green gentian herb
Ubai	*Prunus mume*	Fructus Pruni mumis	Wu Mei (Rou)	Wu Mui (Yuk)	Black plum fruit
Ukon	*Curcuma longa, C. aromatica*	Tuber Curcumae	Yu Jin	Yuk Gam	Turmeric tuber
Ukyukompi	*Sapium sebiferum*	Cortex radicis Sapii sebiferi	Wu Jiu (Mu) Gen Pi	Wu Kau Muk Gan Pei	Chinese tallow tree root bark
Urajirokashi	*Quercus salicina, Q. myrsinaefolium*	Folium Querci	Zhu Zi Ye	Jyu Ji	Oak leaf
Ushoda	*Zaocys dhumnades*	Zaocys	Wu Shao She	U Sau Se	Black grass-snake
Uyaku	*Lindera strychnifolia*	Radix Linderae	Wu Yao, Tai Wu	Wu Yeuk, Toi Wu	Lindera root
Uyoryo	*Limonitum*	Limonitum	Yu Liang Shi	Yu Leung Sek	Clay ironstone
Uzu	*Aconitum carmichaeli*	Radix Aconiti carmichaeli	Chuan Wu Wu Tou	Chyun Wu, Wu Tau	Prepared Sichuan aconite root tuber
Yakan	*Belamcanda chinensis*	Rhizoma Belamcandae	She Gan	Se Gon	Leopard flower root
Yakoto	*Polygonum multiflorum*	Caulis Polygoni multiflori	Ye Jiao Teng	Ye Gou Tang	Flowery knotweed stem
Yakuchinin	*Alpinia oxyphylla*	Fructus Alpiniae oxyphyllae	Yi Zhi Ren	Yik Ji Yan	Sharp-leaf galangal berry
Yakumoso	*Leonorus heterophyllus, L. japonicus, L. sibiricus* and spp	Herba Leonori	Yi Mu Cao, Chong Wei	Yik Mou Chou, Chong Wai	Asian motherwort herb
Yamyosha	*Vespertilium murinum*	Excrementum Vespertilii	Ye Ming Sha	Ye Ming Sa	Bat dropping
Yokuinin	*Coix lachryma-jobi* var. *Ma-yuen*	Semen Coicis	Yi Yi Ren	San Yi Mai, Yi Yi Yan	Job's-tears seed
Yonyu, Shiyojin	*Codonopsis lanceolata*	Radix Codonopsis lanceolatae	Yang Ju, Shi Ye Shen	Yang Guk, Sei Yip Sam	Goat's-tit bellflower root
Yuo	*Realgar*	Realgar	Xiong Huang	Song Wong	Realgar

JAPANESE	SCIENTIFIC	PHARMACEUTICAL	MANDARIN	CANTONESE	ENGLISH
Yutan	*Ursus arctos* and spp	Fel Ursi	Xiong Dan	Hung Daam	Bear gallbladder
Zenkatsu	*Buthus Martensi*	Buthus	Quan Xie	Chyun Kit	Scorpion
Zenko	*Peucedanum praeruptorum, P. decursivum*	Radix Peucedani	Qian Hu	Chin Wu	Asian masterwort root
Zokudan	*Dipsacus japonica*	Radix Dipsaci japonicae	Xu Duan	Juk Dyun	Japanese teasel root
Zokuzuishi	*Euphorbia lathyris*	Semen Euphorbiae lathyris	Qian Jin Zi	Chin Gam Ji	Caper spurge seed
Zukani	*Eriocheir sinensis, E. japonicus*	Eriocheir	Jin Xie	Jeun Haai	Tianjin crab

Cross Index of English Remedy Names

ENGLISH	SCIENTIFIC	PHARMACEUTICAL	MANDARIN	CANTONESE	JAPANESE
Abalone shell	*Haliotis diversicolor, H. gigantea* and spp	Concha Haliotis	Shi Jue Ming	Sek Kyut Ming	Sekketsumei
Acronychia heartwood	*Acronychia laurifolia*	Lignum Acronychiae	Sha Tang Mu, Jiang Xiang	Sa Tong Muk	
Actinidia gall	*Actinidia polygama*	Galla fructi Actinidiae	Mu Tian Lian	Muk Tin Lin	Mokutenryo
Actinolite	*Actinolitum*	Actinolitum	Yang Qi Shi	Yeung Hei Sek	
Actinostemma leaf and seed	*Actinostemma lobata*	Folium et semen Actinostemmae	He Zi Cao	Hap Ji Chou	
Adder's tongue herb	*Ophioglossum vulgatum*	Herba Ophioglossi	Ping Er Xiao Cao	Ping Yi Siu Chou	
Adenosma herb	*Adenosma glutinosum*	Herba Adenosmae glutinosi	Mao She Xiang	Mou Se Heung	
Adenostemma herb	*Adenostemma lavenia*	Herba Adenostemmae	Ma Zhi Hu, Feng Qi Cao	Ma Ji Wu, Fung Hei Chou	
Aduki bean	*Phaseolus calcaratus, P. angularis*	Semen Phaseoli calcarati	Chi Xiao Dou	Chek Siu Dau	Sekishozu
Aeginetia herb	*Aeginetia indica*	Herba Aeginetiae	Guan Zhen Huang, Ye Gu	Gwon Jam Wong, Ye Gu	
Aerial fig root	*Ficus microcarpa, F. retusa*	Radix Fici microcarpae seu retusae	Lao Gong Xu, Rong Shu Xu	Lou Gung Chuk	
African marigold flower	*Tagetes erecta*	Flos Tagetis	Wan Shou Ju	Maan Sau Guk	
Agate	*Agate*	Agate	Ma Nao		
Agave leaf	*Agave americana*	Folium Agavis americanae	Jin Bian Long She Lan	Gam Bin Lung Sit Laan	
Aizoon stonecrop herb	*Sedum aizoon*	Herba Sedi aizoonis	Jing Tian San Qi	Ging Tin Saam Chat	
Akebia fruit	*Akebia quinata*	Fructus Akebiae	Ba Yue Zha, Yu Zhi Zi	Baat Yut Jaat, Yu Ji Ji	
Akebia stem	*Akebia quinata, A. trifoliata*	Caulis Akebiae	Mu Tong, Bai Mu Tong	Baak Muk Tong	Mokutsu
Alangium root	*Alangium chinense*	Radix Alangii	Ba Jiao Feng	Baat Gok Fung	
Algae	*Laminaria* spp	Herba Laminariae	Hai Dai	Hoi Daai	
Alligator Alternanthera herb	*Alternanthera philoxeroides*	Herba Alternantherae	Kong Xiu Lian Zi Cao	Hung Sam Lin Ji Chou	
Alocasia root	*Alocasia odora*	Rhizoma Alocasiae	Guang Lang Du, Hai Yu	Hoi Wu	
Aloe resin	*Aloe vera* var. *chinensis*	Resina Aloidis	Lu Hui	Lou Wui	
Aloeswood	*Aquilaria agallocha, A. sinensis*	Lignum Aquilariae	Chen Xiang	Cham Heung	Jinko
Altai anemone root	*Anemone altaica*	Rhizoma Anemoni altaicae	Jiu Jie Chang Pu	Gau Jit Cheung Pou	Arutai ginrenkon
Alum	*Alumen*	Alumen	Ming Fan	Ming Faan	Myoban
Amber resin	*Pinus succinifera*	Resina Pini succiniferae (Succinum)	Hu Po	Fu Po	

ENGLISH	SCIENTIFIC	PHARMACEUTICAL	MANDARIN	CANTONESE	JAPANESE
American ginseng root	*Panax quinquefolius*	Radix Panacis quinquefolii	Xi Yang Shen	Fa Kei Sam, Sei Yang Sam	Seiyojin
Amethyst orchid root	*Bletilla striata*	Rhizoma Bletillae	Bai Ji	Baak Gap	Byakukyu
Amorpho-phallus root	*Amorphophallus rivieri, A. sinensis, A. knojac*	Rhizoma Amorphophalli	Ju Ruo	Geui Yeuk	
Amur adonis herb	*Adonis amurensis*	Herba Adonis	Fu Shou Cao	Fuk Sau Chou	
Amur corydalis corm	*Corydalis ambigua* var. *amurensis*	Rhizoma Corydalis ambiguae	Yan Hu Suo, Dong Bei Yan Hu Suo	Yin Wu Sok, Dung Bak Yin Wu Sok	
Amur grape root	*Vitis amurensis*	Radix Vitis amurensis	Shan Teng Teng Yang	Saan Tang Tang Yeung	
Androsaca herb	*Androsaca umbellata*	Herba Androsacae	Dian Di Mei		
Anemone root	*Anemone raddeana*	Rhizoma Anemonis raddeanae	Liang Tou Jian	Leung Tau Jim	
Anisodus root or seed	*Anisodus tanguticus*	Redix seu semen Anisodi	Zang Qie	Jong Ke	
Annual copperleaf herb	*Acalypha australis*	Herba Acalyphae	Tie Xian (Cai)	Tit Yin	
Annual sowthistle herb	*Sonchus oleraceus*	Herba Sonchi	Ku Cai	Fu Choi	
Annual wormwood herb	*Artemisia annua*	Herba Artemisiae annuae	Huang Hua Hao Qing Hao	Wong Fa Hou, Ching Hou	
Anomalous wormwood herb	*Artemisia anomala*	Herba Artemisiae anomalae	Liu Ji Niu	Lau Gei Nou	Ryukido
Antelope horn	*Saiga tatarica*	Cornu Saigae	Ling Yang Jiao	Ling Yeung Gok	Reiyokaku
Aralia bark	*Aralia elata, A. elata* var. *suninermis*	Cortex Araliae elatate	Ci Lao Ya Pi	Chu Lou Nga	Taranoki
Ardisia root	*Ardisia gigantifolia*	Rhizoma Ardisiae gigantifoliae	Zou Ma Tai	Jau Ma Toi	
Arhat fruit	*Momordica grosvenori*	Fructus Momordicae grosvenorii	Luo Han Guo	Lou Haan Kwo	Rakanka
Arhat leaf	*Momordica grosvenori*	Folium Momordicae grosvenorii	Luo Han Ye	Lou Haan Yip	Rakankayo
Arnebia root	*Arnebia euchroma, A. guttata*	Radix Arnebiae	Zi Cao, Xin Jiang Zi Cao	Ji Chou, San Geung Ji Chou	Shikon
Aromatic madder herb	*Elsholtzia splendens, E. stauntonii*	Herba Elsholtziae	Xiang Ru (Cao)	Heung Yu (Chou)	Koju
Asafoetida resin	*Ferula foetida*	Resina Ferulae (Asafoetidae)	A Wei	A Ngai	Agi
Asian birch bark	*Betula platyphylla*	Cortex Betulae	Hua Mu Pi	Wa Muk Pei	
Asian Buddleia root	*Buddleia asiatica*	Radix Buddleiae asiaticae	Bai Pu Jiang	Baak Pou Geung	
Asian buplever root	*Bupleurum chinense, B. falcatum, B. longiradiatum* and spp	Radix Bupleuri	Chai Hu	Chaai Wu	Saiko

ENGLISH	SCIENTIFIC	PHARMACEUTICAL	MANDARIN	CANTONESE	JAPANESE
Asian cantharides	*Mylabris*	Mylabris	Ban Mao	Ban Mou	Hanmyo
Asian celandine herb	*Chelidonium majus* var. *asiaticum*	Herba Chelidonii	Bai Qu Cai	Baak Wat Choi	Hakkutusai
Asian coral tree bark	*Erythrina variegata* var. *orientalis*	Cortex Erythrinae	Hai Tong Pi	Hoi Tung Pei	Kaitohi
Asian corydalis corm	*Corydalis yanhusuo*	Rizoma Corydalis yanhusuoidis	Yan Hu Suo, Yuan Hu	Yin Wu Sok, Yun Wu	Engosaku
Asian dittany root bark	*Dictamnus dasycarpus*	Cortex radicis Dictamni	Bai Xian Pi	Baak Sin Pei	Hakusempi
Asian dodder seed	*Cuscuta chinensis , C. japonica*	Semen Cuscutae	Tu Si Zi	Tou Si Ji	Toshishi
Asian fieldmint herb	*Mentha arvensis*	Herba Menthae arvensis	Bo He	Bok Ho	Hakka
Asian ginseng flower	*Panax ginseng*	Flos Panacis ginsengis	Ren Shen Hua	Yan Sam Fa	
Asian ginseng leaf	*Panax ginseng*	Folium Panacis ginsengis	Ren Shen Ye	Yan Sam Yip	Ninjinyo
Asian ginseng neck	*Panax ginseng*	Rhizoma Panacis ginsengis	Ren Shen Lu	Yan Sam Lu	Ninjinro
Asian ginseng root	*Panax ginseng*	Radix Panacis ginsengis	Ren Shen	Yan Sam	Ninjin
Asian green gentian root	*Swertia pseudochinensis* and spp	Radix Swertiae	Dang Yao	Dong Yeuk	
Asian hawthorn berry	*Crataegus pinnatifida, C. cuneata* and spp	Fructus Crataegi	Shan Zha (Rou)	Saan Ja (Yuk)	Sanzashi
Asian leek seed	*Allium tuberosum*	Semen Alii tuberosi	Jiu Cai Zi	Gau Choi Ji	Kyushi
Asian masterwort root	*Peucedanum praeruptorum, P. decursivum*	Radix Peucedani	Qian Hu	Chin Wu	Zenko
Asian mistletoe twig	*Loranthus parasiticus, L. yadorici* and spp	Ramulus Loranthi	Sang Ji Sheng	Song Gei Sang	Sokisei
Asian mistletoe twig	*Taxillus yadoriki, T. chinensis*	Ramulus Taxilli	Shi Ji Sheng	Chi Gei Sang	
Asian mistletoe twig	*Viscum liquidambaricum*	Ramulus Visci liquidambarici	Bian Ji Sheng	Bin Gei Sang	
Asian moneywort herb	*Lysimachia christinae, L. hemsleyana*	Herba Lysimachiae	Jin Qian Cao, Guo Lu Huang	Gam Chin Chou, Gwo Lou Wong	Kinsenso
Asian motherwort herb	*Leonorus heterophyllus, L. japonicus, L. sibiricus* and spp	Herba Leonori	Yi Mu Cao, Chong Wei	Yik Mou Chou, Chong Wai	Yakumoso
Asian motherwort seed	*Leonorus heterophyllus* and spp	Semen Leonori	Chong Wei Zi	Chong Wai Ji	
Asian mugwort leaf	*Artemisia argyi*	Folium Artemisiae argyi	Ai Ye	Ngaai Yang, Ngaai Yip	Gaiyo
Asian olive fruit	*Canarium album*	Fructus Canarii	Gan Lan, Jing Guo	Gaam Laam	
Asian pasqueflower root	*Pulsatilla chinensis, P. cernua, P. turczaninovii, P. ambigua* and spp	Radix Pulsatillae	Bai Tou Weng	Baak Tau Yung	Hakutoo

ENGLISH	SCIENTIFIC	PHARMACEUTICAL	MANDARIN	CANTONESE	JAPANESE
Asian plantain leaf	*Plantago asiatica, P. depressa* and spp	Folium Plantaginis	Che Qian Cao	Che Chin Chou	Shazenso
Asian plantain seed	*Plantago asiatica, P. depressa* and spp	Semen Plantaginis	Che Qian Zi	Che Chin Ji	Shazenshi
Asian poke root	*Phytolacca acinosa, P. esculenta*	Radix Phytolaccae acinosae	Shang Lu	Seung Luk	Shoriku
Asian rosewood	*Dalbergia odorifera*	Lignum Dalbergiae odoriferae	Jiang Xiang	Geung Heung	
Asian soft-shell turtle shell	*Amyda sinensis, Trionix sinensis*	Carapax Amydae seu Trionis	Bie Jia	Bit Gaap	Bekko
Asian toddalia root	*Toddalia asiatica*	Radix Toddaliae	Fei Long Zhang Xue	Fei Lung Jeung Hyut	
Asian trumpetcreeper flower	*Campsis grandiflora*	Flos Campsis grandiflorae	Ling Xiao Hua	Ling Siu Fa	
Asian trumpetcreeper root	*Campsis grandiflora*	Radix Campsis grandiflorae	Ling Xiao Gen	Ling Siu Gan	Ryoshoka
Asian venus clam shell	*Meretrix meretrix*	Concha Metretris	Wen Ge	Man Gap	
Asian violet root and herb	*Viola yedoensis, V. japonica*	Radix et herba Violae yedoensis	Zi Hua Di Ding	Ji Fa Dei Ding	Shikajicho
Asian wild ginger root and herb	*Asarum sieboldii, A. heterotropoides* and spp	Radix et herba Asari	Xi Xin	Sai San	Saishin
Asian wintergreen root and herb	*Pyrola rotundifolia subsp. chinensis, P. Japonica*	Radix et herba Pyrolae	Lu Xian Cao, Lu Ti Cao	Luk Haam Chou, Luk Tai Chou	Rokuteiso
Asian wisteria gall	*Wisteria sinensis, W. floribunda*	Galla Wisteriae	Zi Teng Zi, Teng Liu	Ji Tang Ji, Tang Lau	Figikobu
Asparagus root	*Asparagus officinalis*	Rhizoma Asparagi officinalis	Shi Diao Bai	Sek Diu Baak	
Ass hide glue	*Equus asinus* and spp	Gelatinum corii Equi asini	E Jiao	O Gaau	Akyo
Assam crotalaria seed or herb	*Crotalaria assamica*	Semen seu herba Crotalariae assamicae	Da Zhu Shi Dou, Zi Xiao Rong	Daai Ju Si Dau	
Assam indigo leaf	*Baphicacanthus cusia*	Folium Baphicacanthi	Ma Lan Ye	Ma Laam Yip	Banranyo
Assam indigo root	*Baphicacanthus cusia*	Radix Baphicacanthi	Ma Lan Gen	Ma Laam Gan	Banrankon
Astilbe root	*Astilbe chinensis*	Rhizoma Astilbis	Luo Xin Fu	Lok San Fu	
Astragalus root	*Astragalus membranaceus, A. mongholicus* and spp	Radix Astragali	Huang Qi	Wong Kei, Paak Kei	Ogi
Atalantia root	*Atalantia buxifolia*	Radix Atalantiae	Dong Feng Ju Gen	Dung Fung Gwat Gan	Tofukitsu
Auricle dogbane root	*Cynanchum auriculatum*	Radix Cynanchi auriculati	Bai Shou Wu, Niu Pi Xiao	Baak Sau Wu, Ngau Pei Siu	
Baikal skullcap root	*Scutellaria baicalensis, S. viscidula, S. amoena*	Radix Scutellariae baicalensis	Huang Qin	Wong Sam	Ogon
Balloonflower root	*Platycodon grandiflorum*	Radix Platycodonis	Jie Geng, Ku Jie Geng	Gat Gan	Kikyo
Bamboo fern herb	*Coniogramme japonica*	Herba Coniogrammis	Huo Xue Lian	Fo Hyut Lin	

ENGLISH	SCIENTIFIC	PHARMACEUTICAL	MANDARIN	CANTONESE	JAPANESE
Bamboo grass leaf	*Lopatherum gracile*	Folium Lopatheri	Dan Zhu Ye	Daam Juk Yip	Tanchikuyo
Bamboo grass root	*Lopatherum gracile*	Radix Lopatheri	Dan Zhu Gen	Daam Juk Gan	
Barbed skullcap root and herb	*Scutellaria barbata, B. rivularis*	Radix et herba Scutellariae barbatae	Ban Zhi Lian	Bun Ji Lin	
Barberry wood	*Berberis thunbergii*	Lignum Berberis thunbergii	Xiao Nie	Siu Maak	Megi
Barley malt sugar	*Hordeum vulgare*	Saccharum Hordei	Yi Tang, Jiao Yi	Yi Tong	
Basil herb	*Ocimum basilicum*	Herba Ocimi	Jiu Ceng Ta, Luo Le	Lo Lak	
Basil seed	*Ocimum Basilicum*	Fructus Ocimi	Guang Ming Zi	Gwong Ming Ji	
Bat dropping	*Vespertilium murinum*	Excrementum Vespertilii	Ye Ming Sha	Ye Ming Sa	Yamyosha
Bauhinia stem	*Bauhinia championi*	Caulis bauhiniae championi	Jiu Long Teng, Wu Teng	Gaau Lung Tang, Lung Sou Tang	
Bead tree root bark	*Melia azedarach, M. toosendan*	Cortex radicis Meliae	Ku Lian (Gen) Pi	Fu Lin (Gan) Pei	Kurenkombi
Bear gallbladder	*Ursus arctos* and spp	Fel Ursi	Xiong Dan	Hung Daam	Yutan
Beard lichen thallus	*Usnea diffracta* and spp	Thallus Usneae	Song Luo	Chung Lo	
Beautiful galangal berry	*Alpinia zerumbet*	Fructus Alpiniae zerumbetsis	Da Cao Kou	Daai Chou Kau	
Beeswax	*Apis cerana* and spp	Cera flava	Feng La	Fung Laap	
Beggartick herb	*Bidens bipinnata*	Herba Bidentis bipinnatae	Gui Zhen Cao	Gwai Jam Chou	
Begonia herb	*Begonia crassirostris*	Herba Begoniae crassirostris	Hong Ban Bian Lian	Hung Bun Bin Lin	
Begonia herb	*Begonia fimbristipula*	Herba Begoniae fimbristipulae	Zi Bei Tian Kuei Hong Tian Kui	Ji Mai Tin Kwai, Hung Tin Kwai	
Bengal dayflower herb	*Commelina benghalensis*	Herba Commelinae	Tang Shi Song	Tong Sek Chung	
Benzoin	*Styrax benzoin*	Benzoinum	An Xi Xiang	Ngon Sik Heung	Ansokuko
Betel husk	*Areca catechu, A. dicksonii*	Pericarpium Arecae	Da Fu Pi	Daai Fuk Pei	Daifukuhi
Betel nut	*Areca catechu, A. dicksonii*	Semen Arecae catechu	Bing Lang	Ban Long	Binroji
Betel nut flower	*Areca catechu, A. dicksonii*	Flos Arecae catechu	Bing Lang Hua	Ban Long Fa	Binroka
Betel pepper leaf	*Piper betle*	Folium Piperis betlis	Ju Jiang Ye, Qing Lou Ye	Geui Jeung Yip	
Birthwort root or stem	*Aristolochia moupiensis*	Radix seu caulis Aristolochiae moupiensis	Huai Tong	Waai Tung	
Bistort root	*Polygonum bistorta*	Radix Polygoni bistortae	Quan Shen	Kyun Sam	
Bitter apricot kernel	*Prunus armeniaca* and var.	Semen Pruni armeniacae	Xing Ren, Ku Xing Ren	Baak Hang Yan	Kyonin
Bitter bamboo leaf	*Pleioblastus amarus*	Folium Pleioblasti	Ku Zhu Ye	Fu Juk Yip	
Bitter evodia root	*Evodia lepta*	Radix Evodiae leptae	San Ya Ku (Gen)	Sam Nga Fu (Gan)	

ENGLISH	SCIENTIFIC	PHARMACEUTICAL	MANDARIN	CANTONESE	JAPANESE
Bitter melon fruit	*Momordica charantia*	Fructus Momordicae charantiae	Ku Gua (Gan)	Fu Gwa (Gam)	
Bittersweet stem	*Solanum dulcamara*	Caulis Solani dulcamari	Ku Qie	Fu Ke	
Black atractylodes root	*Atractylodes lancea, A. sinensis* and spp	Rhizoma Atractylodis lanceae	Cang Zhu, Mao Cang Zhu	Chong Seut, Mau Chong Seut	Sojutsu
Black bamboo leaf	*Phyllostachys nigra* var. *henonis* and spp	Folium Phyllostachis	Zhu Ye	Juk Yip	
Black bamboo root	*Phyllostachys nigra* var. *henonis* and spp	Radix Phyllostachis	Zi Zhu Gen	Ji Juk Gan	
Black bamboo sap	*Phyllostachys nigra* var. *henonis* and spp	Succus Phyllostachis	Zhu Li	Juk Lai	Chikureki
Black bamboo shaving	*Phyllostachys nigra* var. *henonis* and spp	Caulis Phyllostachis in taeniis	Zhu Ru	Juk Yu	Chikujo
Black ferric oxide	*Ferrum*	Pulvis ferri	Chen Sha	San Sa	
Black figwort root	*Scrophularia ningpoensis, S. buergeriana*	Radix Scrophulariae ningpoensis	Xuan Shen, Yuan Shen	Yun Sam, Yun Sam	Genjin
Black grass-snake	*Zaocys dhumnades*	Zaocys	Wu Shao She	U Sau Se	Ushoda
Black henbane seed	*Hyoscyamus niger*	Semen Hyoscyami	Tian Xian Zi	Tin Sin Ji	
Black iron oxide	*Ferrum*	Pulvis ferri	Chen Sha	Chan Sa	
Black jujube berry	*Zizyphus jujuba* var. *inermis*	Fructus Zizyphi jujubae	Da Zao	Daai Jou	Taiso
Black pepper corn	*Piper nigrum*	Fructus Piperis nigri	Hu Jiao, Hei Hu Jiao	Wu Jiu, Mai Wu Jiu	Kosho
Black pepper root	*Piper nigrum*	Radix Piperis nigri	Hu Jiao Gen	Wu Jiu Gan	
Black plum flower	*Prunus mume*	Flos Pruni mumis	Lu Er Mei, Lu Mei Hua	Lat Mui Fa	
Black plum fruit	*Prunus mume*	Fructus Pruni mumis	Wu Mei (Rou)	Wu Mui (Yuk)	Ubai
Black sesame seed	*Sesamum indicum*	Fructus Sesami	Hei Zhi Ma Hu Ma Ren	Hak Ji Ma	
Blessed thistle herb	*Silybum marianum*	Herba Silybi	Shui Fei Ji	Seui Fei Gai	
Bogbean leaf	*Menyanthes trifoliata*	Folium Menyanthis	Shui Cai Ye	Seui Choi Yip	Suisayo, Meisai
Boiler or chimney soot		Pulvus fumi carbonisati	Bai Cao Shuang	Baak Chou Sheung	
Boneknit root	*Davallia divaricata*	Rhizoma Davalliae	Gu Sui Bu	Gwat Seui Bou	Kotsusaiho
Boneknit root	*Drynaria fortunei* and spp	Rhizoma Drynariae	Gu Sui Bu	Gwat Seui Bou	Kotsusaiho
Boneknit root	*Pseudodrynaria fortunei, D. baronii*	Rhizoma Pseudodrynariae	Gu Sui Bu	Gwat Seui Bou	Kotsusaiho
Boor's mustard herb	*Thlaspi arvense*	Herba Thlaspis	Xi Ming	Sik Ming	
Borax	*Borax*	Borax	Peng Sha	Pang Sa	Hosha
Borneo camphor	*Dryobalanops camphora*	Borneolum	Bing Pian	Bing Pin	Ryuno
Boss fern root	*Cyrtomium fortunei*	Rhizoma Cyrtomi	Guan Zhong, Hun Ji Tou,	Gwun Jung, Fan Gai Tau	

ENGLISH	SCIENTIFIC	PHARMACEUTICAL	MANDARIN	CANTONESE	JAPANESE
Bottle gourd fruit	*Lagenaria siceraria*	Fructus Lagenariae	Hu Lu Ke	Wu Lok Hok	
Bottlegourd herb	*Desmodium pseudotriquetrum, D. triquetrum*	Herba Desmodii pseudotriquetrii	Long Shi Huang	Lung Sek Wong	
Brachypode aconite root	*Aconitum brachypodum* and spp	Radix Aconiti brachypodi	Xue Shang Yi Zhi Yao	Syu Seung Yat Ji Hou	
Bractless spurge root	*Euphorbia ebracteolata*	Radix Euphorbiae ebracteolatae	Lang Du, Yue Xian Da Ji	Long Duk, Yu Sin Daai Gik	
Breynia tip	*Breynia fruticosa*	Cacumen Breyniae	Hei Mian Ye	Haak Min Yip	
Bright bugleweed herb	*Lycopus lucidus*	Herba Lycopi	Ze Lan	Jaak Laan	Takuran
Bright bugleweed root	*Lycopus lucidus*	Rhizoma Lycopi lucidi	Di Sun	Dei Seun	
Bright changium root	*Changium smyrnioides*	Radix Changii	Ming Dang Shen	Ming Dong Sam	Mintojin
Broad-leaf liriope root	*Liriope platyphylla*	Radix Liriopis platyphyllae	Mai Men Dong	Mak (Mun) Dung	
Broadleaf holly leaf	*Ilex latifolia*	Folium Ilicis latifoliae	Ku Ding Cha	Fu Ding Cha	
Brown's lily bulb	*Lilium brownii* var. *colchesteri*	Bulbus Lilii	Bai He	Baak Hap	Hyakugo
Brown's lily flower	*Lilium brownii* var. *colchesteri*	Flos Lilii	Bai He Hua	Baak Hap Fa	
Brown's lily root	*Lilium brownii* var. *colchesteri*	Radix Lilii	Bai He Gen	Baak Hap Gan	
Brucea berry	*Brucea javanica*	Fructus Bruceae	Ya Dan Zi	Nga Daan Ji	Atanshi
Buckwheat root	*Fagopyrum cymosum*	Rhizoma Fagopyri	Jin Qiao Mai Gen	Gam Kiu Mak Gan	
Buddleia flower and bud	*Buddleia officinalis*	Flos Buddleiae	Mi Meng Hua	Mat Mung Fa	Mitsumoka
Buddleia root	*Buddleia lindleyana*	Radix Buddleiae lindleyanae	Qi Li Xiang	Chat Lei Heung	
Bugleweed herb	*Ajuga decumbens*	Herba Ajugae	Bai Mao Xia Ku Cao, Jing Gu Cao	Baak Mou Ha Fu Chou, Gan Gwat Chou	
Bulrush flower	*Juncus effusus*	Flos Junci	Deng Xin Hua	Ding Sam Fa	
Bulrush pith	*Juncus effusus*	Medulla Junci	Deng Xin Cao	Dang Sam Chou	Toshinso
Bung's Clerodendron leaf	*Clerodendron bungei*	Folium Clerodendronis bungeis	Chou Mu Dan	Chau Maau Daan	
Bur-reed root	*Sparganium simplex, S. stoloniferum, S. stenophyllum*	Rhizoma Sparganii	San Leng	Saam Ling	
Burdock seed	*Arctium lappa*	Fructus Arctii	Niu Bang Zi	Ngau Pong Ji	Goboshi
Burma boxwood twig and leaf	*Murraya paniculata*	Ramulus et folium Murrayae	Jiu Li Xiang	Gau Lei Heung	
Bush cherry kernel	*Prunus japonica*	Semen Pruni japonicae	Yu Li Ren	Yuk Lei Yan	Ikurinin
Caesalpinia seed	*Caesalpinia minax*	Semen Caesalpiniae minacis	Ku Shi Lian (Zi)	Fu Sek Lin (Ji)	
Cairo morning-glory herb	*Ipomoea cairica*	Herba Ipomoeae cairicae	Wu Zhao Long	Ng Jaau Lung	
Cajeput leaf	*Melaleuca leucadendron*	Folium Melaleucae leucadendronis	Bai Qian Ceng	Baak Chin Chang	

ENGLISH	SCIENTIFIC	PHARMACEUTICAL	MANDARIN	CANTONESE	JAPANESE
Calamine	*Calamina, Smithsonitum*	Calamina, Smithsonitum	Lu Gan Shi	Lou Gam Sek	Rokanseki
Calcined dragon bone	*Stegodon orientalis et al.*	Os Stegodontis calcinatum	Duan Long Gu, Shu Long Gu	Taan Lung Gwat	
Calcined oyster shell	*Ostrea gigas*	Concha Ostreae calcinati	Duan Mu Li	Taan Mou Lai	
Calcite	*Calcitum*	Calcitum	Han Shui Shi, Fang Jie Shi	Hon Seui Sek	Kansuiseki
Calcium hydroxide	*Calcaria*	Calcaria	Chen Shi Hui	Chan Sek Wei	
Callicarpa leaf	*Callicarpa pedunculata*	Folium Callicarpae pedunculatae	Zi Zhu Ye	Ji Jyu Yip	Jijuso
Calomel	*Calomelas*	Calomelas	Qing Fen	Ching Fan	Keifun
Caltrop fruit	*Tribulus terrestris*	Fructus Tribuli	Bai Ji Li	Baak Jat Lai	Byakishitsuri
Camphor flake	*Cinnamomum camphora*	Camphora	Zhang Nao	Jeung Naau	Shono
Camphor plant	*Blumea balsamifera*	Herba Blumeae balsamiferae	Ai Na Xiang, Da Feng Cao	Ngaai Naap Heung	Daifuso
Camphor wood	*Cinnamomum camphora*	Lignum Cinnamomi camphorae	Zhang Mu	Jeung Muk	
Canna lily root	*Canna indica*	Rhizoma Cannae	Mei Ren Jiao (Gen)	Mei Yan Jiu (Gan)	Dandoku
Cannabis seed	*Cannabis sativa*	Semen Cannabis	Huo Ma Ren	Fo Ma Yan	Mashinin
Cantaloupe seed	*Cucumis melo*	Semen Cucumis	Tian Gua Zi	Tim Gwa Ji	
Cantharides	*Cantharis vosicatoria*	Cantharis	Ban Mao	Ban Mou	Hanmyo
Canton sanchi leaf	*Gynura segetum*	Folium Gynurae	San Qi Cao, Ju San Qi	Sam Chat Chou	
Caper spurge seed	*Euphorbia lathyris*	Semen Euphorbiae lathyris	Qian Jin Zi	Chin Gam Ji	Zokuzuishi
Capparis berry	*Capparis masaikai*	Semen Capparis	Ma Bin Lang	Ma Ban Long	Kuttokei
Caragana flower	*Caragana sinica* and spp	Flos Caraganae	Jin Que Hua	Gam Jeuk Fa	
Caragana root	*Caragana sinica, C., microphylla* and spp	Radix Caraganae	Jin Ji Er	Gam Jik Yi	
Carambola flower	*Averrhoa carambola*	Flos Averrhoae	Yang Tao Hua	Yeung Tou Fa	
Carambola fruit	*Averrhoa carambola*	Fructus Averrhoae	Yang Tao	Yeung Tou	
Carbonized mogera	*Mogera robusta* and spp., *Scaptochirus moschatus*	Mogera carbonisatus	Yan Shu Shuang	Yim Syu Seung	Ensosu
Carp	*Cyprinus carpio*	Cyprinus	Li Yu	Lei Yu	
Cassia Cinnamon bark	*Cinnamomum cassia*	Cortex Cinnamomi cassiae	Rou Gui (Pi)	Yuk Gwai (Pei)	Nikkei
Cassia cinnamon inner bark	*Cinnamomum cassia*	Cortex intimum Cinnamomi cassiae	Rou Gui Xin	Yuk Gwai San	
Cassia cinnamon twig	*Cinnamomum cassia*	Ramulus Cinnamomi cassiae	Gui Zhi , Rou Gui Zhi	Gwai Ji	Keishi
Castor bean	*Ricinus communis*	Semen Ricini	Bi Ma Zi	Bei Ma Ji	
Cat thorn holly leaf	*Ilex cornuta*	Folium Ilicis cornutae	Gou Gu Ye	Gau Gwat Yip	
Catalpa bark	*Catalpa bungei*	Cortex Catalpae	Zi Bai Pi, Qiu Mu Pi	San Baak Pei, Chau Muk Pei	

ENGLISH	SCIENTIFIC	PHARMACEUTICAL	MANDARIN	CANTONESE	JAPANESE
Catalpa fruit	*Catalpa ovata*	Fructus Catalpae	Zhi Shi	San Sat	Kisasage
Catechu paste	*Acacia catechu*	Pasta Acaciae seu Uncariae	Er Cha	Yi Cha	Asenyaku
Catechu paste	*Uncaria gambir* and spp	Pasta Uncaria seu Acaciae	Er Cha	Yi Cha	
Cattail pollen	*Typha latifolia, T. angustifolia* and spp	Pollen Typhae	Pu Huang, Xiang Pu	Pou Wong, Heung Pou	Hoo
Cayratia herb	*Cayratia japonica*	Herba Cayratiae	Wu Lian Mei	Wu Lin Mui	
Cedrela root bark	*Cedrela sinensis*	Cortex radicis Cedrelae	Chun Gen Bai Pi	Jung Gan Baak Pei	
Celery wormwood herb	*Artemisia apiacea*	Herba Artemisiae apiaceae	Qing Hao	Ching Hou	Seiko
Celestial hemp corm	*Gastrodia elata*	Rhizoma Gastrodiae	Tian Ma	Tin Ma	Temma
Centipeda herb	*Centipeda minima*	Herba Centipedae	E Bu Shi Cao	Ngo Bat Sik Chou	Sekikozui, Gabusho-kuso
Centipede	*Scolopendra subspinipes mutilans*	Scolopendra	Wu Gong	Ng Gung	Gosho
Central China schisandra berry	*Schizandra sphenantera*	Fructus Schisandrae sphenanterae	Wu Wei Zi, Hua Zheng Wu Wei Zi	Ng Mei Ji, Wa Jung Ng Mei Ji	Gomishi
Cereus flower	*Hylocereus undatus*	Flos Hylocerei	Jian Hua, Ba Wang Hua	Gim Fa	
Cerulean passionflower herb	*Passiflora coeruleae*	Herba Passiflorae coeruleae	Xi Fan Lian	Sai Faan Lin	
Cerusite	*Cerussa*	Cerussa	Qian Fen	Yun Fan	
Ceylon cinnamon bark	*Cinnamomum zeylanicum*	Cortex Cinnamomi zeylanici	Rou Gui, Xi Lan Rou Gui	Yuk Gwai, Sek Laan Yuk Gwai	
Ceylon leadwort	*Plumbago zeylanicum*	Herba Plumbaginis	Hei Mian Ma, Bai Hua Dan	Baak Fa Daan	
Chain-fern root	*Woodwardia japonica, W. unigemmata*	Rhizoma Woodwardiae	Guan Zhong, Gou Ji Guan Zhong	Gwun Jung, Gau Jek Gun Jung	
Charred Asian hawthorn berry	*Crataegus pinnatifida, C. cuneata* and spp	Fructus Crataegi carbonisatus	Shan Zha Tan	Saan Ja Tan	
Charred cattail pollen	*Typha latifolia, T. angustifolia* and spp	Pollen Typhae carbonisatus	Pu Huang Tan	Pou Wong Taan	
Charred human hair	*Homo sapiens*	Crinis carbonisatus Hominis	Xue Yu Tan	Hyut Yu Taan	
Charred windmill palm petiole	*Trachycarpus excelsa, T. fortunei*	Fibra Stipulae Trachycarpi carbonisata	Zong Lu Pi Tan	Jung Leui Pei Daan	
Chaulmoogra seed	*Hydnocarpus anthelmintica, H. hainanensis*	Semen Hydnocarpi	Da Feng Zi	Daai Fung Ji	Daifushi
Cherokee rosehip	*Rosa laevigata*	Fructus Rosae laevigatae	Jin Ying Zi	Gam Ying Ji	Kinoshi
Chicken dung vine root and stem	*Paederia scandens*	Radix et caulis Paederiae	Ji Shi Teng	Gai Niu Tang	Hakumokeis hito
Chicken egg membrane	*Gallus gallus domesticus*	Membrana follicularis ovi	Feng Huang Yi		

ENGLISH	SCIENTIFIC	PHARMACEUTICAL	MANDARIN	CANTONESE	JAPANESE
Chicken gizzard lining	*Gallus gallus domesticus*	Endothelium corneum gigeriae Galli	Ji Nei Jin	Gai Na Gam	Keinaikin
China jute seed	*Abutilon theophrastii*	Semen Abutili theophrasti	Qing Ma (Zi)	King Ma (Ji)	
Chinese aralia root	*Aralia chinensis*	Radix Araliae chinensis	Song Mu Bai Pi	Sung Muk Baak Pei	
Chinese caterpillar mushroom	*Cordyceps sinensis* and host larvae *Hepialus armoricanus or Holotrichia koraiensis*	Sclerotium Cordycepsis	Dong Chong Xia Cao	Dung Chung Ha Chou	Tochukaso
Chinese chestnut	*Castanea mollissima*	Fructus Castaneae	Li Zi, Feng Li Gu	Leut Ji	Furitsukaku
Chinese chive bulb	*Allium macrostemon*	Bulbus Allii macrostemonis	Xie Bai	Se Baak	Gaihaku
Chinese cinquefoil herb	*Potentilla chinensis*	Herba Potentillae chinensis	Wei Ling Cai	Wai Ling Choi	
Chinese clematis root	*Clematis chinensis, C. hexapetala* and spp	Radix Clematis chinensis	Wei Ling Xian	Wai Ling Sin	Ireisen
Chinese elder stem and leaf	*Sambucus chinensis* and spp	Caulis et folium Sambuci chinensis	Shuo Zhuo	Sok Dik	
Chinese elm bark	*Ulmus parvifolia*	Cortex Ulmi parvifoliae	Lang Yu Pi	Long Yu Pei	
Chinese gelsemium	*Gelsemium elegans*	Radix Gelsemii	Gou Wen	Au Man	
Chinese greenbrier root, China root	*Smilax china*	Rhizoma Smilacis chinensis	Jin Gang Teng, Ba Qi	Gam Gong Tang, Bat Kai	
Chinese gymnocladus berry	*Gymnocladus chinensis*	Fructus Gymnocladi	Fei Zao Jia	Fei Jou Choi	
Chinese horse chestnut	*Aesculus wilsonii, A. chinensis*	Fructrus Aesculi	Suo Luo Zi	So Lo Ji	
Chinese indigo herb	*Polygonum tinctorium*	Herba Polygoni tinctorii	Lan Shi	Laam Sat	
Chinese knotweed herb	*Polygonum chinense*	Herba Polygoni chinensis	Huo Tan Mu (Cao), Qing Fan Teng	Fo Tan Mou (Chou)	
Chinese lantern calyx or fruit	*Physalis alkekengi* (var. *franchetii)*	Calyx seu fructus Physalis	Suan Jiang, Jing Deng Long	Syun Jeung, Ching Dang Lung	
Chinese lantern root	*Physalis alkakengi* (var. *franchetii)*	Rhizoma Physalis	Suan Jiang Gen	Syun Jeung Gan	
Chinese lizardtail herb	*Saururus chinensis*	Herba Saururi	San Bai Cao	Saam Baak Chou	
Chinese lovage root	*Ligusticum sinense, L. jeholense*	Radix Ligustici sinensis	Gao Ben	Gou Bun	Kohon
Chinese osbeckia herb	*Osbeckia chinensis*	Herba Osbeckiae	Tian Xiang Lu, Jin Shi Lu	Tin Heung Lou	
Chinese parasol tree seed	*Firmiana simplex*	Semen Firmianae	Wu Tong Zi	Ng Tung Ji	
Chinese paris root	*Paris chinensis*	Rhizoma Paris chinensis	Zhong Lou, Qi Ye Yi Zhi Hua	Jung Lau, Chat Yip Yat Ji Pa	
Chinese pear rind	*Pyrus betulaefolia*	Pericarpium Pyri	Li Pi	Lei Pei	

ENGLISH	SCIENTIFIC	PHARMACEUTICAL	MANDARIN	CANTONESE	JAPANESE
Chinese pearltwist herb	*Spiranthes sinensis*	Herba Spiranthis	Pan Long Shen	Pun Lung Sam	
Chinese pink herb	*Dianthus chinensis*	Herba Dianthi chinensis	Qu Mai, Shi Zhu	Geui Mak, Sek Juk	
Chinese quince fruit	*Chaenomeles lagenaria*	Fructus Chaenomelis lagenariae	Mu Gua, Chuan Mu Gua	Muk Gwa, Chyun Muk Gwa	Mokka
Chinese quince fruit	*Chaenomeles sinensis*	Fructus Chaenomelis sinensis	Mu Gua, Ming Za	Muk Gwa	
Chinese raspberry fruit	*Rubus chingii*	Fructus Rubi chingii	Fu Pen Zi	Fuk Pun Ji	Fukubonshi
Chinese redbud bark	*Cercis chinensis*	Cortex Cercis	Zi Jing Pi	Ji Ging Pei	
Chinese redbud bark	*Kadsura peltigera*	Cortex Kadsurae peltigerae	Zi Jing Pi	Ji Ging Pei	
Chinese sacred lily bulb	*Narcissus tazetta* var. *chinensis*	Bulbus Narcissi	Shui Xian Gen	Seui Sin Gan	
Chinese sacred lily seed	*Narcissus tazetta* var. *chinensis*	Fructus Narcissi	Shui Xian Zi	Seui Sin Ji	
Chinese sage root and herb	*Salvia chinensis*	Radix et herba Salviae chinensis	Shi Jian Chuan, Chai Shen, Zi Shen	Sek Gin Chyun, Toi Sam, Ji Sam	
Chinese St. John's wort herb	*Hypericum chinense*	Herba Hyperici Chinensis	Jin Si Tao		
Chinese stephania stem	*Stephania sinica*	Caulis Stephaniae sinicae	Jin Bu Huan	Gam Bat Wun	
Chinese sumac bark	*Rhus chinensis*	Cortex Rhudis chinensis	Yan Fu Mu	Yim Fo Muk	Gobaishi
Chinese sumac gallnut	*Rhus sinensis* and spp, *Schlechtendaria chinensis*	Galla Rhudis sinensis	Wu Bei Zi	Ng Pan Ji	
Chinese sumac root	*Rhus chinensis*	Radix Rhudis chinensis	Pu Yan Pian	Pou Yim Pin	
Chinese tallow tree root bark	*Sapium sebiferum*	Cortex radicis Sapii sebiferi	Wu Jiu (Mu) Gen Pi	Wu Kau Muk Gan Pei	Ukyukompi
Chinese tamarisk tip	*Tamarix chinensis*	Cacumen Tamaricis	Xi He Liu	Sei Ho Lau	Seikaryu
Chinese teasel fruit	*Dipsacus chinensis* and spp	Fructus Dipsaci	Ju Sheng Zi	Geui Sing Ji	
Chinese tinospora stem	*Tinospora sinensis*	Caulis Tinosporae sinensis	Kuan Jin Teng	Gwan Gam Tang	Kankinto
Chinese tulip bulb	*Tulipa edulis*	Rhizoma et radix Tulipae	Shan Ci Gu, Guang Ci Gu	San Chi Gu, Gwong Chi Gu	
Chinese water pine tip	*Glyptostrobus pensilis*	Cacumen Glyptostrobi	Shui Song Mao	Seui Chung Ma	
Chlorite schist	*Chloris*	Chloris	Qing Meng Shi	Ching Mein Sek	
Chrysanthemum flower	*Chrysanthemum x morifolium*	Flos Chrysanthemi	Ju Hua, Gan Ju Hua	Guk Fa	
Cicada fungus	*Cordyceps scotianus* and *host Cryptotympana atrata* and spp	Sclerotium Cordycepsis scotianus	Chan Hua, Jin Chan Hua	Sim Fa, Gam Sim Fa	
Cicada slough	*Cryptotympana atrata* and spp	Periostracum Cryptotympanae	Chan Tui	Sim Teui, Sim Tyut	Sentai
Cinchona bark	*Cinchona succiruba* and spp	Cortex Cinchonae	Jin Ji Le, Jin Ji Na Pi	Gam Gai Laak	
Cinnabar	*Cinnabarum*	Cinnabarum	Zhu Sha	Ju Sa	Shusha

ENGLISH	SCIENTIFIC	PHARMACEUTICAL	MANDARIN	CANTONESE	JAPANESE
Cinnabar sage root	*Salvia miltiorrhiza*	Radix Salviae miltiorrhizae	Dan Shen	Daan Sam	Tanjin
Cinnamon bark	*Cinnamomum japonicum, C. zeylanicum, C. obtusifolium*	Cortex Cinnamomi japonici	Gui Pi	Gwai Pei	
Cissus stem	*Cissus pteroclada*	Caulis Cissi	Kuan Jin Teng	Gwan Gam Tang	
Citron fruit	*Citrus medica, C. wilsonii*	Fructus Citri medicae	Xiang Yuan, Gou Yuan	Heung Yun	
Citron rind	*Citrus medica, C. wilsonii*	Pericarpium Citri medicae	Xiang Yuan Pi, Gou Yuan Pi	Heung Yun Pei, Gau Yun Pei	
Citrus fibre	*Citrus* spp	Fasciculus vascularis Citri, Endocarpium Citri	Ju Luo, Ju Bai	Gwat Lok	
Citrus flower	*Citrus grandis* and spp	Flos Citri grandi	Ju Hong Hua	Gwat Heung Fa	
Citrus leaf	*Citrus* spp.	Folium Aurantium	Ju Ye	Gwat Yip	
Clam shell	*Cyclina sinensis*	Concha Cyclinae	Hai Ge Ke, Ke Li	Hoi Gap Hok	Kaigokaku
Clay ironstone	*Limonitum*	Limonitum	Yu Liang Shi	Yu Leung Sek	Uyoryo
Cleavers herb	*Galium aparine*	Herba Galii aparinis	Ba Xian Cao, Zhu Yang Yang	Baat Sin Chou	
Cleistolcalyx bud	*Cleistocalyx operculatus*	Gemma Cleistocalycis	Shui Weng Hua	Seui Yung Fa	
Climbing hops flower	*Humulus scandens*	Herba Humuli scandentis	Lu Cao	Leut Chou	
Climbing nightshade herb	*Solanum lyratum*	Herba Solani lyrati	Bai Ying, Shu Yang Quan, Bai Mao Teng	Baak Ying, Baak Mou Tang	
Climbing ragwort herb	*Senecio scandens*	Herba Senecionis scandens	Qian Li Guang	Chin Lei Gwong	
Clinopodium herb	*Clinopodium confine*	Herba Clinopodii	Jian Dao Cao	Jin Dou Chou	
Clove bud	*Eugenia caryophyllata*	Gemma Eugeniae	Ding Xiang	Ding Heung	Choko
Clove strip herb	*Jussiaea repens*	Herba Jussiaeae	Kuo Tang She	Gwo Tong Se	
Clubmoss herb	*Lycopodium clavatum*	Herba Lycopodi	Shen Jin Cao	Sam Gam Chou	
Cluster cardamom flower	*Amomum cardamomum*	Flos Amomi cardamomi	(Bai) Dou Kou Hua	(Baak) Dau Kau Fa	Byakuzu-kuka
Cluster cardamom pod	*Amomum cardamomum*	Fructus Amomi cardamomi	Bai Dou Kou	Baak Dau Kau	Byakuzuku
Cnidium seed	*Cnidium monnieri*	Fructus Cnidii	She Chuang Zi	Se Chong Ji	Jashoshi
Cochin bitter melon seed	*Momordica cochinchinensis*	Semen Momordicae cochinchinensis	Mu Bie Zi	Muk Bit Ji	Mokubesshi
Cochin cardamom fruit	*Amomum tsao-ko*	Fructus Amomi tsao-konis	Cao Guo (Ren)	Chou Gwat (Yan)	Soka
Cochin cudrania root	*Cudrania cochinchinensis*	Radix Cudraniae cochinchinensis	Chuan Po Shi	Chyun Po Sek	
Cock'scomb herb	*Celosia cristata*	Herba Celosiae cristatae	Ji Guan Hua	Gai Gun Fa	
Cocklebur cardamom pod	*Amomum xanthioides*	Fructus Amomi xanthioidis	Sha Ren, Suo Sha Mi	Sa Yan, Suk Sa Mat	
Cockle shell	*Arca inflata* and spp	Concha Arcae	Wa Leng Zi	Nga Ling Ji	Garyoshi

ENGLISH	SCIENTIFIC	PHARMACEUTICAL	MANDARIN	CANTONESE	JAPANESE
Cockroach	*Eupolyphaga sinensis*	Eupolyphaga	Tu Bie Chong	Dei Bit Chung	Shachu
Coffee senna seed	*Cassia occidentalis*	Semen Cassiae occidentalis	Wang Jiang Nan Zi	Mong Gong Naam	Banshashi
Coin-leaf desmodium herb	*Desmodium styracifolium*	Herba Desmodii	Guang Dong (Jin) Qian Cao	Gwong Dung (Gam) Chin Chou	Kinsenso
Collina violet root and herb	*Viola collina*	Radix et herba Violae collinae	Di He Tao	Dei Hat Tou	
Coltsfoot flower	*Tussilago farfara*	Flos Tussilaginis	Kuan Dong Hua	Fun Dung Fa	Kantoka
Common camellia flower	*Camellia japonica*	Flos Camelliae japonicae	Shan Cha Hua	Saan Cha Fa	
Common dayflower herb	*Commelina communis*	Herba Commelinae	Ya Zhi Cao	Ngaap Jek Chou	
Common dysosma root	*Dysosma versipellis*	Rhizoma Dysosmae versipellis	Gui Jiu	Gwai Kau	
Common harebell root	*Adenophora trachelioides, A. remotifolia*	Radix Adenophorae trachelioidis	Ji Ni	Chai Ni	
Common trumpetcree-per flower	*Campsis radicans*	Flos Campsis radicantis	Ling Xiao Hua, Mei Jou Ling Xiao	Ling Siu Fa, Mei Jau Ling Siu	
Conessi bark	*Holarrhenia antidysenterica*	Cortex Holarrheniae	Zhi Xie Mu Pi	Ji Se Muk Pei	
Copper rust	*Malachitum*	Malachitum	Tong Lu	Tung Luk	
Coral skeleton	*Porites nigrescens*	Os Poritis	Shi Hua	Sek Fa	
Coralberry root	*Ardisia crenata, A. bicolor*	Radix Ardisiae crenatae	Da Lo San, Zhu Sha Gen	Jyu Sa Gan	Shushakon
Coriander herb	*Coriandrum sativum*	Herba Coriandri	Hu Sui	Wu Sai	
Coriander seed	*Coriandrum sativum*	Fructus Coriandri	Yan Sui Zi	Yun Sai Ji	
Coriaria leaf	*Coriaria sinica*	Folium Coriariae	Ma Sang Ye	Ma Song Yip	
Corn cob	*Zea mays*	Medulla Zeae	Yu Mi Xin	Yuk Mai Sam	
Corn grain	*Zea mays*	Fructus Zeae	Yu Shu Shu	Yuk Suk Syu	
Cornsilk style	*Zea mays*	Stylus Zeae	Yu Mi Xu, Yu Mi Rui	Yuk Mai So, Yuk Mai Yeui	Gyokuma-ishu
Cotton root bark	*Gossypium hirsutum, G. herbaceum*	Cortex radicis Gossypii	Mian Hua Gen	Min Fa Gan	
Cotton rose flower	*Hibiscus mutabilis*	Flos Hibisci mutabili	Fu Rong Hua	Fu Yung Fa	
Cotton rose leaf	*Hibiscus mutabilis*	Folium Hibisci mutabilis	Fu Rong Ye	Fu Yung Yip	
Cotton seed	*Gossypium hirsutum, G. herbaceum*	Semen Gossypii	Mian Hua Zi	Min Fa Ji	
Country mallow herb	*Abutilon indicum*	Herba Abutilonis indici	Mo Pan Cao, Mi Lan Cao	Mo Bun Chou	
Cowcockle seed	*Vaccaria segetalis*	Semen Vaccariae	Wang Bu Liu Xing	Wong Bat Lau Hang	Ofurugyo
Cowrie shell	*Cypraea moneta, C. macula* and spp	Concha Cypraeae	Bei Zi	Chan Bu Chi	
Cratoxylon leaf	*Cratoxylon ligustrinum*	Folium Cratoxyli	Huang Niu Cha	Wong Ngau Cha	
Creeping fig fruit	*Ficus pumila*	Fructus Fici pumilae	Bi Li, Mu Man Tou	Bai La	
Creeping rostellularia herb	*Rostellulariae procumbens*	Herba Rostellulariae	Jue Chuang	Jeuk Chong	

ENGLISH	SCIENTIFIC	PHARMACEUTICAL	MANDARIN	CANTONESE	JAPANESE
Cremastra corm	*Cremastra variabilis*	Rhizoma et radix Cremastrae	Shan Ci Gu	Saan Chi Gu	
Crepe jasmine herb	*Ervatamia divaricata, E. hainaensis*	Herba Ervatamiae	Gou Ya Hua	Gaau Nga Fa	
Cricket	*Gryllulus chinensis, G. mitratus, Gampsocleis buergeri*	Gryllulus	Xi Shuai	Sik Seut	
Crisp ardisia herb	*Ardisia crispa*	Herba Ardisiae crispae	Bai Liang Jin	Baak Leung Gam	
Crossosteph-ium herb	*Crossostephium chinense*	Herba Crossostephii	Fu Rong	Fu Yung	
Croton seed	*Croton tiglium*	Semen Crotonis	Ba Dou	Ba Dau	
Cruciate bluehart herb	*Buchnera cruciata*	Herba Buchnerae	Gui Yu Jian	Gwai Yu Jin	
Crystallized blue vitriol	*Chalcanthitum*	Chalcanthitum	Dan Fan, Shi Dan	Daan Faan	Tanban
Cubeb peppercorn	*Litsea cubeba*	Fructus Litseae	Bi Cheng Qie	Bat Ching Ke	
Cubeb root and stem	*Litsea cubeba*	Radix et caulis Litseae	Dou Chi Jiang	Dau Chek Geung	Toshikyo
Cudrania heartwood	*Cudrania tricuspidata*	Lignum Cudraniae tricuspidatae	Da Ding Huang, Zhe Mu	Je Muk	
Cudweed herb	*Gnaphalium affine*	Herba Gnaphalii	Shu Qu Cao	Syu Guk Chou	
Cuttlefish bone	*Sepia esculenta, Sepiella maindroni*	Os Sepiae seu Sapiellae	Hai Piao Xiao, Wu Zei Gu	Hoi Piu Seui	
Cyathea root	*Cyathea spinulosa*	Rhizoma Cyatheae	Guan Zhong	Gwun Jung	
Cymbidium orchid herb and root	*Cymbidium ensifolium*	Herba et radix Cymbidii	Jian Lan Hua	Gin Laan Fa	
Cymbidium orchid leaf	*Cymbidium ensifolium*	Folium Cymbidii	Jian Lan Ye	Gin Laan Yip	
Cymbidium orchid root	*Cymbidium ensifolium*	Radix Cymbidii	Jian Lan Gen	Gin Laan Gan	
Cymose knotweed Root	*Polygonum cymosum*	Radix et rhizoma Polygoni cymosi	Kai Jin Suo	Hoi Gam So	
Cymose rose root bark	*Rosa cymosa*	Cortex radicis Rosae cymosae	Hong Ci Teng, Hong Gen, Xiao Jin Ying	Hung Chi Teng, Siu Gam Ying	
Daemonorops root	*Daemonorops margaritae*	Radix Daemonoropsis	Huang Teng Gen	Wong Tang Gan	
Dahurian pasqueflower root	*Pulsatilla dahurica*	Radix Pulsatillae dahuricae	Bai Tou Weng, Xing An Bai Tou Weng	Baak Tau Yung, Ing On Baak Tau Yung	
Dahurian rising hemp root	*Cimicifuga dahurica*	Radix Cimicifugae dahuricae	Sheng Ma, Xing An Sheng Ma	Sing Ma, Hing On Sing Ma	Shoma
Dalmatia pellitory flower	*Pyrethrum cinerariifolium*	Flos Pyrethri	Chu Chong Ju	Cheui Chung Guk	
Daurian rhododendron leaf	*Rhododendron dauricum, R. mariesii*	Folium Rhododendri daurici	Man Shan Hong	Mun Saan Hung	
Day lily root	*Hemerocallis thunbergii*	Rhizoma et radix Hemerocallis thunbergii	Li Lu	Lai Lou	

ENGLISH	SCIENTIFIC	PHARMACEUTICAL	MANDARIN	CANTONESE	JAPANESE
Decumbent corydalis herb	*Corydalis decumbens*	Herba Corydalis decumbensis	Xia Tian Wu	Ha Tin Mou	
Dehydrated gypsum	*Gypsum fibrosum*	Gypsum dehydratum	Shu Shi Gao	Chek Sek Gou	
Dentate-leaf corydalis corm	*Corydalis turtschaninovii*	Rhizoma Corydalis	Yan Hu Suo, Chi Ban Yan Hu Suo	Yin Wu Sok, Chi Faan Yin Wu Sok	Engosaku
Dichondra herb	*Dichondra repens*	Herba Dichondrae	Ma Di Jin	Ma Dei Jing	Kinsenso
Discolored cinquefoil herb	*Potentilla discolor*	Herba Potentillae discoloris	Fan Bai Cao	Faan Baak Chou	
Distant lemongrass herb	*Cymbopogon distans*	Herba Cymbopogonis distansis	Yun Xiang Cao	Yun Heung Chou	
Divaricate typhonium root	*Typhonium divaricatum*	Rhizoma Typhonii divaricatii	Li Tou Jian	Lai Tau Jim	
Dogbane root and herb	*Apocynum lancifolium, A. venetum, A. hendersonii*	Radix et herba Apocyni	Luo Bu Ma	Lo Bou Ma	
Dogspine root	*Cibotium barometz*	Rhizoma Cibotii	Gou Ji	Gau Jek	Kuseki
Dolomite	*Ophicalcitum*	Ophicalcitum	Hua Rui Shi	Fa Yeui Sek	Kazuiseki
Dong quai head	*Angelica sinensis, A. acutiloba*	Caput Angelicae sinensis	Dang Gui Tou	Dong Gwai Tou	Tokito
Dong quai root	*Angelica acutiloba*	Radix Angelicae acutilobae	Dang Gui	Dong Gwai	
Dong quai root	*Angelica sinensis*	Radix Angelicae sinensis	Dang Gui	Dong Gwai	Toki
Dong quai tail	*Angelica sinensis, A. acutiloba*	Extremas radicis Angelicae sinensis	Dang Gui Wei	Dong Gwai Mai	Tokio
Downy bellflower root	*Codonopsis pilosula, C. tangshen, C. nervosa*	Radix Codonopsis	Dang Shen	Fong Dong Sam	Tojin
Downy rosemyrtle root	*Rhodomyrtus tomentosa*	Radix Rhodomyrti	Shui Duo Nian, Shan Nian Gen	Seui Do Lin, San Nim Gan	
Downy wormwood herb	*Artemisia capillaris, A. scoparia*	Herba Artemisiae capillaris	Yin Chen (Hao), Mian Yin Chen	Yan Chan (Hou), Min Yan Chan	Inchinko
Dragon bone	*Stegodon orientalis, S. rhinocerus sinensis, Hipparion*	Os Stegodontis	Long Gu	Lung Gwat	Ryukotsu
Dragon tooth	*Stegodon orientalis et al.*	Dens Stegodontis	Long Chi	Lung Ji	
Dragon's-blood resin	*Daemonorops draco*	Resina Daemonoropsis (Sanguis draconis)	Xue Jie	Hyut Kit	Kekketsu
Dried Asian ginseng root	*Panax ginseng*	Radix Panacis ginsengis	Sheng Shai Shen	Sang Sai Sam	
Dried ginger root	*Zingiber officinalis*	Rhizoma Zingiberis	Gan Jiang	Gaan Geung	Kankyo
Dry-fried Job's-tears seed	*Coix lachryma-jobi* var. *Ma-yuen*	Semen Coicis preparatae	Shu Yi Ren	Suk Yi Mai	
Duckweed herb	*Lemna minor*	Herba Lemnae	Fu Ping	Fau Ping	
Duckweed herb	*Spirodela polyrrhiza*	Herba Spirodelae	Fu Ping	Fau Ping	

ENGLISH	SCIENTIFIC	PHARMACEUTICAL	MANDARIN	CANTONESE	JAPANESE
Dung beetle	*Catharsius molossus, Xylotrupes dichotomus*	Catharsius seu Xylotrupes	Jiang Lan Chong	Jeung Long Chung	
Dwarf cherry kernel	*Prunus humilis*	Semen Pruni humili	Yu Li Ren, Ou Li	Yuk Lei Yan, Ngao Lei	
Dwarf lilyturf root	*Ophiopogon japonicus*	Radix Ophiopogonis	Mai (Men) Dong	Mak (Mun) Dung	Bakumondo
Dyer's yam root	*Dioscorea cirrhosa*	Rhizoma Dioscoreae cirrhosae	Shu Liang	Syu Leung	
Earthworm	*Pheretima aspergillum, Allolobophora caliginosa*	Pheretima seu Allolobophora	Di Long	Dei Lung	Jiryu
Egg yolk	*Gallus gallus domesticus*	Vitellus Galli	Ji Zi Huang	Gai Ji Wong	
Eggplant root	*Solanum melongena*	Radix et rhizoma Solani melongenae	Qie Gen	Ke Gan	
Elecampane flower	*Inula japonica, I. brittanica, I. linariaefolia*	Flos Inulae	Xuan Fu Hua	Syun Fuk Fa	Sembukuka
Elecampane herb	*Inula japonica, I. brittanica, I. linariaefolia*	Herba Inulae	Jin Fei Cao	Gam Fai Chou	Kinfutsuso
Elecampane root	*Inula helenium*	Radix Inula helenii	Tu Mu Xiang	Tou Muk Heung	
Eleuthero ginseng root	*Eleutherococcus senticosus*	Radix seu cortex radicis Eleutherococci senticosi	Ci Wu Jia (Gen Pi)	Chi Ng Ga (Gan Pei)	
Emodi's podophyllum root	*Podophyllum emodii*	Rhizoma Podophylli emodii	Tao Er Qi	Tou Yi Chat	
Ephedra root	*Ephedra sinica*	Radix Ephedrae	Ma Huang Gen	Ma Wong Gan	Maokon
Ephedra stem	*Ephedra sinica*	Herba Ephedrae	Ma Huang	Ma Wong	Mao
Ephemerantha stem	*Ephemerantha fimbriata*	Herba Ephemeranthae	Shi Hu	Sek Hap	Sekkoku
Ericerus worm	*Ericerus pela*	Ericerus	Chong Bai La	Chung Baak Laap	
Erycibe root and stem	*Erycibes obtusifolia*	Radix et caulis Erycibis	Ding Gong Teng	Ding Gung Tang	
Eucalyptus leaf	*Eucalyptus globulus*	Folium Eucalypti globuli	An Ye	Ngon Yip	
Eucommia bark	*Eucommia ulmoides*	Cortex Eucommiae	Du Zhong	Dou Jung	Tochu
Eucommia leaf	*Eucommia ulmoides*	Folium Eucommiae	Du Zhong Ye	Dou Jung Yip	
European water clover leaf	*Marsilea quaddrifolia*	Folium Marsileae	Ping	Ping	
Evodia berry	*Evodia rutaecarpa*	Fructus Evodiae rutecarpae	Wu Zhu Yu	Ng Jyu Yu	Goshuyu
False hellebore root	*Veratrum nigrum* and spp	Radix et rhizoma Veratri	Li Lu	Lai Lou	Riro
Fameflower root	*Talinum paniculatum*	Radix Talini	Tu Ren Shen	Tou Yan Sam	
Fan palm seed	*Livistona chinensis*	Semen Livistonae	Kui Shu Zi	Kwai Sat Ji	
Fangchi birthwort root	*Aristolochia fangchi, A. westlandii*	Radix Aristolochiae fangchis	Fang Ji, Guang Fang Ji	Fong Gei, Gwong Fong Gei	

ENGLISH	SCIENTIFIC	PHARMACEUTICAL	MANDARIN	CANTONESE	JAPANESE
Felt fern leaf	*Pyrrosia lingua, P. petiolosa* and spp	Folium Pyrrosiae	Shi Wei	Sek Wai	
Fennel seed	*Foeniculum vulgare*	Fructus Foeniculi	Xiao Hui Xiang	Siu Wui Heung	Shouikyo
Fenugreek seed	*Trigonella foenum-graecum*	Semen Trigonellae	Hu Lu Ba	Wu Lou Ba	
Fermented Pinellia corm	*Pinellia ternata*	Rhizoma Pinelliae fermentatae	Ban Xia Qu	Bun Ha Chau	
Fermented rice with red yeast	*Oryza sativa* and *Monascus purpureus*	Fructus Oryzae fermentatus cum Monasco	Hong Qu Mi	Hung Ju Mai	
Fermented soybean	*Glycine max*	Semen Glycinis preparatum	Dan Dou Chi	Taam Dau Si	Tantoshi
Feverflower leaf	*Dichroa febrifuga*	Folium Dichroae	Shu Qi	Suk Chat	Shokushitsu
Feverflower root	*Dichroa febrifuga*	Radix Dichroae	Chang Shan	Seung Saan	Joszan
Field lotus herb	*Eclipta prostata, E. alba*	Herba Ecliptae	Han Lian Cao, Mo Han Lian	Hon Lin Chou	Kanrenso
Field thistle herb and root	*Cephalanoplos segetum*	Radix et herba Cephalanoplis	Xiao Ji	Siu Gai	
Fig flower	*Ficus carica*	Flos Fici	Wu Hua Guo	Wu Fa Gwat	
Fimbriate orostachys herb	*Orostachys fimbriatus*	Herba Orostachis	Wa Song	Nga Chung	
Finger lemon flower	*Citrus medica* var. *sarctodactylus*	Flos Citri sarctodactylis	Fo Shou (Gan) Hua	Fut Sao Fa	Bushukan
Finger lemon fruit	*Citrus medica* var. *sarcodactylis*	Fructus Citri medicae	Fo Shou (Gan)	Fut Sau (Gam)	
Fischer's spurge root	*Euphorbia fischeriana*	Radix Euphorbiae fischerianae	Lang Du, Lang Du Da Ji	Long Duk, Long Duk Daai Gik	
Fish airbladder	*Acipenser sinensis, Miichthys* spp	Colla piscis	Yu Biao Jiao	Yu Biu Gaau	
Fish otolith	*Pseudosciaena crocea, P. polyactis, Sciaena schlegeli*	Otozithum Sciaenae	Yu Nao Shi	Yu Nou Sek	
Fishwort herb	*Houttuynia cordata*	Herba Houttuyniae	Yu Xing Cao	Yu Seng Chou	Juyakuso
Fissistigma herb	*Fissistigma glaucescens*	Herba Fissistigmae	Wu Gu Teng	Wu Gwat Tang	
Five additions root bark	*Acanthopanax gracilistylus*	Cortex radicis Acanthopanacis gracilistylus	Wu Jia Pi, Xi Zhu Wu Jia	Ng Ga Pei, Sai Chu Ng Ga	
Five additions root bark	*Acanthopanax gracilistylus, A. spinosus, A. sessiliflorus* and spp	Cortex radicis Acanthopanacis	Wu Jia Pi	Ng Ga Pei	Gokahi
Five-leaf chastetree berry	*Vitex negundo* var. *cannabifolia*	Fructus Viticis negundonis	Mu Jing Zi	Maau Ging Ji	
Five-leaf chastetree leaf	*Vitex negundo* var. *cannabifolia*	Folium Viticis negundonis	Mu Jing Ye	Maau Ging Yip	
Flat milkvetch seed	*Astragalus complanatus* and spp	Semen Astragali complanati	Sha Yuan Zi, Sha Yuan Ji Li	Sa Yun Ji, Sa Yun Jek Lai	Saenshi, Toshitsuri
Flax seed	*Linum usitatissimum*	Semen Lini	Ya Ma Zi	A Ma Ji	

ENGLISH	SCIENTIFIC	PHARMACEUTICAL	MANDARIN	CANTONESE	JAPANESE
Fleshy broomrape herb	*Cistanche salsa* and spp	Herba Cistanchis	Rou Cong Rong	Yuk Chung Yung	Nikujuyo
Flexuose grape root	*Vitis flexuosa*	Radix Vitis flexuosis	Ge Lei Zhi Gen	Got Leui Jap Gan	
Flower (bee) pollen	*Pollen*	Granum floris pollinis	Feng Hua Fen	Fung Fa Fan	
Flowering clematis herb	*Clematis florida*	Herba Clematis floridae	Tie Xian Lian	Ti Chik Lin	
Flowering quince fruit	*Chaenomeles speciosa*	Fructus Chaenomelis speciosae	Mu Gua, Tie Geng Hai Tang	Muk Gwa, Tip Gang Hoi Teng	
Flowery knotweed root	*Polygonum multiflorum*	Radix Polygoni multiflori	He Shou Wu	Ho Sau Wu	Kashuu
Flowery knotweed stem	*Polygonum multiflorum*	Caulis Polygoni multiflori	Ye Jiao Teng	Ye Gou Tang	Yakoto
Full-flowered lysimachia	*Lysimachia congestiflora*	Herba Lysimachiae congestiflorae	Xiao Guo Lu Huang	Siu Gwo Lou Wong	
Flying squirrel dropping	*Trogopterus xanthipes* and spp, *Pteromys volans* and spp	Excrementum Trogopteri seu Pteromi	Wu Ling Zhi	Ng Ling Ji	
Foraha resin	*Calophyllum inophyllum*	Resina Calophylli	Hu Tong Lei	Ng Tung Leui	
Forbes' wild ginger root	*Asarum forbesii*	Rhizoma Asari forbesii	Du Heng	Dou Hang	
Forked glorybower leaf	*Clerodendron trichotomum*	Folium Clerodendronis trichotomi	Chou Wu Tong (Ye)	Chau Ng Tung (Yip)	
Formosa lady' slipper herb	*Cypripedium formosanum*	Herba Cypripedii	Yi Dian Hong	Yut Dim Hung	
Forsythia valve	*Forsythia suspensa*	Fructus Forsythiae	Lian Qiao	Lin Kiu	Rengyo
Foxnut	*Euryale ferox*	Semen Euryalis	Qian Shi	Him Sat	Kenjitsu
Fragrant Solomon's seal root	*Polygonatum odoratum* var. *pluriflorum, P. plurifolium*	Rhizoma Polygonati odorati	Yu Zhu	Yuk Juk	Gyokuchiku
Frangipani flower	*Plumeria rubra* var. *acutifolia*	Flos Plumeriae	Ji Dan Hua	Gai Daan Fa	
Frankincense resin	*Boswellia carterii* and spp.	Resina Boswelliae	Ru Xiang	Yu Heung	Nyuko
French hydrangea flower	*Hydrangea macrophylla*	Flos Hydrangeae	Ba Xian Hua	Baat Sin Fa	
Fresh ginger root	*Zingiber officinalis*	Rhizoma Zingiberis recentis	Sheng Jiang	Saang Geung	Shokyo
Fresh ginger root skin	*Zingiber officinalis*	Rhizoma Zingiberis	(Sheng) Jiang Pi	Saang Geung Pei	
Fresh radish root	*Raphanus sativus*	Radix Raphani recentis	Luo Bo Gen	Lo Ba Gan	
Fresh Rehmannia root	*Rehmannia glutinosa*	Radix Rehmanniae	Sheng Di (Huang)	Sang Dei (Wong)	Shojio
Fresh scallion bulb	*Allium fistulosum*	Bulbus Allii fistulosi	Cong Bai	Chung Baak	
Frogfruit herb	*Lippia nodiflora*	Herba Lippiae	Peng Lai Cao, Ya She Huang	Fung Loi Chou, Ngaap Sit Wong	
Fujian kadsura pepper stem	*Piper hancei* var. *squamiglandiferu m*	Caulis Piperis squamiglandiferi	Hai Feng Teng, Xian Lin Ju	Hoi Fung Tang	

ENGLISH	SCIENTIFIC	PHARMACEUTICAL	MANDARIN	CANTONESE	JAPANESE
Furry agrimony herb	*Agrimonia pilosa* var. *japonica*	Herba Agrimoniae pilosae	Xian He Cao	Sin Hok Chou	Senkakuso
Furry agrimony winter bud	*Agrimonia pilosa* var. *japonica*	Gemma Agrimoniae pilosae	He Cao Ya	Hok Chou Nga	
Furry holly root	*Ilex pubescens*	Radix Ilicis pubescentis	Mao Dong Qing	Mou Dung Ching	Motosei
Gadfly	*Tabanus bivittatus*	Tabanus	Meng Chong	Mung Chung	
Galanga root	*Kaempferia galanga*	Rhizoma Kaempferiae	Shan Nai, Sha Jiang	Saan Noi	
Galangal root	*Alpinia officinarum*	Rhizoma Alpiniae officinari	Gao Liang Jiang	Gou Leung Geung	Koryokyo
Gambir vine twig	*Uncaria rhynchophylla, U. hirsuta, U. macrophylla* and spp	Ramulus et uncus Uncariae	Gou Teng	Ngau Tang, Sheung Ngau (Tang)	Choto
Gamboge resin	*Garcinia morella*	Resina Garciniae	Teng Huang	Tang Wong	
Gan Xi cinnabar sage root	*Salvia przelwalskii*	Radix	Dan Shen, Gan Xi Shu Wei	Daan Sam, Gam Sai Syu Mei	
Garden balsam flower	*Impatiens balsamina*	Flos Impatiensis	Ji Xing Hua	Jek Chin Fa	
Garden balsam herb	*Impatiens balsamina*	Herba Impatientis	Tou Gu Cao	Tau Gwat Chou	
Garden balsam seed	*Impatiens balsamina*	Semen Impatiensis	Ji Xing Zi	Jek Chin Ji	Kyuseishi
Gardenia pod	*Gardenia jasminoides*	Fructus Gardeniae	Zhi Zi Shan Zhi Zi	Ji Ji, Saan Ji Ji	Sanshishi
Garlic bulb	*Allium sativum*	Bulbus Allii sativi	Da Suan	Daai Syun	Taisan
Gendarussa herb	*Gendarussa vulgaris*	Herba Gendarussae	Bo Gu Dan	Bok Gwat Daam	
Geranium herb	*Geranium wilfordii, G. thunbergii*	Herba Geranii	Lao He Cao	Lou Hap Chou	Gennoshio-uko
Gigantic spurge root	*Euphorbia nematocypha*	Radix Euphorbiae nematocyphae	Lang Du, Da Lang Du	Long Duk, Daai Long Duk	
Ginkgo leaf	*Ginkgo biloba*	Folium Ginkgoidis	Yin Xing Ye, Bai Guo Ye	Ngan Hang Yip, Baak Gwo Yip	Ginkyoyo
Ginkgo nut	*Ginkgo biloba*	Fructus Ginkgoidis	Bai Guo, Yin Xing He	Baak Gwo, Ngan Hang Wat	Ginkyo
Giraldi's daphne bark	*Daphne giraldii, D. tangutica, D. retusa*	Cortex Daphnis giraldii	Zu Shi Ma	Jou Si Ma	
Glabrous greenbrier root	*Smilax glabra*	Rhizoma Smilacis glabrae	Tu Fu Ling	Tou Fuk Ling	
Glauber's salt, Pure mirabilite	*Mirabilitum*	Mirabilitum purum	Xuan Ming Fan	San Ming Fun	Bosho
Globe amaranth flower	*Gomphrena globosa*	Flos Gomphrenae	Qian Ri Hong	Jin Yat Hung	
Globe thistle root	*Echinops latifolius, E. gmelinii*	Radix Echinopsis	Lou Lu	Lau Lou	
Glorybower leaf	*Clerodendron inerme*	Folium Clerodendronis inermis	Shui Hu Man	Seui Wu Mun	

ENGLISH	SCIENTIFIC	PHARMACEUTICAL	MANDARIN	CANTONESE	JAPANESE
Glossy privet berry	*Ligustrum japonicum, L. lucidum*	Fructus Ligustri	Nu Zhen Zi	Neui Jing Ji	Joteishi
Goat horn	*Naemorrhedis*	Cornu Naemorrhedis	Shan Yang Jiao	San Yeung Gok	Sanyokaku
Goat's-tit bellflower root	*Codonopsis lanceolata*	Radix Codonopsis lanceolatae	Yang Ju, Shi Ye Shen	Yang Guk, Sei Yip Sam	Yonyu, Shiyojin
Goatear herb	*Inula cappa*	Herba Inulae cappae	Bai Niu Dan, Bai Mian Feng	Baak Ngau Daam	
Gold foil	*Aurum*	Folium Auri	Jin Bo	Gam Bok	
Golden eye-grass root	*Curculigo orchioides*	Rhizoma Curculigonis	Xian Mao	Sin Maau	Sembo
Golden Hair grass	*Pogonatherum crinitum*	Herba Pogonatheri	Bi Zi Cao	Bat Jai Chou	
Golden larch root bark	*Pseudolarix amabilis. P. kaempferi*	Cortex radicis Pseudolaricis	Tu Jing Pi	Tou Ging Pei	
Goldenrod herb	*Solidago virgaurea, S. derurrens*	Herba Solidaginis	Yi Zhi Huang Hua, Liu Zhi Huang	Yat Ji Wong Fa, Lau Ji Wong	
Goldthread root	*Coptis chinensis, C. omeiensis* and spp	Rhizoma Coptis	Huang Lian, Chuan Lian	Wong Lin, Chyun Wong Lin	Oren
Gotu kola leaf	*Centella asiatica*	Folium Centellae	Ji Xue Cao, Peng Da Wan	Jik Syut Chou, Pang Daai Yan	
Great burnet root	*Sanguisorba officinalis*	Radix Sanguisorbae	Di Yu	Dei Yu	Jiyu
Greater galangal berry	*Alpinia galanga*	Fructus Alpiniae Galangae	Hong Dou Kou	Hung Dau Kau	
Greater galangal root	*Alpinia galanga*	Radix Alpiniae galangae	Da Liang Jiang	Daai Leung Geung	
Green bauhinia herb	*Bauhinia paraglauca*	Herba Bauhiniae paraglaucae	Hu Die Cao		
Green birthwort capsule	*Aristolochia contorta, A. debilis*	Fructus Aristolochiae	Ma Dou Ling	Ma Dau Ling	Batorei
Green birthwort root	*Aristolochia contorta, A. debilis*	Radix Aristolochiae	Qing Mu Xiang, Ma Dou Ling Gen	Ching Muk Heung	Seimokko
Green birthwort stem	*Aristolochia contorta, A. debilis*	Caulis Aristolochiae	Tian Xian Teng	Tin Sin Tang	Tensendo
Green vitriol	*Melanteritum*	Melanteritum	Zao Fan, Lu Fan	Jou Faan	
Green-white clerodendron leaf	*Clerodendron cyrtophyllum*	Folium Clerodendronis cyrtophylli	Da Qing Ye	Daai Cheng Yip	
Ground ivy herb	*Glechoma hederacea, G. longituba*	Herba Glechomae	Lian Qian Cao	Ling Chin Chou	
Guangxi turmeric root	*Curcuma kwangsiensis*	Rhizoma Curcumae kwangsiensis	E Zhu, Guang Xi Er Zhu	Ngo Seut, Gwong Sai Ngo Seut	
Guava leaf	*Psidium guajava*	Folium Psidii	Fan Shi Liu Gan Ye	Faan Sek Lau Gon Yip	
Gymnema stem and root	*Gymnema sylvestre* and spp	Caulis et radix Gymnemae	Wu Xue Teng	Mou Heu Tang	
Gynostemma herb	*Gynostemma pentaphyllum*	Herba Gynostemmae	Jiao Gu Lan	Gaan Gu Laam	
Gypsophyla root	*Gypsophyla oldhamiana*	Radix Gypsophylae	Yin Chai Hu	Ngan Chaai Wu	
Gypsum	*Gypsum fibrosum*	Gypsum	Shi Gao	Sek Gou	Sekko

ENGLISH	SCIENTIFIC	PHARMACEUTICAL	MANDARIN	CANTONESE	JAPANESE
Hainan cardamom pod	*Amomum longiligulare*	Fructus Amomi longiligularis	Sha Ren, Hai Nan Sha Ren	Sai Yan, Hoi Naam Sa Yan	
Hairy angelica Root	*Angelica pubescens, A. laxiflora* and spp	Radix Angelicae pubescentis	Du Huo	Duk Wut	Dokkatsu
Hairy beggartick herb	*Bidens pilosa*	Herba Bidentis pilosae	San Ye Gui Zhen Cao	Sam Yip Gwai Jam Chou	
Hairy beggartick herb	*Bidens pilosa* var. *minor* and spp	Herba Bidentis pilosae	Xian Feng Cao	Heun Fung Chou	
Hairy siegesbeckia herb	*Siegesbeckia pubescens, S. orientalis, S. glabrescens*	Herba Siegesbeckiae	Xi Xian Cao	Hei Lim Chou	
Happy tree root bark	*Camptotheca acuminata*	Cortex radicis Camptothecae	Xi Shu	Hei Syu	
Happy tree seed	*Camptotheca acuminata*	Fructus Camptothecae	Xi Shu Guo	Hei Syu Gwo	
Hawksbill turtle shell	*Eretmochelys imbricata*	Plastrum Eretmochelis	Dai Mao	Doi Mou	Taimai
Heart-leaf aralia root	*Aralia cordata*	Radix Araliae cordatae	Tu Dang Gui	Tou Dong Gwai	
Heart-leaf madder root	*Rubia cordifolia*	Radix Rubiae cordifoliae	Qian Cao Gen	Sin Chou Gan	Seisokon
Heart-leaf madder stem	*Rubia cordifolia*	Caulis Rubiae cordifoliae	Lu Gu Dan	Lu Gwat Daan	
Heart-thread lotus leaf	*Andrographis paniculata*	Folium Andrographis	Chuan Xin Lian	Chyun Sam Lin	Senshinren
Hedgehog fungus	*Hericium erinaceus*	Fructification Hericii	Hou Gu		
Hedgehog hide	*Erinaceaus europoeus, Hemichianum dauricus*	Corium Erinacei	Ci Wei Pi	Chi Wai Pei	
Hedysarum root	*Hedysarum polybotrys* and spp	Radix Hedysari polybotris	Huang Qi, Hong Qi	Wong Kei	
Helicteres herb	*Helicteres angustifolia*	Herba Helicteres	Shan Zhi Ma	Saan Ji Ma	
Heliotrope herb	*Heliotropium indicum*	Herba Heliotropi	Da Wei Yao, Er Gou Cao	Daai Mei Yiu	
Helmintho-stachys root	*Helminthostachys zeylanica*	Rhizoma Helminthostachys	Di Wu Song	Dei Ng Gung	
Hematite	*Haematitum*	Haematitum	Dai Zhe Shi	Doi Jyu Sek	Taishaseki
Hemsleya tuber	*Hemsleya amabilis, H. macrosperma* and spp.	Radix Hemsleyae	Xue Dan	Hat Daam	
Hens-and-chickens herb	*Orostachys japonica, O. fimbriatus*	Herba Orostachis	Wa Song	Nga Chung	
Heraclean rising hemp root	*Cimicifuga heracleifolia*	Radix Cimicifugae heracleifoliae	Sheng Ma, Ta San Ye Sheng Ma	Sing Ma, Da Sam Yip Sing Ma	Shoma
Heteroclite kadsura stem	*Kadsura heteroclita*	Caulis Kadsurae heteroclitae	Hai Feng Teng	Hoi Fung Tang	
Hoelen fungus	*Poria cocos*	Sclerotium Poriae	Fu Ling	(Wong) Fuk Ling, Waan Ling	Bukuryo
Hoelen skin	*Poria cocos*	Cortex Poriae	Fu Ling Pi	Wong Ling Pei, Fuk Ling Pei	Bukuryoshi

ENGLISH	SCIENTIFIC	PHARMACEUTICAL	MANDARIN	CANTONESE	JAPANESE
Hoelen spirit	*Poria cocos*	Sclerotium Poriae paradicis	Fu Shen	Pou Fuk Sam	Bukushin
Holly-leaf acanthus root	*Acanthus ilicifolius*	Radix Acanthi ilicifolii	Lao Shu Le	Lou Syu Laak	
Homalomena root	*Homalomena occulta*	Rhizoma Homalomenae	Qian Nian Jian	Chin Nin Gin	Sennenken
Honey	*Apis cerana* and spp	Mel	Feng Mi	Fung Mat	
Honey mushroom	*Armillaria mellea*	Sclerotium Armillariae	Mi Huan Jun		
Honey-preserved jujube berry	*Zizyphus jujuba* var. *inermis*	Fructus Zizyphi jujubae praeparatae	Mi Zao	Mat Jou	
Honey-fried licorice root	*Glycirrhiza uralensis, G. glabra* and spp	Radix Glycirrhizae preparatae	Zhi Gan Cao	Jek Gam Chou	Shakanzo
Honeylocust fruit	*Gleditsia sinensis* and spp.	Semen Gleditsiae	Zao Jiao Zi	Jou Gok Ji	
Honeylocust pod	*Gleditsia sinensis* and spp	Fructus Gleditsiae	Zao Jiao, Zao Jia	Jou Gok, Jou Gaap	Sokaku
Honeylocust spine	*Gleditsia sinensis* and spp	Spina Gleditsiae	Zao Jiao Ci	Jou Gok Chi	Sokakushi
Hookweed root	*Cyathula officinalis,. C. officinalis*	Radix Cyathulae	Chuan Niu Xi	Chyun Ngau Sat	
Hops flower	*Humulus lupulus*	Flos Humuli lupuli	Pi Jiu Hua	Be Jau Fa	
Hornet nest	*Polistes mandarinus, Parapolybia varia*	Nidus Polistis seu Parapolybiae	Lu Feng Fang	Lou Fun Fong	
Horny goat weed leaf	*Epimedium saggitatum, E. macranthum* and spp	Folium Epimedii	Yin Yang Huo, Xian Ling Pi	Yam Yeung Fok, Sin Ling Pei	Inyokaku
Horse bezoar	*Equus caballos*	Calculus Equi	Ma Bao	Ma Bou	
Horsetail herb	*Equisetum hiemale*	Herba Equiseti hiemalis	Mu Zei	Muuk Chaak	Mokuzoku
House lizard	*Gecko chinensis, G. japonicus* and spp	Gecko chinensis	Shou Gong, Bi Hu	Sau Gung, Bik Fu	
Hovenia seed and fruit	*Hovenia dulcis*	Semen et fructus Hoveniae	Zhi Ju Zi	Ji Gwat Ji	
Hubei anemone herb	*Anemone hupehensis*	Herba Anemonis hupehensis	Da Po Wan Hua Hua	Da Po Wun Fa Fa	
Hubei fritillary bulb	*Fritillaria hupehensis*	Bulbus Fritillariae hupehensis	Hu Bei Bei Mu	Wu Bak Bui Mou	
Human placenta	*Homo sapiens*	Placenta Hominis	Zi He Che	Ji Ho Je	Shikasha
Human urine	*Homo sapiens*	Urina Hominis	Ren Niao	Yan Niu	
Human urine sediment	*Homo sapiens*	Sedimen urinae Hominis	Ren Zhong Bai, Qiu Shi Dan	Yan Jung Baak	
Hupei rosewood	*Dalbergia hupeana*	Folium Dalbergiae hupeanae	Tan Gen	Taan Gan	
Hyacinth bean	*Dolichos lablab*	Semen Dolichis	Bai Bian Dou	Baak Bin Dau	Hakuhenzu
Hyacinth bean bud	*Dolichos lablab*	Gemma Dolichis	Bian Dou Hua	Bin Dau Fa	Henzuka
Hyacinth bean capsule	*Dolichos lablab*	Testa Dolichoris	Bian Dou Yi	Bin Dau Yi	
Hyacinth bean root	*Dolichos lablab*	Radix Dolichoris	Rou Dou Gen	Yuk Dau Gan	
Ice vine root	*Cissampelos pareira*	Radix Cissampeli	Xi Sheng Teng	Sak Sang Tang	

ENGLISH	SCIENTIFIC	PHARMACEUTICAL	MANDARIN	CANTONESE	JAPANESE
Immature trifoliate orange fruit	*Poncirus trifoliata*	Fructus Ponciri immaturi	Lu Yi Zhi Qiao, Gou Yuan	Luk Ji Ji Hok, Gau Yun	
India skullcap herb	*Scutellaria indica*	Herba Scutellariae indicae	Han Xin Cao	Hon Sam Chou	
Indian aster herb	*Aster indicus* and spp	Herba Asteris indici	Ma Lan	Ma Laan	
Indian heliotrope herb	*Heliotropium indicum*	Herba Heliotropi	Er Gou Cao	Yi Ngau Chou	
Indian oleander leaf	*Nerium indicum*	Folium Nerii	Jiao Zhu Tao Ye	Gap Juk Tou Yip	
Indian sorrel herb	*Oxalis corniculata*	Herba Oxalis	Cu Jiang Cao	Chou Jeung Chou	
Indian spikenard root	*Nardostachys jatamansi, N. chinensis*	Radix Nardostachis	Gan Song	Gam Chung	
Indigo leaf	*Indigofera tinctoria*	Folium Indigoferae	Mu Lan Ye	Muuk Laam Yip	
Iphigenia bulb	*Iphigenia indica*	Bulbus Iphigeniae	Shan Ci Gu	San Chi Gok	
Iron filing/cinder	*Ferrum*	Frusta Ferrum	Sheng Tie Luo	Sang Tit Lo	
Iron pyrite	*Pyritum rotundum*	Pyritum rotundum	She Han Shi		
Isodon herb	*Isodon japonicus*	Herba Isodonis	Ye Ming Cao	Yin Ming Chou	Enmeiso
Ixeris herb	*Ixeris denticulata*	Herba Ixeris	Mu Dou Hui	Mou Tau Wui	
Ixora root	*Ixora chinensis*	Radox Ixorae	Long Chuan Hua Gen	Lung Syun Fa Gan	
Japanese black Atractylodes root	*Atractylodes japonica*	Rhizoma Atractylodis japonicae	Cang Zhu, Guan Cang Zhu	Chong Seut, Gwan Chong Seut	
Japanese butterbur flower	*Petasites japonicus*	Flos Petasitis	Feng Dou Cai	Fung Dau Choi	
Japanese buttercup root and herb	*Ranunculus japonicus*	Radix et herba Ranunculi japonicae	Mao Gen	Maau Gan	
Japanese catnip herb	*Schizonepeta tenuifolia*	Herba Schizonepetae	Jing Jie	Ging Gaai	Keigai
Japanese climbing fern herb	*Lygodium japonicum*	Herba Lygodii	Hai Jin Sha Teng	Hoi Gam Sa Tang	Kaikinshato
Japanese climbing fern spore	*Lygodium japonicum*	Spora Lygodii	Hai Jin Sha	Hoi Gam Sa	Kaikinsha
Japanese creeper stem	*Parthenocissus tricuspidata*	Caulis Parthenocissi	Pa Shan Hu, Di Jin	Pa San Fu, Dei Gam	
Japanese dock root	*Rumex japonicus, R. nepalensis*	Radix Rumicis japonici	Yang Ti	Yeung Tai	
Japanese dogwood berry	*Cornus officinalis*	Fructus Corni	Shan Zhu Yu, Shan Yu Rou	San Jyu Yu, San Yu Yuk	Sanshuyu
Japanese elder bark	*Sambucus japonicus*	Cortex Sambuci japonici	Lu Ying		Rakutokuda
Japanese flowering fern root	*Osmunda japonica*	Rhizoma Osmundae	Guan Zhong, Zi Qi Guan Zhong	Gwun Jung, Ji Kei Gwun Jung	Tohoku-kanju
Japanese ginseng root	*Panax japonicus*	Radix Panacis japonici	Zhu Jie (Ren) Shen	Juk Jit (Yan) Sam	Tikusetu-ninjin
Japanese green gentian herb	*Swertia japonica, S. pseudochinensis*	Herba Swertiae	Dang Yao Cao	Dong Yeuk Chou	Toyaku

ENGLISH	SCIENTIFIC	PHARMACEUTICAL	MANDARIN	CANTONESE	JAPANESE
Japanese honeysuckle flower	*Lonicera japonica*	Flos Lonicerae japonicae	Jin Yin Hua, Ren Dong Hua	Gam Ngan Fa Yan Dung Fa	Kinginka
Japanese honeysuckle stem and leaf	*Lonicera japonica*	Ramus et folium Lonicerae japonicae	Jin Yin Teng, Ren Dong Teng	Gam Ngan Tang, Yan Dung Tang	
Japanese Knotweed root and leaf	*Polygonum cuspidatum*	Radix et folium Polygoni cuspidati	Hu Zhang	Fu Jeung	
Japanese mahonia root	*Mahonia japonica*	Radix Mahoniae japonicae	Shi Da Gong Lao Gen	Sap Daai Gung Lou Gan	
Japanese masterwort root	*Peucedanum japonicum*	Radix Peucedani japonici	Fang Gui	Fong Kwai	
Japanese milkwort herb	*Polygala japonica*	Herba Polygalae japonicae	Gua Zi Jin	Gwa Ji Gam	
Japanese morning glory seed	*Pharbitis nil, P. purpurea* and spp	Semen Pharbitis	Qian Niu Zi	Hin Ngau Ji	
Japanese pagoda tree bud	*Sophora japonica*	Gemma Sophorae japonicae	Huai (Hua) Mi	Waai (Fa) Mai	
Japanese pagoda tree flower	*Sophora japonica*	Flos Sophorae japonicae	Huai Hua	Waai Fa	
Japanese pagoda tree fruit	*Sophora japonica*	Fructus Sophorae japonicae	Huai Jiao (Zi)	Wai Jiu (Ji)	
Japanese pearlwort herb	*Sagina japonica*	Herba Saginae	Qi Gu Cao	Chat Gu Chou	
Japanese peppervine root	*Ampelopsis japonica*	Radix Ampelopsis	Bai Lian	Baak Lim	Byakuran
Japanese red star lily bulb	*Lilium concolor*	Bulbus Liliii concoloris	Shan Dan	Saan Daan	
Japanese rose flower	*Rosa rugosa*	Flos Rosae rugosae	Mei Gui Hua	Mui Gwai Fa	Maikaika
Japanese rosehip	*Rosa rugosa*	Fructus Rosae rugosae	Mei Gui Zi	Mui Gwai Ji	
Japanese St. John's wort herb	*Hypericum japonicum*	Herba Hyperici japonici	Tian Ji Huang, Di Er Cao	Tin Jik Wong, Dei Yi Chou	
Japanese stemona root	*Stemona japonia*	Radix Stemonae japonicae	Bai Bu, Man Sheng Bai Bu	Baak Bou, Maan Sang Baak Bou	Hyakubu
Japanese stephania stem	*Stephania japonica*	Caulis Stephaniae japonicae	Qian Jin Teng	Chin Gam Tang	
Japanese teasel root	*Dipsacus japonica*	Radix Dipsaci japonicae	Xu Duan	Juk Dyun	Zokudan
Japanese thistle herb	*Cirsium japonicum*	Herba Cirsii japonici	Da Ji	Daai Gai	Taikei
Japanese torreya nut	*Torreya grandis, T. nucifera*	Semen Torreyae	Fei Zi	Fei Ji	
Japanese violet root and herb	*Viola japonica*	Radix et herba Violae japonicae	Li Tou Cao	Lai Tau Chou	
Japanese yam root	*Dioscorea japonica*	Rhizoma Dioscoreae japonicae	Feng Che Er	Fung Che Yi	
Jasmine flower	*Jasminum officinale* var. *grandiflorum*	Flos Jasmini officinalis	Su Xin Hua	Sou Hing Fa	

ENGLISH	SCIENTIFIC	PHARMACEUTICAL	MANDARIN	CANTONESE	JAPANESE
Jasmine sambac flower	*Jasminum sambac*	Flos Jasmini sambacis	Mo Li Hua	Mut Lei Fa	
Jasmine sambac root	*Jasminum sambac*	Radix Jasmini sambacis	Mo Li Gen	Mut Lei Gan	
Java bellflower root	*Campanumoea javanica*	Radix Campanumoeae	Tu Dang Shen	Tou Dong Sam	
Java elder stem and leaf	*Sambucus javanica*	Caulis et folium Sambuci javanici	Shuo Diao	Sok Duk	
Jellyfish tentacle	*Rhopilema esculenta*	Tentaculum Rhopilema	Hai Zhe	Hoi Jit	
Jellywort herb	*Mesona chinensis*	Herba Mesonae	Xian Cao, Liang Fen Cao	Heun Chou, Leung Fan Chou	
Jimsonweed flower	*Datura metel*	Flos Daturae	Yang Jin Hua	Yeung Gam Fa	
Job's-tears root	*Coix lachryma-jobi* var. *Ma-yuen*	Radix Coicis	Yi Yi Gen	Yi Yi Gan	
Job's-tears seed	*Coix lachryma-jobi* var. *Ma-yuen*	Semen Coicis	Yi Yi Ren	San Yi Mai, Yi Yi Yan	Yokuinin
June beetle grub (larva)	*Holotrichia diomphalia*	Holotrichia	Qi Cao	Chai Chou	
Justicia herb	*Justicia procumbens*	Herba Justiciae	Jue Chuang Cao, Shu Wei Huang	Jeuk Chong, Syu Mei Wong	
Kadsura pepper stem	*Piper hancei*	Caulis Piperis hanceis	Hai Feng Teng	Hoi Fung Tang	
Kalopanax bark	*Kalopanax septemlobus*	Cortex Septemlobi	Chuan Tong Pi	Chyun Tung Pei	
Katsumada's galangal seed	*Alpinia katsumadai*	Semen Alpiniae katsumadis	Cao Dou Kou	Chou Dau Kau	Sozuku
Keiskeana mugwort seed	*Artemisia keiskeana*	Fructus Artemisiae keiskeanae	An Lu Zi	Am Leui Ji	
Kelp seaweed	*Laminaria japonica* and spp	Thallus Laminariae	Kun Bu	Gwan Bou	Kombu
Kirilow's ragwort herb	*Senecio kirilowii*	Herba Senecionis kirilowii	Kou She Cao	Gau Sit Chou	
Kite-tail iris root	*Iris tectorum*	Rhizoma Iris tectoris	Yuan Wei	Yun Mei	
Kiwi fruit	*Actinidia chinensis*	Fructus Actinidiae chinensis	Mi Hou Tao, Teng Li	Nei Hau Tou	
Kiwi root	*Actinidia chinensis*	Fructus Actinidiae chinensis	Teng Li Gen	Tang Li Gan	
Knotgrass herb	*Polygonum aviculare*	Herba Polygoni avicularis	Bian Xu	Bin Chuk	Henchiku
Knotty pine wood shaving	*Pinus tabulaeformis, P. massoniana, P. yunnannensis*	Lignum Pini nodi	Song Jie, You Song Jie	Chung Jit, Yao Chung Jit	Shosetsu
Knotweed herb	*Polygonum lapathifolium*	Herba Polygoni lapathifolii	La Liao Cao	La Lou Chou	
Know mother root	*Anemarrhena asphodeloides*	Radix Anemarrhenae	Zhi Mu	Ji Mou	Chimo
Knoxia root	*Knoxia valerianoides*	Radix Knoxiae	Hong Da Ji	Hung Daai Gik	Kogataigeki
Kochia seed	*Kochia scoparia*	Semen Kochiae	Di Fu Zi	Dei Fu Ji	Jibushi
Korean ash bark	*Fraxinus rhynchophyllae, F. bungeana, F. chinensis* and spp	Cortex Fraxini	Qin Pi	Cheun Pei	
Korean raspberry fruit	*Rubus coreanus*	Fructus Rubi coreani	Dao Sheng Gen	Dou Sang Gan	

ENGLISH	SCIENTIFIC	PHARMACEUTICAL	MANDARIN	CANTONESE	JAPANESE
Kudzu flower	*Pueraria lobata, P. omeiensis* and spp	Flos Puerariae	Ge Hua	Got Fa	
Kudzu root	*Pueraria lobata, P. omeiensis* and spp	Radix Puerariae	Ge Gen	Got Gan	Kakkon
Kyllinga herb	*Kyllinga brevifolia*	Herba Kyllingae	Shui Wu Gong	Seui Ng Gung	
Lacquer	*Rhus verniciflua*	Succus exsiccatus Rhudis	Gan Qi	Gon Chat	
Lance-leaf lily bulb	*Lilium lancifolium*	Bulbus Liliii lancifolii	Bai He, Juan Duan	Baak Hap, Gyun Daan	
Lance-leaf liriope root	*Liriope spicata*	Radix Liriopis spicatae	Mai (Men) Dong, Hu Bei Mai Men Dong	Mak (Mun) Dung, Wu Ba Mak Dung	
Large flower wild ginger herb	*Asarum maximum*	Herba Asari maximi	Ta Hua Xi Xin	Daai Fa Sai San	
Large-leaf Callicarpa leaf	*Callicarpa macrophylla*	Folium Callicarpae macrophyllae	Zi Zhu Ye, Ta Ye Zi Zhu	Ji Jyu Yip, Daai Yip Ji Jyu	
Large-leaf gentian root	*Gentiana macrophylla, G. tibetica, G. dahurica* and spp	Radix Gentianae macrophyllae	Qin Jiao	Cheun Gau	Jingyo
Lawn (water) pennywort herb	*Hydrocotyle sibthorpioides*	Herba Hydrocotylis	Tian Hu Sui	Tin Wu Seui	
Leather-leaf mahonia leaf	*Mahonia bealei*	Folium Mahoniae bealei	Shi Da Gong Lao Ye, Kuo Ye Shi Da Gong Lao Ye	Sap Daai Gung Lou Yip, Fut Yip Sap Daai Gung Lou Yip	Judaikoro
Leech	*Hirudo nipponia, Whitmania pigra* and spp	Hirudo seu Whitmania	Shui Zhi	Seui Jik	
Lemongrass herb	*Cymbopogon citratus*	Herba Cymbopogonis	Xiang Mao	Heung Maau	
Leontice root	*Leontice robustum*	Radix Leonticis	Hong Mao Qi	Hung Mou Chat	
Leopard bone	*Panthera*	Os Leopardis	Bao Gu		
Leopard flower herb	*Belamcanda chinensis*	Herba Belamcandae	She Gan Miao	Se Gon Miu	
Leopard flower root	*Belamcanda chinensis*	Rhizoma Belamcandae	She Gan	Se Gon	Yakan
Leucas herb	*Leucas mollissima*	Herba Leuci	Bai Hua Zi Cao, Hu Yao Huang	Baak Fa Ji Chou, Fu Ngao Wong	
Licorice bean herb	*Abrus precatorius, A. cantoniensis*	Herba Abri	Ji Gu Cao	Gai Gwat Chou	
Licorice bean root	*Abrus precatorius, A. cantoniensis*	Radix Abri	Xiang Si Zi Gen	Seung Si Ji Gan	
Lilac daphne flower	*Daphne genkwa*	Flos Daphnis genkwae	Yuan Hua	Yun Fa	Genka
Limnophila herb	*Limnophila sessiliflora*	Herba Limnophilae	Shuang Liu Huang	Seung Lan Wong	
Linden flower	*Tilia cordata*	Flos Tiliae	Duan Shu Hua		
Lindera root	*Lindera strychnifolia*	Radix Linderae	Wu Yao, Tai Wu	Wu Yeuk, Toi Wu	Uyaku
Lindernia herb	*Lindernia anagallis*	Herba Linderniae	Ding Jing Cao	Ding Ging Chou	
Lindley's eupatorium herb	*Eupatorium lindleyanum* var. *tripartum*	Herba Eupatorii	Ye Ma Zhui, Jian Pei Lan	Ye Ma Jeui, Jim Pui Laan	

ENGLISH	SCIENTIFIC	PHARMACEUTICAL	MANDARIN	CANTONESE	JAPANESE
Lindley's eupatorium herb	*Eupatorium lindleyanum*	Herba Eupatorii lindleyani	Cheng Gan Sheng Ma	Ping Gon Sing Ma	
Litharge	*Lithargyrum*	Lithagyrum	Mi Tuo Seng	Muk Toi Sang	Mitsudaso
Lizardtail leaf	*Sauropus rostratus, S. changianus*	Folium Sauropi	Long Li Ye	Lung Lei Yip	
Lock yang stem	*Cynomorium songaricum*	Herba Cynomorii	Suo Yang	Soi Yeung	Sayo
Long pepper fruit spike	*Piper longum*	Fructus Piperis longis	Bi Ba	Bat Pa	Hihatsu
Long yam root	*Dioscorea hypoglauca*	Rhizoma Dioscoreae hypoglaucae	Bi Xie, Fen Bi Xie, Bei Xie	Bei Gaai, Fan Bei Gaai	Hikai
Long-leaf oxknee root	*Achyranthes longifolia*	Radix Achyranthis longae	Tu Niu Xi	Tou Ngau Sat	
Long-stalk kadsura root	*Kadsura longipedunculata*	Radix Kadsurae longipedunculatae	Hong Mu Xiang	Hung Muk Heung	
Longan flower	*Euphoria longan*	Flos Euphoriae	Long Yan Hua	Lung Ngaan Fa	
Longan fruit pulp	*Euphoria longan*	Arillus Euphoriae	Long Yan Rou	Lung Ngaan Yuk	Ryuganniku
Longan fungus	*Fomes applanatus* and *host fruit Euphoria longana*	Sclerotium Fomis	Long Yan Gu	Lung Ngan Gu	
Longan seed	*Euphoria longan*	Semen Euphoriae	Long Yan He	Lung Ngaan Ho	
Loosestrife herb	*Lythrum salicaria*	Herba Lythri salicariae	Qian Cu Cai	Jin Wat Choi	
Loquat fruit	*Eriobotrya japonica*	Fructus Eriobotryae	Pi Pa	Pei Pa	
Loquat leaf	*Eriobotrya japonica*	Folium Eriobotryae	Pi Pa Ye	Pei Pa Yip	Biwayo
Lotus flower	*Nelumbo nucifera*	Flos Nelumbinis	Bai Lian Hua	Baak Lin Fa	
Lotus leaf	*Nelumbo nucifera*	Folium Nelumbinis	He Ye, Lian Lie	Ho Yip	Kayo
Lotus plumule	*Nelumbo nucifera*	Plumula Nelumbinis	Lian Xin	Lin Sam	
Lotus receptacle	*Nelumbo nucifera*	Receptaculum Nelumbinis	Lian Fang	Lin Fong	Renshin
Lotus root node	*Nelumbo nucifera*	Rhizoma nodi Nelumbinis	Ou Jie	Ngau Jit	
Lotus seed	*Nelumbo nucifera*	Semen Nelumbinis	Lian Zi	Lin Ji	Renshi
Lotus seed heart	*Nelumbo nucifera*	Epicentrum seminis Nelumbinis	Lian Zi Xin	Lin Ji Sam	
Lotus stamen	*Nelumbo nucifera*	Stamen Nelumbinis	Lian Xu	Lin Sou	Renshu
Lotus stem	*Nelumbo nucifera*	Ramulus Nelumbinis	Lian Geng	Lin Gang	
Lovage root	*Ligusticum levisticum*	Radix Ligustici levistici	Ou Dang Gui	Au Dong Gwai	
Luffa skin	*Luffa cylindrica, L. acutangula*	Pericarpium Luffae	Si Gua Pi	Si Gwa Pei	
Lunathyrum fern root	*Lunathyrum vegetius, L. giraldii*	Rhizoma Lunathyri	Guan Zhong	Gwun Jung	
Lychee rind	*Litchi chinensis*	Pericarpium Litchis	Li Zhi Ke	Lai Ji Hok	
Lychee seed	*Litchi chinensis*	Semen Litchis	Li Zhi He	Lai Ji Ho	
Lycopodium pollen	*Lycopodium serratum* and spp	Pollen Lycopodii	Qian Cang Ta, Pu Di Wu Gong, Guo Jiang Long, Yu Bai	Jin Jang Tap	

ENGLISH	SCIENTIFIC	PHARMACEUTICAL	MANDARIN	CANTONESE	JAPANESE
Lyonia herb	*Lyonia ovafolia, L. neziki*	Herba Lyoniae	Nan Zhu	Naam Juk	
Lysimachia herb	*Lysimachia sikokiana*	Herba Lysimachiae sikokianae	Ling Ling Xiang	Ling Ling Heung	
Lysimachia root or herb	*Lysimachia capillipes*	Rhizoma seu herba Lysimachiae capillipis	Man Shan Xiang	Mun Sam Heung	
Lysionotus herb	*Lysionotus pauciflora*	Herba Lysinoti	Shi Diao Lan	Sek Diu Laan	
Macaque bezoar	*Macaca mulatta*	Calculus Macacae	Hou Zao	Hau Jou	Koso
Macaque gel	*Macaca mulatta*	Gelatinum Macacae	Hou Jiao	Hao Gaau	
Macrotomia root	*Macrotomia euchroma*	Radix Macrotomiae	Zi Cao	Ji Chou	Shikon
Mactra shell	*Mactra sulcataria*	Concha Mactrae	Ge	Hok	Jiseki
Madagascar periwinkle root and herb	*Catharanthus roseus*	Radix et herba Catharanthi	Chang Chun Hua	Cheung Cheun Fa	
Maggot	*Chrysomyia megacephala* and spp	Larva Chrysomyiae	Wu Gu Chong	Ng Guk Chung	
Magnetite	*Magnetitum*	Magnetitum	Ci Shi	Chi Sek	
Magnolia bark	*Magnolia officinalis, M. biloba, M. obovata*	Cortex Magnoliae officinalis	Hou Po Chuan Po	Hau Pok, Chyun Pok	Koboku
Magnolia flower	*Magnolia officinalis, M. biloba, M. obovata*	Flos Magnoliae officinalis	Hou Po Hua	Hau Pok Fa	Koboka, Kobokuka
Mahonia leaf	*Mahonia fortunei*	Folium Mahoniae fortunei	Shi Da Gong Lao Ye, Xi Ye Shi Da Gong Lao Ye	Gung Lou Yip, Sai Yip Sap Daai Gung Lou Yip	Judaikoro
Maitake, Hen of the woods mushroom	*Grifola frondosa*	Sclerotium Grifolae frondosae			Maitake
Malay padauk wood, Burma rosewood	*Pterocarpus indicus*	Lignum Pterocarpi	Zi Tan	Ji Taan	
Male deer genitals	*Cervus nippon* and spp	Testes et penis Cervi	Hua Lu Shen	Fa Luk Sam	
Male dog genitals	*Canis*	Testes et penis canis	Guang Gou Shen	Gwong Gau Sam	Kujin
Manchurian birthwort stem	*Aristolochia manshuriensis, A. moupinensis*	Caulis Aristolochiae manshuriensis	Guan Mu Tong	Gwaan Muk Tung	
Manchurian lilac bark	*Syringa manchuriensis*	Cortex Syringae	Bao Ma Zi		
Manganite	*Manganitum*	Manganitum	Wu Ming Yi	Mon Ming Yi	
Mango seed	*Mangifera indica*	Semen Mangiferae	Mang Guo Zi	Man Gou Wat	
Marlberry root and herb	*Ardisia japonica*	Radix et herba Ardisiae japonicae	Zi Jin Niu, Jin Niu Cao	Ji Gam Ngau	
Marsdenia herb	*Marsdenia tenacissima*	Herba Marsdeniae	Wu Gu Teng	Wu Gwat Tang	
Mature deer antler	*Cervus nippon* and spp	Cornu Cervi	Lu Jiao	Luk Gok	Rokkaku
Mature deer antler glue	*Cervus nippon* and spp	Colla cornu Cervi	Lu Jiao Jiao	Luk Gok Gaau	Rokkakukyo
Mature deer antler powder	*Cervus nippon* and spp	Cornu Cervi degelatinatum	Lu Jiao Shuang, Rong Mo	Luk Gok Shuen	Rokkakuso
Mature deer tail	*Cervus nippon* and spp	Cauda Cervi	Lu Wei Ba	Luk Mei Ba	

ENGLISH	SCIENTIFIC	PHARMACEUTICAL	MANDARIN	CANTONESE	JAPANESE
Mauritius jujube seed	***Zizyphus mauritiana***	Semen Zizyphi mauritianae	Mian Zao Ren	Mai Jou Yan	
Meadow rue herb	***Thalictrum foliolosum***	Herba Thalictri	Tang Song Cao		
Medicated leaven		Massa fermentata	Shen Qu	Sam Chau	Shinkiku
Medicated leaven tea		Massa fermentata	Shen Qu Cha	Sam Chau Cha	
Melastoma herb	***Melastoma candidum***	Herba Melastomae candidae	Ye Mu Dan	Ye Maau Daan	
Melodinus fruit	***Melodinus suaveolens***	Fructus Melodini	Shan Chen, Qu Tou Ji	Saan Chaang	
Melothria root	***Melothria mederospatana***	Radix Melothriae mederospatanae	Diao Jin Zhong	Diu Gam Jung	
Mercury	***Hydragyrum***	Hydragyrum	Shui Yin	Seui Yin	
Mercury chloride	***Hydragyrum chloratum***	Compositum hydragyrum chloratum	Bai Jiang Dan	Baak Geung Dun	
Mercury oxide (crude)	***Hydragyrum chloratum***	Compositum hydragyrum oxydatum crudum	San Xian Dan	Baak Gong Daan	
Metaplexis fruit	***Metaplexis japonica***	Fructus Metaplexis	Tian Qiang Ke	Tin Cheung Hok	
Metaplexis herb	***Metaplexis japonica***	Herba Metaplexis	Guo Lu Huang, Luo Mo	Lo Mo	
Mezerum flower	***Daphne odora***	Flos Daphnis odorae	Rui Xiang Hua	Seui Heung Fa	
Mica schist	***Chloris***	Chloris	Jin Meng Shi	Gam Mein Sek	
Mica, Chlorite schist	***Mica, Chloritum***	Mica, Chloritum	Meng Shi, Jin Meng Shi	Mung Sek, Ching Mung Sek	
Microcos leaf	***Microcos paniculata***	Folium Microcotis	Bu Zha Ye	Bou Jai Yip	
Microsorium herb	***Microsorium hancockii, M. dilatatum***	Herba Microsorii	Lu Ji Wei	Luk Gai Mei	
Millet grain	***Setaria italica***	Fructus Setariae	Xiao Mi	Suk Mai	
Millettia root	***Millettia philipinensis***	Radix Millettiae philipinensis	Niu Da Li	Ngao Daai Lik	
Millettia root and stem	***Millettia dielsiana, M. reticulata, M. nitida***	Radix et caulis Millettiae dielsianae	Ji Xue Teng	Gai Yut Tang	Keiketto
Millettia root and stem	***Millettia reticulata***	Radix et caulis Millettiae reticulatae	Ji Xue Teng, Kun Ming Ji Xue Teng	Kwan Ming Gai Yut Tang	
Mimosa bark	***Albizzia julibrissin, A. lebbak*** and spp	Cortex Albizziae	He Huan Pi	Hap Fun Pei	Gokanhi
Mimosa flower	***Albizzia julibrissin, A. lebbek*** and spp	Flos Albizziae	He Huan Hua	Hap Fun Fa	Gokanka
Mimosa herb	***Mimosa pudica***	Herba mimosae pudicae	Han Xiu Cao	Ham Sau Chou	
Mioga ginger root	***Zingiber mioga***	Rhizoma Zingiberis miogae	Rang He	Yeung Ho	
Mirabilite	***Mirabilitum***	Mirabilitum	Mang Xiao	Mong Seu	Bosho
Miscanthus herb	***Miscanthus sinensis***	Herba Miscanthi	Mang Jing	Mong Hong	
Mock strawberry herb	***Duchesnea indica***	Herba Duchesneae	She Mei	Se Mui	

ENGLISH	SCIENTIFIC	PHARMACEUTICAL	MANDARIN	CANTONESE	JAPANESE
Moellendorf's spikemoss herb	*Selaginella moellendorfii*	Herba Selaginella moellendorfii	Jiang Nan Juan Bai	Gong Naam Kyun Paap	
Moghania root	*Moghania macrophylla, M. philippinensis*	Radix Moghaniae	Yi Tiao Gen	Yat Tiu Gan	
Mongolian dandelion root and herb	*Taraxacum mongolicum*	Radix et herba Taraxaci	Pu Gong Ying	Pou Gung Ying	Hokoei
Mongolian thyme herb	*Thymus mongolicus*	Herba Thymi mongolici	Di Jiao	Dei Jiu	
Moonseason rose bud	*Rosa chinensis*	Gemma Rosae chinensis	Yue Ji Hua	Yut Gwai Fa	Gekkika
Moonseason rose root	*Rosa chinensis*	Radix Rosae chinensis	Yue Ji Gen	Yut Gwai Gan	
Morinda root	*Morinda officinalis*	Radix Morindae	Ba Ji Tian	Ba Gik Tin	Hagekiten
Mother of pearl shell	*Pteria margaritifera* and spp	Concha Pteriae	Zhen Zhu Mu	Chan Ju Mou	
Mountain clematis stem	*Clematis montana, C. armandii*	Caulis Clematis montanae	Chuan Mu Tong	Chyun Muk Tong	
Mountain licorice stem and leaf	*Mussaenda pubescens, M. parviflora*	Caulis et folium Mussaendae	Shan Gan Cao	Saan Gam Chou	
Mountain yam root	*Dioscorea opposita, D. batatas*	Rhizoma Dioscoreae oppositae	Shan Yao Shu Yu	Wai Saan, Saan Yeuk	Sanyaku
Mucuna root and stem	*Mucuna birdwoodiana, M. sempervirens*	Radix et caulis Mucunae	Ji Xue Teng, Chang Chun You Ma Teng	Gei Hat Tang, Seung Cheun Yao Ma Tang	
Mulberry fruit	*Morus alba*	Fructus Mori	Sang Shen (Zi)	Song Sam (Ji)	Sojin
Mulberry leaf	*Morus alba*	Folium Mori	Sang Ye	Song Yip	Soyo
Mulberry root bark	*Morus alba*	Cortex radicis Mori	Sang Bai Pi	Song Baak Pei	Sohakuhi
Mulberry twig	*Morus alba*	Ramulus Mori	Sang Zhi	Song Ji	Soshi
Multibanded krait	*Agkistrodon acutus* and *Bungarus multicinctus*	Agkistrodon seu Bungarus	Bai Hua She	Baak Fa Se	Hakkada
Mung bean	*Phaseolus radiatum*	Semen Phaseoli radiati	Lu Dou	Luk Dau	Ryokuzu
Mung bean flower	*Phaseolus mungo*	Flos Phaseoli	Lu Dou Hua	Luk Dau Fa	
Mung bean husk	*Phaseolus radiatum*	Testa Phaseoli radiatae	Lu Dou Yi	Luk Dau Yip	
Muscovite	*Muscovitum*	Muscovitum	Yun Mu Shi	Wan Mou Sek	
Musk	*Moschus berezovskii* and spp	Secretio Moschi	She Xiang	Se Heung	Jako
Musk mallow seed	*Malva verticillata*	Semen Malvae	Dong Kui Zi	Dung Kwai Ji	
Mussel	*Mytilus crassitesta* and spp	Mytilus	Dan Cai	Daam Choi	
Myrobalan fruit	*Terminalia chebula* and var.	Fructus Terminaliae	He Zi (Rou)	Ho Ji (Yuk)	Kashi
Myrrh resin	*Commiphora myrrha*	Resina Commiphorae	Mo Yao	Mut Yeuk	Motsuyaku
Nasturtium herb	*Rorippa montana, R. indica*	Herba Rorippae	Han Cai	Hon Choi	

ENGLISH	SCIENTIFIC	PHARMACEUTICAL	MANDARIN	CANTONESE	JAPANESE
Native peppervine root	*Melothria heterophylla*	Radix Melothriae heterolphyllae	Tu Bai Lian	Taou Baak Lin	
Negundo chastetree berry	*Vitex negundo*	Fructus Viticis negundonis	Huang Jing Zi	Wong Ging Ji	
Nepalese ivy leaf	*Hedera nepalensis* var. *sinensis*	Herba Hederae nepalensis	Chang Chun Teng	Seung Cheun Tang	
Nervilia herb	*Nervilia fordii*	Herba Nerviliae	Qing Tian Kui	Ching Tin Kwai	
Nippon yam root	*Dioscorea nipponica*	Rhizoma Dioscoreae nipponicae	Chuan Shan Long	Chyun Saan Lung	
North China iris seed	*Iris pallasii* var. *chinensis*	Semen Iris pallasii	Ma Lin Zi	Ma Leun Ji	
Northern sandroot	*Glehnia littoralis*	Radix Glehniae	Bei Sha Shen	Mai Sa Sam	Shajin
Northern wild ginger root	*Asarum heterotropoides*	Herba Asari heterotropoidis	Xi Xin, Bei Xi Xin	Bak Sai San	
Northern wormwood herb	*Artemisia scoparia*	Herba Artemisiae scopariae	Bei Yin Chen	Bak Yan Chan	
Notopterygium root	*Notopterygium incisum, N. forbesii, N. francherii*	Rhizoma et radix Notopterigii	Qiang Huo	Geung Wut	Kyokatsu
Nutmeg seed	*Myristica fragrans*	Semen Myristicae	Rou Dou Kou	Yuk Dau Kau	Nikuzuku
Oak fruit	*Quercus acutissima*	Fructus Querci acutissimae	Xiang Shi	Jeung Sat	
Oak gall	*Quercus infectoria*	Galla Querci	Mo Shi Zi	Mut Sik Ji	
Oak leaf	*Quercus salicina, Q. myrsinaefolium*	Folium Querci	Zhu Zi Ye	Jyu Ji	Urajirokashi
Oak twig and bark	*Quercus dentata, Q. acutissima*	Ramulus et cortex Querci	Pu Suo	Pok Sau	Bokuso
Oldham's eleagnus root	*Eleagnus oldhamii*	Radix Eleagni oldhamii	Yi Wu Gen	Yi Ng Gan	
Onosma root	*Onosma paniculatum*	Radix Onosmae	Zi Cao	Ji Chou	
Opium poppy husk	*Papaver somniferum*	Pericarpium Papaveris	Ying Su Ke	Ngang Suk Hok	Ozokukoku
Orchid tree bark	*Bauhinia variegata*	Cortex Bauhiniae variegatae	Lao Bai Hua Pi	Lou Baak Fa Pei	
Orchid-grass herb	*Eupatorium fortunei*	Herba Eupatorii fortunei	Pei Lan	Pui Laan	Haikan
Oregano herb	*Origanum vulgare*	Herba Origani vulgaris	Tu Yin Chen, Tu Xiang Ru	Tou Gam Chan, Tou Heung Yu	
Oriental arborvitae berry	*Biota orientalis*	Semen Biotae orientalis	Bai Zi Ren	(Baak) Ji Yan	Hakushinin
Oriental arborvitae tip	*Biota orientalis*	Cacumen Biotae orientalis	Ce Bai Ye	Jak Paak Yip	Sokuhakuyo
Oriental hammock fern root	*Blechnum orientale*	Rhizoma Blechni	Guan Zhong, Wu Mao Jue Guan Zhong, Dong Fang Wu Mao Jue Ye	Gwun Jung, Dung Fong Wu Mou Kyut Yip	Kanju
Oriental paperbush flower	*Edgeworthiae chrysantha*	Flos Edgeworthiae chrysanthae	Jie Xiang Hua, Meng Hua	Git Heung Fa, Mung Fa	

ENGLISH	SCIENTIFIC	PHARMACEUTICAL	MANDARIN	CANTONESE	JAPANESE
Orobanche herb	*Orobanche caerulescens* and spp	Herba Orobanchis	Lie Dang	Lit Dong	
Oroxylum seed	*Oroxylum indicum*	Semen Oroxyli	Mu Hu Die	Muk Wu Dip	Mokukocho
Orpiment	*Orpimentum*	Orpimentum	Ci Huang, Xiong Huang	Chi Wong	
Orthosiphon herb	*Clerodendranthus spicatus*	Herba Clerodendranthi	Mao Xu Cao	Maau Sao Chou	
Orthosiphon herb	*Orthosiphon aristatus, O. grandiflorus*	Herba Orthosiphonis	Mao Xu Kao, Hua Shi Cao	Maau Sou Chou, Fa Sek Chou	
Osmanthus twig bark	*Osmanthus fragrans*	Cortex ramuli Osmanthi	Gui Hua Pi	Gwai Fa Pei	
Ostrich-feather fern root	*Matteucia struthiopteris*	Rhizoma Matteuciae	Guan Zhong, Jia Guo Jue Guan Zhong	Gwun Jung, Ying Gwo Kyut Gwun Jung	
Otter liver	*Lutra lutra*	Jecur Lutrae	Ta Gan	Taap Gon	
Ox gallbladder	*Bos taurus domesticus, Bubalis bubalis*	Vesica fellae Bovis	Niu Dan	Ngau Daam	Gyutan
Ox gallstone	*Bos taurus domesticus, Bubalis bubalis*	Calculus Bovis	Niu Huang	Ngau Wong	Goo
Ox hide	*Bos taurus domesticus, Bubalis bubalis*	Corium Bovis	Niu Pi	Ngau Pei	
Oyster shell	*Ostrea gigas* and spp	Concha Ostreae	Mu Li	Mou Lai	Borei
Pale-flower fritillary bulb	*Fritillaria pallidiflora*	Bulbus Fritillariae pallidiflorae	Yi Bei Mu	Yi Bui Mou	
Pangolin scale	*Manis pentadactyla*	Squama manis	Chuan Shan Jia	Chyun San Gaap	Senzanko
Panicled clerodendron root	*Clerodendron paniculatum*	Radix Clerodendronis paniculati	Bai Long Chuan Gen	Baak Lung Chyun Gan	
Panicled dogbane root and herb	*Cynanchum paniculatum*	Radix et herba Cynanchi paniculati	Xu Chang Qing, Liao Diao Zhu	Cheui Cheung Hing	
Paniculate swallowwort herb	*Pycnostelma paniculatum*	Herba Pycnostelmae	Shan Diao Zhu, Xu Chang Jing	Cheui Cheung Hing	
Paper mulberry fruit	*Broussonetia papyrifera*	Fructus Broussonetiae	Chu Shi Zi	Chyu Sat Ji	
Paris root	*Paris polyphylla, P. chinensis, P. formosana* and var.	Rhizoma Paris	Qi Ye Yi Zhi Hua, Zao Xiu	Chak Yip Jek Ji Fa, Sat Yau	Kenjin
Parmelia thallus	*Parmelia tinctorum, P. reticulata*	Thallus Parmeliae	Shi Er		
Patchouli herb	*Pogostemon cablin*	Herba Pogostemis	Guang Huo Xiang	Gwong Fok Heung	
Patrinia herb and root	*Patrinia scabiosaefolia, P. villosa*	Herba et rhizoma Patriniae	Bai Jiang Cao	Baai Jeung Chou	Haishoso
Patrinium violet herb	*Viola patrinii*	Herba Violae patriniae	Hua Tou Cao	Wa Tau Chou	
Paulownia flower	*Paulownia tomentosa*	Flos Paulowniae	Pao Tong Hua	Pau Tung Fa	
Pavetta herb	*Pavetta hongkongiensis*	Herba Pavettae	Man Tian Xing	Mun Tin Sing, Daai Sa Yip	

ENGLISH	SCIENTIFIC	PHARMACEUTICAL	MANDARIN	CANTONESE	JAPANESE
Peach kernel	*Prunus persica* and spp	Semen Pruni persicae	Tao Ren	Tou Yan	Tonin
Peanut skin	*Arachis hypogaea*	Pericarpium Arachis	Hua Sheng Pi	Fa Sang Pei	Kashohi
Pearl	*Pteria margaritiferae*	Fructus conchae Pteriae	Zhen Zhu	Chan Ju	Shinju
Pearl ginseng root	*Panax major, P. repens*	Radix Panacis majoris	Zhu Er Shen	Ju Yi Sam	
Pedatisect pinellia corm	*Pinellia pedatisecta*	Rhizoma Pinelliae pedatisectae	Zhang Ye Ban Xia, Wu Zhang Nan Xing	Jeung Yip Bun Ha, Fu Jeung Lam Sing	
Peeled Tripterygium root	*Tripterygium hypoglaucum*	Radix Tripterygii hypoglauci decorticati	Kun Ming Shan Hai Tang, Diao Mao Cao	Kwan Ming Saan Hoi Tong	
Peking spurge root	*Euphorbia pekinensis*	Radix Euphorbiae pekinensis	Jing Da Ji	Ging Daai Gik	Taigeki
Peregrine speedwell herb and root	*Veronica peregrina*	Herba et radix Veronicae	Jie Gu Xian Tao	Jip Gwat Sin Tou	
Perennial lespedeza herb	*Lespedeza cuneata*	Herba Lespedezae	Ye Guan Men	Ye Gwaan Mun	
Perfoliate knotweed herb	*Polygonum perfoliatum*	Herba Polygoni perfoliati	Gang Ban Gui, Guan Ye Liao	Gong Bun Gwai, Gwan Yip Lou	
Perilla leaf	*Perilla frutescens*	Folium Perillae	Zi Su Ye	Sou Yip	Shisoyo
Perilla seed	*Perilla frutescens*	Fructus Perillae	Zi Su Zi	Sou Ji	Soshi
Perilla stem	*Perilla frutescens*	Ramulus Perillae	Zi Su Geng	Sou Gan	
Persimmon calyx	*Diospyros kaki*	Calyx Diospyri	Shi Di	Chi Dai	Shitei
Persimmon frost	*Diospyros kaki*	Saccharum Diospyris	Shi Bing Shuang	Chi Beng Sheung	
Persimmon frosted fruit	*Diospyros kaki*	Fructus Diospyri	Shi Shuang Bing	Chi Shuen Bing	
Persimmon leaf	*Diospyros kaki*	Folium Diospyri	Shi Ye	Chi Yip	
Peru lantern herb	*Physalis peruviana*	Herba Physalis peruvianae	Deng Long Cao	Dang Lung Chou	
Peruvian thevetia leaf and seed	*Thevetia peruviana*	Folium et semen Thevetiae	Huang Hua Jia Zhu Tao (Ye)	Wong Fa Gaap Juk Tou (Yip)	
Phlogopite, Red mica	*Phlogopitum*	Phlogopitum	Jin Meng Shi	Gam Mung Sek	
Phoenix-tail fern	*Pteris multifida* and spp	Herba Pterii	Feng Wei Cao	Fung Mei Chou	
Photinia stem or leaf	*Photinia serrulata*	Caulis et folium Photiniae	Shi Nan Teng, Shi Nan Ye	Sek Naam Tang, Sek Naam Yip	
Picrorrhiza root	*Picrorrhiza kurroa*	Radix Picrorrhizae	Hu Huang Lian	Wu Wong Lin	Kooren
Pig gallbladder	*Sus scrofa domestica*	Fel Suidis	Zhu Dan	Ju Daam	
Pigeon pea seed	*Cajanus cajan*	Semen Cajani	Mu Dou Zi	Muk Dau Ji	
Pigeon-pea root	*Sophora subprostata*	Radix Sophorae subprostatae	Shan Dou Gen	Saan Dau Gan	
Pine kernel	*Pinus tabulaeformis* and spp	Semen Pini	Song Zi	Chung Ji	
Pine pollen	*Pinus massoniana, P. tabulaeformis* and spp	Pollen Pini	Song Hua Fen	Chung Fa Fan	

ENGLISH	SCIENTIFIC	PHARMACEUTICAL	MANDARIN	CANTONESE	JAPANESE
Pine resin	*Pinus massoniana, P. tabulaeformis* and spp, *Larix* spp	Resina Pini preparatae, Colophonium	Song Xiang	Chung Heung	
Pipefish	*Solenognathus* spp., *Syngnathoides biaculeatus*	Solenognathus	Hai Long	Hoi Lung	
Pipewort herb	*Eriocaulon buergerianum, E. sieboldianum*	Herba Eriocaulonis	Gu Jing Cao	Guk Jing Chou	Kokuseiso
Pipewort seed	*Eriocaulon buergerianum, E. sieboldianum*	Fructus Eriocaulonis	Gu Jing Zi	Guk Jing Ji	
Pistachio leaf	*Pistacia chinensis*	Folium Pistaciae	Huang Lian Ya	Wong Lin Nga	
Pitcher plant herb	*Nepenthes mirabilis*	Herba Nepenthis	Zhu Long Cao	Jyu Lung Chou	
Pittosporum root	*Pittosporum pentandrum*	Radix Pittospori	Qi Li Xiang	Chat Lei Heung	
Plebeian sage herb and root	*Salvia plebeia*	Herba et radix Salviae plebeiae	Li Zhi Cao	Lai Jik Chou	
Pleianth dysosma root	*Dysosma pleiantha*	Rhizoma Dysosmae pleianthae	Ba Jiao Lian	Baat Gok Lin	
Pleianth podophyllum root	*Podophyllum pleianthum*	Rhizoma Podophylli pleianthi	Ba Jiao Lian	Ba Gok Lin	
Pleione corm	*Pleione bulbocodioides*	Rhizoma Pleionis	Shan Ci Gu	Saan Chi Gu	
Plum poppy herb	*Macleaya cordata*	Herba Macleayae	Bo Luo Hui	Bok Lok Wui	
Plum tree bark	*Prunus jamasakura, P. yedoensis*	Cortex Pruni	Ying Pi	Ying Pei	Ouhi
Plum yew twig and leaf	*Cephalotaxus sinensis*	Ramulus et folium Cephalotaxi sinensis	Tu Xiang Fei	Tou Heung Fei	
Polyanth rose root	*Rosa polyantha* and spp.	Radix Rosae polyanthae	Qiang Wei Gen		
Polypody herb	*Polypodium hastatum*	Herba Polypodii	Qi Xing Cao	Chat Sing Chou	
Pomegranate husk	*Punica granatum*	Pericarpium Punicae	Shi Liu Pi	Sek Lau Pei	Sekiryuhi
Pomegranate root bark	*Punica granatum*	Cortex Radicis Punicae	Shi Liu Gen Pi	Sek Lau Gan Pei	Sekiryu-kombi
Pomelo leaf	*Citrus grandis*	Folium Citri grandi immaturi	You Ye	Yau Yip	
Pomelo rind	*Citrus grandis*	Pericarpium Citri grandi immaturi	You Pi (Ju Hong), Hua Ju Hong	Yau Pei (Gwat Hung), Fa Gwat Hung	
Pomelo seed	*Citrus grandis*	Semen Citri grandi immaturi	You He	Yau Hat	
Poplar resin	*Populus euphratica* and spp	Resina Populi	Hu Tong Lei	Wu Tung Leui	
Porphyra herb	*Porphyra tenera*	Herba Porphyrae	Zi Cai	Ji Choi	
Potassium nitrate	*Niter*	Niter	Xiao Shi	Siu Sek	Shoseki
Potato yam tuber	*Dioscorea bulbifera*	Rhizoma Dioscoreae bulbiferae	Huang Yao Zi	Wong Yeuk Ji	Oyakushi

ENGLISH	SCIENTIFIC	PHARMACEUTICAL	MANDARIN	CANTONESE	JAPANESE
Powdered dragon arum corm with ox bile	*Arisaema consanguineum, A. amurense* and spp	Pulvis Arisaemae cum felle Bovis	Dan Nan Xing	Daam Naam Sing	Tannansho
Praying mantis egg case	*Paratenodera sinensis* and *augustipennis, Hierodula patellifera, Mantis religiosa, Statilia maculata*	Paratenodera seu Hierodula seu Mantis seu Statilia	Sang Piao Xiao	Song Piu Seu	
Prepared alum	*Alumen*	Alumen praeparatum	Ku Fan	Gu Faan	
Prepared dragon arum corm	*Arisaema consanguineum, A. amurense* and spp	Rhizoma Arisaemae preparatae	Tian Nan Xing, Zhi Nan Xing	Tin Naam Sing, Jek Naam Sing	
Prepared flagellate typhonium root	*Typhonium flagelliforme*	Rhizoma Typhonii flagelliformis preparata	Shui Ban Xia	Seui Bun Ha	
Prepared giant typhonium root	*Typhonium giganteum*	Rhizoma Typhonii gigantei preparata	Bai Fu Zi, Yu Bai Fu	Baak Fu Ji	Byakubushi
Prepared Korean aconite root	*Aconitum coreanum*	Rhizoma Aconiti coreani	Bai Fu Zi, Guan Bai Fu	Baak Fu Ji, Gwan Baak Fu Ji	
Prepared pinellia corm	*Pinellia ternata*	Rhizoma Pinelliae ternatae preparatae	Ban Xia Fa Ban Xia	Bun Ha, Faat Bun Ha	Hange, Kohange
Prepared Rehmannia root	*Rehmannia glutinosa*	Radix Rehmanniae preparatae	Shu Di (Huang)	Suk Dei (Wong)	Jukujio
Prepared Sichuan aconite root	*Aconitum carmichaeli*	Radix lateralis Aconiti carmichaeli praeparatae	Fu Zi	Fu Ji	Bushi
Prepared Sichuan aconite root tuber	*Aconitum carmichaeli*	Radix Aconiti carmichaeli	Chuan Wu Wu Tou	Chyun Wu, Wu Tau	Uzu
Prepared vomit nut	*Strychnos pierrana, S. nux-vomica* and spp	Semen Strychnotis preparatae	(Zhi) Ma Qian Zi	Ma Chin Ji	Basenshi
Prepared wild aconite root tuber	*Aconitum chinense, A. kusnezoffii* and spp	Radix Aconiti chinensis	Cao Wu, Bei Wu Tou	Chou Wu, Mai Wu Tau	So-u
Prickly ash berry	*Zanthoxylum planispinum*	Fructus Zanthoxyli planispini	Zhu Ye Jiao	Juk Yip Jiu	
Prickly ash root	*Zanthoxylum avicennae*	Radix Zanthoxyli avicennae	Niao Bu Su, Bai Ma Niao	Niu Bat Suk	
Prickly nightshade fruit	*Solanum xanthocarpum*	Herba Solani xanthocarpi	Huang Shui Qie	Wong Seui Ke	
Prickly pear root	*Opuntia dillenii* and spp	Rhizoma Opuntiae	Xian Ren Zhang	Sin Yan Jeung	
Prickly spurge herb	*Euphorbia milii*	Herba Euphorbiae milii	Ci Peng Hua	Chi Fung Fa	
Prime white root	*Cynanchum stauntoni, C. glaucescens*	Radix et rhizoma Cynanchi stauntoni	Bai Qian	Baak Chin	Byakuzen
Prince ginseng root	*Pseudostellaria heterophylla*	Radix Pseudostellariae	Tai Zi Shen	Yi Sam, Taai Ji Sam	Taishijin
Prince's feather berry	*Polygonum orientale*	Fructus Polygoni orientalis	Shui Tong Hua Zi	Seui Tung Fa Ji	

ENGLISH	SCIENTIFIC	PHARMACEUTICAL	MANDARIN	CANTONESE	JAPANESE
Prince's feather herb	*Polygonum orientale*	Herba Polygoni orientalis	Shui Tong Hua Cao Hong Cao	Seui Tung Fa Chou Hung Chou	
Prinsepia seed	*Prinsepia uniflora*	Semen Prinsepiae	Rui Ren (Rou)	Seui Yan (Yuk)	
Prolific spurge root	*Euphorbia prolifera*	Radix Euphorbiae proliferae	Lang Du, Ji Chang Lang Du	Long Duk, Gai Cheung Long Duk	
Protohermes larva	*Protohermes grandis*	Vermiculus Protohermis	Sun Tai Lang Chun	Syun Taai Long Chung	Magotaro-mushi
Proud pink herb	*Dianthus superbus, D. chinensis*	Herba Dianthi	Qu Mai	Geui Mak	Kubaku
Pseudoginseng flower	*Panax notoginseng*	Flos Panacis notoginsengis	San Qi Hua	Saam Chat Fa	Sanshishika
Pseudoginseng root	*Panax notoginseng*	Radix Panacis notoginsengis	San Qi Tian Qi	Saam Chat Tin Chat	Sanshishi
Pterospermum root	*Pterospermum heterophyllum*	Radix Pterospermi	Ban Feng He Gen	Bun Fung Ho Gan	
Puffball mushroom	*Lasiosphaera fenslii* and spp, *Calvatia lilacina, C. fenzlii, C. gigantea*	Sclerotium Lasiosphaerae seu Calvatiae	Ma Bo	Ma But	Babotsu
Pumice	*Pumus*	Lapis Pumicis	Fu Hai Shi	Fau Hoi Sek	Kaifuseki
Purple willow twig	*Salix purpurea*	Ramulus Salicis purpureae	Shui Yang Zhi	Seui Yeung Ji	
Puqi fritillary bulb	*Fritillaria puqiensis*	Bulbus Fritillariae puqiensis	Hu Bei Bei Mu, Pu Qi Bei Mu	Wu Bak Bui Mou, Pou Kei Bui Mou	
Purple fluorite	*Fluoritum*	Fluoritum	Zi Shi Ying	Ji Sek Ying	
Purple groomwell flower	*Lithospermum erythrorhizon*	Flos Lithospermi	Zi Cao Rong	Ji Chou Yan	
Purple groomwell root	*Lithospermum erythrorhizon*	Radix Lithospermi	Zi Cao	Ji Chou	Shikon
Purple nutsedge root	*Cyperus rotundus*	Rhizoma Cyperi	Xiang Fu	Heung Fu	Kobushi
Purslane herb	*Portulacca oleracea*	Herba Portulaccae	Ma Chi Xian	Ma Chi Yin	Bashiken
Pyrite	*Pyritum*	Pyritum	Zi Ran Tong	Ji Yin Tung	Shizendo
Pyrolusite	*Pyrolusitum*	Pyrolusitum	Wu Ming Zi	Mou Ming Ji	
Quassiawood bark	*Picrasma quassioides*	Cortex Picrassiae	Ku Shu Pi	Fu Syu Pei	
Quassiawood twig and leaf	*Picrasma quassioides*	Ramulus et folium Picrasmae	Ku (Shu) Mu	Fu (Syu) Muk	
Quick-fried ginger root	*Zingiber officinalis*	Rhizoma Zingiberis	Pao Jiang	Bou Geung	Hokyo
Quinate chasteberry root	*Vitex quinata*	Radix Viticis quinatae	Pu Jiang Gen	Pou Geung Gan	
Rabbit dropping	*Lepus* spp	Excrementum Lepi	Wang Yue Sha	Mong Yut Sa	
Rabdosia herb	*Rabdosia rubescens* and spp	Herba Rabdosiae	Dong Ling Cao	Dun Ling Chou	
Racemose elecampane root	*Inula racemosa*	Radix Inulae racemosae	Tu Mu Xiang, Zong Zhuang Tu Mu Xiang	Tou Muk Heung, Chung Ching Tou Muk Heung	
Radish leaf	*Raphanus sativus*	Folium Raphani	Luo Bo Ye	Lo Ba Yip	
Radish root	*Raphanus sativus*	Radix Raphani	Di Gu Luo		
Radish seed	*Raphanus sativus*	Semen Raphani	Lai Fu Zi	Loi Fuk Ji	

ENGLISH	SCIENTIFIC	PHARMACEUTICAL	MANDARIN	CANTONESE	JAPANESE
Rambutan fruit	*Nephelium lappaceum*	Fructus Nephelii	Shao Zi	Siu Ji	
Ramie root	*Boehmeria nivea*	Radix Boehmeriae	Zhu Ma Gen	Chyu Ma Gan	
Ramose horsetail herb	*Equisetum ramosissimum*	Herba Equiseti ramosissimi	Bi Tong Cao	Bat Tung Chou	
Rangoon creeper nut	*Quisqualis indica*	Fructus Quisqualis	Shi Jun Zi	Si Gwan Ji	Shikunshi
Rattlesnake orchid root	*Pholidota chinensis*	Radix Pholidotae	Shi Xian Tao Gen	Sek Sin Tou Gan	
Rauvolfia root	*Rauvolfia verticillata, R. yunnanensis, R. latifrons, R. serpentina* and spp	Radix Rauvolfiae	Luo Fu Mu	Lo Fu Mou	
Raw pinellia corm	*Pinellia ternata*	Rhizoma pinelliae ternatae	Sheng Ban Xia	Sang Bun Ha, So Bun Ha	Shohange
Realgar	*Realgar*	Realgar	Xiong Huang	Song Wong	Yuo
Red bayberry bark	*Myrica rubra*	Cortex Myricae rubrae	Yang Mei Pi	Yeung Miu Pei	
Red cicada	*Huechys sanguinea, H, philaemata*	Huechys	Hong Niang Zi	Hung Leung Ji	
Red citrus outer rind	*Citrus grandis* and spp	Exocarpium rubrum Citri	Ju Hong (Pi), Hua Ju Pi	Gwat Heung (Pei), Fa Gwat Pei	
Red cured Asian ginseng root	*Panax ginseng*	Radix Panacis ginsengis praeparatae	Hong Ren Shen	Hung Yan Sam	Koninjin
Red gypsum	*Gypsum rubrum*	Gypsum rubrum	Han Shui Shi, Hong Shi Gao	Hon Seui Sek, Hung Sek Gau	
Red hoelen	*Poria cocos*	Sclerotium Poriae rubrae	Chi Fu Ling	Chek Fuk Ling	Sekibikuryo
Red jujube berry	*Zizyphus jujuba* var. *inermis*	Fructus Zizyphi jujubae	Hong Zao	Hung Jou	Koso
Red kaolin	*Halloysitum rubrum*	Halloysitum	Chi Shi Zhi	Chek Sek Chi	Shakusek-ishi
Red lead oxide	*Minium*	Minium	Qian Dan, Huang Dan	Chin Daan, Wong Daan	Entan
Red modelwood flower	*Adina rubella*	Flos Adinae	Shui Yang Mei	Seui Yeung Mui	
Red peony root	*Paeonia lactiflora, P. obovata, P. veitchii*	Radix Paeoniae rubrae	Chi Shao (Yao)	Chek Cheuk (Yeuk)	Sekishaku-(yaku)
Red spiderlily corm	*Lycoris radiata*	Rhizoma Lycoris	Shi Suan	Sek Syun	
Red squash seed	*Cucurbita moschata*	Semen Cucurbitae	Nan Gua Zi	Naam Gwa Ji	Nankashi
Red stonecrop flower	*Sedum erythrosticum*	Flos Sedi erythrostici	Jing Tian Hua	Ging Ting Fa	
Red stonecrop herb	*Sedum erythrostictum*	Herba Sedi erythrosticti	Jing Tian (San Qi)	Ging Tin	
Red tasselflower herb	*Emilia sonchifolia*	Herba Emiliae	Yang Ti Cao	Yeung Tai Chou	
Reishi mushroom	*Ganoderma lucidum, G. sinense, G applanatum* and spp	Sclerotium Ganodermae	Ling Zhi (Cao)	Ling Ji (Chou)	Reishi

ENGLISH	SCIENTIFIC	PHARMACEUTICAL	MANDARIN	CANTONESE	JAPANESE
Resurrection plant herb	*Selaginella tamariscina*	Herba Selaginellae tamariscinae	Juan Bai	Kyun Paap	
Rhinoceros horn	*Rhinoceros unicornis, R. bicornis*	Cornu Rhinoceri	Xi Jiao	Sai Gok	
Rhodea herb	*Rhodea japonica*	Herba Rhodeae	Wan Nian Xing		
Rhubarb root	*Rheum palmatum, R. tanguticum, R. officinale*	Rhizoma Rhei	Da Huang	Daai Wong	Daio
Rice grain	*Oryza sativa*	Fructus Oryzae	Jing Mi	Gang Mai	
Rice malt (syrup)	*Oryza sativa*	Saccharum Oryzae			Koi
Rice paper pith	*Tetrapanax papyrifera*	Medulla Tetrapanacis	Tong Cao	Tong Chou, Bai Tong Chou	Toso
Ringworm bush leaf	*Cassia alata*	Folium Cassiae alatae	Dui Ye Dou Ye	Deui Yip Dau Yip	
Ripe bitter orange fruit	*Citrus aurantium* var. *amara*	Fructus Citri aurantii amarae	Zhi Ke, Zhi Qiao, Dai Dai Hua Zhi Qiao	Ji Hok, Doi Doi Fa Ji Hok	Kikoku
Ripe tangerine rind	*Citrus reticulata, C. tangerina, C. erythrosa*	Pericarpium Citri reticulatae	Chen Pi, Ju Pi	Chan Pei, Gwat Pei	Chimpi
Rising hemp root	*Cimicifuga foetida*	Radix Cimicifugae foetidae	Sheng Ma	Sing Ma	Shoma
Roasted borax	*Borax*	Borax	Shu Peng Sha	Syu Pang Sa	
Roasted red kaolin	*Halloysitum rubrum*	Halloysitum	Shu Chi Shi	Chek Sek Ji	
Roasted sour jujube seed	*Zizyphus spinosa*	Semen Zizyphi spinosae preparatae	Chao Suan Zao Ren	Syu Jou Yan	
Rock candy cured Asian ginseng root	*Panax ginseng*	Radix Panacis ginsengis praeparatae	Bai Shen	Baak Sam	Hakujin
Rock candy cured Asian ginseng root tail	*Panax ginseng*	Extremas radicis Panacis ginsengis praeparatae	(Ren) Shen Xu	(Yan) Sam Son	
Rock salt	*Halitum*	Halitum	Da Qing Yan	Daai Ching Yim	
Rock sweetflag root	*Acorus gramineus*	Rhizoma Acori graminei	Shi Chang Pu	Sek Cheung Pou	
Rooting lobelia herb and root	*Lobelia chinensis*	Herba et radix Lobeliae chinensis	Ban Bian Lian	Bau Bin Ling	Hanbanren
Rose geranium herb	*Pelargonium graveolens*	Herba Pelargonii	Xiang Ye	Heung Yip	
Rose of Sharon flower	*Hibiscus syriacus*	Flos Hibisci syriaci	Mu Jin Hua	Mut Gan Fa	
Rose of Sharon root bark	*Hibiscus syriacus*	Cortex radicis Hibisci syriacus	Mu Jin Pi	Mut Gan Pei	
Rosemary herb	*Rosmarinus officinalis*	Herba Rosmarini	Mi Die Xiang	Mai Dit Heung	
Rosemyrtle seed	*Rhodomyrtus tomentosa*	Semen Rhodomyrti	Shan Ren Zi	Saan Nam Ji	
Rough elephant's foot herb	*Elephantopus scaber*	Herba Elephantopi	Di Dan Tou, Ku Di Dan, Tu Gong Ying	Fu Dei Daam	
Rough holly leaf and root	*Ilex asprella*	Folium et radix Ilicis asprellae	Gang Mei (Gen), Wang Dian Jing	Gong Mui Gan, Maan Dim Gam	

ENGLISH	SCIENTIFIC	PHARMACEUTICAL	MANDARIN	CANTONESE	JAPANESE
Rough oxknee root	*Achyranthes aspera*	Radix Achyranthis asperae	Wei Niu Xi, Ju Niu Xi, Dou Kou Cao	Wai Ngau Sat, Dou Kau Chou	
Round-leaf holly leaf	*Ilex rotunda*	Folium Ilicis rotundis	Jiu Bi Ying	Gau Bit Ying	
Rue herb	*Ruta graveolens*	Herba Rutae	Chou Cao	Chau Chou	
Rugose giant hyssop herb	*Agastache rugosa*	Herba Agastachis	Huo Xiang	Fok Heung	Kakko
Rungia herb	*Rungia pectinata*	Herba Rungiae	Hai Er Cao	Haai Yi Chou	
Ryukyu banana root	*Musa basjoo*	Caudex Musae	Ba Jiao Gen	Ba Jiu Gan	
Sabia twig	*Sabia japonica*	Ramulus Sabiae	Qi Feng Teng	Ching Fung Tang	
Sacred bamboo fruit	*Nandina domestica*	Fructus Nandinae	(Nan) Tian Zhu Zi	(Naam) Tin Juk Ji	
Sacred bamboo leaf	*Nandina domestica*	Folium Nandinae	(Nan) Tian Zhu Ye	(Naam) Tin Juk Yip	
Sacred bamboo root and stem	*Nandina domestica*	Radix et caulis Nandinae	(Nan) Tian Zhu Gen	(Naam) Tin Juk Gan	
Safflower	*Carthamus tinctorius*	Flos Carthami tinctorii	Hong Hua	Hung Fa	Koka
Saffron stigma	*Crocus sativus*	Stigma Croci	Xi Hong Hua, Fan Hong Hua	Fun Hung Fa	Bankoka
Sago palm leaf	*Cycas revoluta*	Folium Cycadis	Tie Shu	Tit Syu	
Sago palm seed	*Cycas revoluta*	Semen Cycadis	Su Tie Zi	Sou Tit Ji	
Salmiac, Sal ammoniac	*Salammonitum* and *Halitum*	Salmiacum	Nao Sha	Lou Sa	
Salsola root and herb	*Salsola collina, S. ruthenica, S. richteri*	Radix et herba Salsolae	Zhu Mao Cai	Jyu Mou Choi	
Sandalwood	*Santalum album*	Lignum Santalum	Tan Xiang	Taan Heung	
Sappanwood	*Caesalpinia sappan*	Lignum Caesalpiniae	Su Mu	Sou Muk	Soboku
Sargassum seaweed	*Sargassum fusiforme* and spp	Herba Sargassi	Hai Zao	Hoi Chou	Kaiso
Sargentodoxa stem	*Sargentodoxa cuneata*	Caulis Sargentodoxae	Da Xue Teng	Daai Hyut Tang	
Saxifrage herb	*Saxifraga stolonifera*	Herba Saxifragae stoloniferae	Hu Er Cao	Fu Yi Chou	
Scabrous gentian root	*Gentiana scabra, G. triflora, G. manshurica*	Radix Gentianae scabrae	Long Dan Cao	Lung Daam Chou	Ryutan
Scallion seed	*Allium fistulosum*	Semen Allii fistulosi	Cong Zi	Chung Ji	Sohaku
Scarlet kadsura stem	*Kadsura coccinea*	Caulis Kadsurae coccineae	Fan Tuan Teng	Faan Tyun Tang	
Scarlet pimpernel herb	*Anagallis arvensis*	Herba Anagallis	Jian Feng Hong	Gin Fung Hung	
Schisandra berry	*Schisandra chinensis*	Fructus Schisandrae	Wu Wei Zi	Ng Mei Ji	Gomishi
Schizophragma root bark	*Schizophragma integrifolium*	Cortex radicis Schizophragmae	Zuan Di Feng	Jyun Dei Fung	
Scoparia root	*Scoparia dulcis*	Radix Scopariae	Ye Gan Cao, Zhu Cai Cao Gen	Ye Gam Chou, Chu Jai Chou Gan	
Scorpion	*Buthus Martensi*	Buthus	Quan Xie	Chyun Kit	Zenkatsu
Scurf pea berry	*Psoralea corylifolia*	Fructus Psoraleae	Bu Gu Zhi	Bou Gwat Ji	Hokotsushi
Sea buckthorn berry	*Hippophae rhamnoides*	Fructus Hippophae	Sha Ji	Sa Jik	
Sea cucumber	*Stichopus japonicus*	Stichopus	Hai Shen	Hoi Sam	

ENGLISH	SCIENTIFIC	PHARMACEUTICAL	MANDARIN	CANTONESE	JAPANESE
Sea horse	*Hippocampus kellogiand* spp	Hippocampus	Hai Ma	Hoi Ma	Kaiba
Seal genitals	*Callorhinus ursinus, Phoca vitulina*	Testes et penis Callorhini seu Phocae	Hai Gou Shen	Hoi Gau Sam	Kaikujin
Seashore chastetree berry	*Vitex rotundifolia, V. trifolia*	Fructus Viticis rotundifoliae	Man Jing Zi	Maan Ging Ji	Mankeishi
Securinega shoot and root	*Securinega suffruticosa*	Gemma et radix Securinegae	Yi Ye Qiu	Yat Yip Chau	
Selenite	*Selenitum*	Selenitum	Xuan Jing Shi	San Ching Sek	
Selfheal spike	*Prunella vulgaris*	Spica Prunellae	Xia Ku Cao	Ha Fu Chou	Kagoso
Semiaquilegia herb	*Semiaquilegia adoxoides*	Herba Semiaquilegiae	Tian Kui	Tin Kwai	
Semiaquilegia root	*Semiaquilegia adoxoides*	Radix Semiaquilegiae	Tian Kui	Tin Kwai	
Senna leaf	*Senna acutifolia, S. angustifolia*	Folium Sennae	Fan Xie Ye	Faan Sie Yip	
Serrate-leaf chloranthus	*Chloranthus serratus*	Radix Chloranthi	Ji Ji	Kap Gei	
Serrated clubmoss	*Lycopodium serratum* and *varieties*	Herba Lycopodii serrati	Jin Bu Huan	Gam Bat Wun	
Serratula root	*Serratula chinensis*	Radix Serratulae	Guang Dong Sheng Ma	Gwong Dung Jing Ma	
Sessile stemona root	*Stemona sessilifolia*	Radix Stemonae sessilifoliae	Bai Bu, Zhi Li Bai Bu	Baak Bou, Chek Lap Baak Bou	
Seven-lobe yam root	*Dioscorea septemloba*	Rhizoma Dioscoreae septemlobae	Bi Xie, Mian Bi Xie	Bei Gaai, Min Bei Gaai	
Sharp-leaf galangal berry	*Alpinia oxyphylla*	Fructus Alpiniae oxyphyllae	Yi Zhi Ren	Yik Ji Yan	Yakuchinin
Shearer's felt fern leaf	*Pyrrosia sheareri*	Folium Pyrrosiae sheareri	Shi Wei, Lu Shan Shi Wei	Sek Wai, Lou San Sek Wai	Sekii
Shepherd's purse herb	*Capsella bursa-pastoris*	Herba Capsellae	Ji Cai	Chai Choi	Seisai
Shield fern root	*Dryopteris crassirhizoma*	Rhizoma Dryopteris	Guan Zhong, Mian Ma Guan Zhong	Gwun Jung, Min Ma Gwun Jung	Tohoku-kanju
Shield-leaf yam root	*Dioscorea zingiberensis*	Rhizoma Dioscoreae zingiberis	Dun Ye Shu Yu	Teun Yip Syu Yu	
Shiitake mushroom	*Lentinula edodes*	Sclerotium Lentinulae	Xiang Gu	Heung Gu	Shiitake
Shiny asparagus root	*Asparagus cochinchinensis*	Rhizoma Asparagi cochinensis	Tian (Men) Dong	Tin (Mun) Dung	Tenmondo
Shiny bramble root	*Zanthoxylum nitidum*	Radix Zanthoxyli nitidi	Ru Di Jin Niu, Liang Mian Zhen	Yap Dei Gam Ngau	
Shoe flower	*Hibiscus rosa-sinensis*	Flos Hibisci rosa-sinensis	Fu Sang Hua	Fu Song Fa	
Siberian cocklebur	*Xanthium sibiricum, X. strumarium*	Fructus Xanthii	Cang Er Zi	Chong Yi Ji	Sojishi
Siberian cork tree bark	*Phellodendron amurense, P. chinense*	Cortex Phellodendris	Huang Bai Chuan Bai	Wong Paak Chyun Paak	Obaku
Siberian milkwort root	*Polygala sibirica*	Radix Polygalae sibiricae	Tian Yuan Zhi	Tin Yun Ji	
Siberian moonseed root	*Menispermum dauricum*	Radix Menispermi	Bei Dou Gen	Pan Dau Gan	

ENGLISH	SCIENTIFIC	PHARMACEUTICAL	MANDARIN	CANTONESE	JAPANESE
Siberian Solomon's-seal root	*Polygonatum sibiricum, P. cyrtonema, P. kingianum*	Rhizoma Polygonati	Huang Jing	Wong Jing	Osei
Sichuan bead tree berry	*Melia toosendan*	Fructus Meliae toosendanis	Chuan Lian Zi	Chyun Lin Ji	
Sichuan bellflower root	*Codonopsis tangshen*	Radix Codonopsis tangshenis	Dang Shen, Chuan Dang Shen	Chyun Dong Sam	
Sichuan Dolomiaea root	*Dolomiaea souliei*	Radix Dolomiaeae souliei	Chuan Mu Xiang	Chyun Muk Heung	
Sichuan fritillary bulb	*Fritillaria cirrhosa*	Bulbus Fritillariae cirrhosae	Chuan Bei Mu	Chyun Bui Mou	Senbaimo
Sichuan lovage root	*Ligusticum walichii*	Radix Ligustici walichii	Chuan Xiong, Xiong Qiong	Chyun Gung	Senkyu
Sichuan peppercorn	*Zanthoxylum bungeanum*	Fructus Zanthoxyli bungeani	Chuan Jiao, Hua Jiao	Chyun Jiu, Fa Jiu	Shokusho
Sichuan peppercorn	*Zanthoxylum simulans*	Fructus Zanthoxyli simulansis	Ye Hua Jiao	Ye Fa Jiu	
Sichuan teasel root	*Dipsacus asperoides*	Radix Dipsaci asperoides	Xu Duan, Chuan Duan	Juk Dyun, Chyun Dyun	
Sickle senna seed	*Cassia tora, C. obtusifolia* and spp	Semen Cassiae torae	Jue Ming Zi, Cao Jue Ming	Kyut Ming Ji, Chou Kyut Ming	Ketsumeishi
Siebold's wild ginger herb	*Asarum sieboldii*	Herba Asari sieboldii	Xi Xin, Hua Xi Xin	Wa Sai San	
Silk cotton tree flower	*Gossampinus malabarica*	Flos Gossampini	Mu Mian Hua	Muk Min Fa	
Silk vine root bark	*Periploca sepium*	Cortex radicis Periplocae	Gang Liu Pi, Xiang Liu Pi	Gong Lau Pei, Heung Lau Pei	
Silkworm dropping	*Bombyx mori*	Excrementum Bombicis	Can Sha	Chaam Sa	Sansha
Silkworm larva	*Bombyx mori artificially* infected with *Beauveria bassiana*	Bombyx beauveriatus	Jiang Yong	Geung Yung	
Silkworm larva	*Bombyx mori* infected with *Beauveria bassiana*	Bombyx beauveriatus	Jiang Can	Geung Chaam	
Silkworm slough	*Bombyx mori*	Periostracum Bombycis	Ma Ming Dui	Ma Ming Teui	
Silver ear mushroom	*Tremella fuciformis*	Sclerotium Tremellae fucimormis	Bai Mu Er	Baak Muk Yi	Hakumokuji
Silver quail-grass seed	*Celosia argentea*	Semen Celosiae argenteae	Qing Xiang Zi	Ching Seung Ji	Seisoshi
Single-bract fritillary bulb	*Fritillaria unibracteata*	Bulbus Fritillariae unibracteatae	Chuan Bei Mu, An Zi Bei Mu	Chyun Bui Mou, Am Ji Bui Mou	
Sinnate desmodium herb	*Desmodium sinnatum*	Herba Desmodii sinnati	Guo Lu Huang, Nian Ren Hua	Lim Yan Fa	
Sinomenium root	*Sinomenium acutum*	Radix Sinomenii	Qing Feng Teng	Ching Fung Tang	
Six god flower	*Spilanthes acmella* var. *oleracea*	Flos Spilanthis	Liu Shen Hua	Lau Sam Fa	
Six-petal clematis root	*Clematis hexapetala*	Radix Clematis hexapetalae	Wei Ling Xian, Mian Tuan Tie Xian Lian	Wai Ling Sin, Min Tyun Ti Chik Lin	

ENGLISH	SCIENTIFIC	PHARMACEUTICAL	MANDARIN	CANTONESE	JAPANESE
Skimmia stem and leaf	***Skimmia reevesiana, S. japonica***	Caulis et folium Skimmiae	Yin Yu	Yan Wu	
Slug	***Limax agrestic***	Limax	Guo Yu	Gwat Kut	
Small-leaf raspberry leaf	***Rubus parvifolius***	Folium Rubi parvifolii	Mao Mei, Hao Tian Biao	Mau Mui	
Smooth sarcandra herb	***Sarcandra glabra***	Herba Sarcandrae	Jiu Jie Feng	Gau Jit Fung	
Snail	***Eulota peliomphala***	Eulota	Gua Niu	Wo Ngau	
Snake grape root and leaf	***Ampelopsis brevipedunculata***	Radix et folium Ampelopsis brevipedunculatae	She Pu Tao, Shan Pu Tao	Se Pou Tou, Saan Pou Tou	
Snakegourd fruit	***Trichosanthes kirilowii, T. japonica, T. uniflora***	Fructus Tricosanthis	Gua Lou (Shi)	Kwut Lau	Karo
Snakegourd rind	***Trichosanthes kirilowii, T. japonica, T. uniflora***	Pericarpium Tricosanthis	Gua Lou Pi	Kwut Lau Pei	Karohi
Snakegourd root	***Trichosanthes kirilowii, T. japonica, T. uniflora***	Radix Trichosanthis	Tian Hua Fen	Tin Fa Fun	Tenkafun
Snakegourd seed	***Trichosanthes kirilowii, T. japonica, T. uniflora***	Semen Trichosanthis	Gua Lou Ren	Kwut Lau Yan	Karonin
Snakeskin slough	***Elephe taeniurus*** and spp, ***Dinodon rufozonatum***	Periostracum/Exuviae Elephis	She Tui (Pi)	Se Teui (Pei)	Dataihi
Snaketongue grass herb	***Oldenlandia diffusa***	Herba Oldenlandiae	Bai Hua She She Cao	Baak Fa Se Sit Chou	Byakkaja-zesso
Snow lotus herb	***Saussurea laniceps, S. involucrata*** and spp	Herba Saussureae lanicepsis	Xue Lian Hua	Hat Ling Fa	
Snow lotus root	***Saussurea laniceps, S. involucrata*** and spp	Radix Saussureae lanicepsis	Xue Lian Gen	Hat Ling Gan	
Soapnut seed, Bodhi seed	***Sapindus mukorossi***	Semen Sapindi	Wu Huan Zi, Mu Huan Zi	Mou Waan Ji	
Soapnut tree root	***Sapindus mukorossi***	Radix Sapindi	Wu Huan Gen, Mu Huan Gen	Mou Waan Gan	
Soda-apple nightshade herb	***Solanum surratense***	Herba Solani surattensis	Ye Dian Jie	Ye Din Ke	
Soft birthwort herb	***Aristolochia mollissima***	Herba Aristolochiae mollissimae	Xun Gu Feng, Mian Mao Ma Dou Ling	Cham Gwat Fung, Min Mou Ma Dou Ling	
Sour jujube seed	***Zizyphus spinosa***	Semen Zizyphi spinosae	Suan Zao Ren, Jin Zao Ren	Syun Jou Yan	Sansonin
South China St. John's wort herb	***Hypericum sampsonii***	Herba Hyperici sampsonii	Yuan Bao Cao	Yun Bou Chou	
Southern cinnabar sage root	***Salvia bowleyana***	Radix Salviae bowleyanae	Dan Shen, Nan Dan Shen	Daan Sam, Naam Dam Sam	
Soybean husk	***Glycine max***	Pericarpium Glycinis	Hei Dou Yi	Haak Dau Yi	

ENGLISH	SCIENTIFIC	PHARMACEUTICAL	MANDARIN	CANTONESE	JAPANESE
Spatholobus gel	*Spatholobus suberectus*	Gelatinum Spatholobi	Ji Xue Teng Jiao	Gai Yut Tang Gaau	
Spatholobus stem	*Spatholobus suberectus*	Caulis Spatholobi	Ji Xue Teng, Mi Hua Dou	Gai Yut Tang, Mat Fa Dau	
Spearmint herb	*Mentha spicata*	Herba Menthae spicatae	Xiang Hua Cai, Liu Lan Xiang	Heung Fa Choi, Lou Laan Heung	
Speranskia herb	*Speranskia tuberculata*	Herba Speranskiae	Tou Gu Cao	Tau Gwat Chou	
Spikemoss herb	*Selaginella doederleinii, S. involvens*	Herba Selaginellae	Shi Shang Bai	Sek Song Paap	
Spongegourd	*Luffa cylindrica, L. acutangula*	Fasciculus vascularis Luffae	Si Gua Luo	Si Gwa Lou	Shikaraku
Spreading violet root and herb	*Viola diffusa*	Radix et herba Violae diffusae	Di Bai Cao	Dei Baak Chou	
Sprouted barley grain	*Hordeum vulgare*	Fructus germinatus Hordei	Mai Ya	San Man Nga	Bakuga
Sprouted millet grain	*Setaria italica*	Fructus germinatus Setariae	Su Ya	Suk Nga	
Sprouted rice grain	*Oryza sativa*	Fructus Oryzae germinatus	Gu Ya	Gu Nga	Kokuga
Sprouting soybean	*Glycene max*	Semen Glycinis germinati	Dou (Huang) Juan	Dau (Wong) Geun	
St. John's wort	*Hypericum ascyron*	Herba Hyperici ascyronis	Hong Han Lian	Hung Hon Lin	
Stalactite tip	*Stalactitum, Balanophylla* spp.	Stalactitum	E Guan Shi, Shi Zhong Ru	Ngo Gun Sek	
Star anise fruit	*Illicium verum*	Fructus Illicii	Ba Jiao Hui Xiang	Baat Gok Wui Heung	
Star jasmine stem	*Trachelospermum jasminoides*	Caulis Trachelospermi	Luo Shi Teng	Lok Sek Tang	Chikusekito
Starwort fuit or seed	*Carpesium abrotanoides*	Fructus seu semen Carpesii	He Shi	Hok Sat	Kakushitsu
Starwort herb	*Carpesium abrotanoides*	Herba Carpesii	Tian Ming Jing	Tin Ming Jing	
Statice root	*Statice sinensis*	Radix Staticis	Hong Mao Cha	Hung Maau Cha	
Stellara root	*Stellera chamaejasme*	Radix Stellerae	Hong Lang Du, Lang Du	Hung Long Duk, Long Duk	
Stellaria root	*Stellaria dichotoma* var. *lanceolata*	Radix Stellariae	Yin Chai Hu	Ngan Chaai Wu	Ginsaiko
Stephania root	*Stephania tetrandra*	Radix Stephaniae tetrandrae	Han Fang Ji, Fang Ji	Haan Fong Gei Fong Gei	Kamboi
Sterculia seed	*Sterculia staphigera, S. lychnophera*	Semen Sterculiae	Pang Da Hai	Bun Daai Hoi	Bantaikai
Stinkbug	*Aspongopus*	Aspongopus	Jiu Xiang Chong	Gau Heung Chung	
Stinking elm fruit paste	*Ulmus macrocarpa*	Praeparatio fructus Ulmi	Wu Yi	Mon Yi	Bui
Stone ear mushroom	*Umbilicaria esculenta*	Sclerotium Umbilicariae	Shi Er	Sek Yi	
Stonebushel stem	*Dendrobium chrysanthum*	Herba Dendrobii chrysanthi	Shi Hu, Shu Hua Shi Hu	Sek Wu, Chuk Fa Shi Hu	
Stonebushel stem	*Dendrobium fimbriatum*	Herba Dendrobii fimbriati	Shi Hu, Ma Bian Shi Hu	Sek Wu, Ma Bin Sek Wu	
Stonebushel stem	*Dendrobium loddigesii*	Herba Dendrobii loddigesii	Shi Hu, Wan Cao Shi Hu	Sek Wu, Waan Chou Sek Wu	

ENGLISH	SCIENTIFIC	PHARMACEUTICAL	MANDARIN	CANTONESE	JAPANESE
Stonebushel stem	*Dendrobium moniliforme*	Caulis Dendrobii miniliformis	Xi Jing Shi Hu, Xiao Wan Chai	Sai Ging Sek Wu	
Stonebushel stem	*Dendrobium nobile*	Herba Dendrobii nobilis	Shi Hu, Jin Sha Shi Hu	Sek Wu, Gam Ja Sek Wu	
Stonebushel stem	*Dendrobium nobile, D. linawianum, D. officinale* and spp	Herba Dendrobii	Shi Hu	Sek Wu	Sekkoku
Stonebushel stem	*Dendrobium officinalis*	Herba Dendrobii officinalis	Shi Hu, Tie Pi Shi Hu	Sek Wu, Tit Pei Sek Wu	
Storax resin	*Liquidambar orientalis*	Resina Liquidambaris (Styrax liquidis)	Su He Xiang	Sou Hap Heung	Sogoko
Storksbill or cranesbill herb	*Erodium stephaniarum, Geranium* spp	Herba Erodii seu Geranii	Lao Guan Cao	Lou Gwun Chou	
Strap flower	*Loropetalum chinense*	Flos Loropetali	Ji Hua	Gai Fa	
Strap flower bark	*Loropetalum chinense*	Cortex Loropetali	Ji Mu	Gai Muk	
Strawberry-leaf cinquefoil root	*Potentilla fragarioides*	Radix Potentillae fragarioidis	Mei Ye Wei Ling Cai	Mui Yip Wai Ling Choi	
Stringy stonecrop root and herb	*Sedum sarmentosum*	Radix et herba Sedi sarmentosi	Chui Pen Cao	Chai Pan Chou	
Strobilanthes root	*Strobilanthes flaccidifolius*	Radix Strobilanthis	Ma Lan Gen	Ma Laam Gan	
Strophanthus seed	*Strophanthus divaricatus*	Semen Strophanthi	Yang Jiao Yao	Yeung Gok Aau	
Subglobular bellflower root	*Codonopsis subglobosa*	Radix Codonopsis subglobosae	Dang Shen, Qiu Hua Dang Shen	Dong Sam, Kau Fa Dong Sam	
Sulphur	*Sulphurum*	Sulphurum	Liu Huang, Shi Liu Huang	Lau Wong, Sek Lau Wong	Io
Sundew herb	*Drosera burmanni*	Herba Droserae	Jin Di Luo	Gam Dei Lo	
Sunflower receptacle	*Helianthus annuus*	Receptaculum Helianthi	Xian Ji Gui Hua Pan	Heung Yat Kwai Fa Bun	
Sunspurge herb	*Euphorbia helioscopia*	Herba Euphorbiaeheliosc opiae	Ze Qi	Jaak Chat	Takushitsu
Supplejack root	*Berchemia lineata*	Radix Berchemiae	Tie Bao Jin	Tit Bau Gam	
Swallow-wort root	*Cynanchum atratum, C. versicolor*	Radix Cynanchi atrati	Bai Wei	Baak Mei	Byakubi
Sweet apricot kernel	*Prunus armeniaca* and var.	Semen Pruni armeniacae dulcis	Tian Xing Ren, Nan Xing Ren	Tim Hang Yan, Naam Hang Yan	
Sweet ladybell root	*Adenophora trachelioides*	Radix Adenophorae trachelioidis	Gan Jie Geng	Gam Gaat Gan, Ai Ji Sam	
Sweet orange fruit	*Citrus sinensis*	Fructus Citri sinensis	Tian Chen	Tim Chaang	
Sweet rice	*Oryza sativa*	Fructus Oryzae	Nuo Mi	Lo Mai	
Sweet rice root	*Oryza sativa*	Radix Oryzae	Nuo Dao Gen (Xu)	No Du Gan	Jubeikon
Sweet spurge root	*Euphorbia kansui*	Radix Euphorbiae kansui	Gan Sui	Gam Seui	Kansui
Sweet tea leaf	*Hydrangea serrata* var. *thunbergii*	Folium Hydrangeae	Gan Cha	Gam Cha	Amatya, Dochouzan

ENGLISH	SCIENTIFIC	PHARMACEUTICAL	MANDARIN	CANTONESE	JAPANESE
Sweetflag root	*Acorus calamus*	Rhizoma Acori calami	Shui Chang Pu, Bai Chang Pu	Seui Cheung Pou, Baak Cheung Pou	Shobu
Swiss centaury root	*Rhaponticum uniflorum*	Radix Rhapontici	Lou Lu	Lau Lou	Roro
Swordbean seed	*Canavalia gladiata, C. ensiformis*	Semen Canavaliae	Dao Dou	Dou Dau	
Tabasheer	*Phyllostachys nigra* var. *henonis* and spp	Concretio silicea bambusae	Tian Zhu Huang	Tin Juk Wong	
Taipei fritillary bulb	*Fritillaria taipaiensis*	Bulbus Fritillariae taipaiensis	Chuan Bei Mu, Tai Bai Bei Mu	Chyun Bui Mou, Taai Baak Bui Mou	
Taiwan elder stem and leaf	*Sambucus formosana/taiwaniana*	Caulis et folium Sambuci formosanae	Mao Gu Xiao	Mon Gwat Siu	
Taiwan maple fruit	*Liquidambar taiwaniana*	Fructus Liquidambaris	Lu Lu Tong	Lou Lou Tung	Rorotsu
Taiwan maple fruit resin	*Liquidambar taiwaniana*	Resina Liquidambaris taiwaninanae	Bai Jiao Xiang	Baak Gaau Heung	
Taiwan mistletoe twig	*Scurrula ritozanensis*	Ramulus Scurrulae	Tai Wan Ji Sheng	Toi Waan Ji Sang	
Taiwan schefflera leaf and stem	*Schefflera arboricola, S. kwangsiensis, S. venulosa*	Folium et caulis Schefflerae	Qi Ye Lian	Chat Yip Lin	
Talc	*Talcum*	Talcum	Hua Shi	Wat Sek	Kasseki
Tangerine seed	*Citrus reticulata, C. tangerina, C. erythrosa*	Semen Citri reticulatae	Ju He	Gwat Hat	
Tansy mustard seed	*Descurainia sophia*	Semen Descurainiae	Ting Li Zi	Ting Lai Ji	Teirekishi
Taro root	*Colocasia esculenta*	Radix Colocasiae	Yu Tou Gen	Wu Tau Gan	
Tartary aster root	*Aster tataricus*	Radix Asteris tatarici	Zi Wan	Ji Yun	Shion
Tatarinow's sweetflag root	*Acorus tatarinowii*	Rhizoma Acori tatarinowii	Jie Chang Pu	Jik Cheung Pou	
Tawny day lily flower	*Hemerocallis fulva*	Flos Hemerocallis	Xuan Cao Hua	Syun Chou Fa	
Tawny day lily root	*Hemerocallis fulva*	Radix Hemerocallis	Xuan Cao (Gen)	Syun Chou Gan	
Tea leaf	*Camellia sinensis*	Folium Camelliae sinensis	Cha Ye	Cha Yip	Fujucha, Chayo
Ternate buttercup root	*Ranunculus ternatus*	Radix Ranunculi	Mao Zhao Cao, Mao Zhua Cao	Maau Jau Chou	
Tetragonia herb	*Tetragonia tatragonoides*	Herba Tetragoniae	Fan Xing	Faan Haang	Bankyo, Mantsai
Thick-leaf croton root	*Croton crassifolius*	Radix Crotonis crassifolii	Ji Gu Xiang	Gai Gwat Heung	
Thick-leaf Dolomiaea root	*Dolomiaea berardioidea*	Radix Dolomiaea berardioidea	Hou Ye Chuan Mu Xiang	Hau Yip Chyun Muk Heung	
Thin-leaf buplever root	*Bupleurum scorzonerifolium*	Radix Bupleuri scorzonerifolii	Chai Hu, Xia Ye Chai Hu	Chaai Wu, Hap Yip Chaai Wu	
Thin-leaf glossgyne herb	*Glossogyne tenuifolia*	Herba Glossogyne	Shan Shen Zi	Saan Sam Jai	
Thin-leaf milkwort root	*Polygala tenuifolia*	Radix Polygalae	Yuan Zhi	Yun Ji	Onji
Thin-leaf rattlebox herb	*Crotalaria sessiliflora*	Herba Crotalariae	Ye Bai He	Ye Baak Hap	

ENGLISH	SCIENTIFIC	PHARMACEUTICAL	MANDARIN	CANTONESE	JAPANESE
Thladiantha fruit	*Thladiantha dubia*	Fructus Thladianthae	Zhi Pao	Chek Pau	
Thorny eleagnus leaf	*Eleagnus pungens*	Folium Eleagni pungensis	Hu Tui (Zi) Ye	Wu Teui (Ji) Yip	
Three-leaf acanthopanax root bark	*Acanthopanax trifoliatus*	Cortex radicis Acanthopanacis trifoliati	Wu Jia Pi, Bai Le	Ng Ga Pei, Baak Lak	
Three-leaf cocculus root	*Cocculus trilobus*	Radix Cocculi	Mu Fang Ji	Muk Fong Gei	
Three-needle barberry root	*Berberis sargentiana, B. wilsonae, B. vernae* and spp	Radix Berberis sargentianae	San Ke Zhen	Saam Gwo Jam	
Thunder ball fungus	*Mylitta lapidescens*	Sclerotium Mylittae	Lei Wan	Leui Yun	
Tianjin crab	*Eriocheir sinensis, E. japonicus*	Eriocheir	Jin Xie	Jeun Haai	Zukani
Tiger bone	*Panthera*	Os tigris	Hu Gu	Fu Gwat	Kokotsu
Tinospora root	*Tinospora sagittata, T. capillipes*	Radix Tinosporae	Jin Guo Lan	Gam Gwo Laam	Kinkaran
Toad venom	*Bufo gargarizans, B. melanostictus*	Secretio Bufonis	Chan Su	Sim Sou	Senjo
Toad-headed lizard	*Gecko gecko, G. verticilatus*	Gecko	Ge Jie	Gap Gaai	Gokai
Tobacco nightshade root	*Solanum verbascifolium*	Radix Solani verbascifolii	Ye Yan Ye Gen, Tu Yen Tou	Ye Yin Yip Gan, Tou Yin Tau	
Tortoise shell	*Chinemys reevesii*	Plastrum Chinemis	Gui Ban	Gwai Baan	Kiban
Tortoise shell gel	*Chinemys reevesii*	Gelatinum carapaxis Chinemis	Gui Ban Jiao	Gwai Baan Gaau	
Tree of heaven bark	*Ailanthus altissima*	Cortex Ailanthi	Chun (Bai) Pi	Chan (Baak) Pei	
Tree of heaven fruit	*Ailanthus altissima*	Fructus Ailanthi	Feng Yen Cao	Fung Ngaan Chou	
Tree of heaven root bark	*Ailanthus altissima*	Cortex radicis Ailanthi	Chun Gen Pi	Chan Gan Pei	
Tree peony root bark	*Paeonia suffruticosa*	Cortex radicis Paeoniae suffruticosae	Mu Dan Pi, Dan Pi	Maau Daan Pei, Daan Pei	Botanpi
Trichosporum herb	*Trichosporum acuminatum*	Herba Trichospori	Bai Mian Feng	Baak Ming Fung	
Trifoliate orange fruit	*Poncirus trifoliata*	Fructus Ponciri	Gou Ju	Gau Gwat	
Tuberous stemona root	*Stemona tuberosa*	Radix Stemonae tuberosae	Bai Bu, Dui Ye Bai Bu	Baak Bou, Deui Yip Baak Bou	
Tung seed	*Aleurites fordii*	Semen Aleuritis	You Tong Zi	Yau Tung Ji	
Turkey tail mushroom	*Coriolus versicolor (syn. Trametes versicolor)*	Sclerotium Corioli versicolori	Yun Zhi	Wan Ji	
Turmeric root	*Curcuma longa. C. aromatica*	Rhizoma Curcumae	Jiang Huang	Geung Wong	Kyoo
Turmeric tuber	*Curcuma longa, C. aromatica*	Tuber Curcumae	Yu Jin	Yuk Gam	Ukon
Twining psychotria herb	*Psychotria serpens*	Herba Psychotriae serpentis	Chuan Gen Teng, Bo Gu Cao	Chyun Gen Tang	
Twist-leaf fritillary bulb	*Fritillaria tortifolia*	Bulbus Fritillariae tortifoliae	Yi Bei Mu, Tuo Li Bei Mu	Yi Bui Mou, Tok Lei Bui Mou	

ENGLISH	SCIENTIFIC	PHARMACEUTICAL	MANDARIN	CANTONESE	JAPANESE
Typhonium root	*Typhonium giganteum*	Radix Typhonii	Du Jiao Lan	Duk Gok Lin	
Umbel desmodium flower	*Desmodium umbellatum*	Flos Desmodii umbellati	Gu Su Hua	Gu Sou Fa	
Umbel polypore mushroom	*Polyporus umbellatus*	Sclerotium Polypori	Zhu Ling	Ju Ling	Chorei
Umbilical cord	*Homo sapiens*	Funis umbilici Hominis	Qi Dai	Chi Daai	
Umbrella tree bark	*Schefflera octophylla*	Cortex Schefflerae octophyllae	Ya Jiao Mu Pi	Ngaap Geuk Muk Pei	
Unripe bitter orange fruit	*Citrus aurantium, C. wilsonii*	Fructus Citri aurantii immaturi	Zhi Shi	Ji Sat	Kijitsu
Unripe citrus fruit	*Citrus grandis* and spp.	Fructus Citri grandi immaturi	Ju Hong Zhu	Gwat Heung	
Unripe myrobalan fruit	*Terminalia chebula* and var.	Fructus Terminaliae immaturi	Cang Qing Guo		
Unripe peach fruit	*Prunus persica, P. davidiana*	Fructus persicae immaturi	Bi Tao Gan		
Unripe prepared black plum	*Prunus mume*	Fructus Mumis immaturis preparatae	Bai Mei	Baak Mui	
Unripe tangerine rind	*Citrus reticulata, C. tangerina, C. erythrosa*	Pericarpium Citri reticulatae viride	Qing Pi	Ching Pei	Johi
Upright ladybell root	*Adenophora stricta, A. capillaris, A. tetraphylla* and spp	Radix Adenophorae strictae	Nan Sha Shen	Naam Sa Sam	Nanshajin
Ural licorice root	*Glycirrhiza uralensis, G. glabra* and spp	Radix Glycirrhizae	Gan Cao	Gam Chou	Kanzo
Uraria herb	*Uraria lagopodioides*	Herba Urariae	Hu Li Wei, Tong Tian Cao	Tung Tin Chou	
Urine-prepared licorice root	*Glycirrhiza uralensis, G. glabra* and spp	Radix Glycirrhizae preparatae cum urino	Ren Zhong Huang	Yan Chung Wong	
Valerian root	*Valeriana officinalis, V. hardwickii*	Rhizoma Valerianae	Xie Cao	Kit Chou	
Vanieria stem	*Vanieria cochinchinensis*	Caulis Vanieriae	Huang Jin Kui, Chuan Po Shi	Wong Jin Kwai	
Velvet deer antler	*Cervus nippon* and spp	Cornu cervi parvum	Lu Rong, Rong Tou, Nen Lu Rong	Luk Yan	Rokujo
Ventilago root and stem	*Ventilago leiocarpa*	Radix et rhizoma Ventilaginis	Xue Feng Teng, Qing Pi Mao	Hyut Fung Tang	
Vernonia herb	*Vernonia cinerea*	Herba Vernoniae	Yi Zhi Xiang	Yat Ji Heung	
Vervain herb	*Verbena officinalis*	Herba Verbenae	Ma Bian Cao	Ma Bin Chou	
Viper	*Agkistrodon halys*	Agkistrodon	Fan Bi	Faan Bei	
Viper gallbladder	*Naja naja atra, Bungarus fasciatus, Elaphe radiata*	Fel Najae seu Bungari seu Elaphis	She Dan	Se Daam	
Walnut leaf	*Juglans regia*	Folium Juglandis	Hu Tao Ye	Wu Tou Yip	
Walnut meat	*Juglans regia*	Semen Juglandis	Hu Tao Ren	Wu Tou Yan	Kotoniku
Walnut twig	*Juglans regia*	Ramulus Juglandis	Hu Tao Zhi	Wu Tou Ji	

ENGLISH	SCIENTIFIC	PHARMACEUTICAL	MANDARIN	CANTONESE	JAPANESE
Wampi fruit	*Clausenia lansium*	Pericarpium Clauseniae	Huang Pi Guo	Wong Pei Gwo	
Wampi leaf	*Clausenia lansium*	Folium Clauseniae	Huang Pi Ye	Wong Pei Yip	
Wampi seed	*Clausenia lansium*	Semen Clauseniae	Huang Pi He	Wong Pei Ho	
Water buffalo horn	*Bubalus bubalis*	Cornu Bubali	Shui Niu Jiao	Seui Ngau Gok	
Water caltrop fruit	*Trapa bispinosa, T. bicornis*	Fructus Trapae	Ling Qiao	Ling Gok	
Water chestnut herb	*Heleocharis plantaginea*	Herba Heleocharis	Bi Qi	But Chai	Bossai
Water chickweed herb	*Stellaria aquatica*	Herba Stellariae aquaticae	Cha Chi Huang	Cha Si Wong	
Water clove herb	*Ludwigia prostata*	Herba Ludwigiae	Shui Ding Xiang	Seui Ding Heung	
Water dropwort	*Oenanthe javanica*	Herba Oenanthis	Shui Qin	Seui Kan	
Water pepper fruit	*Polygonum hydropiper*	Fructus Polygoni hydropiperis	Liao Shi	Lou Sek	
Water pepper herb and root	*Polygonum hydropiper*	Herba et radix Polygoni hydropiperis	Shui Liao	Seui Liu	
Water plantain root	*Alisma orientalis*	Rhizoma Alismae	Ze Xie	Jaak Se	Takusha
Water-reed root	*Phragmites communis*	Radix Phragmitis	Lu Gen	Lou Gan	Rokon
Water-reed twig	*Phragmites communis*	Ramulus Phragmitis	Wei Jing	Lou Ging	
Watermelon fruit	*Citrullus vulgaris*	Fructus Citrulli	Xi Gua	Sai Gwa	Seika
Watermelon rind	*Citrullus vulgaris*	Pericarpium Citrulli	Xi Gua Pi	Sai Pa Pei	
Waxgourd fruit rind	*Benincasa hispida*	Epicarpium Benincasae	Dong Gua Pi	Dung Gwa Pei	Tokahi
Waxgourd seed	*Benincasa hispida*	Semen Benincasae	Dong Gua Ren	Dong Gwa Yan	Tokanin
Wedelia herb	*Wedelia chinensis*	Herba Wedeliae	Ma Lan Jin, Peng Qi Ju	Paang Kei Guk	
Weeping willow twig	*Salix babylonica, S. gracilistyla*	Folium Salicis	Liu Ye	Lau Yip	
Weeping willow twig	*Salix babylonica, S. gracilistyla*	Ramulus Salicis	Liu Zhi	Lau Ji	
Western mistletoe herb	*Viscum coloratum, V. album*	Herba Visci	Hu Ji Sheng	Wu Gei Sang	
Wheat berry	*Triticum aestivum*	Fructus Tritici	Fu Xiao Mai	Fau Siu Mak	Fushobaku
White angelica Root	*Angelica dahurica, A. anomala, A. taiwaniana*	Radix Angelicae dahuricae	Bai Zhi	Baak Ji	Byakushi
White arsenic	*Arsenicum album*	Arsenolitum	Pi Shi, Xin Shi		
White atractylodes root	*Atractylodes macrocephala*	Rhizoma Atractylodis macrocephalae	Bai Zhu	Baak Seut	Byakujutsu
White champac flower	*Michelia alba*	Flos Micheliae	Bai Lan Hua	Baak Laan Fa	
White cow parsnip root	*Heracleum candicans*	Radix Heraclei candicantis	Du Huo	Duk Wut	

ENGLISH	SCIENTIFIC	PHARMACEUTICAL	MANDARIN	CANTONESE	JAPANESE
White elm bark	*Ulmus pumila*	Cortex Ulmi pumilae	Yu Qian	Yu Chin	
White kaolin	*Halloysitum album*	Halloysitum album	Bai Shi Zhi	Baak Sek Ji	
White lysimachia herb	*Lysimachia candida*	Herba Lysimachiae candidae	Dan Tian Cao	Daan Tiu Chou	
White mustard seed	*Sinapis alba*	Semen Sinapis albae	Bai Jie Zi	Baak Gaai Ji	
White oxknee Root	*Achyranthes bidentata*	Radix Achyranthis	Niu Xi, Huai Niu Xi	Ngau Sat, Wai Ngau Sat	Goshitsu
White oxknee root	*Cuccubala baccifer*	Radix Cuccubalae bacciferis	Bai Niu Xi	Baak Ngao Sat	
White peony root	*Paeonia lactiflora*	Radix Paeoniae lactiflorae	Bai Shao (Yao)	Baak Cheuk (Yeuk)	Byakushaku (yaku)
White spurge root	*Euphorbia pallasii, E. abracteolatae, E. fischerianae*	Radix Euphorbiae pallasii seu ebracteolatae	(Bai) Lang Du	(Baak) Long Duk	
Wikstroemia flower	*Wikstroemia chamaedaphne*	Flos Wikstroaemiae chamaedaphnis	Rao Hua	Iu Fa	
Wikstroemia root	*Wickstroemia indica*	Radix Wickstroemiae	Liao Ge Wang (Gen)	Liu Go Wong	Ryokao
Wild chrysanthe-mum flower	*Chrysanthemum indicum*	Flos Chrysanthemi indici	Ye Ju Hua	Gam Guk Fa, Ye Guk Fa	Nogikuka
Wild Asian ginseng	*Panax ginseng*	Radix Panacis ginsengis	Ye Shan Shen	Gam San Sam	
Wild cardamom flower	*Amomum villosum*	Flos Amomi villosi	Sha Ren Hua, (Yang) Chun Sha Hua	Sa Yan Fa, (Yeung) Chyun Sa Fa	Saninka
Wild cardamom pod (fruit)	*Amomum villosum*	Fructus Amomi villosi	Sha Ren, (Yang) Chun Sha Ren	Sa Yan, (Yeung) Chyun Sa Yan	Sanin
Wild cardamom seed	*Amomum villosum*	Semen Amomi villosi	Guang Sha Ren	Gwong Sa Yan	
Wild cardamom shell	*Amomum villosum*	Pericarpium Amomi villosi	Sha Ren Ke	Sa Yan Hok	
Wild carrot seed	*Daucus carota*	Fructus Dauci	Nan He Zao	Naam Hok Sat	
Wild grape root	*Vitis thunbergii* and spp	Radix Vitis	Ye Pu Tao	Ye Pou Tou	
Wild hawthorn berry	*Crataegus cuneata*	Fructus Crataegus cuneatae	Ye Shan Zha	Ye Saan Ja	
Wild honeysuckle flower	*Lonicera confusa*	Flos Lonicerae confusae	Tu Yin Hua, Shan Yin Hua	Tou Ngan Fa	
Wild pepper twig	*Piper wallichii*	Ramulus Piperis wallichii	Shi Nan Teng	Sek Naam Tang	
Wild rose root	*Rosa multiflora*	Radix Rosae multiflorae	Ye Qiang Wei Gen	Ye Cheung Mei Gan	
Wild sage herb	*Lantana camara*	Herba Lantanae	Wu Se Mei	Ng Sik Mui	
Willow plum root bark	*Prunus salicina*	Cortex radicis Pruni salicinae	Li Gen Bai Pi	Lei Gan Baak Pei	
Wind-protector root	*Ledebouriella divaricata, L. seseloides*	Radix Ledebouriellae	Fang Feng	Fong Fung	Bofu
Windmill palm seed	*Trachycarpus excelsa, T. fortunei*	Fructus Trachycarpi	Zong Lu Zi	Jung Leui Ji	

ENGLISH	SCIENTIFIC	PHARMACEUTICAL	MANDARIN	CANTONESE	JAPANESE
Winged spindletree twig	*Euonymus alata*	Ramulus Eunymi alati	Gui Jian Yu	Gwai Jin Yu	
Winter cherry herb	*Solanum nigrum*	Herba Solani nigri	Long Kui	Lung Kwai	
Wintergreen holly leaf	*Ilex chinensis*	Folium Ilicis chinensis	Si Ji Qing, Dong Qing Ye	Sei Gwai Ching, Dung Ching Yip	
Wintersweet flower	*Chimonanthus praecox*	Flos Chimonanthi	La Mei Hua	Laap Mui Fa	Sakubaika
Witchweed herb	*Striga asiatica*	Herba Strigae	Du Jiao Gan	Duk Geuk Gam	
Woad leaf	*Isatis indigotica*	Folium Isatis indigoticae	Song Lan Ye	Song Laan Yip	
Woad leaf	*Isatis tinctoria*	Folium Isatis tinctoriae	Da Qing Ye	Daai Ching Yip	
Woad pigment	*Isatis tinctoria* and *spp, Baphicacanthus cusia, Indigofera suffruticosa, Polygonum tinctorium*	Indigo pulverata levis	Qing Dai	Ching Doi	
Woad root	*Isatis tinctoria, I. indigotica*	Radix Isatis tinctoriae	Ban Lan Gen	Baan Laam Gan	
Wolf'smilk herb	*Euphorbia humifusa*	Herba Euphorbiae humifusae	Di Jin Cao	Dei Gam Chou	
Wolfberry	*Lycium chinense, L. barbarum*	Fructus Lycii	Gou Qi Zi	Gau Gei Ji, Gei Ji	Kukoshi
Wolfberry leaf	*Lycium chinense, L. barbarum*	Folium Lycii chinensis	Gou Qi Ye	Gau Ji Yip	
Wolfberry root bark	*Lycium chinense*	Cortex radicis Lycii	Di Gu Pi	Dei Gwat Pei	Jikoppi
Wood aromatic root	*Saussurea lappa*	Radix Saussureae lappae	Mu Xiang, Yun Mu Xiang	Muk Heung	Mokko
Wood ear mushroom	*Auricularia auricula*	Sclerotium Auriculariae	Mu Er	Muk Yi	Kikurage
Wood louse	*Armadillidium vulgare, Porcellio scaber*	Armadillidium	Shu Fu	Syu Fu	
Wood stove clay		Terra flava usta, Bolus usta	Fu Long Gan	Fuk Lung Gon	Bukuryukan
Wood whitlow grass seed	*Lepidium apetalum, L. virginicum*	Semen Lepidii	Ting Li Zi	Ting Lai Ji	Teirekishi
Woolly grass flower	*Imperata cylindrica* var. *major*	Flos Imperatae	Bai Mao Hua	Baak Maau Fa	
Woolly grass root	*Imperata cylindrica* var. *major*	Rhizoma Imperatae	Bai Mao Gen	Baak Maau Gan	Bokon
Wormseed herb	*Chenopodium ambrosioides*	Herba Chenopodii ambrosioidis	Tu Jing Jie	Tou Ging Gai	
Xinjiang peony root	*Paeonia sinjiangensis*	Radix Paeoniae sinjiangensis	Xin Jiang Bai Shao (Yao)	San Geung Chek Cheuk	
Yellow azalea flower	*Rhododendron molle*	Flos Rhododendri mollis	Nao Yang Hua, Huang Du Juan	Naau Yeung Fa, Wong Dou Gun	
Yellow azalea fruit	*Rhododendron molle*	Fructus Rhododendris mollis	Ba Li Ma	Baat Lei Ma	
Yellow dock root	*Rumex crispus*	Radix Rumicis crispi	Niu Er Da Huang	Ngau Yi Daai Wong	

ENGLISH	SCIENTIFIC	PHARMACEUTICAL	MANDARIN	CANTONESE	JAPANESE
Yellow ear mushroom	*Tremella mesenterica*	Sclerotium Tremellae mesentericae	Huang Mu Er	Wong Muk Yi	
Yellow pagoda tree berry	*Sophora flavescens*	Fructus Sophorae flavescentis	Ku Shen Zi	Fu Sam Ji	
Yellow pagoda tree root	*Sophora flavescens*	Radix Sophorae flavescentis	Ku Shen	Fu Sam	
Yellow pond lily root	*Nuphar japonicum, N. pumilum*	Rhizoma Nupharis	Ping Peng Cao Gan	Ping Fung Chou Gan	Senkotu
Yellow vine root pith	*Tripterygium wilfordii*	Medulla radicis Tripterygii	Lei Gong Teng	Leui Gung Tang	
Yew twig and leaf	*Cephalotaxus fortunei*	Ramulus et folium Cephalotaxi	San Jian Shan	Saam Jim Chaam	
Young cantaloupe stalk	*Cucumis melo*	Caulis Cucumis	Tian Gua Di	Tim Gwa Dai	Katei
Yulan magnolia bud	*Magnolia liliflora, M. denudata, M. yulan* and spp	Gemma Magnoliae	Xin Yi Hua	San Yi Fa	Shinika
Yumin fritillary bulb	*Fritillaria yuminensis*	Bulbus Fritillariae yuminensis	Yi Bei Mu, Yu Min Bei Mu	Yi Bui Mou, Yu Man Bui Mou	
Yunnan paris root	*Paris yunnanensis*	Rhizoma Paris yunnanensis	Zhong Lou, Yun Nan Zhong Lou	Jung Lau, Wan Laam Jung Lau	
Zedoary root	*Curcuma zedoaria, C. aeruginosa* and spp	Rhizoma Curcumae zedoariae	E Zhu, Peng Er Zhu	Ngo Seut, Fung Ngo Seut	Gajutsu
Zhejiang fritillary bulb	*Fritillaria thunbergii*	Bulbus Fritillariae thunbergii	Zhe Bei Mu	Chit Bui Mou	Setsubaimo
Zhejiang prickly ash bark	*Zanthoxylum ailanthoides*	Cortex Zanthoxyli ailanthoidis	Zhe Tong Pi	Jit Tung Pei	

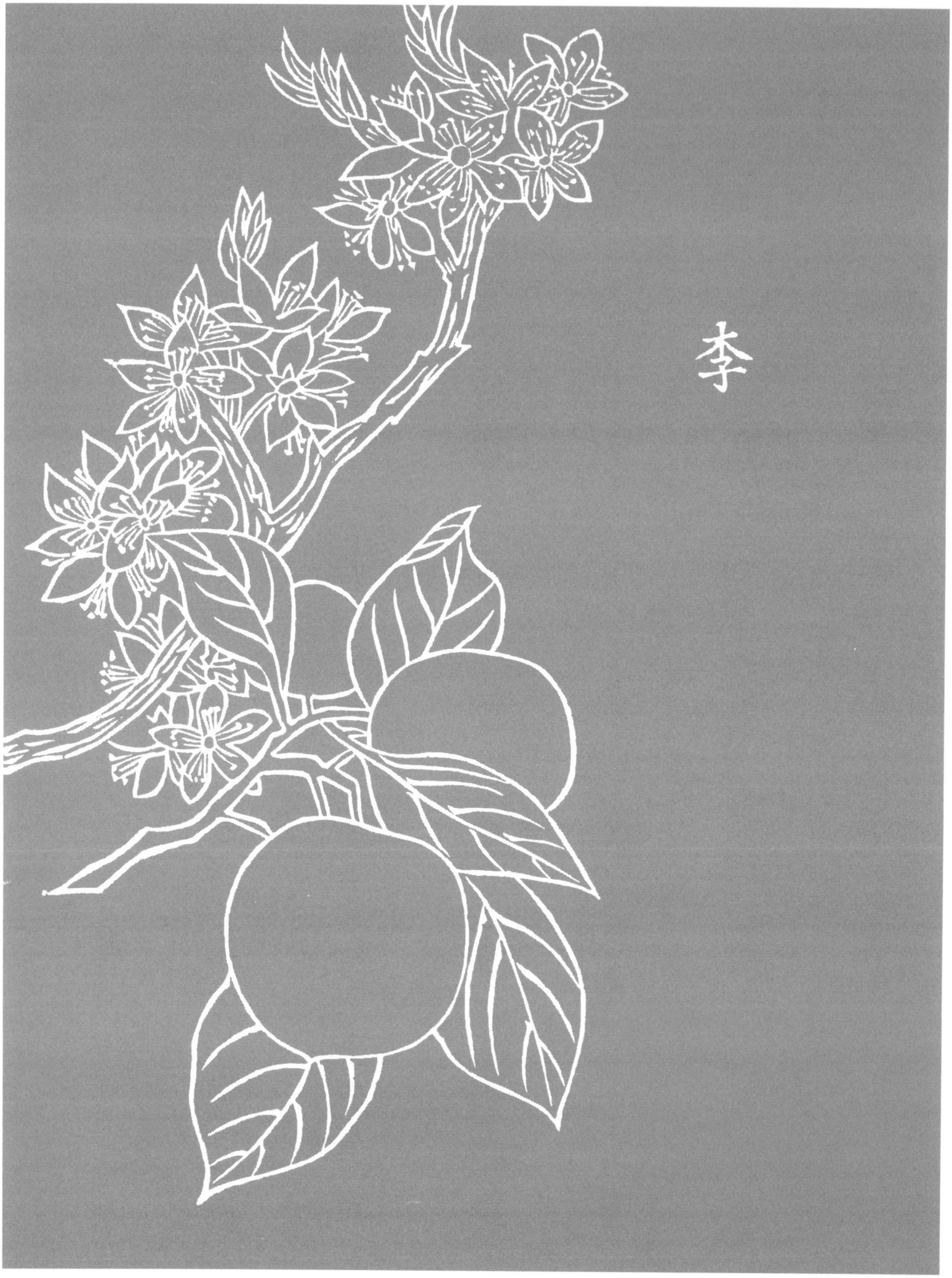
李

Glossary of Herbal Medicine Terms

Items in italics denote remedy actions.

adaptogenic — enhances adaptation response to stress
Air body — one of the four bodies, dealing with movement and response, having the nervous system as its main substrate
alterative — promotes systemic changes
analeptic — revives from shock or poisoning
analgesic — relieves pain internally
anesthetic — deadens local sensation or pain
anhydrotic — stops sweating
anodyne — relieves pain
antacid — reduces gastric acid
anthelmintic — treats worms
antiabortive — prevents miscarriage
antiaging — retards aging
antiallergic — treats allergies or hypersensitivities
antiarthritic — treats arthritis
antiasthmatic — treats asthma
antibacterial — treats bacteria
anticatarrhal — reduces catarrh
anticoagulant — prevents blood clotting
anticonvulsant — reduces convulsions
antidepressant — relieves depression
antidiarrheal — treats diarrhea
antidyskratic — rebalances the fluids in the presence of a fluids dyskrasia (disharmony)
antiemetic — reduces or stops vomiting
antienuretic — treats enuresis (involuntary urination)
antifungal — treats fungus or yeast
antigenic — reduces antibody production
anti-infective — treats infection
anti-inflammatory — reduces inflammation
antileucorrheal — treats leucorrhea
antilipemic — lowers blood lipid levels in the presence of hyperlipidemia
antilithic — prevents or dissolves and flushes out stones
antineoplastic — treats neoplasm or cancer
antioxidant — reduces oxidation by inhibiting free radical formation
antiparasitic — treats parasites

antipruritic — relieves skin itching
antipyretic — reduces fever by lowering temperature
antirheumatic —treats rheumatism
antisecretory — reduces secretions
antiseptic — topically prevents or restrains infection or putrefaction
antispasmodic — relieves spasms or cramps
antitumoral — treats tumors
antitussive — relieves coughing
antiviral — treats viruses
aperitive — stimulates the appetite
aphrodisiac — promotes sexuality
astriction — a tightening effect
astringent — astricts or tightens tissue
bioenergies — natural forces that create and sustain living things
biotype — an individual psychosomatic type; in Greek medicine a manifestation of a person's *physis* (natural condition) according to their *krasis* (quality) and fluid balance
Blood — structive physiological force grounded in the blood fluid; also known in Chinese medicine as *xue*
bronchodilatant — dilates the bronchi
cardiac — relating to the heart
carminative — relieves intestinal flatus
coagulant — promotes blood clotting
cholagogue — promotes bile flow
choleretic — enhances bile quality and quantity
cicatrisant — promotes tissue repair and reduces scarring
cold — one of the four qualities; a qualitative concept used in pharmacognosy, diagnostics and pathology to designate an effective quality; in pathology it defines a condition with insufficient objective or subjective warmth, as in hypothermia with feeling cold
congestion — a pathological condition involving stasis of one of the fluids, i.e. blood, mucous, interstitial or other fluid
constraint — a pathological condition involving mental or emotional, and therefore nervous, tension.
contraceptive — prevents conception
counterirritant — irritates to cause derivation
damp — one of the four qualities; a qualitative concept used in pharmacognosy, nosology and pathology to mean an effective quality; in pathology defining a condition caused by a stagnation of one of the pure or impure fluids, and therefore often qualified, e.g. mucous damp, water damp, phlegm damp; if unqualified, then usually referring to excessive mucous secretion (catarrh)
decongestant — relieves fluid or blood congestion
deficiency — a pathological condition presenting a functional or structural insufficiency or weakness
demulcent — soothes the mucous membrane
depressant — reducing mental/cerebral functions
derivation — a therapeutic technique that uses counterirritation to draw blood away from an area of disease to another body part, usually through the methods of cupping or bloodletting, or the topical use of *rubefacient, vesicant* or *pustulant* remedies
dermal — relating to the skin
dermatropic — having a tropism for the skin
detergent — cleans and disinfects wounds
detumescent — reduces swelling

detoxicant — resolves and clears toxin(s)
diaphoretic — promotes sweating
diathesis — an individual tendency or predisposition for disharmony inherent in an individual's *physis* (natural condition) or terrain
digestant — promotes digestion
discutient — resolves tumors
dissolvent — promotes solution (dissolving) of hard deposits, tissues or exudates
diuretic — promotes increased urination
draining diuretic — relieves fluid congestion (edema) and increases urination
dryness — one of the four qualities; a qualitative concept used in pharmacognoscy, diagnostics and pathology to denote an effective quality; in pathology designating a condition with insufficient mucous or other fluid secretion present
effective qualities — qualitative aspects of the nature of any substance—mineral, herbal, animal or human; applied to remedies, they consist of taste, warmth and moisture; they are effective because they produce physiological therapeutic effects (see four qualities below).
eliminant — promotes elimination through an excretory channel
emetic — causes vomiting
emmenagogue — promotes menstrual discharge
emollient — soothes and moistens the skin
Essence — an etheric or vital force governing growth, regeneration and reproduction; known as *jing* in Chinese medicine
excess — a pathological condition presenting a redundancy of function or substance
expectorant — promotes phlegm expulsion
external — (also exterior); a pathological condition at the initial or alarm stage of the three stages of general adaptation to stressors, and at the Tai Yang phase of the Chinese six disease stages; external conditions occur on the superficial body levels and present acute symptoms.
febrifuge — reduces fever
fetal relaxant — relaxing or calming to the fetus and therefore reducing abnormal fetal movement
Fluid body — one of the four bodies, dealing with metabolic (i.e. transformative) activities and mediated by the body fluids
four bodies — four physiological systems corresponding to the four elements: the Warmth, Air, Fluid and Physical bodies. Each is housed and regulated by certain organ systems, having specific qualities and functions, and dealing with specific forms of energy.
four fluids — also known as four humors; in Greek medicine the four basic fluid substances responsible for maintaining balance (or *eukrasia,* literally "good mixture"); they are phlegm, yellow bile, black bile and blood; when imbalanced they cause a dyskrasia, or poor (fluid) mixture, synonymous with disharmony
four level stages — the Chinese medical theory of the progression of disease according to four levels, namely the Defensive, Qi, Blood and Nutritive levels
four qualities — energetic, dynamic, effective qualities used to describe substances and processes such as remedies (pharmacognosy) and pathological conditions (pathology); hot/cold, dry/damp are the four qualities
free radical inhibitor — reduces free radicals
galactagogue — produces milk flow
ground — the place where disease occurs, whether the whole person, constitution or particular tissue; synonymous with terrain
heat — (also hot); one of the four qualities; a qualitative concept used in pharmacology, diagnostics and pathology; in pathology designating a condition with excessive warmth response, such as fever or inflammation, as well as subjective feelings of excessive warmth, and properly known as injurious heat.
hemogenic — builds blood (cells)

hemolytic — destroys blood (cells)
hemostatic — stops bleeding
hydragogue — expells water through the bowels
hydrogenic — retains fluids
hypertensive — increases blood pressure
hypnotic — calming the mind and spirit
hypoglycemiant — lowers blood sugar levels
hypotensive — reduces blood pressure
immune enhancer — enhances immune potential
immune potential — the potential of the immune system for effective response to pathogens
immune regulator — regulates immunity in hypersensitivity (i.e. allergic and autoimmune) disorders
immunostimulant — stimulates immune functions
interferon inducent — produces interferon
internal — (also interior); a pathological condition at the exhaustion phase of adaptation to stressors, and at any of the three Yin phases of the Chinese six meridian stages of disease (Tai Yin, Jue Yin, Shao Yin); internal conditions occur in the internal organs or systems and manifest chronic or degenerative symptoms
laxative — promotes gentle bowel movement
lenify — to soothe or mitigate
lenitive — reduces irritation
leukocytogenic — increases white blood cells
lymphocyte stimulant — increases T-lymphocytes and lymphocyte transformation rate
mucogenic — produces mucus
mucolytic — softens hardened bronchial sputum or intestinal mucus
mucostatic —stops mucus production and catarrhal discharge
mucus — mucosal fluid
nervine — having an affinity for the nervous system
nutritive — promotes nutrition or provides nourishment
optitropic — having a tropism for the eyes and vision
oxytocic — promotes labor contractions by releasing oxytocin hormone
parasiticide — kills parasites
parturient — promotes labor
pattern of disharmony — a syndrome, consisting of a complex of specific signs and symptoms
phagocyte stimulant — enhances phagocyte functions
pharmacognosy — the study of the nature of remedies
pharmacology — the study of the physiological effects of remedies
phenomenology — the study of empirically observed phenomena
phlegm — bronchial mucous
physical bodies — one of the four bodies; physical body tissue as a whole
puerperal — relating to childbirth
purgative — promotes copious bowel movement
pustulant — causes pustules
Qi — a Chinese medical term denoting active physiological energy
rash-promoting — promoting eruptions in eruptive fever
refrigerant — promotes a cooling down and clears heat
relaxant — promotes relaxation
resolvent — resolves toxicosis
resorbant — promotes catabolic resorption
restorative — restores and strengthens
righteous Qi —a Chinese medical term denoting the sum of "righteous" (*zheng*) Qi available to a

person. It is also defined by its opposite, "injurious" or "pathogenic" (*xie*) Qi. In practice it can be reconciled with the Greek medical concept of vital spirit(s).

rubefacient — causes skin reddening through hyperemia

secretory — promotes secretions

sedative — reduces activity

simple — a single remedy

six channel stages — the Chinese medical theory of stages of disease according to the six channel pairs; exogenous illness begins in the Tai Yang stage and progresses to the Yang Ming, Shao Yang, Tai Yin, Shao Yin and Jue Yin stages

spasmolytic — reduces spasm or cramp in the smooth or striped muscles

spermicidal — kills sperm

stages of adaptation — the theory of the three stages of adaptation to stressors, being the alarm, resistance and exhaustion stages; also known as the general adaptation syndrome

stages of disease — the theory of the four stages of disease according to vital activity; illness begins in the acute stage and progresses to the subacute, chronic and degenerative

Stagnation — a pathological condition denoting a slowing down of normal processes and buildup of injurious or toxic substances (e.g. mucus, sputum, endotoxins, fatty and mineral deposits, etc.)

stimulant — increases activity and promotes warmth

structive — producing substance and form; the opposite/complementary of active

styptic — stops bleeding through topical application

syndrome — a specific complex of signs and symptoms presenting a symptom picture; synonymous with "pattern of disharmony"

temperament — krasis (which see)

teratogenic — injures the fetus

tonic — restores and strengthens

toxicosis — (also "autotoxicosis"); a pathological condition involving the accumulation of endogenous or exogenous toxins

toxins — injurious (pathological) substances generated internally or accumulated from the environment

trophorestorative — nourishes and builds tissue

tropism — the property of a remedy of having an affinity or bias for treating certain organs, systems or body parts

vasoconstrictor — tightens blood vessels

vasodilator — expands blood vessels

vermicide — kills internal parasites

vermifuge — expels intestinal parasites

vesicant — causes watery blisters

vulnerary — promotes tissue healing

Warmth body — one of the four bodies, dealing with warmth responses, such as inflammation, fever or dislike of heat; or a lack of these, as in hypothermia or fear of cold

Yang — physiological energies of the Yang type

Yin — physiological energies of the Yin type

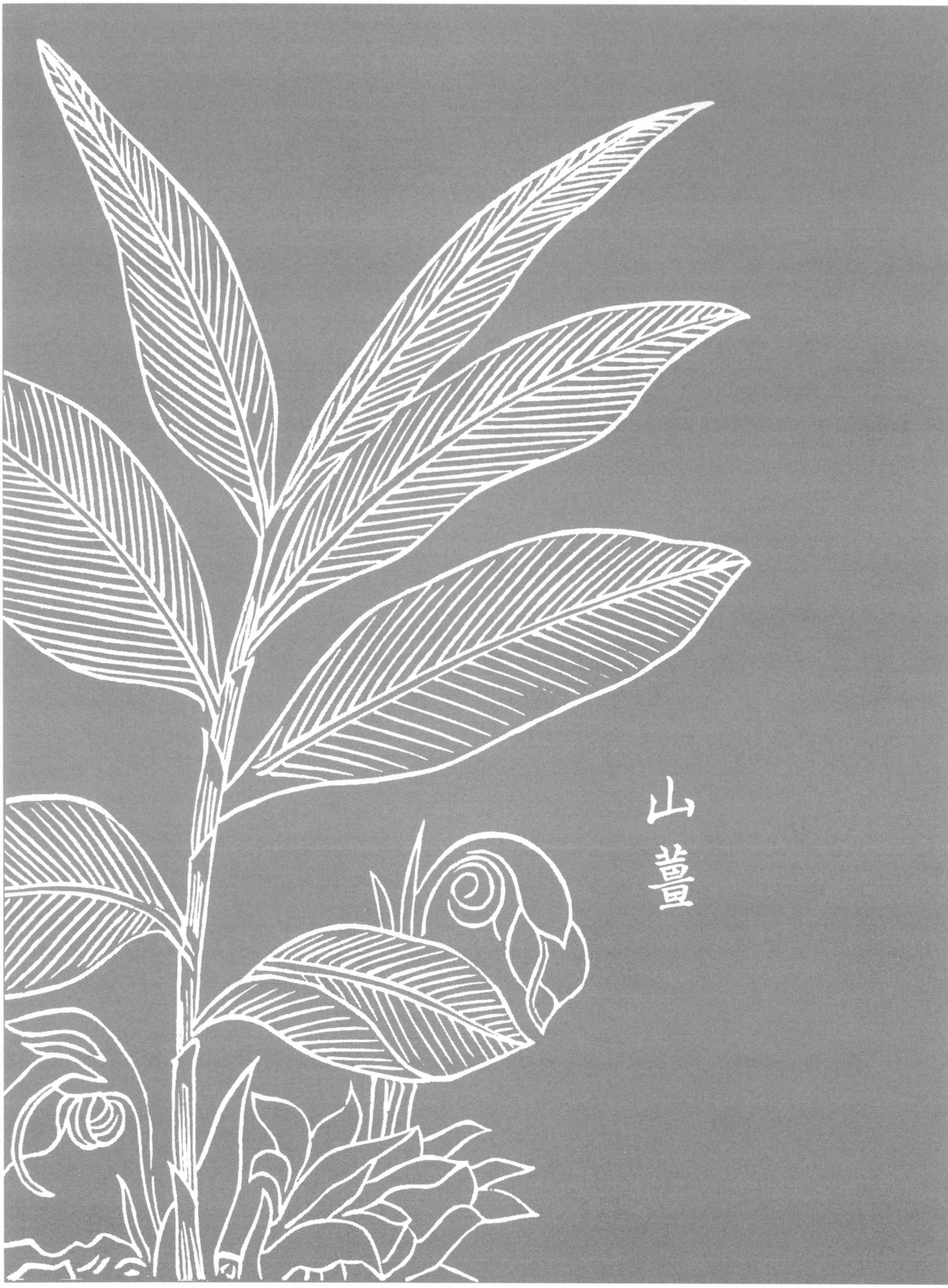
山薑

Glossary of Latin Pharmaceutical Terms

Latin Term	Remedy Part
arillus	flesh
bombyx	larva
bulbus	bulb
cacumen	tip, end twig
calculus	stone
calyx	calyx
carapax	dorsal shell
caudex	stalk
caulis	stem
cinis	ash
colla	glue
concha	shell
concretio	hard secretion
cornu	horn
cortex	bark
cortex radicis	root bark
endothelium	inner lining
excrementum	dropping or stool
exocarpium	outer rind
exuvia	slough
farina	flour
fel	gallbladder
flos	flower
folium	leaf
fructificatio	mushroom
fructus	fruit
galla	gall
gelatinum	glue
gemma	bud
herba	herb
lamina	blade
lichen	lichen
lignum	wood
medulla	pith
nodus	node, protuberance
oleum	oil
oleum aethereum	essential oil
ootheca	egg case
os	bone
pedicellus	pedicel
pericarpium	rind, husk
periostracum	slough
placenta	placenta
plastrum	ventral shell
plumula	plumule
pollen	pollen
radix	root
ramulus	twig
ramus	branch
resina	resin
rhizoma	rhizome
scapus	scapus
sclerotium	mushroom
secretio	secretion
semen	seed
spica	spike
spina	spine
spora	spore
squama	scale
staminus	stamen
stigma	stigma
succus	juice, sap
terra	clay, earth
thallus	thallus
tuber	tuber
turio	shoot, sprout
uncus	thorn
venenum	venom

Glossary of Mandarin Pronunciation

Initials

b -	as in *mob*
p -	as in *pin* but more aspirated
m -	as in *may*
f -	as in *far*
d -	as in *day* but less voiced
t -	as in *tall* but more aspirated
n -	as in *no*
l -	as in *lay*
z -	as in *Zen*
c -	as in *its,* but with more aspiration and the tongue farther foreward
s -	as in *see,* but with the tongue farther foreward
zh -	as in *jungle,* but pronounced more with the teeth
ch -	as in *chair,* but with the tongue curled far back on the palate
sh -	as in *wash,* but with the tongue curled far back on the palate
r -	as in *ran,* but with the tongue curled back on the palate
j -	as in *jeans,* but with the tongue tip on the lower teeth
q -	as in *cheese,* but with the tongue tip on the lower teeth
x -	between the *s* in *saw* and the *sh* in *shawl*
y -	as in *yen,* but softer
g -	as in *guy,* but less voiced
k -	as in *kite,* but more aspirated
h -	like *ch* in the average Swiss German pronounciation of *nach*

Finals

- a	as in *father*
- o	as in the American pronunciation of *awe* or the French *lors*
- e	like the *er* in *dinner* in the American pronunciation
- i	after simple initials: as in *seem.* After silibant initials and after retroflex initials, the *- i* is not pronounced
- er	as in the American pronunciation of *stir*
- ai	as in *my*
- ei	as in *say*
- ao	as in *now,* but more in the lips
- ou	as in *mow,* but with lips more pursed, as in the Scottish pronunciation
- an	similar to the American pronunciation of *John,* or as in the German *Bahn*
- en	as in the German *können*
- ang	as in *dung,* but more nasal and guttural
- eng	as as in *urn* + *ng,* very nasal
- ong	as in the German *Zeitung*
- ia	as in the German *ja*
- iao	as in *meeow*
- ie	as in *yes*
- iu	as in *pew*
- ian	like the *ee* in *seem* and the *un* in *fun*
- in	as in *seen* or the German *hin*
- iang	like the *ee* in *seem* and the *ung* in *dung*
- ing	as in the Chinese final *eng* with a *y -* at the beginning (*y* + *urn* + *ng*), very nasal and guttural
- iong	like the *ee* in *seem* plus the *ong* of *gong* in the British pronunciation
- u	as in *moon* or the German *Mut*

- *ua*	as in *guava*
- *uo*	somewhat as in the British pronunciation of *worry*
- *uai*	like the *ui* in *quiet*
- *uei*	as in *way*
- *uan*	as in *wand*
- *un*	as in the Spanish *uno*
- *uang*	as in *w* plus *ung* (as in *hung*)
- *ü*	like the German *ü*
- *üe*	like the German *ü* plus the *e* in *yes*
- *üan*	like the German *ü* plus the *un* in *unto*
- *ün*	as in the German *dünn*
- *ui*	as in *we* or the French *oui*

Notes

• All the finals from - *ia* onwards are actually combinations of two finals, or an initial and a final.

• The system of transliteration used in this text is the widely-adopted Pinyin system.

Glossary of Cantonese Pronunciation

Initials

p -	as in *pull*
t -	as in *tall*
k -	as in *kitten*
ch -	as in *chip,* but with the tongue nearer the teeth and more explosive
kw -	as in *queen*
b -	as in *bay*
d -	as in *day*
g -	as in *gay*
j -	between the *j* of *june* and the *dds* of *adds*
gw -	as in *guava*
m -	as in *ma*
n -	as in *no*
ng -	as in *sing*
f -	as in *far*
l -	as in *lay*
h -	as in *how*
s -	between the *s* of *see* and the *sh* of *she*
y -	as in *yet*
w -	as in *wet*

Finals

- a	as in *father*
- aai	as in *my* but longer, as in the German *Laib*
- ai	as in *my*
- aau	as in *now* but longer, as in the German *Frau*
- au	as in *now*
- aam	as in *some* but longer, as in the German *Rahm*
- am	as in *some*
- aan	as in the British pronunciation of *aunt* or the German *Mahn*
- an	as in *done*
- aang	as in *dung* but longer, as in the German *Hahn*
- ang	as in *dung*
- aap	as in *up* but longer, as in the French *âpre*
- ap	as in *cup*
- aat	as in *nut* but longer, as in the German *Naht*
- at	as in *cut*
- aak	as in *duck* but longer, as in the German *mag*
- ak	as in *duck* or the French *tac*
- e	as in *let* but longer, as in the French *aime*
- eng	as in length but longer, as in the German *längst*
- ek	as in *deck* but longer
- ei	as in *say*
- eu	as in the British pronunciation of *fur* or the French *seul*
- eung	as in *urn* + *ng*
- euk	as in *quirk* but shorter
- eui	as in the French *seuil*
- eun	as in the German *können*
- eut	as in the German *löten,* but shorter, as in the Turkish *sit*
- i	as in *ease* or the German *hin*
- iu	as in *pew*
- im	as in *seem* or the German *ihm*
- in	as in *keen* or the German *ihn*
- ip	as in *jeep* but shorter, as in the French *Philippe*

- *it*	as in *meet* or the German *Lied*
- *ing*	as in *sing* or the German *singen*
- *ik*	as in *lick* or the German *fickerig*
- *o*	as in the American pronunciation of *awe* or the French *lors*
- *oi*	as in *joy*
- *on*	as in the British pronunciation of *on*
- *ong*	as in the British pronunciation of *gong*
- *ot*	as in the British pronunciation of *hot*
- *ok*	as in the British pronunciation of *lock*
- *ou*	as in *mow* but with lips more pursed, as in the Scottish pronunciation
- *u*	as in *moon* or the German *Mut*
- *ui*	as in *we* or the French *oui*
- *un*	as in *moon*
- *ut*	as in the German *Mutter*
- *ung*	as in the German *Zeitung*
- *uk*	as in *look* or the German *guck*
- *yu*	as in the German *Lüge*
- *yun*	as in the German *günstig*
- *yut*	as in the German *Jütland*

Notes

• When *p, k* and *t* are final consonants, they are not pronounced. Instead of being explosive as in Western languages, they are silent. With *p, k* and *t,* the lips, teeth and throat respectively make a silent final to the preceeding vowel or diphthong.

For example, the final - *ap* is pronounced as in *cup,* but the *p* is silent as the lips simply close without letting any air out (the explosive). The same goes for the final - *at,* in which the tongue hits the inside top front teeth without any explosive sound. Likewise the final - *ak* ends with the throat closing up silently.

• All - *u* finals are prononounced with a soft *w* sound in front of them. The *w* sound is generated with pursed lips.

• All three - *yu* finals are pronounced with a flat *ü* sound (as in the German *Lüge*), i.e., without any *y* sound (as in *yam*) produced by the tongue.

• The system of transliteration used in this text is the widely-adopted Yale system.

• Like Mandarin Chinese, Cantonese Chinese has a system of tones, only more complex. It comprises a total of nine tones. For reasons of simplicity, the Cantonese tones have been omitted from this text.

• When working out the correct Cantonese pronunciation of remedies, or when comparing an herbalist's pronunciation with the one given in this text, keep in mind that many Cantonese doctors pronounce them differently than the correct or official way given in this text. This is because Cantonese itself comprises several dialects, just as German does, none of which are phonetically written down.

• When two or more Cantonese remedy names are listed in the materia medica, it is not because one is the official pronunciation and the other a dialectic variant. It is because the remedy has other distinct names that are commonly used by Cantonese doctors. Sometimes, but not always, these other names correspond to the remedy's other Mandarin names. For example, the most common Cantonese name for the remedy Astragalus Huang Qi is Baak Kei. This corresponds to its Mandarin name Bei Qi. In Mandarin however, the name Huang Qi is more commonly used.

A similar but more complex example is seen with the Cantonese name for the remedy Codonopsis Dang Shen. Its main Cantonese name is Fong Dong Sam, corresponding to the archaic, now rarely used Mandarin name Fang Dang Shen. Cantonese remedy names thereby often preserve older or regional names now rarely used in the mainstream Mandarin.

Syndrome and Disease

Syndrome or Symptom Picture

- the systemistic approach to illness
- symptom picture definition is based on the spatial-circular logic of synchronicity and correspondence
- the older, traditional method of defining illness used in vitalistic medical systems such as Chinese medicine, Greek medicine, Homeopathy and Eclectic herbal medicine
- also known as syndrome, pattern of disharmony, specific symptomatology, etc.
- is seen as a condition of on-going dynamic change in the individual's vital force, which presents ever-changing patterns of signs and symptoms
- relies for its definition primarily on naked observation of the patient as a whole person
- signs and symptoms have various origins
- the signs and symptom presentation is simultaneously the cause and effect of the illness
- the phenomena of signs and symptoms themselves define the symptom picture
- signs and symptoms may be physiological, emotional and/or mental
- signs and symptoms are fundamentally an expression of the individual vital force or *qi*
- the diagnosis of signs and symptoms is mainly functional
- treatment aims to re-establish homeostasis in the whole individual by improving his or her vital force or *qi,* thereby promoting a resolution of the syndrome
- <u>examples</u>: Lung phlegm cold, kidney dryness, venous blood stagnation, coronary blood deficiency

Disease

- the reductionistic approach to illness
- disease definition is based on the temporal-linear logic of cause and effect
- the more contemporary method of defining illness initially developed by Greek medicine and developed in modern times by allopathic Western medicine since the sixteenth century
- is seen as a fixed biological and taxonomical entity that runs a predetermined course in humans
- relies for its definition primarily on scientifc analysis of the patient's pathogenic tissues or structures
- signs and symptoms have a single origin (shown by arrow)
- signs and symptoms are seen to be caused by specific endogenous or exogenous pathogens
- the mechanisms of pathogenesis underlying the signs and symptoms define the disease
- signs and symptoms are primarily physiological
- signs and symptoms are mainly an expression of the pathogens at work
- diagnosis of signs and symptoms is mainly morphological
- treatment aims to remove the offending pathogens or correct the mechanical dysfunction in order to end the disease
- <u>examples</u>: flu, bronchitis, candidiasis, herpes

The Four Remedy Actions

stimulants

pungent, dry, warm/hot

essential oils, glycosides

- stimulate arterial circulation - *arterial stimulants*
- promote sweating - *diaphoretics*
- promote urination - *diuretics*
- promote bowel movement - *laxatives*
- promote expectoration - *expectorants*
- stimulate organ functions – *respiratory/digestive/urinary/reproductive/musculoskeletal/central nervous stimulants*

restoratives

sweet, moist, warm

saponins, other glycosides, trace minerals

- provide moisture - *demulcents*
- nourish the blood - *hemogenics & nutritives*
- restore organ & gland functions - *coronary/digestive/liver/urinary/musculoskeletal/central nervous/endocrine restoratives*

astringent, dry, cool

tannins, flavonoids, saponins

- promote astriction - *astringents, venous decongestants*
- stop bleeding - *hemostatics, anticoagulants*

relaxants

pungent, cool

essential oils, alkaloids, glycosides

- reduce smooth muscle spasms - *spasmolytics*
- reduce convulsions - *anticonvulsants*
- relax organ functions - *respiratory/criculatory/digestive/urinary/musculoskeletal/central nervous relaxants*

sedatives

bitter, dry, cool/cold

alkaloids, essential oils, organic acids

- reduce inflammation - *anti-inflammatories*
- reduce fever - *antipyretics*
- reduce infection - *anti-infectives*
- reduce toxicosis - *detoxicants*
- relieve pain - *analgesics*

Key

- main remedy action
- main effective qualities
- main chemical constituents
- main therapeutic actions

See p. 66 for a discussion of the four remedy actions.

The Phytogeographic Regions of China and Important Remedies Produced

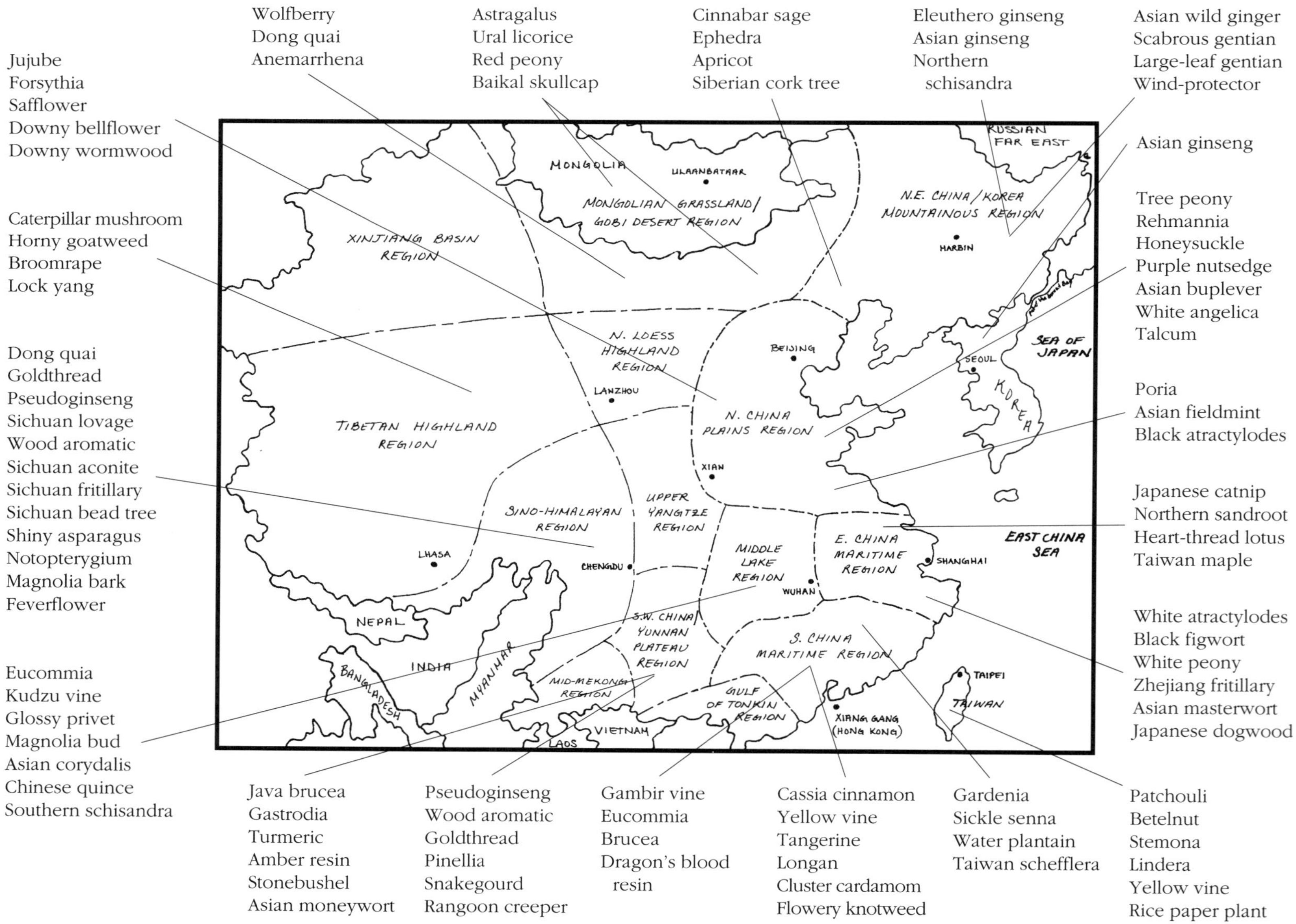

Resource Guide

Suppliers of Chinese Remedies in Bulk — North America

Kwok Shing Import-Export, Inc.
1818 Harrison St
San Francisco, CA 94103
Tel 415/861-1668
800/326-1668

North-South China Herbs
1556 Stockton St.
San Francisco, CA 94133
Tel 415/421-4907
Fax 415/421-5576

Mayway Corp.
1338 Mandela Parkway
Oakland, CA 94607
Tel 510/208-3113
800/262-9929
Fax 510/208-3069
800/909-2828

Tai Sang Trading Co.
1018 Stockton St.
San Francisco, CA 94108
Tel 415/981-5364
Fax 415/981-2032

Suppliers of Chinese Remedies in Bulk — Europe

AcuMedic
101-105 Camden High St.
London W1 7JN, England
Tel 171/388-5783/6704
Fax 171/387-5766

17 Carlisle Rd
London NW9 0HD, England
Tel 181/201-3688
Fax 181/201-3633

Mayway Corp.
43 Waterside Trading Estate
Trumpers Way
London W7 2QD, England
Tel 181/893-6873
Fax 181/893-6874

Selected Bibliography

Works on Chinese Herbal Medicine

Primary Sources: Chinese and Japanese Language Books

Academy of Traditional Chinese Medicine and the Guangdong College of Traditional Chinese Medicine. *Zhong Yi Ming Ci Shu Yu Ci Dian [Dictionary of Chinese Medical Terminology and Nomenclature]*. Hong Kong, 1975

Akamatsu, Kaneyoshi. *Shintei Wakanyaku [Newly Revised Oriental Remedies]*. Tokyo, 1980

Anon. *Ming Yi Bie Lu [An Eminent Physician's Reference Work]*. 502-557

Anon. *Pin Hui Jing Yao [The Essential Qualities of Medicinal Plants]*. n.d.

Anon. *Shennong Ben Cao Jing [Shennong's Herbal]*. before 25 B.C. Repr. Hong Kong, 1955

Beijing Traditional Medical College, eds. *Zhong Yao Fang Ji Xue [The Prescriptions of Traditional Chinese Remedies]*. Beijing, 1971

Canton Department of Hygiene. *Chang Yong Zhong Cao Yao Jou Zi [Manual of the Most Commonly Used Medicinal Plants and Remedies]*. Beijing, 1969

Chang, H.T. *Lapidarum Sinicum*. Beijing, 1921

Chen Qin-ming. *Dang Dai Zhong Yao Xue [Modern Chinese Materia Medica]*. Taipei, 1977

Chen Ren-shan. *Yao Wu Chu Chan Pien [Herb Differentiation according to Habitat]*. 1930. Repr. Taipei 1977

Chen Zhang-qi. *Ben Cao Shi Yi [Supplement to the Newly Revised Herbal]*. 739

Chengdu College of Traditional Chinese Medicine. *Zhong Yao Xue [Chinese Herbal Medicine]*. Shanghai, 1977

Cheung, Siu-cheong, and Li, Ning-hon, eds. *Xiang Gang Zhong Cao Yao [Chinese Medicinal Herbs of Hong Kong]* (5 vols). Hong Kong, 1978

Chiu Chen-po. *Zhong Yao Xin Bian [A New Manual of Chinese Materia Medica]*. Shanghai, 1955

Cui Shu-De. *Zhong Yao Da Quan [Great Compendium of Chinese Materia Medica]*. Harbin, 1989

Da Ming (Se Ming). *Zhi Hua Zi Zhu Jia Ben Cao [Zhi Hua Zi School Herbal]*. 960-1279

Department of Hygiene, Peking, Lanzhou, Zhenyang, Xinjiang. *Pei Fang Chang Cao Yao Jou Zi [Handbook of Medicinal Plants and Remedies Most Commonly Used in Temperate China]*. Beijing, 1971

Gansu Provincial Academy of New Medicine. *Zhong Yao Xue [Chinese Materia Medica]*. Beijing, 1982

Gu Ming et al. *Han Ying Chang Yong Zhong Yi Ci Hui [Chinese-English Glossary of Common Terms in Traditional Chinese Medicine]*. Hong Kong, 1982

Guangdong College of Traditional Chinese Medicine. *Zhong Yi Fang Yao Xue [Traditional Chinese Medical Prescriptions and Substances]*. Guangzhou, 1973

Huang Xian-kai et al. *Han Ying Chang Yong Yi Xue Ci Hui [Chinese-English Collection of Common Medical Terminology]*. Beijing, 1982

Hsu, Hong-yen. *Taiwan Ti Chu Chan ZhongYao Cao Cai Tu Chien [Illustrated Guide to the Medicinal Plants of Taiwan]*. Taipei, 1972

Institute of Chinese Materia Medica, Academy of Traditional Chinese Medicine. *Quan Guo Zhong Cao Yao Hui Bian [All China Traditional and Herbal Remedies]* (2 vols). Beijing 1975-78

Institute of Present-Day Chinese Medicine. *Ling Nan Cai Yao Lou [Compendium of the Southern Materia Medica]* (2 vols.). Hong Kong, 1964

Jiangxi College of Traditional Chinese Medicine. *Zhong Cao Yao [Chinese Materia Medica]*. Beijing, 1978

Jiangsu New Medical College, eds. *Zhong Yao Da Ci Dian [Encyclopedia of the Traditional Materia Medica]* (3 vols.). Shanghai 1976

Kaibara Ekiken (Ekken). *Yamato Honso [Materia Medica of Japan]*. 1708

Lan Mao. *Tien Nan Ben Cao [Southern Yunnan Herbal]*. 1397-1476. Repr. Kunming, 1975

Li Shi-zhen. *Ben Cao Gang Mu*. 1578. Repr. in 2 vols. Beijing, 1957

Li Xun. *Hai Yao Ben Cao [Herbal from the Sea]*. 618-906

Lin, Chi-sou. *Zhong Cao Yao Cheng Fen Hua Xue [The Chemistry of Chinese Remedy Constituents]*. Taipei, 1977

Ling Yi-kui. *Zhong Yao Xue [Chinese Materia Medica]*. Shanghai, 1984

Liu Han. *Kai Bao Ben Cao [Kai Bao Herbal]*. c. 973

Liu, Wen-tao et al. *Ben Cao Pin Hui Qing Yao [Essential Remedies of Chinese Materia Medica]*. 1505

Lou, Z.C, Xiao, P.G and Xu, G.J, eds. *Zhong Yao Zhi [Chinese Materia Medica]* (4 vols.). Beijing, 1980-87

Lu Gui-seng. *Zhong Yao Ko Xue Hua Da Zi Dian [Compendium of Scientific Studies of Chinese Medicine*. 1954

Miao, W.W. *Zhong Cao Yao De Gu Shi [Stories of Remedies and Herbs]*. Beijing, 1981

Murakoshi Michio. *Yakuyo Shyokubutsu Jiten [Dictionary of Medicinal Plants]*. Tokyo, 1958

Namba, Tsuneo. *Genshoku Wakanyaku Zukan [Color Illustrations of Crude Remedies]*. Tokyo, 1980

Nanjing Institute of Materia Medica. *Yao Cai Xue [Study of Chinese Remedies]*. Hong Kong

Pei Jian and Zhou Tai-yen. *Zhong Guo Yao Yong Zhe Wou Zhe [Medicinal Plants Used in Pharmacology]* (2 vols.). Beijing, 1956

People's Hygiene Agency. *Chang Yong Zhong Cao Yao Di Ren Bie [Manual of the Most Frequent Confusions Among Chinese Medicinal Plants]*. Shanghai, 1972

Pharmaceutics Institute of the Academy of Medicine, Beijing, et al. *Zhong Yao Chi [New Chinese Materia Medica]*. Beijing, 1961

Pharmacopeia Committee of the Ministry of health. *Zhong Hua Ren Min Gong He Guo Yao Dian [Pharmacopeia of the People's Republic of China]*. Beijing, 1985

Ren Ren-an, et al. *Zhong Yao Yang Ding Xue [Pharmacognoscy of Chinese Remedies]*. Shanghai, 1986

Shanghai College of Traditional Chinese Medicine. *Zhong Cao Yao Xue [Chinese Materia Medica]*. Hong Kong, 1975

Shu Xue-zhong, Chen Da-shun and He Yon-shun. *Han Ying Shuang Jie Chang Yong Zhong Yi Ming Ci Shu Yu [Chinese-English Terminology of Traditional Chinese Medicine]*. Changsha, 1981

Su Jing. *Tang Ben Cao [Tang Herbal]*. 659

Su Song. *Tu Jing Ben Cao [Illustrated Herbal]*. 1064

Takagi, Keijiro et al. *Wakan Yakubutsugaku [Pharmacology of East Asian Medicinal Plants]*. Tokyo, 1982

Tang Shen-wei. *Zheng Lei Ben Cao [Herbal Arranged According to Patterns]*. 1098-1107

Terajima Lioan. *Wakan Sansai Zukan [Illustrated Book of Japanese Herbs]*. 1712

Wang Ji. *Ben Cao Hui Bian*.

Wu Yi-lo. *Ben Cao Zong Xin [Revision of Ben Cao Pei Yao]*. 1757. Repr. Shanghai, 1958

Wu Jia-jing. *Tu Jie Zhong Yao Yao Wu Xue [Illustrated Pharmacology of Chinese Remedies]*. 1973

Wu Jin-xie. *Zhong Guo Yi Xue Da Ci Dian [Comprehensive Dictionary of Chinese Medicine]*. Shanghai, 1981

Xu Guo-Jun, ed. *Zhong Cao Yao Cai Shi Tu Pu [Coloured Illustrations of Chinese Traditional and Herbal Drugs]*. Fujian Science and Technology Publishing Co. Fuzhou, 1990

Xu Jiao-mu and Jiu Nian-yong. *Tai Wan Yao Cai Fu Cha Tu [The Illustrated Medicinal Plants of Taiwan]*. Taipei, 1980

Xu Jiao-mu and Jiu Nian-yong. *Tai Wan Ke Chi Ye Sheng Zhi Wu [The Illustrated Edible Wild Plants of Taiwan]*. Taipei, 1980

Yan Kuen-yin, ed. *Han Fang Yi Xue Li Lun [Medical Theory of Chinese Herbal Formulas]*. Taipei, 1974

———. *Bing Zhen Bu Fang Ji Tu Jie [Formulas Illustrated by Signs and Symptoms]*. Taipei, 1974

Yen Kun-ying. *Zhong Guo Cao Yao Fu Cha Tu Tian Jan—Yi Liao [Illustrated Chinese Materia Medica, Crude Remedies]*. Taipei, 1980

———. *Zhong Guo Cao Yao Fu Cha Tu—Jia Gong Yi Liao [Illustrated Chinese Materia Medica, Prepared Remedies]*. Taipei, 1980

Zai Ke-min et al. *Chang Yong Zhong Yao De Yao Li He Ying Yong [Pharmacology and Application of Frequently Used Chinese Remedies]*. Suzhou, 1981

Zhang En-qin, ed. *The Chinese Materia Medica*. Shanghai, 1989

———. *Rare Chinese Materia Medica*. Shanghai, 1989

———. *Chinese Medicated Diet*. Shanghai, 1989

———. *Prescriptions of Traditional Chinese Medicine*. Shanghai, 1989

Zhang Zhong-jing. *Shang Han Lun [Treatise on Hot Diseases]*. 219

Zhao Xue-min. *Wai Tai Bi Yao*. 752. Repr. Beijing, 1958

Zhong Shan Medical School. *Zhong Yao Lin Chuang Ying Yong [Clinical Applications of Chinese Materia Medica]*. Guangdong, 1976

Primary Sources: Chinese and Japanese Language Journal Articles

Bian Chun-fu, Zhang Da-he and Wang Jian-hua. "Chinese Medicines Used in Anesthesia." ACME 2(1), 1988

Chen Ke-ji and Zhang Wen-pen. Advances on Anti-Ageing Herbal Medicines in China. ACME 1(2), 1987

Chen Fa-chun. "Progress in the Studies on Natural Antilipemic Compounds." Chinese Traditional and Herbal Drugs 20(4), 1989

Ding Guang-sheng. "Anti-Arrhythmia Agents in Traditional Chinese Medicines." ACME 1(2), 1987

Du Yu-mao and Chen Ren-hou. "Mechanism of Chinese Medicines in Prevention and Treatment of AIDS." Journal of Shaanxi College of Traditional Chinese Medicine 13(1), 1990

Han De-wu, Xu Rui-ling and Yeung Shen Chang-shing. "Chinese Medicines for the Prevention and Treatment of Viral Hepatitis." ACME 2(1), 1988

Hsu Hong-yen, editor. Oriental Healing Arts International Bulletin. Oriental Healing Arts Institute, Long Beach.

Hsu Hong-yen. Advances of Research on Medicinal Plants in Taiwan. ACME 1(3), 1988

Hu Bi and But, Paul Pui-hay. "Chinese Materia Medica for Radiation Protection." ACME 1(3), 1987

Hu Xi-ming, editor. Journal of Traditional Chinese Medicine. Beijing

Huang Jiao-cheng. "Biopharmaceutical Studies on Active Components of Chinese Traditional Drugs." ACME 2(1), 1988

Kohda, A. et al. Nihon Yakurigaku Zasshi 78(31), 1982

Lee Kuo-hsiung and Yamagishi Takashi. "Antineoplastic Terpenoids from Chinese Medicinal Plants." ACME 1(4), 1987

Leung Wing-nang and Tso Wung-wa. "Gossypol—A Potential Male Contraceptive." ACME 2(2), 1988

Li Zhong. "Pharmacology of Polysaccharides from Chinese Drugs." Chinese Pharmaceutical

Bulletin 23 (8), 1988
Lu Lan-xun. "Antilipemic Chinese Medicines." Shaanxi Journal of Chinese Traditional Medicine, 1987
Mao Xiao-juan et al. "Effects of the Polysaccharides of Astragalus Membranaceus and Hedysarum Polybotrys on Humoral Immunity in Mice." Chinese Journal of Immunology 4(3), 1988
Mo Li-li, Li Xiu-ting and Liang Song-min. "Chinese Drugs for Atherosclerosis." ACME 3(1), 1989
Qin Wan-zhang. "Progress in the Treatment of Autoimmune Diseases by Traditional Chinese Medicine." Journal of Clinical Dermatology, 1988
Qiu Gang and Wu An-ran. "Chinese Materia Medica with Anti-Atopy Effect." ACME 1(1), 1986
Sun San-sheng et al. "Survey on the Botanical Origin of Varieties of the Crude Drug Huang Qi and their Identification." Chinese Pharmaceutical Journal 25(11), 1990
Tang Wei-ci. "Chinese Medicinal Materials from the Sea." ACME 1(4), 1987
Tang Xiao-shan, Chen Hong-shan, and Zheng Xing-quan. "Inhibition of Human Immunodeficiency Virus Reverse Transcriptase in Vitro by Extracts of Chinese Medicinal Herbs." Acta Academiae Medicinae Sinica 12 (6), 1990
Wan Jia-zhen and Huang Yue-hua. "Studies on Semen Zizyphi Spinosae in Preventing Acute Altitude Sickness." Pharmacology and Clinics of Chinese Materia Medica, 1986
Wu He-ping and Yao Ming-qi. "Chinese Crude Drugs Having Immunological Actions." Shanghai Journal of Traditional Chinese Medicine (9), 1989
Xu Chang-zao, Zhou Shu-li, et al. "Determination of Metallic Elements in some Blood Activating Chinese Drugs and a Discussion of their Mechanisms of Action." Trace Elements (2), 1989
Xu Guo-jun and Wang Zheng-tao. "Advances of Pharmacognoscy in China from 1985-1988." ACME 3(4), 1989
Xu Guo-jun and But, Paul Pui-Hay. "Recent Advances of Pharmacognosy in China." ACME 1(1)
Xu Yue-lin and Kang Ke-fei. "Progress in the Research on Tripterygium wilfordii." Shanghai Medical Journal 11(3), 1988
Zhang Shu-lan et al. "Effects of Natural Cordyceps and the Cultured Mycelia of Cordyceps Sinensis on Murine Immune Organs and Functions of Mononuclear Phagocyte Systems." Shanghai, 1985
Zhao Min-fen, Yang Kai and Yu Su-qin. "Determination of Trace Elements in 44 Antiviral Chinese Herbs by Atomic Emission Spectropnotometry." Trace Elements (2), 1989
Zhu Da-yuan. "Recent Advances on the Active Components in Chinese Medicines." ACME 1(2), 1987

Secondary Sources: Western Language Books and Articles

Beijing Medical College, eds. *Dictionary of Traditional Chinese Medicine*. Hong Kong, 1984
Bensky, Dan, and Gamble, Andrew, comp. and trans. *Chinese Herbal Medicine: Materia Medica*. Seattle, 1986
Bensky, Dan, and Barolet, Randall, comp. and trans. *Chinese Herbal Medicine: Formulas and Strategies*. Seattle, 1991
Braquet, P., ed. Ginkgolides—*Chemistry, Pharmacology and Clinical Perspectives*. Barcelona, 1988
Braun, R. *List of Medicines Exported from the Yangtze Ports*. Chinese Maritime Customs. Shanghai, 1909
Brekhman, I.I. et al., eds. *New Data on Eleutherococcus*. Vladivostok 1984
But, Paul Pu-hai, Hu, S.Y. and King, C.Y. "Vascular Plants Used in Chinese Medicine." Fitoterapia 51(5). 1980
Chang Hson-mou, and But, Paul Pui-hai, eds. *Pharmacology and Applications of Chinese Materia Medica* (2 vols.). Singapore, 1986
Chang Hson-mou, Yeung, H.W., Tso, W.W. and Koo, A. *Advances in Chinese Medicinal Materials Research*. Singapore, 1985
Chang, S.S., and Chang, P.S. "Pharmacological actions of Cordyceps chinensis Zacc." Acta Pharm.

Sinica 6(3), 1958
Cheung, C.S., and U Aik-kaw, comp. and trans. *Synopsis of The Pharmacopeia*. San Francisco, 1984
Cheung, Siu-cheong, and Li, Ning-hon, eds. *Chinese Medicinal Herbs of Hong Kong* (5 vols). Hong Kong 1978
China Maritime Customs. *List of Chinese Medicines*. Shanghai, 1889
Cleyer, Andreas. *Medicamenta Simplicia Chinensium*. Frankfurt, 1682
Couling, S. *The Encyclopedia Sinica*. Shanghai, 1917
Dabry. *La médecine chez les chinois*. Paris, 1853
Daumas, C. *Médecins et médecine en Chine*. Grasse, 1858
Debeaux. *Pharmacie et matiere médicale chinoises*. Paris, 1865
Douthwaite, A.W. "Notes on Chinese Materia Medica." China Medical Journal 3(53). 1889
Duke, James A., and Ayensu, Edward S. *Medicinal Plants of China* (2 vols.). Algonac, 1985
Dymock, W. *Pharmacographica Indica* (3 vols.). Bombay, 1890-93
———. *The Vegetable Materia Medica of Western India*. Bombay
Ehling, Dagmar. *The Chinese Herbalist's Handbook*. Santa Fe, 1994
Foster, Steven, and Yue Chong-xi. *Herbal Emissaries*. Rochester, 1992
Fulder, Steven. *The Tao of Medicine: Ginseng and other Chinese Herbs for Inner Equilibrium and Immune Power*. Rochester, VT, 1990
Gauger, G. "Chinesische Roharzneiwaaren." Repertorium fuer Pharmacie und Praktische Chemie in Russland, Vol. VII. 1848
Gimlette, J.D., and Thomson, H.W. *A Dictionary of Malayan Medicine*. London, 1939
Halstead, Bruce, and Hood, Loretta L. *Eleutherococcus senticosus*. Los Angeles, 1984
Hanbury, Daniel. "Notes on Chinese Materia Medica." Pharmaceutical Journal. 1860-61
Hooper, D. "Chinese Drugs in Malaya." The Gardner's Bulletin (6). Strait Settlements, 1929
Hsu Hong-yen, Chen, Yuh-pan and Hong, Mina. *The Chemical Constituents of Oriental Herbs* (2 vols.). Los Angeles, 1982
———. *Oriental Materia Medica: A Concise Guide*. Los Angeles, 1980
———. *Treating Cancer with Chinese Herbs*. Los Angeles, 1982
———, and Preacher, W.G., eds. *Shang Han Lun: The Great Classic of Chinese Medicine*. Long Beach, 1981
———, and Wang, S.Y., trans. *Chin Kuei Yao Lueh: Prescriptions from the Golden Chest*. Long Beach, 1983
Hu, Shiu-ying. *An Enumeration of Chinese Materia Medica*. Hong Kong, 1980
———. "A Contribution to our Knowledge of Ginseng." American Jouirnal of Chinese Medicine 5(1-23). 1977
———. "History of the Introduction of Exotic Elements into Traditional Chinese Medicine." Journal of the Arnold Arboretum 71. 1990
Huebotter, Bruno. *Die Chinesische Medizin zu Begin*. Leipzig, 1929
Huebotter, F. *Beitraege zur Kenntnis der Chinesischen sowie der Tibetisch-Mongolischen Pharmacologie*. Berlin 1923
Hunan Health Committee. *ABarefoot Doctor's Manual*. London, 1978
Hunter, S.A. *A Manual of Therapeutics and Pharmacy*. Shanghai, 1890
Jeanselme. *Pratique medicale en Chine*. Paris, 1901
Johnson, O.S. *A Study of Chinese Alchemy*. Shanghai, 1928
Kariyone, T., and Kimura, Y. *Japanese-Chinese Medicinal Plants*. 1949
Kariyone, T., and Koiso, Y. *Atlas of Medicinal Plants*. Osaka, 1971
Keys, John. *Chinese Herbs: Their Botany, Chemistry and Pharmacodynamics*. Tokyo, 1976
Kirtikar and Basu. *Indian Medicinal Plants* (4 vols.). Allahabad, 1935
Kleiweg de Zwaan, J.P. *Heilkunde der Chinesen und Haarlem*. 1917
Kong, Y.C., and But, Paul Pui-hai, comp. and trans. *An Enumeration of Chinese Materia Medica*. Hong Kong, 1980

Kubota, S. and Okanishi, T. *Folia Pharmacorum Sinicorum [Chinese Materia Medica]*. Mukden, 1931
Laufer, Berthold. *Sino-Iranica: Chinese Contributions to the History of Civilization in Ancient Iran.* Chicago, 1919
Lien, E.J. and Li, W.Y. *Structure Activity Relationship Analysis of Anticancer Chinese Drugs and Related Plants*. Long Beach, 1985
Liu, Frank, and Liu Wan-mau. *Chinese Medical Terminology*. Hong Kong, 1980
Lockhart. *The Medical Missionary in China.*
Lu, Henry C. *Correspondence Course in Chinese Herbal Medicine.* Vancouver, 1977
Nadkarni, K.M. *Indian Materia Medica*. Bombay, 1927
National Academy of Sciences. *Herbal Pharmacology in the People's Republic of China.* Washington, 1975
National Institute for the Control of Pharmaceutical and Biological Products, ed. *Color Atlas of Chinese Traditional Drugs*. Beijing, 1987
Perrot, E., and Hurrier, P. *Matiere medicale et pharmacopee sino-annamites* Paris, 1907
Perry, Lily May. *Medicinal Plants of East and Southeast Asia*. Cambridge, 1980
Petelot, Alfred. *Les plantes médicinales du Cambodge, du Laos et du Vietnam* (4 vols.). Saigon, 1952-54
Porkert, Manfred. *Klassische Chinesische Pharmakologie.* Heidelberg, 1978
Porter Smith, Frederick. *Contributions towards the Materia Medica and Natural History of China.* Shanghai, 1871
Quisumbing, Eduardo. *Medicinal Plants of the Philippines*. Manila, 1951
Read, Bernard E. *Chinese Medicinal Plants from the Pen Ts'ao Kang Mu*. Shanghai, 1936, 1977
———. *Chinese Materia Medica: Insect Drugs, Dragon and Snake Drugs, and Fish Drugs.* Shanghai 1934, 1939, 1941, 1977
———. *Chinese Materia Medica: Turtle and Shellfish Drugs, Avian Drugs, and a Compendium of Minerals and Stones*. Shanghai 1932, 1937, 1977
———. *Chinese Materia Medica: Animal Drugs*. Beijing, 1931, 1977
Regnault, Jules. *La medecine des chinois*. Hanoi, 1902
———. *Medecine et pharmacie chez les chinois et chez les annamnites*. Paris, 1899
Roi, Jacques. *Traité des plantes médicinales chinoises.* Paris, 1955
Soubeyran, J. Leon. *La matiere médicale chez les chinois*. Paris, 1873
Stuart, G.A. *Chinese Materia Medica, Vegetable Kingdom*. Shanghai, 1911
Tang, W., and Eisenbrand, G. *Chinese Drugs of Plant Origin.* New York, 1992
Tsung Pi-kwang. *Immune System and Chinese Herbs.* Irvine, 1989
Unschuld, Paul U. *Medicine in China: History of Pharmaceutics*. Berkeley, 1987
Watt, George. *Dictionary of the Economic Products of India.* 1897
Wee Yeow-chin and Hsuan Keng. *Illustrated Dictionary of Chinese Medicinal Herbs*. Hong Kong, 1992
Willard, Terry. *Reishi Mushroom: Herb of Spiritual Potency.* Washington, 1990
Wiseman, Nigel. *A Complete Chinese Materia Medica.* Watertown, 1997
Wong Ming. *La médecine chinoise par les plantes*. Paris, 1980
Xu, G.J. *A Glossary of Chinese-Latin-English Names of Chinese Traditional and Herbal Drugs.* Nanjing, 1986
Yen Kun-ying. *Illustrated Chinese Materia Medica*. Hong Kong, 1993
Yeung Him-che. *Handbook of Chinese Herbs and Formulas* (2 vols.). Los Angeles, 1985
Zhou Jin-huang, Liu Gan-zhong and Chen Ji-nui. *Recent Advances in Chinese Herbal Drugs: Actions and Uses*. Hong Kong, 1994
Zhu Liang-feng et al. *Aromatic Plants and Essential Constituents.* Hong Kong, 1993
Zwaan, J.P. Kleiweg de. *Heilkunde der Chinesen und Japaner.* Haarlem, 1917

Works on Oriental Botany

Academia Sinica, Commercial Ministry and Institute of Botany. *Flora of Economic Plants of China.* Beijing, 1961

Anon. Taiwan Chih Wu Chih *[Flora of Taiwan].* Taipei, 1979

Botanical Institute of Academia Sinica. *Zhong Guo Gao Deng Zhe Wu Tu Jian (Iconographia Cormophytorum Sinicorum)* (5 vols.). Shanghai, 1971

Bretschneider, Emil V. *Botanicon Sinicum* (3 vols.). Shanghai, 1881 and 1895

———. *History of European Botanical Studies in China* (2 vols.). 1898. repr. Leipzig, 1981

Burkill, I. H. *A Dictionary of the Economic Products of the Malay Penninsula* (2 vols). London, 1935

Chang Mei-chen, Miao Bo-mao, Lu Rui-ling, Qiu Lian-qing, Wei Zhi and Li Ping-tao. *Flora Reipublicae Popularis Sinicae.* Beijing, 1992

Chun, W.Y. *Chinese Economic Trees.* Shanghai, 1921

Delectis Florae Reipublicae Popularis Sinicae. *Flora Reipublicae Popularis Sinicae.* Beijing, 1959

Edy, Harry H. *Ferns of Hong Kong.* Hong Kong, 1977

Forbes, Frances B., and Hemsley, William B. *Index Florae Sinensis.* 1888

Geerts. *Produits de la nature japonaise et chinoise.*

Henry, A. *A List of Plants from Formosa...* Trans. Asiatic Society of Japan 24 (Suppl.)

How, F.C. *Zhong Guo Zhong Zi Zhi We Ke Shu Ci Dian [A Dictionary of the Families and Genera of Chinese Seed Plants].* Beijing, 1982

———, *Flora of Guangzhou.* Beijing, 1956

Hsieh Wen-hwa. *Taiwan Tzu Sheng Yu Yung Chung Yao Yuan I Chi Wu Tu Shuo [Illustrations of Selected Wild and Cultivated Plants of Taiwan].* Taipei, 1960

Hu, Shiu-ying. "An Enumeration of the Food Plants of China with their Vernacular Names in Chinese." Flora of China project of the Arnold Arboretum.

Institute of Chinese Materia Medica. *Medicinal Plants in China.* Manila, 1989

Iwasaki, Kan'en. *Honzo Zufu [Medicinal Plant Illustrations].* 1884

Kaempfer, Engelberth. *Amaenitates Exoticae.* Paris, 1712

Kaibara Ekiken (Ekken). *Ekiken Yojo Kun.* c. 1660

Kitagawa, M. *Neo-Lineamenta Florae Manshuricae or Enumeration of the Spontaneous Vascular Plants Hitherto Known from Manchuria.* Vaduz, 1979

Kunming Institute of Botany, Academy of Sciences, eds. *Index Florae Yunnanensis* (2 vols.). Kunming, 1984

Laufer, Berthold. "Sino-Iranica." Field Museum of Natural History, Publication 201, Anthropological Series 15(3). Chicago, 1919

Li, H.L. "The Vegetables of Ancient China." Economic Botany 23. 1969

———, Liu, T.S., Huang, T.C., Koyama, T. and De Vol, C.E., eds. *Flora of Taiwan* (6 vols.). Taipei, 1975-79

Liu, Tang-shui. *A List of Economic Plants in Taiwan.* Taipei, 1952

———. *Taiwan Mu Ben Zhi Wu Tu Zhi [Illustrations of Native and Ligneous Plants of Taiwan].* Taipei, 1960

Loureiro, Joao de. *Flora cochinchinensis.* Lisbon, 1788

Makino, Tomitaro. *Shin Nihon Shokubutsu Zukan [New Illustrated Flora of Japan].* Tokyo, 1965

Matsumura, J. Nippon Shokubutsumeii: *Nomenclature of Japanese Plants in Latin, Japanese and Chinese.* Tokyo, 1884

Merill, E.D. and Walker, E.H. *A Bibliography of Eastern Asiatic Botany.* Jamaica Plain, MA, 1938

Murukosa, Michio. *Naigai Shokubutsu Dai Zukan [Complete Illustrations of Native and Imported Plants].* n.p.n.d.

Needham, Joseph. *Science and Civilisation in China* (6)1. Cambridge, 1986

Ohwi, J. *Flora of Japan.* Washington, 1965

Oka Koyoku. *Moshi Himbutsu Zuko.* 1785
Okuyama Haruki (ed.). *Nihon Shokubutsu Zufu [Japanese Plants Illustrated].* Tokyo, 1977
Peking Academy of Sciences. *Zhong Guo Zhe Wu Ming Cheng [Nomenclature of Botanical Species].* Beijing, 1954
Siebold, Philipp Franz von. *Flora Japonica* (2 vols.) 1835-44
South China Institute of Botany, Academia Sinica. *Flora Hainanica* (4 vols.). Beijing
———. *Flora of Guangdong* (2 vols.) 1987-91
Sowerby, A. de C. *A Naturalist's Notebook in China.* Shanghai, 1925
———. *The Naturalist in Manchuria.* Shanghai, 1922
Steward, G. A. *Manual of Vascular Plants of the Lower Yangtze Valley, China.* Corvallis, 1958
Tatarinov, A. *Catalogus Medicamentorum Sinensium quae Pekini Comparanda et Determinanda Curavit.* St. Petersburg, 1856
Terasaki, Tomekichi. *Terasaki's Illustrated Flora of Japan.* Tokyo, 1982
Thunberg, Carl Pehr. *Flora Japonica.* Lipsiae, 1784
Walden, B.M. and Hu Shiu-ying. *Wild Flowers of Hong Kong.* Hong Kong 1977
Walker, E.H. *Flora of Okinawa and the Southern Ryukyu Islands.* Washington, 1976
———. *A Bibliography of Eastern Asiatic Botany; Supplement 1.* Washington, 1960
Wilson, E.H. *A Naturalist in China* (2 vols.). London, 1913
Wu Qi-chun. *Zhi Wu Ming Shi Tu Kao.* 1848
Yunnan Institute of Botany. *Economic Plants of Yunnan.* Kunming, 1973

Works on Physiomedical and Eclectic Herbal Medicine

Comfort, J.W. *The Practice of Medicine on Thomsonian Principles.* Philadelphia, 1843
Cook, W.H. *The Science and Practice of Medicine.* 1879
Ellingwood, Finley. *The Eclectic Practice of Medicine.* Chicago, 1910
———. *A Systematic Treatise on Materia Medica and Therapeutics.* Chicago, 1898
Felter, Harvey W. *The Eclectic Materia Medica: Pharmacology and Therapeutics.* Cincinnati, 1922
Priest, A.W., and L.R. Priest. *Herbal Medication.* London, 1981
Scudder, John Milton. *Specific Diagnosis.* 1874
———. *Specific Medication.* 1870
Thurston, J.M. *The Philosophy of Physiomedicalism.* 1900
Webster, Herbert Tracy. *The Principles of Medicine as Applied to Dynamical Therapeutics.* Oakland, 1891
———. *Dynamical Therapeutics.* San Francisco, 1898

Miscellaneous Works

Holmes, Peter. *The Energetics of Western Herbs.* (2 vols). Boulder, 1995
Mowrey, Daniel. *The Scientific Validation of Herbal Medicine.* 1986
Schafer, Edward H. *The Golden Peaches of Samarkand.* Berkeley, 1963
———. *The Vermillion Bird.* Berkeley, 1967
Selye, Hans. *The Stress of Life.* New York, 1976
Unschuld, Paul U. *Medicine in China: A History of Ideas.* Berkeley, 1985

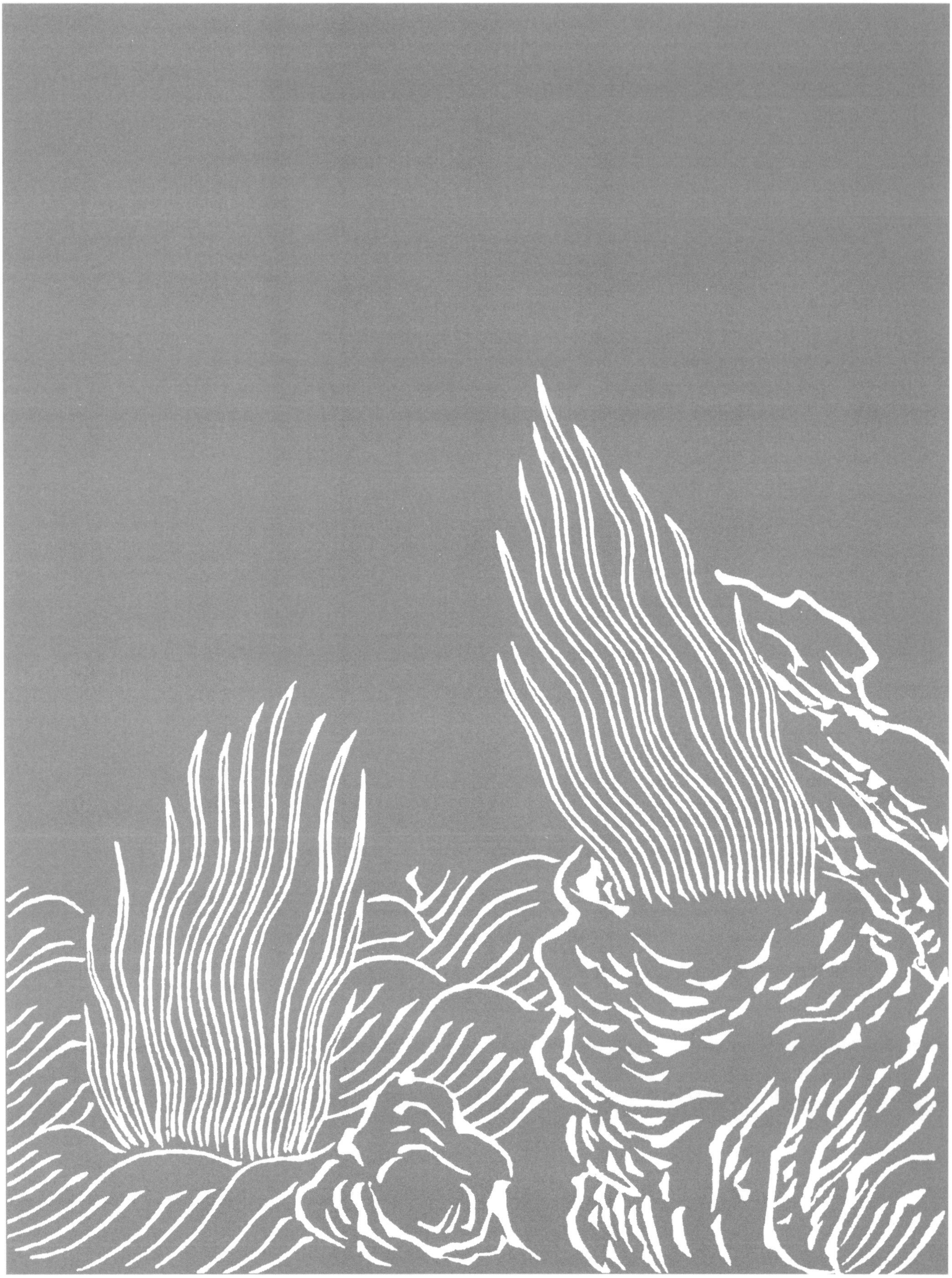

General Index

• Remedy names are listed here by their clinical composite name and their English name. The clinical name is constructed from the remedy's scientific name plus its Mandarin name. To locate a remedy by any other name, such as Mandarin, Cantonese, pharmaceutical or Japanese, refer first to the Cross Indexes that start on p. 637, and find its scientific name. The first half of that scientific name is also the first half of the clinical names in this index.

• Priority has been given to remedy actions rather than symptoms and disease conditions. Although this index does include numerous symptoms and disorders, many will be found with reference to the remedy action that addresses them.

• This index does not include a repertory of symptoms and disorders, but merely lists the page references for these condition. This is why only minimum information is given about the remedy types used for a particular condition. For example, although the entry Otitis media refers to *antiallergics* as the main remedy type indicated for use, this condition may also be treated with *anti-inflammatory* and *anti-infective* remedies, among other possibilities. For repertory information refer to the author's *Energetics of Western Herbs,* Vol. 2.

• Because so many remedies possess stronger or weaker *anti-inflammatory, anti-infective, antipyretic, astringent, detoxicant* and *diuretic* actions, reference is made here only to the most effective and frequently used of these remedies.